Peripheral Neuropathy and Neuropathic Pain

Peripheral Neuropathy and Neuropathic Pain

Edited by Vin Lopez

hayle
medical
New York

Hayle Medical,
750 Third Avenue, 9th Floor,
New York, NY 10017, USA

Visit us on the World Wide Web at:
www.haylemedical.com

ISBN: 978-1-63241-513-4

Printed in China.

Cataloging-in-Publication Data

Peripheral neuropathy and neuropathic pain / edited by Vin Lopez.
p. cm.
Includes bibliographical references and index.
ISBN 978-1-63241-513-4
1. Nerves, Peripheral--Diseases. 2. Neuropathy. 3. Central pain. 4. Neuralgia.
5. Nervous system--Pathophysiology. I. Lopez, Vin.

RC412 .P47 2018
616.856--dc23

Table of Contents

Preface

Peripheral neuropathy is a condition which causes damage to the nerves. Damage to these nerves can affect the movement, sensation and organ function of a person. Whereas, neuropathic pain is a chronic pain which occurs mainly because of injury to the somatosensory nervous system. The usual treatment given to patients suffering from neuropathic pain involves medication like anticonvulsants, antidepressants, dietary supplements, neuromodulators, etc. This book includes some of the vital pieces of work being conducted across the world, on various topics related to peripheral neuropathy and neuropathic pain. It is appropriate for students seeking detailed information in this area as well as for experts.

After months of intensive research and writing, this book is the end result of all who devoted their time and efforts in the initiation and progress of this book. It will surely be a source of reference in enhancing the required knowledge of the new developments in the area. During the course of developing this book, certain measures such as accuracy, authenticity and research focused analytical studies were given preference in order to produce a comprehensive book in the area of study.

This book would not have been possible without the efforts of the authors and the publisher. I extend my sincere thanks to them. Secondly, I express my gratitude to my family and well-wishers. And most importantly, I thank my students for constantly expressing their willingness and curiosity in enhancing their knowledge in the field, which encourages me to take up further research projects for the advancement of the area.

Editor

Intrathecal Infusion of Hydrogen-Rich Normal Saline Attenuates Neuropathic Pain via Inhibition of Activation of Spinal Astrocytes and Microglia in Rats

Yanhu Ge[1,2], Feixiang Wu[1], Xuejun Sun[3], Zhenghua Xiang[4], Liqun Yang[1], Shengdong Huang[5], Zhijie Lu[1], Yuming Sun[1], Wei-Feng Yu[1]*

1 Department of Anesthesiology, Eastern Hepatobiliary Surgery Hospital, Changhai Hospital, Second Military Medical University, Shanghai, China, **2** Department of Anesthesiology, 309th Hospital of CPLA, Beijing, China, **3** Department of Diving Medicine, Faculty of Naval Medicine, Second Military Medical University, Shanghai, China, **4** Department of Neurobiology, Second Military Medical University, Shanghai, China, **5** Department of Cardiothoracic Surgery, Changhai Hospital, Second Military Medical University, Shanghai, China

Abstract

Background: Reactive oxygen and nitrogen species are key molecules that mediate neuropathic pain. Although hydrogen is an established antioxidant, its effect on chronic pain has not been characterized. This study was to investigate the efficacy and mechanisms of hydrogen-rich normal saline induced analgesia.

Methodology/Principal findings: In a rat model of neuropathic pain induced by L5 spinal nerve ligation (L5 SNL), intrathecal injection of hydrogen-rich normal saline relieved L5 SNL-induced mechanical allodynia and thermal hyperalgesia. Importantly, repeated administration of hydrogen-rich normal saline did not lead to tolerance. Preemptive treatment with hydrogen-rich normal saline prevented development of neuropathic pain behavior. Immunofluorochrome analysis revealed that hydrogen-rich normal saline treatment significantly attenuated L5 SNL-induced increase of 8-hydroxyguanosine immunoreactive cells in the ipsilateral spinal dorsal horn. Western blot analysis of SDS/PAGE-fractionated tyrosine-nitrated proteins showed that L5 SNL led to increased expression of tyrosine-nitrated Mn-containing superoxide dismutase (MnSOD) in the spinal cord, and hydrogen-rich normal saline administration reversed the tyrosine-nitrated MnSOD overexpression. We also showed that the analgesic effect of hydrogen-rich normal saline was associated with decreased activation of astrocytes and microglia, attenuated expression of interleukin-1β (IL-1β) and tumor necrosis factor-α (TNF-α) in the spinal cord.

Conclusion/Significance: Intrathecal injection of hydrogen-rich normal saline produced analgesic effect in neuropathic rat. Hydrogen-rich normal saline-induced analgesia in neuropathic rats is mediated by reducing the activation of spinal astrocytes and microglia, which is induced by overproduction of hydroxyl and peroxynitrite.

Editor: Daqing Ma, Imperial College London, Chelsea & Westminster Hospital, United Kingdom

Funding: This work was supported by the grants from the National Natural Science Foundation of China (30901403, 31171013). The funders had no role in study design, data collection and analysis, decision to publish, or preparation of the manuscript.

Competing Interests: The authors have declared that no competing interests exist.

* E-mail: ywf808@sohu.com

These authors contributed equally to this work.

Introduction

Reactive oxygen species (ROS) and reactive nitrogen species (RNS) are key factors in the pathogenesis of central nervous system (CNS) disorders. Studies have shown that ROS and the superoxide byproduct peroxynitrite ($ONOO^-$) are involved in neuropathic pain [1, 2]. Free radical scavengers such as TEMPOL, phenyl-N-tert-butylnitrone (PBN) and vitamin E, could alleviate neuropathic pain [3-6], delivery these agents directly to the sub-arachnoid space produced more potent effects, suggesting that antioxidants exert their anti-allodynic action mainly at the spinal levels [7]. The CNS derives its energy almost exclusively from oxidative metabolism of the mitochondrial respiratory chain, and consumes a disproportionately high amount of the body's O_2 supply. Leakage of high energy electrons along the mitochondria electron transport chain causes the formation of superoxide (O_2^-), hydrogen peroxide (H_2O_2) and peroxynitrite [8-11]. Therefore, in the spinal dorsal horn where signals from primary somatosensory neurons are modulated depending on prior experience, ROS and RNS play an important role in the balance between inhibitory and facilitatory influence.

There is considerable evidence that ROS and RNS contribute to neuropathic pain. However, there remains much uncertainty as to the relative contribution of different types of ROS or RNS molecules. Free radical scavengers indeed alleviate neuropathic pain, but we have not elucidated an antioxidant with no adverse side effects for therapeutic use. Hydrogen has been identified as a ROS scavenger. Ohsawa and colleagues found that hydrogen acts

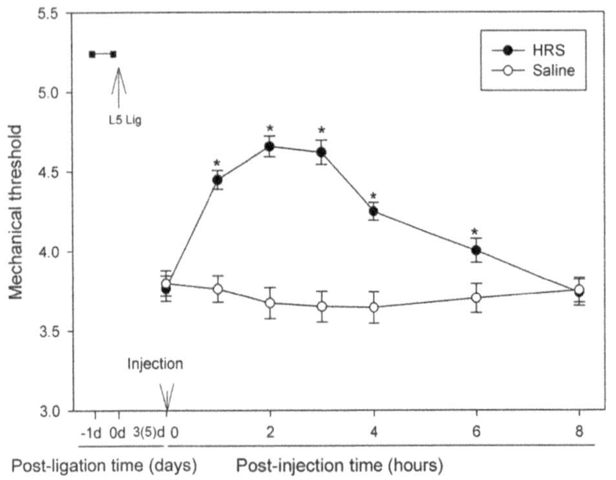

Figure 1. Effects of intrathecal injection of HRS on mechanical thresholds in rat model of neuropathic pain. On the third post-operative (PO) day, the rats were divided into two groups of five, each group receiving either HRS or NS, and behavior tests were done for 8 hrs followed by 48 hrs of rest, and the testing process was repeated. So every rat received all the two treatments followed by behavior testing after each. Thus each point represents the results from ten rats. Note the great increase of mechanical thresholds after HRS injections. Eight hrs after the injection, the thresholds declined to the level of the NS group. Data are expressed as mean±SEM. n = 10. Asterisks indicate significant ($p<0.05$) differences from the NS control group by a two-way repeated ANOVA.

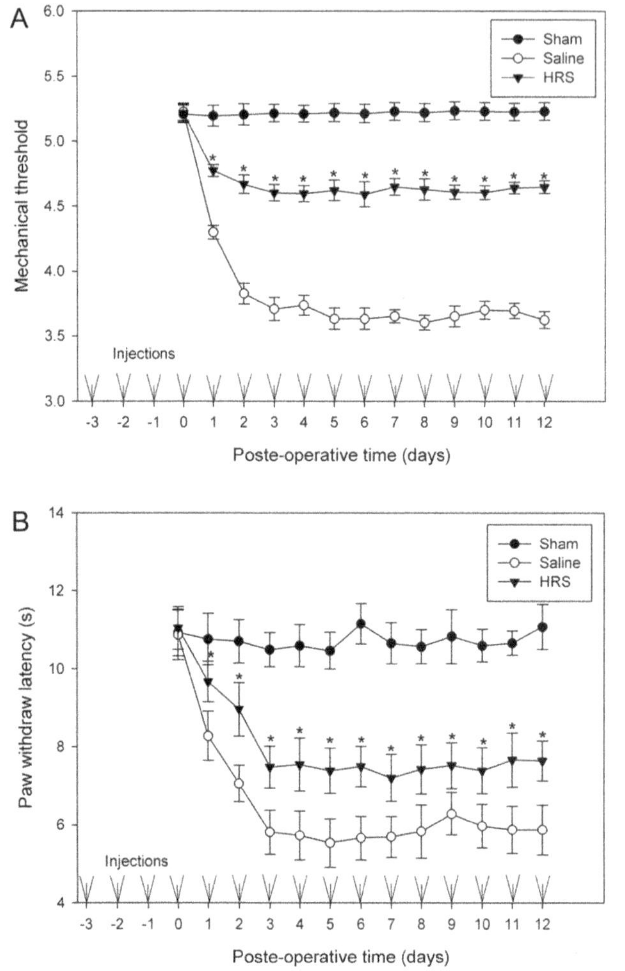

Figure 2. Effects of repeated injection of HRS on mechanical thresholds and paw withdraw latency. Staring 3 days before the lesion, rats of each group received repeated intrathecal injection of HRS or NS respectively at 24 hrs intervals for 15 days. Sham-operation rats received no injection. Mechanical thresholds (A) and PWLs (B) of all rats were determined every 24 hrs. Mechanical thresholds and PWLs of HRS or NS treated rats remained the same levels as the sham rats at the time point of 0 PO day. Note the great increase in mechanical thresholds and PWLs of rats received HRS, and that there is no development of tolerance. Data are expressed as mean±SEM. n = 10 for A and B. Asterisks indicate values significantly ($p<0.05$) different from controls using a two-way repeated ANOVA followed by the Duncan post hoc test.

as an anti-oxidant by selectively reducing hydroxyl (·OH) and peroxynitrite radicals [12]. However, the analgesic efficacy of hydrogen on neuropathic pain is unknown.

Astrocytes are the most abundant cells in CNS and were historically regarded as support cells [13]. Astrocytes contact with neural synapses closely. It is possible that astrocytes not only support the neurons but also modulate the synaptic transmission by regulating the external environment of synapse. Studies have demonstrated that astrocytes contribute to both induction and maintenance of neuropathic pain [14–20]. Microglia are derived from peripheral myeloid precursor cells and penetrate the CNS during embryogenesis [21]. In CNS, microglia are heterogeneously distributed, the spinal cord is one of the areas where microglial density is particularly high [22,23]. The number of microglia dramatically increases after peripheral never injury in pain models. Numerous studies have demonstrated that microglia contribute to neuropathic pain [24–27]. Moreover, a series of studies have implied that the production of ROS in both astrocytes and microglia contribute to neuronal inflammatory process, neuronal death and pain disorders in the CNS [28–32]. Therefore, we speculated that production of ROS and RNS within spinal astrocytes and microglia may be involved in glial activation, leading to central sensitization.

In the present study, we characterized the effect of hydrogen-rich normal saline (HRS) on mechanical and thermal hyperalgesia in a rat model of neuropathic pain, in an attempt to provide evidences to confirm hydroxyl and peroxynitrite as significant mediators of glial activation and proinflammatory cytokine release in neuropathic rats. We hypothesize that elimination of hydroxyl and peroxynitrite within spinal glial cells by HRS will attenuate activation of astrocytes and microglia, prevent proinflammatory cytokine-mediated central sensitization, and thus be a potential therapy for neuropathic pain.

Materials and Method

Sample size, randomization and blinding

The sample size of this study was calculated using G*power 3.1 software (Universität Kiel, Germany). Randomization was performed using a computerized random number generator and animals were assigned to each group by residue method. All the behavior testing and the section analysis were performed by an investigator blinded to the origin of the animal.

Experimental animals

Young adult male Sprague-Dawley rats (3 months old, 300–320 g, Sino-British SIPPR/BK Laboratory Animal Ltd., Shanghai, China) were housed two per cage with free access to food and

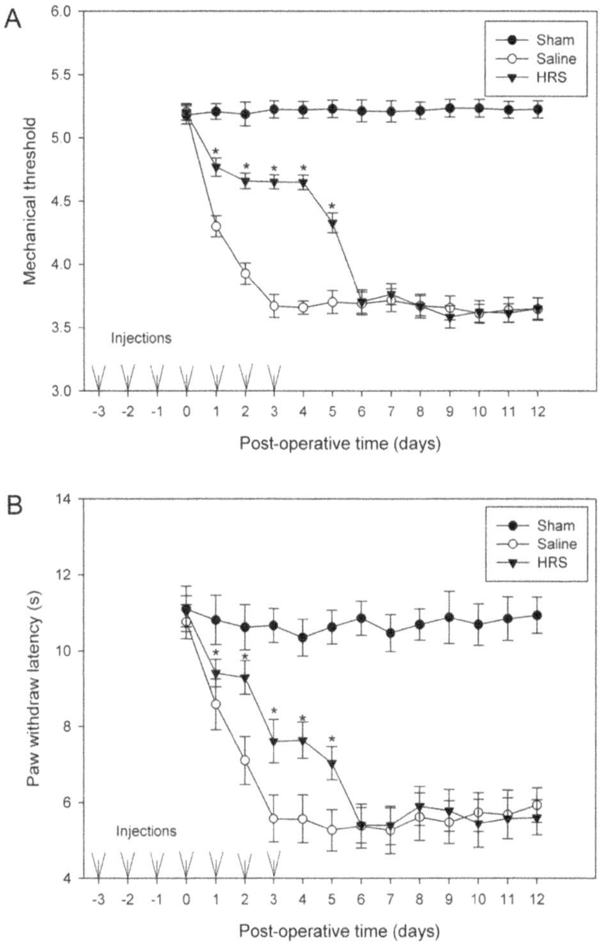

Figure 3. Effects of HRS pretreatment on the development of neuropathic pain behavior. All rats received repeated injection of HRS or NS at 24 hrs intervals for 6 days, on the fourth day after the first dose, L5 spinal nerve was ligated. Note that mechanical thresholds (A) and PWLs (B) were significantly elevated in HRS group as compared to controls, and this effect lasted for 3 days after the administration ceased. Data are expressed as mean±SEM. n = 10 for A and B. Asterisks indicate values significantly ($p<0.05$) different from controls using a two-way repeated ANOVA followed by the Duncan post hoc test.

water. Rats were acclimated for at least 5 days before experimental procedures. Basic foot withdrawal thresholds to mechanical stimuli and paw withdraw latencies (PWLs) to heat stimuli were tested for all rats, animals with abnormal mechanical thresholds or PWLs were excluded. All experimental procedures were approved by the Ethics Committee for Animal Experimentation of the Second Military Medical University. The protocols used in this research project complied with the guidelines for the care and use of laboratory animals of the Second Military Medical University.

Rat model of neuropathic pain (L5 spinal nerve ligation (L5 SNL))

Rats were anesthetized with isoflurane (2% induction, 1.5% maintenance) in O_2, and placed in the prone position. After removing the left L6 vertebral transverse process, the L5 spinal nerve on the left side was separated from the adjacent L4 spinal nerve and the L5 spinal nerve was tightly ligated using 6–0 silk thread [33].

Intrathecal catheterization

Rats were anesthetized with isoflurane and mounted in a conventional stereotaxic frame. A midline incision was made on the skull and the superficial neck muscles were separated by a midline incision. The underlying layer of muscles were separated along the midline by blunt dissection. Next, the muscles were separated from their point of origin on the occipital bone to expose the atlanto-occipital membrane. A small incision was then made on the membrane. A 12.5 cm PE-10 tube (Becton Dickinson and Co., Franklin Lakes, NJ USA) was inserted into the spinal subarachnoid space [34]. The tip of the tube lay in the region of the lumbar enlargement. Before implantation, the tube was sterilized by immersion in 75% ethanol, followed by normal saline (NS) wash, and was filled with NS. The tube was then secured by a loop of suture material around it and through the neck muscle. The external end was sealed with a cap made of a short segment of PE-50 tube (Becton Dickinson and Co., Franklin Lakes, NJ USA) with one end closed. The foot withdrawal thresholds to mechanical stimuli and the PWLs to heat were examined after the surgery, rats developed motor/sensory problems were excluded.

Behavioral testing

The foot withdrawal thresholds to mechanical stimuli were used as an indicator of mechanical sensitivity of the affected paw. The mechanical thresholds were measured using the "up-down" method [35]. Briefly, rats were placed in a plastic chamber (8.0×8.5×20 cm) on the top of a mesh screen platform and habituated for at least 10 min. A set of von Frey monofilaments (von Frey numbers: 3.65, 3.87, 4.10, 4.31, 4.52, 4.74, 4.92 and 5.16; equivalent to 0.45, 0.74, 1.26, 2.04, 3.31, 5.50, 8.32, and 14.45 g, respectively) was chosen. Testing was initiated with filament 4.31 (2.04 g), in the middle of the series, the filaments were applied perpendicular to the ventral surface of the base at the proximal part of the third or fourth toe (this area is the most sensitive site) with sufficient force to bend the filament slightly for 2–3 s. An abrupt withdrawal of the hind paw during stimulation or immediately after stimulus removal was considered as a positive response. If there was a positive response, the next lower filament was used, and if not, the next higher filament was applied. The test was continued until responses to six stimuli had been obtained after the first change in response. The 50% threshold value was calculated using Dixon's formula [36]: 50% threshold $= 10^{(X+\kappa\delta)}/10^4$, where X is the value of the final von Frey hair used (in logarithmic units), κ is the tabular value for the pattern of positive/negative responses, and δ is the mean difference between stimuli in logarithmic units (0.22). In cases where continuous positive or negative responses were observed all the way to the end of the stimulus spectrum, values of 3.54 (0.34 g) or 5.28 (18.72 g) were assigned, respectively.

Thermal hyperalgesia was evaluated using Hargreaves' procedure [37]. Rats were placed in a plastic cage with a glass floor on the day of the experiment. After a 30 min habituation period, the plantar surface (the base at the proximal part of the third or fourth toe) of the hind paw was exposed to a beam of radiant heat delivered with an infrared bulb (Osram halogen-bellaphot bulb; 8V, 50W) through the glass floor. When paw movement interrupted the reflected light, a photoelectric cell turned off the lamp. PWLs were automatically displayed to the nearest 0.1 s, and the cut-off time was 20 s in order to prevent tissue damage. Light intensity was preset to obtain a baseline latency of approximately 11 seconds. The time in seconds between the activation of the heat source and paw withdrawal was recorded. The mean PWL was

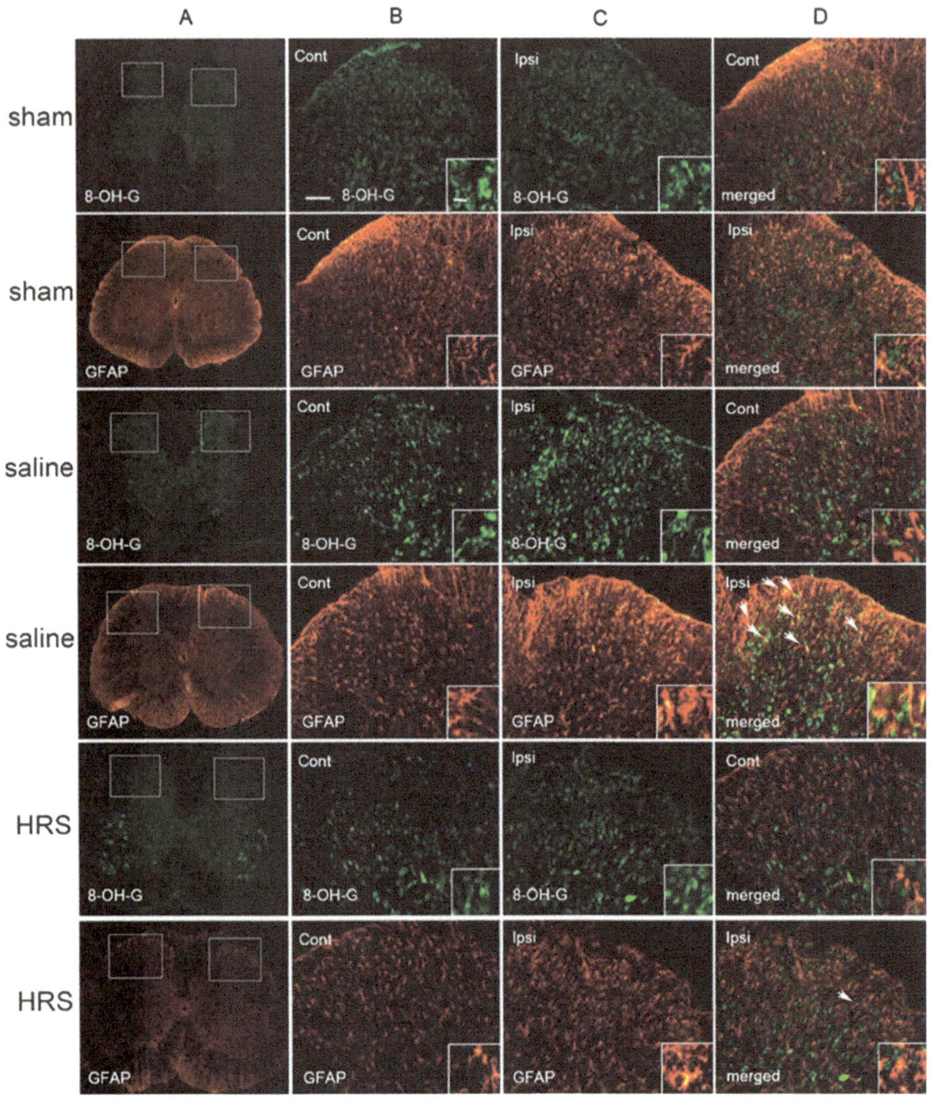

Figure 4. Immunostaining for 8-OH-G and GFAP in sham rats, NS-treated neuropathic rats and HRS-treated neuropathic rats. Pictures in columns B and C are magnification of the insets shown in column A. Enlargements in the insets in columns B, C and D demonstrate the changes in cell shape and expression of 8-OH-G (green) and GFAP (red). Double-staining demonstrate colocalization (arrows) of 8-OH-G and GFAP. Note that an increased number of cells showing immunoreactivity for 8-OH-G and GFAP in neuropathic rats treated with NS as compared to the sham rats. And number of cells showed colocalization of 8-OH-G and GFAP in NS treated neuropathic rats was significantly increased as compared to the sham rats. HRS greatly reversed L5 SNL induced production of 8-OH-G, activation of astrocytes, and increase of 8-OH-G-ir astrocytes. Scale bars, 100 µm and 25 µm in the inset.

calculated from six consecutive trials (each performed every 30 min).

Treatment with HRS

Hydrogen rich normal saline was obtained from the Department of Diving Medicine, the Faculty of Naval Medicine, Second Military Medical University. Normal saline was hydrogenated under 0.4 Mpa ($1\text{Mpa} = 1 \times 10^6$ pascal) for 6 hrs to a supersaturated level, sterilized with gamma radiation and stored under atmospheric pressure (approximately 101325 pascal in Shanghai, China) at 4°C in a sealed aluminum bag with no dead space, and used within a week [38–40]. Hydrogen content was 0.6 mmol/L as measured with gas chromatography [12]. For treatment, 20 ul of HRS was injected intrathecally. Control rats received an equal volume of NS.

Immunostaining

Rats were sacrificed 1 hr after HRS or NS treatment, on the 12th day after L5 SNL or sham operation, when behavioral testing was ended. Catheterized rats received no injection were sacrificed on the 15th day after catheterization. Once rats were anesthetized, the chest was opened and the aorta was perfused with saline, followed by cold fixative (4% paraformaldehyde in 0.1 M phosphate buffer (PB, PH 7.4)). The L4–5 spinal cord segment was removed, post-fixed overnight, and then placed in 30% sucrose until equilibration. The spinal cord was cryosectioned at 16 µm, and the sections were collected in 0.1 M PB. After blocking with 2% normal human serum containing 0.3% Triton X-100 in PB for 1 hr at room temperature, all sections were incubated with a mixture of primary mouse monoclonal antibody against 8-OH-G (1:200 Abcam, Cambridge, MA USA) and goat

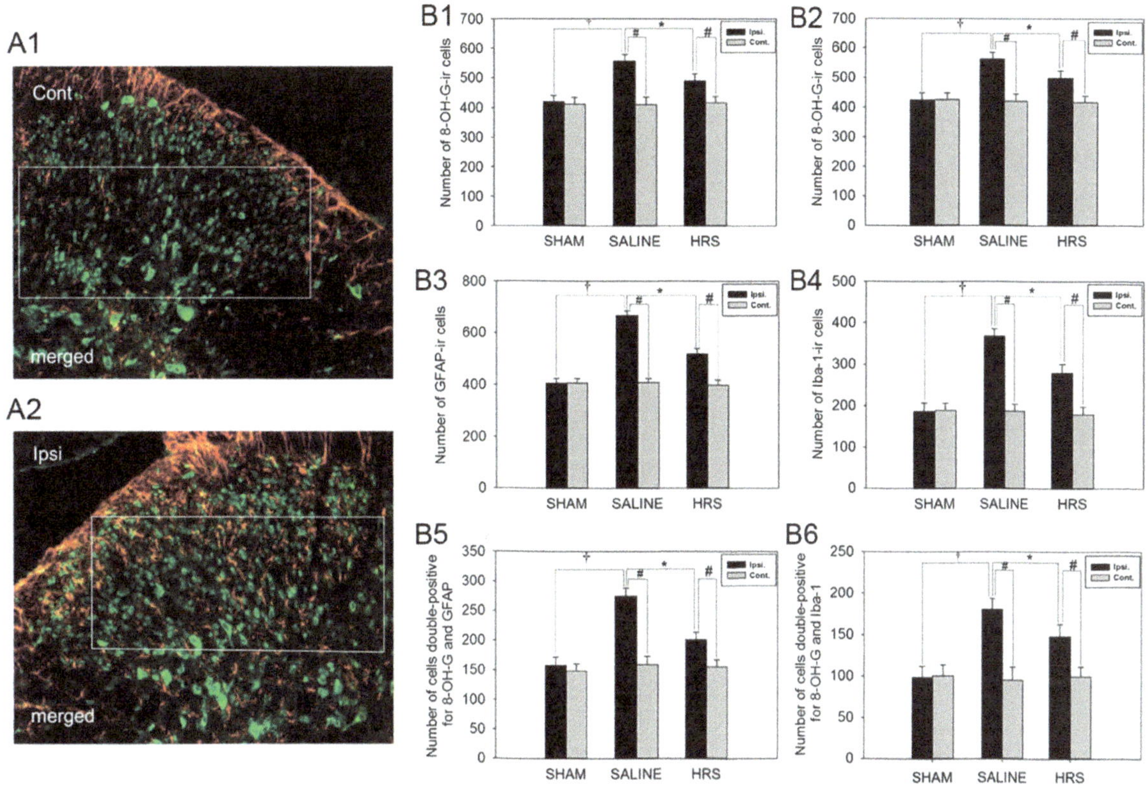

Figure 5. Numbers of cells expressing 8-OH-G, GFAP, Iba-1 and numbers of double-stained cells in all rats. (A1, A2) Merged images of photomicrographs immunostaining for 8-OH-G (green) and GFAP (red) in L5 sections of neuropathic rats treated with NS were taken as example, a rectangular area was manually outlined in the dorsal horn using the rectangular marquee tool, and the size of every selected area is 50 cm×22 cm (2500 μm×1100 μm in the spinal sections). At 20-fold magnification, counts were obtained of the numbers of cells in the areas outlined in the rectangular that were positive for 8-OH-G, GFAP and Iba-1, double staining cells in the areas were also counted. (B1, B2) Number of cells showing immunoreactivity for 8-OH-G in both sides of spinal dorsal horn. (B3, B4) Number of cells showing immunoreactivity for GFAP and Iba-1 in both sides of spinal dorsal horn. (B5, B6) Number of 8-OH-G-ir astrocytes and 8-OH-G-ir microglia in both sides of spinal dorsal horn. Data are expressed as mean±SEM. n = 10 for B1-6. Compared with the sham rats, L5 SNL induced significant production of 8-OH-G, activation of glial cells and increase of 8-OH-G-ir glial cells, †$p<0.01$, by one-way ANOVA. HRS blocked the production of 8-OH-G, glial activation and increase of 8-OH-G-ir glial cells, *$p<0.01$, by one-way ANOVA. Compared to contralateral side, L5 SNL induced significant production of 8-OH-G, activation of glial cells and increase of 8-OH-G-ir glial cells in ipsilateral side. #$p<0.01$, by one-way ANOVA.

polyclonal antibody against GFAP (1:200 Santa Cruz Biotechnology, Santa Cruz, CA USA) or goat polyclonal antibody against Iba 1 (1:200 Abcam, Cambridge, MA USA) for 36–48 hrs at 4°C, followed by a mixture of donkey anti-mouse IgG Fluorescein conjugated and donkey anti-goat IgG cyanine conjugated secondary antibodies (1:300, Jackson ImmunoResearch Laboratories, West Grove, PA, USA) for 2 hrs at room temperature. Sections were then washed, air-dried, and coverslipped with mounting medium. To confirm the specificity of the immunolabeling, some sections were processed as above, but without the primary antibodies. The sections from all animals were processed together in each staining process to minimize staining variability.

Sections were analyzed with a fluorescence microscope (Nikon corporation, Shinjuku, Tokyo Japan), and images were captured with a CCD camera. Consistency was ensured by taking all photographs at the same exposure. Digital images were analyzed using a computer image analysis system (Furi Company, Shanghai China). Ten serial sections (16 μm thick, 150 μm apart) were selected for analysis from each rat. In every image, a rectangular area was manually outlined in the dorsal horn using the rectangular marquee tool, and the size of every selected area was 50 cm×22 cm (2500 μm×1100 μm in the spinal sections). At 20-fold magnification, counts were obtained of the numbers of cells in the areas outlined in the rectangular that were positive for 8-OH-G, GFAP and Iba-1, and double staining cells in the areas were also counted. The average number of positively labeled cells was calculated and presented as data.

Protein extraction

Animals were anesthetized and exanguinated. The lumbar spinal cord was quickly dissected, and immediately frozen. Tissues were stored at −80°C until analysis. Tissue samples (1 g) were homogenized in 5.0 ml extraction buffer (4°C) consisting of phosphate buffered saline (PBS) containing 1mM phenylmethylsulfonyl fluoride. Solubilized extracts were sonicated using a sonifier cell disruptor and centrifuged to remove cellular debris. The protein concentration was assessed using the Bicinchoninic Acid (BCA) Protein Assay method.

Nitrotyrosine immunoprecipitation

Solubilized proteins (2 mg) were incubated with 10 ug mouse monoclonal anti-nitrotyrosine antibody (agarose conjugated, Millipore Corporation, Billerica, MA, USA). Immune complexes were precipitated overnight at 4°C, washed in extraction buffer, resuspended in sample loading buffer (16 mM Tris HCl, PH 6.8/

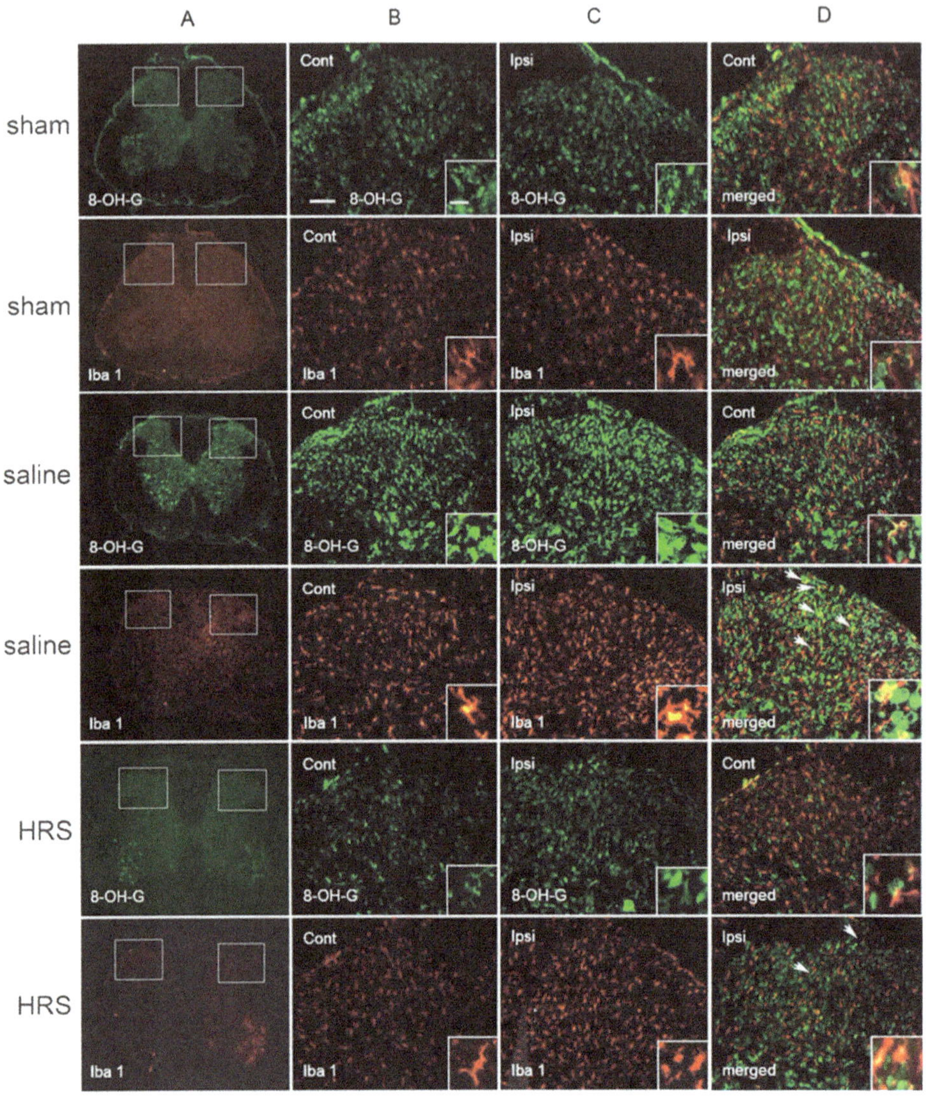

Figure 6. Immunostaining for 8-OH-G and Iba1 in sham rats, NS-treated neuropathic rats and HRS-treated neuropathic rats. Pictures in columns B and C are magnification of the insets shown in column A. Enlargements in the insets in columns B, C and D demonstrate the changes in cell shape and expression of 8-OH-G (green) and Iba-1 (red). Double-staining demonstrate colocalization (arrows) of 8-OH-G and Iba1. Note that an increased number of cells showing immunoreactivity for 8-OH-G and Iba-1 in neuropathic rats treated with NS as compared to the sham rats. And number of cells showed colocalization of 8-OH-G and Iba-1 in NS treated neuropathic rats was significantly increased as compared to the sham rats. HRS greatly reversed L5 SNL induced production of 8-OH-G, activation of microglia, and increase of 8-OH-G-ir microglia. Scale bars, 100 μm and 25 μm in the inset.

2.5% glycerol/0.5% SDS/200 mM 2-mercaptoethanol/0.001% bromophenol blue), heated and immediately fractionated by reducing SDS/PAGE in 12% gels.

Western blot analysis

After separation by SDS/PAGE, proteins were transferred electrophoretically (100 V, 1 hr) to nitrocellulose membranes, which were blocked (1 hr, 20°C) with 5% nonfat milk in 50 mM Tris HCl, PH 7.4/150 mM NaCl/0.05% Tween 20 (TBS/T). For detection of Mn-SOD, blots were incubated (overnight, 20°C) with mouse monoclonal anti-MnSOD antibody (1:1000, Millipore Corporation, Billerica, MA, USA). After three times wash in TBS/T, the immunocomplexed membranes were probed with goat anti-mouse horseradish peroxidase-conjugated secondary antibody (1:10000). Probed membranes were washed three times, and immunoreactive proteins were detected using enhanced chemiluminescence. The integrated optical density (IOD) of lanes resulting from immunoprecipitation was calculated using Image-pro plus analysis (Media Cybernetics Inc., Rockville, MD, USA).

ELISA

Tissue samples were homogenized in a homogenization buffer and centrifugated at 40,000×g for 1 hr. The supernatant was collected, and the. IL-1β and TNF-α levels were assessed by enzyme-linked immunosorbent assay (R&D Systems, Minneapolis, MN, USA) according to the instructions of the manufacturer, and are expressed as picograms per microgram of protein.

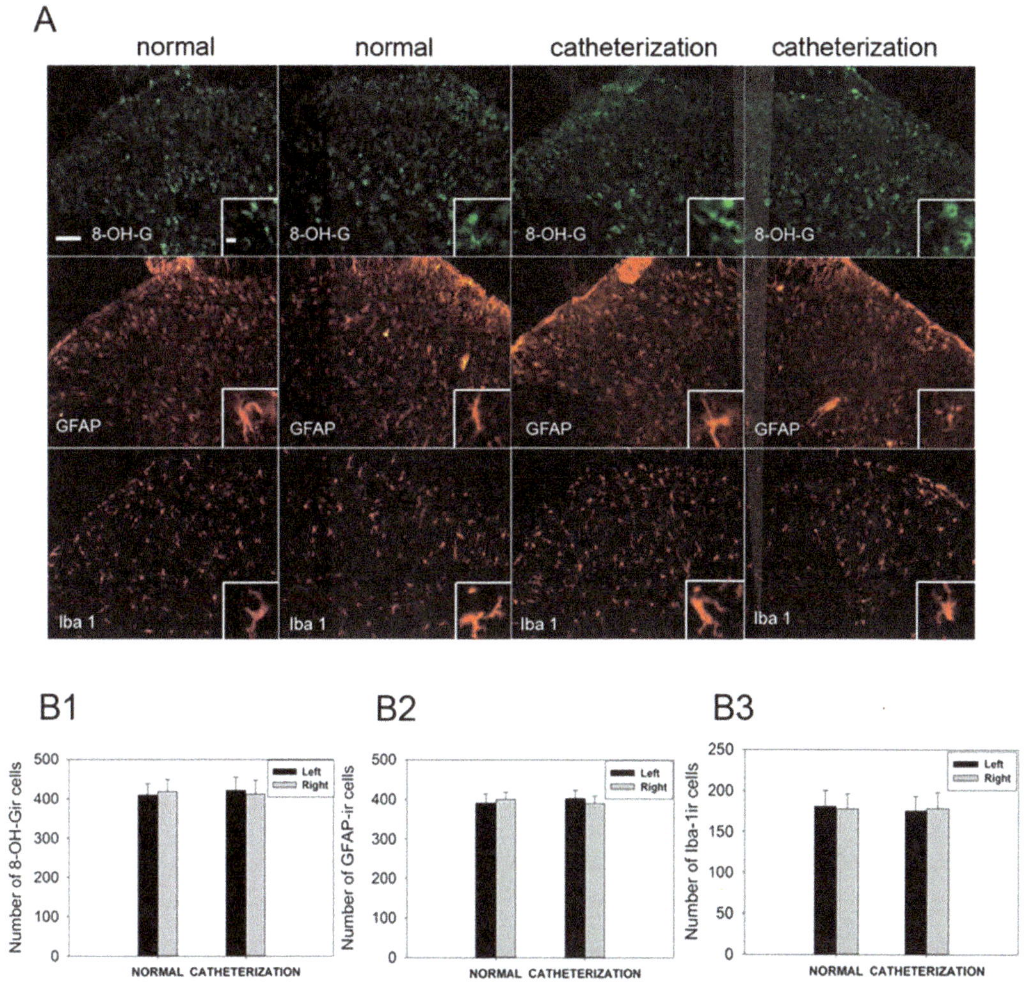

Figure 7. Expression of 8-OH-G, GFAP and Iba-1 in catheterized rats. (A) Photomicrographs of immunostaining for 8-OH-G (green), GFAP (red) and Iba1 (red) in normal rats and catheterized rats. Enlargements in the insets demonstrate the changes in cell shape and expression of 8-OH-G, GFAP and Iba-1. There is no significant difference in number of cells showing immunoreactivity for 8-OH-G, GFAP and Iba-1 between catheterized rats and normal rats. Scale bars, 100 μm and 25 μm in the inset. (B1, B2 and B3) Number of cells showing immunoreactivity for 8-OH-G, GFAP and Iba-1 in both sides of spinal dorsal horn. Data are expressed as mean±SEM. n = 10 for B1-3. Compared to the normal rats, catheterization did not induced significant production of 8-OH-G, activation of glial cells.

Statistics

Data are presented as mean±standard errors of the mean (SEM) and analyzed using the SPSS statistical program. For behavioral responses analysis, two-way repeated ANOVAs were used, followed by post hoc LSD test. Data from image-analysis, immunoprecipitation and ELISA were analyzed by one-way ANOVA analysis. P value of <0.05 was considered to be significant.

Results

The effect of single-dose HRS on mechanical allodynia

Mechanical thresholds of neuropathic rats were evaluated after intrathecal injection of single-dose HRS or NS using a randomized cross-over design [7]. L5 SNL was performed on 10 rats, a procedure that resulted in marked reduction in mechanical thresholds. On the third post-operative (PO) day, the rats were divided into two groups of five, each group receiving either HRS or saline. Mechanical thresholds were determined for all animals at a set of time points (1 hr, 2 hrs, 3 hrs, 4 hrs, 6 hrs, 8 hrs after the injection. The analgesic effect of HRS was short-acting, these time points were chosen to show the pharmacodynamic characters). All animals were then rested for 48 hrs. On the fifth PO day, each group received another injection of HRS or NS, which they did not receive before, followed by the same paradigm of behavioral testing. Figure 1 show the summary of all the testing results and each point represents tests on 10 rats. Note that mechanical thresholds were markedly reduced after nerve ligation, and administration of HRS raised these thresholds for about 8 hrs before the thresholds declined to the level of the NS group.

The long-term effect of HRS treatment on mechanical allodynia and thermal hyperalgesia

To examine long-term effects of HRS, 20 rats were selected and randomly divided into two groups: HRS group and NS group. These 20 rats received intrathecal injection of HRS or saline respectively at 24 hrs intervals for 15 days, on the third day after the first dose, the L5 spinal nerve was ligated. Another 10 rats were selected and underwent a sham operation but received no injection. From the L5 SNL day to 12 days after L5 SNL,

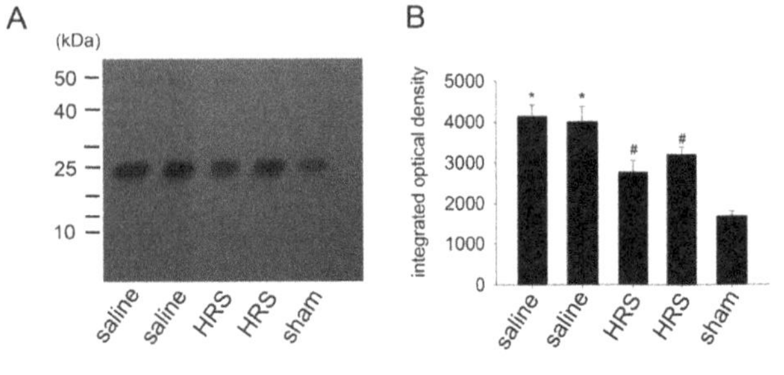

Figure 8. HRS blocks nitrition of MnSOD in spinal cord of neuropathic rats. (A) When compared to the sham group (lane 5), L5 SNL induced significant nitration of MnSOD in neuropathic rats treated with NS (lane 1,2). These events were blocked by HRS treatment (lane 3,4). Approximate sizes (kDa) were estimated using prestained molecular mass markers to the left. (B) The integrated optical density (IOD) of lanes resulted from immunoprecipitation was obtained using Image-pro plus analysis. Data are expressed as mean±SEM (n = 5). Compared to the sham rats, L5 SNL induced significant production of tyrosine-nitrated MnSOD, *p<0.01, by one-way ANOVA. HRS blocked the production of tyrosine-nitrated MnSOD, #p<0.01, by one-way ANOVA.

mechanical thresholds and paw withdraw latencies (PWLs) were determined for all animals at the time points 23–24 hrs after each injection, the first examinations of mechanical threshold and PWL for each rat were done before L5 SNL. Figure 2 shows the results of behavior testing. Note that mechanical thresholds and PWLs of HRS or NS treated rats remained the same levels as the sham rats at the time point of 0 PO day. It was found that mechanical thresholds and PWLs were reduced dramatically after L5 SNL. Mechanical thresholds of neuropathic rats received HRS were increased to a constant level, which was significantly higher than rats received NS (Figure 2 A). Repeated administration of HRS markedly raised PWL of the neuropathic rats, and no significant fluctuations were observed when PWLs reached a latency of 7.5 seconds (on the third PO day). NS injection did not affect the marked decline of mechanical thresholds or PWLs (Figure 2 B). We concluded that no tolerance develops when animals receive repeated treatment of HRS, and injections of HRS do not affect the basal mechanical threshold and PWL in rat without nerve ligation.

The effect of preemptive HRS treatment on mechanical allodynia and thermal hyperalgesia

To examine preemptive analgesic effects, starting 3 days prior to the neuropathic lesion, HRS was administered intrathecally to 10 rats at 24 hrs intervals for 6 days. Additional 10 rats received the same paradigm of saline injection, serving as a control group. On the third day after the first dose, the L5 spinal nerve was ligated. 10 rats that underwent a sham procedure received no injection. From the L5 SNL day to 12 days after L5 SNL, mechanical thresholds and PWLs were determined for all animals at the time points 23–24 hrs after each injection. Figure 3 is a summary of the behavior testing results. Evident is the slow decline in mechanical thresholds after the lesion in rats of the HRS group, and that the thresholds remain at a higher level than saline group for several days after cessation of HRS. Mechanical thresholds in neuropathic rats treated with saline declined sharply, and then became stable when it reached the level of 3.67 (in logarithmic units). Mechanical thresholds in rats of the sham group did not change significantly after the operation (Figure 3 A). The mean PWL was 5.21±0.67 seconds (mean±SD) in rats of sham group

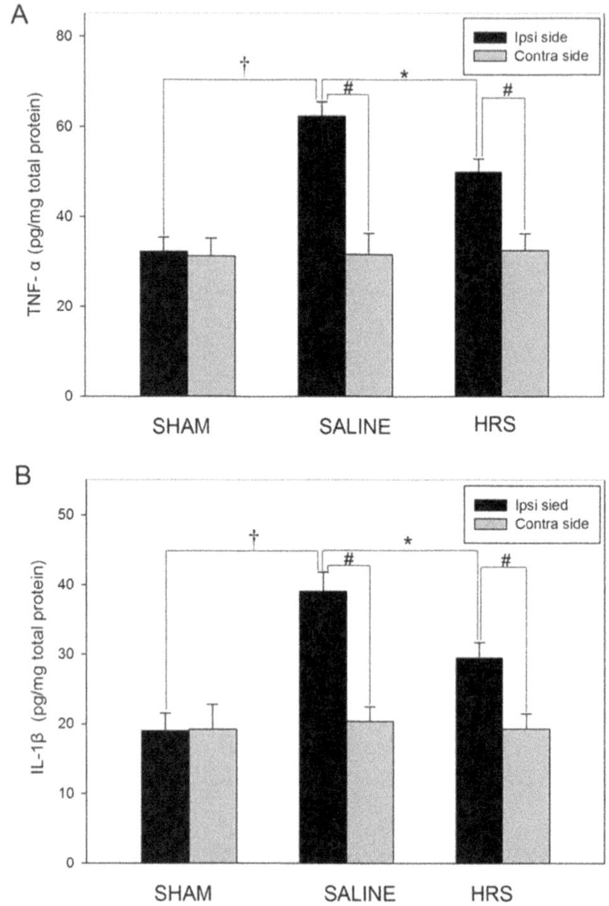

Figure 9. Protein content of TNF-α (A) and IL-1β (B) in both sides of spinal dorsal horn. Data are expressed as mean±SEM. n = 10 for A and B. Compared to the sham rats, L5 SNL induced significant production of TNF-α and IL-1β, †p<0.01, by one-way ANOVA. HRS blocked the production of TNF-α and IL-1β, *p<0.01, by one-way ANOVA. Compared to contralateral side, L5 SNL induced significant production of TNF-α and IL-1β in ipsilateral side. #p<0.01, by one-way ANOVA.

and did not change significantly during the test. Ligation of the spinal nerve caused a significant decrease in PWLs in rats receiving daily NS treatments. PWLs declined much slowly after the lesion in rats receiving daily HRS treatments, and PWLs remain at a higher level than NS group for several days after cessation of HRS (Figure 3 B), indicating that HRS treatment provided a relatively long-lasting preemptive effect.

Astrocytic responses to L5 SNL in NS treated neuropathic rats and HRS treated neuropathic rats

To examine whether HRS could alleviated oxidative stress in the spinal dorsal horn, and reverse the activation of spinal astrocytes, 8-OH-G and glial fibrillary acidic protein (GFAP) immunoreactivities were assessed in the lumbar spinal cord of sham rats, L5 SNL rats treated with HRS and L5 SNL rats treated with NS. To identify whether 8-OH-G was produced in astrocytes, we performed double immunofluorescence staining of 8-OH-G with GFAP. Rats were sacrificed 1 hr after HRS or NS treatment, on the 12th day after L5 SNL or sham operation. In the L4-L5 lumbar dorsal horns of rats in the sham group, low-level 8-OH-G immunostaining was observed. In the neuropathic rats treated with NS, levels of 8-OH-G on the ipsilateral side of spinal dorsal horns were markedly higher, and HRS treated neuropathic rats showed lower production of 8-OH-G in the lumbar dorsal horn compared with NS treated neuropathic rats, as shown in Figure 4 and Figure 5 B1, B2.

In the sham group, the immunostaining of GFAP was low, and the stained astrocytes had extensive processes and were well spaced showing no obvious signs of astrocytic activation. In the neuropathic rats treated with NS, spinal astrocytes on the ipsilateral side were intensely stained and appeared to have an altered shape with long protrusions showing an activated state. In the neuropathic rat treated with HRS, the immunostaining of GFAP was lower, and showed less astrocytic activation, as compared with the neuropathic rats treated with NS (Figure 4 and Figure 5 B3).

Double immunofluorescence staining revealed that spinal astrocytes of sham rats produced a small amount of 8-OH-G. In the spinal cord of neuropathic rats treated with NS, an increased number of astrocytes showed colocalization of 8-OH-G and GFAP on the ipsilateral side. HRS administration lowered the number of astrocytes showing colocalization of 8-OH-G and GFAP (Figure 4 and Figure 5 B5).

Microglial responses to L5 SNL in NS treated neuropathic rats and HRS treated neuropathic rats

The ionized calcium-binding adapter molecule 1 (Iba-1) level in the spinal dorsal horn of sham rats, L5 SNL rats treated with HRS and L5 SNL rats treated with NS were examined to determine whether HRS could alleviate the activation of spinal microglia. Double immunofluorescence staining of 8-OH-G with Iba-1 was also performed to identify whether 8-OH-G was produced in microglia. Rats were sacrificed 1 hr after HRS or NS treatment, on the 12th day after L5 SNL or sham operation. In the sham rats, the Iba-1 immunostaining was low, and microglia stained with Iba-1 showed features of an inactivated state. They had extensive and thinly branched processes and were well spaced. In neuropathic rats treated with NS, microglia on the ipsilateral side were heavily stained and exhibited short, thick processes and enlarged cell bodies, showing characteristics of an activated state. These phenotypic features of resting microglia and activated microglia are consistent with previous studies [41,42]. In neuropathic rats treated with HRS, microglia on the ipsilateral side were activated, but showed fewer features of an activated state than neuropathic rats treated with NS (Figure 6 and Figure 5 B4).

Double immunofluorescence staining revealed that spinal microglia in sham rats produced a small amount of 8-OH-G (Figure 6 and Figure 5 B6). In neuropathic rats treated with NS, the number of microglia on the ipsilateral side of the dorsal horn that showed colocalization of 8-OH-G and Iba-1 was significant larger compared with sham rats. And in neuropathic rats treated with HRS, the number of microglia showing colocalization of 8-OH-G and Iba-1 on the ipsilateral side was larger than that of the sham group, but less than that of the animal treated with saline (Figure 6 and Figure 5 B6).

Rats received catheterization demonstrate normal basal expression of 8-OH-G and normal activation of glial cells in spinal dorsal horn

To exclude the fact that possible over-expression of 8-OH-G and activation of glial cells are caused by catheterization, 8-OH-G, GFAP, and Iba-1 immunoreactivities were assessed in the lumbar spinal cord of normal rats and rats received catheterization 15 days before. In the L4-L5 lumbar dorsal horns, low-level 8-OH-G, GFAP and Iba-1 immunostaining were observed in both normal rats and catheterized rats (Figure 7A). Spinal glial cells had cell bodies that were small and elongated with long protrusions showing no obvious signs of activation. Numbers of cells showing immunoreactivity for 8-OH-G, GFAP and Iba-1 were comparable in normal rats and catheterized rats (Figure 7 B1, B2 and B3).

HRS reverses the elevated tyrosine-nitrated Mn-containing superoxide dismutase (MnSOD) expression in spinal cord of L5 SNL rats

Rats were sacrificed 1 hr after HRS or NS treatment, on the 12th day after L5 SNL or sham operation. Nitration of tyrosine residues in MnSOD of the lumbar dorsal horn was detected by Western blot analysis of SDS/PAGE-fractionated tyrosine-nitrated proteins, which had been immunoprecipitated from total spinal extracts using the monoclonal anti-nitrotyrosine. Immunodetection with monoclonal anti-MnSOD antibody demonstrated low but detectable levels of tyrosine-nitrated MnSOD in sham rats. Neuropathic rats treated with NS exhibited an increased level of immunoreactive tyrosine-nitrated MnSOD, while neuropathic rats treated with HRS exhibited a lower level of tyrosine-nitrated MnSOD as compared with neuropathic rats treated with NS, though it was higher than that in sham rats (Figure 8).

HRS reduces the expression of proinflammatory cytokines in the lumbar spinal cord

To investigate whether the analgesic effect of HRS was associated with the decrease in proinflammatory cytokines production, protein levels of TNF-α and IL-1β on both sides of the spinal cord were assessed using enzyme-linked immunosorbent assay (ELISA). 12 days after nerve ligation, the spinal expressions of both TNF-α and IL-1β on the ipsilateral side of rats treated with NS were up-regulated in comparison with the sham-operated rats (TNF-α: $p<0.01$; IL-1β: $p<0.01$). While HRS reversed the over-expressions (TNF-α: $p<0.01$; IL-1β: $p<0.01$)(Figure 9 A and B). The spinal expressions of TNF-α and IL-1β on the contralateral side of rats treated with saline did not differ from those in the sham group. In comparison with the contralateral side, expressions of TNF-α and IL-1β on the ipsilateral side of the spinal cord of rats treated with NS were found also up-regulated, while HRS reversed the over-expressions (TNF-α: $p<0.01$; IL-1β: $p<0.01$)(Figure 9 A and B).

Discussion

This study showed that intrathecal HRS significantly reduced the behavior signs of allodynia and hyperalgesia in neuropathic rats. Administration of single-dose HRS attenuated mechanical allodynia for about 8 hrs, repeated treatment of HRS ameliorated mechanical allodynia and thermal hyperalgesia without developing tolerance. Preemptive HRS treatment had a long-last effect on mechanical allodynia and thermal hyperalgesia.

In the L4-5 spinal dorsal horn, L5 SNL induced increased production of 8-OH-G, and significantly activated astrocytes and microglia. Intrathecal HRS reduced L5 SNL-induced over-production of 8-OH-G and attenuated activation of glial cells. 8-OH-G production was found in astrocytes and microglia, as indicated by immunostaining. Glial cells activated concurrently when 8-OH-G in glial cells was over-produced, on the contrary, glial activation was attenuated when 8-OH-G was eliminated by HRS. The hydroxyl radical is able to add to double bonds of DNA bases at a second-order, abstracts an H-atom from the methy group and leads to formation of 8-OH-G. Our observation of over-produced 8-OH-G in activated glial cells and reduced 8-OH-G production in less activated glial cells suggests a mechanism of enlargement of pain signals from primary afferent neurons by hydroxyl activated glial cells which play a key role in modulation of pain signals.

Peroxynitrite can nitrate the 3-position of tyrosine residues on MnSOD, indicating that tyrosine-nitrated MnSOD level is directly related to peroxynitrite. We have shown in this study that L5 SNL increased the production of tyrosine-nitrated MnSOD in the lumbar dorsal horn, and intrathecal HRS significantly reduced the over-production of tyrosine-nitrated MnSOD and attenuated allodynia and hyperalgesia. Therefore, we conclude that peroxynitrite contributes to the enhanced processing of nociceptive messages in spinal dorsal horn. Salvemini and coworkers have demonstrated that peroxynitrite plays a key role in nitroxidative regulation of the glutamatergic pathway during nociceptive processing, modulation of glutamate transmission by tyrosine residues nitration, and enhanced neuroimmune activation [43–45]. Our study showed that intrathecal HRS significantly attenuated L5 SNL-induced activation of spinal glial cells, suggesting that spinal peroxynitrite might be involve in the activation of glial cells, and leads to neuropathic pain.

It has been demonstrated that both astrocytes and microglia are capable of releasing proinflammatory factors [46–48]. In the present study, protein levels of TNF-α and IL-1β on both sides of the spinal cord were assessed. 12 days after L5 SNL, expression of TNF-α and IL-1β on the ipsilateral side were significantly up-regulated in comparison with the sham-operated rats, while HRS reversed their over-expression, indicating that changes in levels of proinflammtory factors expression are correlated with the changes in level of hydroxyl and peroxynitrite.

Chronic pain is a state where abnormalities are maintained in both central and peripheral nervous systems [49]. In the spinal cord, there are multiple potential sites where ROS and RNS can exert effects contributing to neuropathic pain, include three mechanisms implicated in central sensitization: alteration in glutamateric neurotransmission, loss of tonic inhibitory controls and glial-neuronal interactions [50], here we focus on glial-neuronal interactions. Under normal conditions, microglia functions as resident macrophages in the CNS. Within hours of peripheral nerve injury, activated microglia accumulates in the superficial dorsal horn. The activated microglial releases proinflammatory cytokines (such as TNF-α, IL-1β and 6), leading to neuronal central sensitization. In the present study, we showed that L5 SNL induced significant activation of microglia mediated by hydroxyl and peroxynitrite and up-regulated the expression of TNF-α and IL-1β on the ipsilateral side. In addition to proinflammatory cytokines, Coull and coworkers demonstrated that activated microglia induced by P2X4 receptors released brain-derived neurotrophic factor (BDNF) [26]. The contribution of astrocytes to central sensitization remains unclear. Many studies showed that activated astrocytes played an important role in central sensitization [51–53], and unlike microglia, astrocyte activation is generally delayed and persists longer, up to several months [50]. Our study showed that L5 SNL induced significant activation of spinal astrocytes mediated by hydroxyl and peroxynitrite.

The selective vulnerability of neural systems to ROS is a common characteristic of age-related degenerative diseases and some painful nerve conditions (including neuropathic pain) [8,54–59]. Knowing pain perception is amplified when noxious stimuli continue and oxidative stress in spinal cells is enhanced in neuropathic conditions [7,60], we postulate that on-going afferent discharges in persistent pain states elevates ROS and RNS production in the spinal cord, and lead to abnormal activation of spinal cells. In the present study, 12 days after L5 SNL, an increased production of ROS and RNS was detected in the spinal dorsal horn, and significant activation of astrocytes and microglia was observed. In the spinal cord of rats treated with HRS, levels of ROS and RNS were lower, and fewer activated glial cells were detected, and the behavior signs of allodynia and hyperalgesia were reduced. Allan and coworkers stated that under persistent pain state, the processes of central sensitization medicated by activated of N-Methyl-D-aspartate (NMDA) receptor are comparable to that implicated in the plastic changes associated with hippocampal long-term potentiation (LTP), a cellular correlate for learning and memory. Jin Mo Chung have demonstrated that ROS were involved in LTP in spinal dorsal horn [61]. In our opinion, ROS and RNS may be key molecules involved in the spinal LTP in neuropathic rats.

Although antioxidants are known to be potentially effective for treatment of neuropathic pain, concerns about their adverse effects, half-life, and tolerance remain. PBN is a potent ROS scavenger, Kim and coworkers showed that PBN ameliorated the behavioral signs of mechanical allodynia in rat model [7]. However, although this compound proved to be a neuroprotective agent, it induced hypothermia and toxicity [62]. Hydrogen gas cannot be produced by the human body since mammalian cells lack the hydrogenase activity [63]. However, it is continuously produced by colonic bacteria in the body and normally circulates in the blood [64]. Studies showed that inhalation of hydrogen gas did not influence physiological parameters such as body temperature, blood pressure, pH, and PO2 in the blood [65]. The half-life of HRS injected intrathecally has not been established yet the analgesic effect persisted for about 8 hrs. Fortunately, no tolerance developed when animals were treated with HRS repeatedly. So, HRS has the following advantages: easy to use, no side effects and no tolerance develops when given continuously, indicating that therapeutic use of HRS may be promising. HRS infusion and H_2 inhalation are most commonly used in clinic hydrogen treatment. Hydrogen administration may not be therapeutic unless enough concentration stays in the spinal cord, so the effective doses needed should be determined before clinical use.

Conclusions

Intrathecal injection of HRS produced analgesic effect in the rat model of neuropathic pain. Preemptive treatments with HRS delayed the development of pain behavior, and no tolerance developed when HRS was given repeatedly. The side effect of HRS seems tenuous as HRS selectively reduces hydroxyl and peroxynitrite. HRS reduced the intracellular levels of hydroxyl and peroxynitrite in the spinal cord, blocked the activation of spinal glial cells, and reduced the expression of proinflammatory factors in the spinal cord. We conclude that abnormal elevation of ROS and RNS plays a key role in central sensitization under neuropathic conditions. HRS has a potentially promising prospect for clinical treatment of neuropathic pain.

Author Contributions

Conceived and designed the experiments: WY. Performed the experiments: YG FW ZX LY SH ZL YS. Analyzed the data: FW XS. Contributed reagents/materials/analysis tools: XS. Wrote the paper: YG.

References

1. Salvemini D, Little JW, Doyle T, Neumann WL (2011) Roles of reactive oxygen and nitrogen species in pain. Free Radic Biol Med 51: 951–966.
2. Hackel D, Pflucke D, Neumann A, Viebahn J, Mousa S, et al. (2013) The connection of monocytes and reactive oxygen species in pain. PLoS One 8: e63564.
3. Kim HK, Kim JH, Gao X, Zhou JL, Lee I, et al. (2006) Analgesic effect of vitamin E is mediated by reducing central sensitization in neuropathic pain. Pain 122: 53–62.
4. Tal M (1996) A novel antioxidant alleviates heat hyperalgesia in rats with an experimental painful peripheral neuropathy. Neuroreport 7: 1382–1384.
5. Lu R, Kallenborn-Gerhardt W, Geisslinger G, Schmidtko A (2011) Additive antinociceptive effects of a combination of vitamin C and vitamin E after peripheral nerve injury. PLoS One 6: e29240.
6. Fidanboylu M, Griffiths LA, Flatters SJ (2011) Global inhibition of reactive oxygen species (ROS) inhibits paclitaxel-induced painful peripheral neuropathy. PLoS One 6: e25212.
7. Kim HK, Park SK, Zhou JL, Taglialatela G, Chung K, et al. (2004) Reactive oxygen species (ROS) play an important role in a rat model of neuropathic pain. Pain 111: 116–124.
8. Coyle JT, Puttfarcken P (1993) Oxidative stress, glutamate, and neurodegenerative disorders. Science 262: 689–695.
9. Hald A, Lotharius J (2005) Oxidative stress and inflammation in Parkinson's disease: is there a causal link? Exp Neurol 193: 279–290.
10. Manczak M, Jung Y, Park BS, Partovi D, Reddy PH (2005) Time-course of mitochondrial gene expressions in mice brains: implications for mitochondrial dysfunction, oxidative damage, and cytochrome c in aging. J Neurochem 92: 494–504.
11. Salvemini D, Neumann W (2010) Targeting peroxynitrite driven nitroxidative stress with synzymes: A novel therapeutic approach in chronic pain management. Life Sci 86: 604–614.
12. Ohsawa I, IIshikawa M, Takahashi K, Watanabe M, Nishimaki K, et al. (2007) Hydrogen acts as a therapeutic antioxidant by selectively reducing cytotoxic oxygen radicals. Nat Med 13: 688–694.
13. Ji RR, Berta T, Nedergaard M (2013) Glia and pain: Is chronic pain a gliopathy? Pain.
14. Watkins LR, Martin D, Ulrich P, Tracey KJ, Maier SF (1997) Evidence for the involvement of spinal cord glia in subcutaneous formalin induced hyperalgesia in the rat. Pain 71: 225–235.
15. Ren K, Dubner R (2010) Interactions between the immune and nervous systems in pain. Nat Med 16: 1267–1276.
16. Okada-Ogawa A, Suzuki I, Sessle BJ, Chiang CY, Salter MW, et al. (2009) Astroglia in medullary dorsal horn (trigeminal spinal subnucleus caudalis) are involved in trigeminal neuropathic pain mechanisms. J Neurosci 29: 11161–11171.
17. Ji RR, Kawasaki Y, Zhuang ZY, Wen YR, Decosterd I (2006) Possible role of spinal astrocytes in maintaining chronic pain sensitization: review of current evidence with focus on bFGF/JNK pathway. Neuron Glia Biol 2: 259–269.
18. Gao YJ, Ji RR (2010) Targeting astrocyte signaling for chronic pain. Neurotherapeutics 7: 482–493.
19. Chiang CY, Sessle BJ, Dostrovsky JO (2012) Role of astrocytes in pain. Neurochem Res 37: 2419–2431.
20. Nakamura Y, Morioka N, Abe H, Zhang FF, Hisaoka-Nakashima K, et al. (2013) Neuropathic pain in rats with a partial sciatic nerve ligation is alleviated by intravenous injection of monoclonal antibody to high mobility group box-1. PLoS One 8: e73640.
21. Ransohoff RM, Perry VH (2009) Microglial physiology: unique stimuli, specialized responses. Annu Rev Immunol 27: 119–145.
22. Lawson LJ, Perry VH, Dri P, Gordon S (1990) Heterogeneity in the distribution and morphology of microglia in the normal adult mouse brain. Neuroscience 39: 151–170.
23. Zhang F, Vadakkan KI, Kim SS, Wu LJ, Shang Y, et al. (2008) Selective activation of microglia in spinal cord but not higher cortical regions following nerve injury in adult mouse. Mol Pain 4: 15.
24. Tsuda M, Shigemoto-Mogami Y, Koizumi S, Mizokoshi A, Kohsaka S, et al. (2003) P2X4 receptors induced in spinal microglia gate tactile allodynia after nerve injury. Nature 424: 778–783.
25. Ji RR, Suter MR (2007) p38 MAPK, microglial signaling, and neuropathic pain. Mol Pain 3: 33.
26. Coull JA, Beggs S, Boudreau D, Boivin D, Tsuda M, et al. (2005) BDNF from microglia causes the shift in neuronal anion gradient underlying neuropathic pain. Nature 438: 1017–1021.
27. Zhang J, Wu D, Xie C, Wang H, Wang W, et al. (2013) Tramadol and propentofylline coadministration exerted synergistic effects on rat spinal nerve ligation-induced neuropathic pain. PLoS One 8: e72943.
28. Kim D, You B, Jo EK, Han SK, Simon MI, et al. (2010) NADPH oxidase 2-derived reactive oxygen species in spinal cord microglia contribute to peripheral nerve injury-induced neuropathic pain. Proc Natl Acad Sci U S A 107: 14851–14856.
29. Yang CM, Hsieh HL, Lin CC, Shih RH, Chi PL, et al. (2013) Multiple factors from bradykinin-challenged astrocytes contribute to the neuronal apoptosis: involvement of astroglial ROS, MMP-9, and HO-1/CO system. Mol Neurobiol 47: 1020–1033.
30. Kim JA, Yun HM, Jin P, Lee HP, Han JY, et al. (2013) Inhibitory effect of a 2,4-bis(4-hydroxyphenyl) but-2-enal diacetate on neuro-inflammatory reactions via inhibition of STAT1 and STAT3 activation in cultured astrocytes and microglial BV-2 cells. Neuropharmacology.
31. Astiz M, Acaz-Fonseca E, Garcia-Segura LM (2013) Sex Differences and Effects of Estrogenic Compounds on the Expression of Inflammatory Molecules by Astrocytes Exposed to the Insecticide Dimethoate. Neurotox Res.
32. Wei H, Gong N, Huang JL, Fan H, Ma AN, et al. (2013) Spinal D-amino acid oxidase contributes to mechanical pain hypersensitivity induced by sleep deprivation in the rat. Pharmacol Biochem Behav 111C: 30–36.
33. Kim SH, Chung JM (1992) An experimental model for peripheral neuropathy produced by segmental spinal nerve ligation in the rat. Pain 50: 355–363.
34. Yaksh TL, Rudy TA (1976) Chronic catheterization of the spinal subarachnoid space. Physiol Behav 17: 1031–1036.
35. Chaplan SR, Bach FW, Pogrel JW, Chung JM, Yaksh TL (1994) Quantitative assessment of tactile allodynia in the rat paw. J Neurosci Methods 53: 55–63.
36. Dixon WJ (1980) Efficient analysis of experimental observations. Annu Rev Pharmacol Toxicol 20: 441–462.
37. Hargreaves K, Dubner R, Brown F, Flores C, Joris J (1988) A new and sensitive method for measuring thermal nociception in cutaneous hyperalgesia. Pain 32: 77–88.
38. Zhang Y, Sun Q, He B, Xiao J, Wang Z, et al. (2011) Anti-inflammatory effect of hydrogen-rich saline in a rat model of regional myocardial ischemia and reperfusion. Int J Cardiol 148: 91–95.
39. Sun Q, Cai J, Liu S, Liu Y, Xu W, et al. (2011) Hydrogen-rich saline provides protection against hyperoxic lung injury. J Surg Res 165: e43–49.
40. Chen H, Sun YP, Li Y, Liu WW, Xiang HG, et al. (2010) Hydrogen-rich saline ameliorates the severity of l-arginine-induced acute pancreatitis in rats. Biochem Biophys Res Commun 393: 308–313.
41. Swartjes M, van Velzen M, Niesters M, Aarts L, Brines M, et al. (2014) ARA 290, a peptide derived from the tertiary structure of erythropoietin, produces long-term relief of neuropathic pain coupled with suppression of the spinal microglia response. Mol Pain 10: 13.
42. Huang ZX, Lu ZJ, Ma WQ, Wu FX, Zhang YQ, et al. (2014) Involvement of RVM-expressed P2X7 receptor in bone cancer pain: Mechanism of descending facilitation. Pain.
43. Little JW, Cuzzocrea S, Bryant L, Esposito E, Doyle T, et al. (2013) Spinal mitochondrial-derived peroxynitrite enhances neuroimmune activation during morphine hyperalgesia and antinociceptive tolerance. Pain 154: 978–986.
44. Chen Z, Muscoli C, Doyle T, Bryant L, Cuzzocrea S, et al. (2010) NMDA-receptor activation and nitroxidative regulation of the glutamatergic pathway during nociceptive processing. Pain 149: 100–106.
45. Muscoli C, Dagostino C, Ilari S, Lauro F, Gliozzi M, et al. (2013) Posttranslational nitration of tyrosine residues modulates glutamate transmission and contributes to N-methyl-D-aspartate-mediated thermal hyperalgesia. Mediators Inflamm 2013: 950947.
46. Hald A (2009) Spinal astrogliosis in pain models: cause and effects. Cell Mol Neurobiol 29: 609–619.
47. Hanisch U-K (2002) Microglia as a source and target of cytokines. Glia 40: 140–155.
48. Abdelmoaty S, Wigerblad G, Bas DB, Codeluppi S, Fernandez-Zafra T, et al. (2013) Spinal actions of lipoxin A4 and 17(R)-resolvin D1 attenuate inflammation-induced mechanical hypersensitivity and spinal TNF release. PLoS One 8: e75543.
49. Woolf CJ, Salter MW (2000) Neuronal plasticity: increasing the gain in pain. Science 288: 1765–1769.
50. Basbaum AI, Bautista DM, Scherrer G, Julius D (2009) Cellular and molecular mechanisms of pain. Cell 139: 267–284.
51. Liu X, Tian Y, Lu N, Gin T, Cheng CH, et al. (2013) Stat3 inhibition attenuates mechanical allodynia through transcriptional regulation of chemokine expression in spinal astrocytes. PLoS One 8: e75804.
52. Lee JY, Choi DC, Oh TH, Yune TY (2013) Analgesic effect of acupuncture is mediated via inhibition of JNK activation in astrocytes after spinal cord injury. PLoS One 8: e73948.
53. Ji XT, Qian NS, Zhang T, Li JM, Li XK, et al. (2013) Spinal astrocytic activation contributes to mechanical allodynia in a rat chemotherapy-induced neuropathic pain model. PLoS One 8: e60733.
54. Balazs L, Leon M (1994) Evidence of an oxidative challenge in the Alzheimer's brain. Neurochem Res 19: 1131–1137.
55. Gotz ME, Kunig G, Riederer P, Youdim MB (1994) Oxidative stress: free radical production in neural degeneration. Pharmacol Ther 63: 37–122.
56. Gerlach M, Ben-Shachar D, Riederer P, Youdim MB (1994) Altered brain metabolism of iron as a cause of neurodegenerative diseases? J Neurochem 63: 793–807.
57. Jenner P (1994) Oxidative damage in neurodegenerative disease. Lancet 344: 796–798.
58. Lewen A, Matz P, Chan PH (2000) Free radical pathways in CNS injury. J Neurotrauma 17: 871–890.

59. Olanow CW (1992) An introduction to the free radical hypothesis in Parkinson's disease. Ann Neurol 32 Suppl: S2–9.
60. Khalil Z, Liu T, Helme RD (1999) Free radicals contribute to the reduction in peripheral vascular responses and the maintenance of thermal hyperalgesia in rats with chronic constriction injury. Pain 79: 31–37.
61. Lee KY, Chung K, Chung JM (2010) Involvement of reactive oxygen species in long-term potentiation in the spinal cord dorsal horn. J Neurophysiol 103: 382–391.
62. Dhainaut A, Tizot A, Raimbaud E, Lockhart B, Lestage P, et al. (2000) Synthesis, structure, and neuroprotective properties of novel imidazolyl nitrones. J Med Chem 43: 2165–2175.
63. Adams MW, Mortenson LE, Chen JS (1980) Hydrogenase. Biochim Biophys Acta 594: 105–176.
64. Reth M (2002) Hydrogen peroxide as second messenger in lymphocyte activation. Nat Immunol 3: 1129–1134.
65. Hayashida K, Sano M, Ohsawa I, Shinmura K, Tamaki K, et al. (2008) Inhalation of hydrogen gas reduces infarct size in the rat model of myocardial ischemia-reperfusion injury. Biochem Biophys Res Commun 373: 30–35.

2

Adenoviral-Mediated Glial Cell Line–Derived Neurotrophic Factor Gene Transfer Has a Protective Effect on Sciatic Nerve Following Constriction-Induced Spinal Cord Injury

An-Kuo Chou[1], Ming-Chang Yang[2,3,4], Hung-Pei Tsai[5], Chee-Yin Chai[6], Ming-Hong Tai[7], Aij-Li Kwan[5,8]*, Yi-Ren Hong[2,3,5]*

1 Department of Anesthesiology, Kaohsiung Chang Gung Memorial Hospital and Chang Gung University College of Medicine, Kaohsiung, Taiwan, R.O.C., **2** Department of Biological Sciences, National Sun Yat-Sen University, Kaohsiung, Taiwan, R.O.C., **3** Department of Biochemistry, Faculty of Medicine, College of Medicine, Kaohsiung Medical University, Kaohsiung, Taiwan, R.O.C., **4** Laboratory of Medical Research, Kaohsiung Armed Forces General Hospital, Kaohsiung, Taiwan, R.O.C., **5** Graduate Institute of Medicine, College of Medicine, Kaohsiung Medical University, Kaohsiung, Taiwan, R.O.C., **6** Department of Pathology, Kaohsiung Medical University Chung-Ho Memorial Hospital, Kaohsiung, Taiwan, R.O.C., **7** Institute of Biomedical Science, National Sun Yat-sen University, Kaohsiung, Taiwan, R.O.C., **8** Department of Neurosurgery, Kaohsiung Medical University Chung-Ho Memorial Hospital, Kaohsiung, Taiwan, R.O.C.

Abstract

Neuropathic pain due to peripheral nerve injury may be associated with abnormal central nerve activity. Glial cell-line-derived neurotrophic factor (GDNF) can help attenuate neuropathic pain in different animal models of nerve injury. However, whether GDNF can ameliorate neuropathic pain in the spinal cord dorsal horn (SCDH) in constriction-induced peripheral nerve injury remains unknown. We investigated the therapeutic effects of adenoviral-mediated GDNF on neuropathic pain behaviors, microglial activation, pro-inflammatory cytokine expression and programmed cell death in a chronic constriction injury (CCI) nerve injury animal model. In this study, neuropathic pain was produced by CCI on the ipsilateral SCDH. Mechanical allodynia was examined with von Frey filaments and thermal sensitivity was tested using a plantar test apparatus post-operatively. Target proteins GDNF-1, GDNFRa-1, MMP2, MMP9, p38, phospho-p38, ED1, IL6, IL1β, AIF, caspase-9, cleaved caspase-9, caspase-3, cleaved caspase-3, PARP, cleaved PARP, SPECTRIN, cleaved SPECTRIN, Beclin-1, PKCσ, PKCγ, iNOS, eNOS and nNOS were detected. Microglial activity was measured by observing changes in immunoreactivity with OX-42. NeuN and TUNEL staining were used to reveal whether apoptosis was attenuated by GDNF. Results showed that administrating GDNF began to attenuate both allodynia and thermal hyperalgesia at day 7. CCI-rats were found to have lower GDNF and GDNFRa-1 expression compared to controls, and GDNF re-activated their expression. Also, GDNF significantly down-regulated CCI-induced protein expression except for MMP2, eNOS and nNOS, indicating that the protective action of GDNF might be associated with anti-inflammation and prohibition of microglia activation. Immunocytochemistry staining showed that GDNF reduced CCI-induced neuronal apoptosis. In sum, GDNF enhanced the neurotrophic effect by inhibiting microglia activation and cytokine production via p38 and PKC signaling. GDNF could be a good therapeutic tool to attenuate programmed cell death, including apoptosis and autophagy, consequent to CCI-induced peripheral nerve injury.

Editor: Yael Abreu-Villaça, Universidade do Estado do Rio de Janeiro, Brazil

Funding: This study was sponsored by National Science Council-96-2314-B-182A-018-MY2, National Science Council-95-2314-B-182A-151, and Chang Gung Memorial Hospital grant CMRP83031 to AKC. The funders had no role in study design, data collection and analysis, decision to publish, or preparation of the manuscript.

Competing Interests: The authors have declared that no competing interests exist.

* E-mail: m835016@cc.kmu.edu.tw (YRH); aijliekwan@yahoo.com.tw (ALK)

Introduction

Neuropathic pain is caused by lesions or diseases of the somatosensory system including peripheral nerve injury and central nerve injury. Spontaneous pain, thermal-mediated hyperalgesia and tactile-evoked allodynia are common neuropathic pain symptoms following peripheral nerve injury, and significantly reduce quality of life and functional status. In clinical observation, neuropathic pain is not confined to the innervation area of the injured nerve, but also affects the adjacent area innervated by other intact nerves. Previous data have shown that sprouting from lamina III into II in neuronal remodeling in the spinal cord might result in the development of persistent tactile allodynia [1,2]. Recent studies have demonstrated that C-fibers appear not to sprout outside their normal laminar distribution after injury [3]. According to current clinical experience, patients with neuropathic pain and visceral pain commonly have poor response to ordinary medication, and usually depend on opioid drugs for pain control [4]. Unfortunately, long-term administration of opiates has well-known side effects including drug addiction and tolerance, immunosuppression, and decreased micturition reflex. New therapeutic approaches such as gene therapy with pain-killer genes may hold promise for treating such patients.

Glial cell line-derived neurotrophic factor (GDNF) is one of the GDNF family of ligands (GFLs). GFLs are important for cell survival, neurite outgrowth, cell differentiation and cell migration, and GDNF promotes the survival of dopaminergic neurons [5]. Nerve injury downregulated GDNF and its receptor, GDNF family receptor alpha-1 (GDNFRa-1), on dorsal root ganglia [6]. Continuous injection of GDNF by osmotic pump promotes regeneration of sensory axons and attenuates neuropathic pain in animal models of nerve injury [7–9]. GDNF has been used as a therapy for neurodegenerative diseases such as Parkinson's disease [10,11] and amyotrophic lateral sclerosis [12,13]. However, the underlying molecular mechanism by which GDNF ameliorates neuropathic pain remains largely unknown. A better understanding of microglial-neuronal interactions in the SCDH will further our understanding of neural plasticity and may also lead to novel therapeutics for chronic pain management.

In this study, we used CCI as neuropathic pain model with adenoviral-mediated GDNF to evaluate the therapeutic effect of GDNF on peripheral nerve injury-induced neuropathic pain, analyzing protein expressions and activations in different aspects including microglia activation (MMP2, MMP9, p38, phospho-p38, IL6 and IL1β), caspase-dependent apoptotic markers (caspase-9, cleaved caspase-9, caspase-3, cleaved caspase-3, PARP, cleaved PARP), caspase-independent apoptotic markers (AIF, SPECTRIN and cleaved SPECTRIN), autophagy marker (Beclin-1), and CCI-induced proinflammatory markers (PKCσ, PKCγ, iNOS, eNOS and nNOS) to determine whether adenoviral-mediated GDNF gene therapy can successfully ameliorate the above gene expression and the different types of associated programmed cell death.

Materials and Methods

Animal model

Male Sprague–Dawley rats weighing (140 to 160 g at the time of surgery (NSC Animal Center, Taiwan) were fed with standard lab rodent chow and water *ad libitum* and housed individually. Rats were anesthetized with an intraperitoneal (i.p.) injection of sodium pentobarbital (Nembutal, 50 mg/kg), and CCI to the right sciatic nerve (SN) was done according to the method of Bennett and Xie (1988) [14], in which the left common sciatic nerves were exposed in the left midthigh and loosely ligated with 4-0 silk thread in three regions at about 1-mm intervals. Animal procedures were performed according to a protocol approved by the Institutional Review Board and Institutional Animal Care and Use Committee of Chang Guang Memorial Hospital.

Gene therapy

Recombinant adenovirus vectors encoding GDNF (Ad-GDNF) or enhanced green fluorescent protein (Ad-GFP) were prepared as described previously [15]. For Ad-GDNF, GDNF cDNA was subcloned into pCA13 to yield the transfer vector, Ad5-GDNF, which was used to transfect 293 cells with pJM17, a plasmid containing the entire adenoviral genome, to generate recombinant virus through homologous recombination by calcium phosphate protocol as described previously [16]. The virus was amplified in 293 cells, purified by two rounds of cesium chloride gradient ultracentrifugation, and dialyzed against buffer containing 10 mM Tris, pH 7.5, 1 mM $MgCl_2$, and 10% glycerol at 48°C. The titer of the virus solution was determined by measuring optical density at a wavelength of 260 nm and plaque-forming assay in 293 cells before storage at −80 °C. Adenovirus vectors [2×10^9 plaque-forming units (pfu) in 100 ml sterile phosphate buffer saline PBS] were administrated via the triceps brachii muscle of anesthetized rats using a disposable insulin syringe equipped with a 27-gauge needle. Injection was performed in a biosafety P2 laboratory, and the care of animals receiving the adenovirus vectors conformed to institutional guidelines.

Tissue preparation

The sciatic nerves were dissected and harvested at 7, 14, or 28 days after the CCI operation and at 28 days after viral injection paired with the CCI operation (six animals for each time point and group). The injured side of the sciatic nerve was cut into two segments from the region of ligation, the adjacent proximal and distal segments. The uninjured contralateral sciatic nerve in each animal was used as the control.

Thermal hyperalgesia

Thermal sensitivity of the plantar hind paws was tested according to Hargreaves' method [17] using a Plantar Test Apparatus (Ugo Basile, Comerio, Italy). Rats were placed unrestrained in individual clear plastic compartments (11 cm×17 cm×14 cm). When the rats were stationary and not attending to the tester or stimulus, an infrared radiant heat source (180 mW) was applied through a glass floor to the middle of the plantar surface of the hind paw, between the foot pads. A photocell automatically stopped the heat source and the timer when the rat lifted its paw. For transected mice that were not capable of hind paw plantar placement, the rats were held gently to assist the plantar placement of the hind paws. Each rat was tested for five trials on each hind paw, with at least 1 min between trials, and the order of testing was randomized to minimize windup or avoidance behaviors. A 20-s maximum cutoff was established to prevent tissue damage.

Allodynia test

The hind paw withdrawal threshold to tactile stimulation was determined using factory-calibrated Touch Test filaments (von Frey, Semmes–Weinstein monofilaments) (Stoelting, Wood Dale, IL, USA). Mice were placed under a small, clear compartment (8 cm×12 cm×5.5 cm) on an elevated wire mesh screen to allow the investigator free access to the plantar surface of the paws. For transected mice that were not capable of hind paw plantar placement, the mice were held gently to assist the plantar placement of the hind paws. Left and right hind paws were tested in a random order using the up-down method when the rat was not attending to the tester or the stimulus.

Hematoxylin/eosin staining

Slides were counterstained with hematoxylin and eosin (H&E) as described elsewhere [18] for tissue examination. Briefly, 6 μm sections were deparaffinized in Xylol (Carl-Roth, Germany) for 10 minutes, rehydrated in a descending ethanol series and rinsed in deionized H_2O for 1 minute. Sections were placed in hematoxylin for 3 minutes, rinsed in tap water for 1 minute to allow stain to develop and then placed in eosin for 1 minute, dehydrated and mounted in Entellan resin (Merck, Germany). The occurrence of clearly detectable eosinophilic spheroids indicative of dystrophic axons [19] was quantified in approximately 90 sections from ipsilateral SCDH so irregular results due to random deviations in spheroid numbers could be ruled out. H&E stained axonal spheroids were generally eosinophilic and round or oval in shape. They varied in diameter (5–50 μm) and sometimes reached a size larger than the nerve cells in SCDH. Morphology and density of

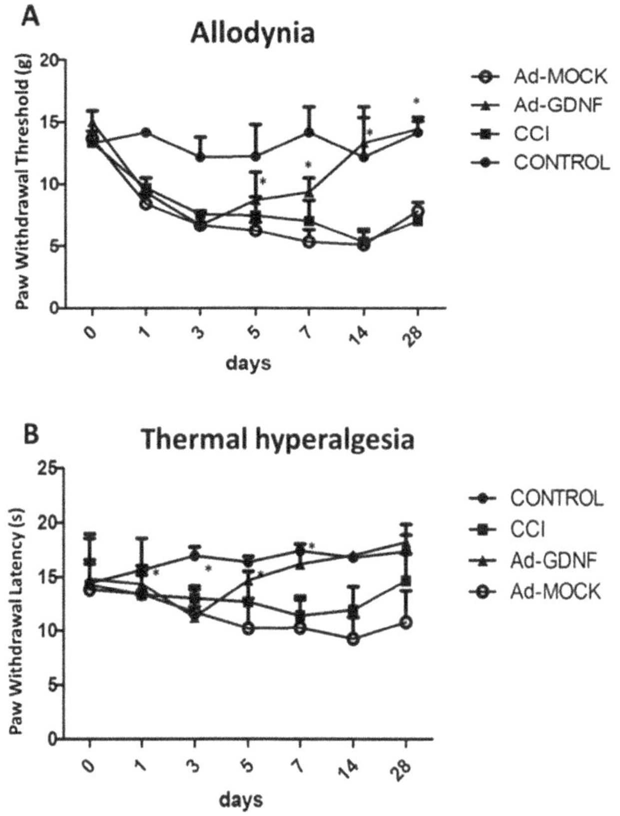

Figure 1. The effect of intramuscular delivery of Ad-GDNF on allodynia (A) and thermal hyperalgesia (B) in the CCI model. *$P<0.05$ compared with the CCI group at each time point.

neurons within the spinal cord were assessed. To avoid examining the same neurons twice, we left more than an 8 μm gap between sections.

Immunohistochemistry

Paraffin embedded samples, after deparaffinization and rehydration, were treated by steam heating for antigen retrieval (30 min) using DAKO antigen retrieval solution (DAKO, Carpenteria, CA). Slides were washed using Tris Buffered Saline (TBS) twice. Endogenous peroxidase was inhibited by immersing the slides in a 3% hydrogen peroxide solution for 10 min. Slides were then washed twice in TBS. The sections were incubated with primary antibody against GDNF 1 hour at room temperature. Slides were washed twice with TBS and consecutively incubated with biotinylated secondary antibody for 30 min. Slides were washed twice with TBS and incubated with DAB for 5 min. Slides were washed twice again with distilled water. Immediately after staining, slides were counterstained with hematoxylin for 1 min. Slides were rinsed for 1 second with distilled water and dehydrated for 1–2 seconds each with 90–100% isopropanol. Finally, samples were immersed in xylene for 10 min each and mounted using Permount (Fisher Scientific, Pittsburg, PA).

Immunofluorescent microscopy

The transversal frozen sections (10 μm) of sciatic nerves were dried and incubated in blocking buffer containing 1.5% normal goat serum and 0.2% Triton X-100 in PBS. The slides were washed twice with PBS, incubated with the primary antibodies (OX-42, phospho-p38, NeuN) at 4°C, 3 days, followed by repeated washing with PBS, and replaced in secondary antibodies conjugated with Alexa 488 or Cy3 for 3 hours at room temperature.

TUNEL test

The mode of cell death induced by CCI was determined by morphological observations done with terminal deoxynucleotidyl transferase (TdT)-mediated dUTP nick end labelling (TUNEL) assay. Briefly, the tissues were fixed with 4% methanol-free paraformaldehyde at 4 °C and washed with phosphate-buffered saline (PBS) for 30 min. An equilibrium buffer (0.1 ml) was added to each of the slides and covered with parafilm for 10 min at 37 °C. A mixture of 1 μl TdT enzyme, 5 μl nucleotide mix and 45 μl equilibrium buffer was prepared in the dark and 50 μl of the mixture was added onto each slide. Slides were incubated in the dark for 1 or 2 h at 37 °C. SSC (2X) was added for 15 min at room temperature to stop the TdT enzyme reaction. The unbound fluorescent-12-dUTP was removed by washing with PBS. The slides were then immersed in propidium iodide for 15 min in the dark to stain the cells. Slides were dried after rinsing with de-ionized water and cover slips were later overlaid on the cell area of the slides.

Western blot

For protein extraction, each single hemi-cord segment was homogenized in protein lysis buffer in the presence of protease inhibitors and incubated on ice for 10 min. Samples were centrifuged at 13,000×rpm for 30 min at 4 °C. Total protein content was determined in the supernatants by the Bio-Rad DC Protein Assay Kit. For Western blot analysis, equal amounts of total protein were separated by sodium dodecyl-sulfate polyacrylamide gel electrophoresis (SDS-PAGE; 12%) and transferred onto PVDF membranes. After blocking for 1 hour at room temperature in Tris-buffered saline containing 0.05% Tween 20 (TBST) and 5% non-fat milk, the membranes were incubated overnight at 4°C with the primary antibody including GDNF (1:100 dilutions; Santa Cruz Biotechnology Inc.); GDNFRa-1(1:100 dilution; R&D Systems Inc.); ERK, p-ERK, p38, phospho-p38, AIF, caspase-3, cleaved caspase-3, caspase-9, cleaved caspase-9, Beclin-1, MMP-2, MMP-9, iNOS, nNOS, eNOS, PARP, cleaved PARP, PKCγ, PKCδ (1: 1,000 dilution; Cell Signaling Technology); ED1, SPECTRIN and cleaved SPECTRIN (1:200 dilutions; Santa Cruz Biotechnology Inc.) directed against the protein of interest. After several washes, an appropriate HRP conjugated secondary antibody (1:5000; Vector Laboratories) was applied for 1 hour at room temperature. Peroxidase activity was visualized using the ECL Western Blotting Detection kit and X-ray films. Quantification of western blots and TUNEL staining were the average band intensities and/or cells with positive staining of chosen antibodies of three independent experiments were determined using ImageJ and plotted.

Data Analyses

Comparisons within groups were made by using one-way analysis of variance (ANOVA). The comparisons across groups were accomplished with one-way ANOVA and, if significant, discrete comparisons were accomplished using Tukey's method for post-hoc testing. A p value of less than 0.05 was considered statistically significant. Data were expressed as mean ± SEM.

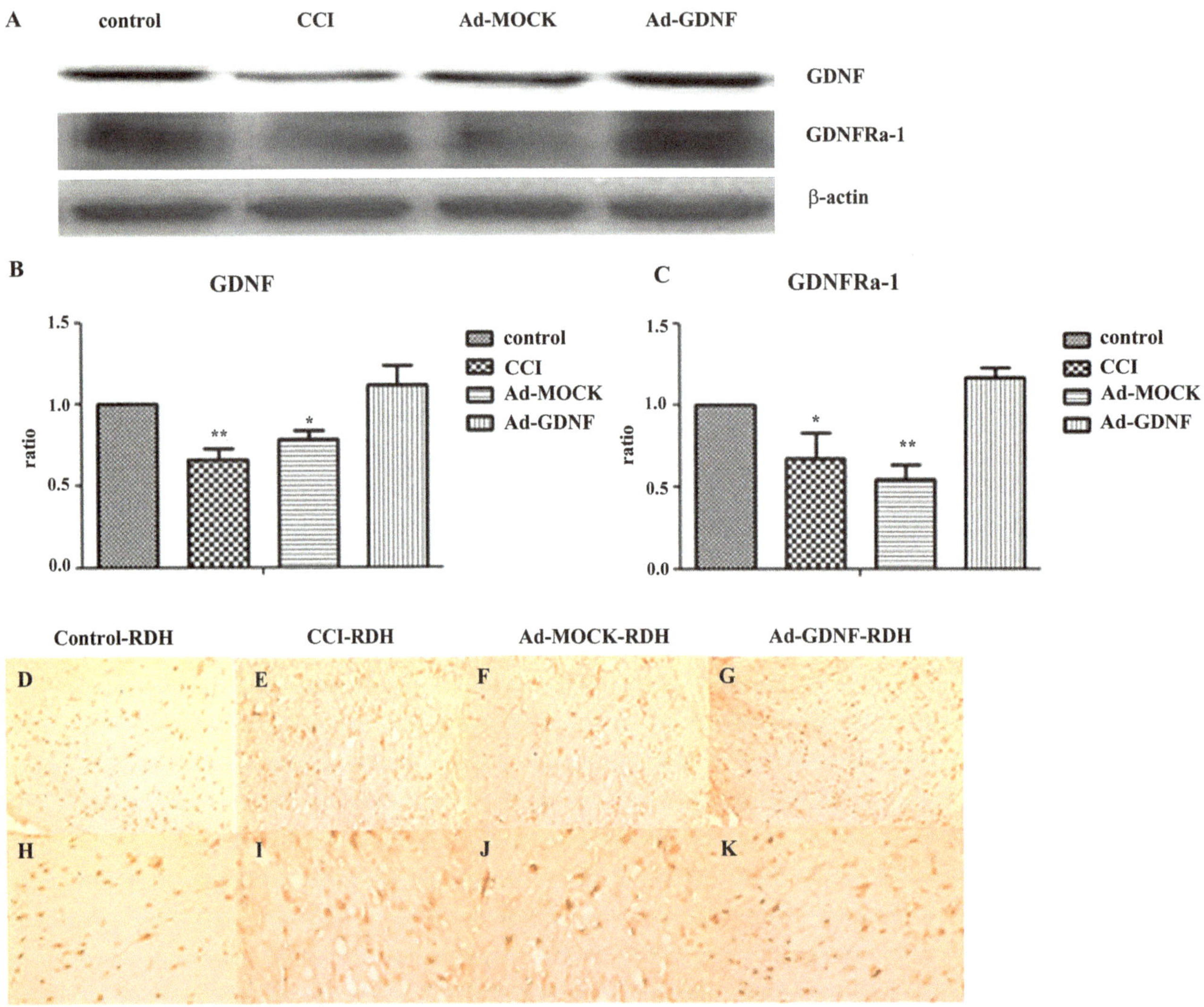

Figure 2. Immunoblotting showing protein expression level with respect to GDNF and its receptor. Western blot analysis showing the expression levels of GDNF and its receptor, GDNFRa-1, under control, CCI, and ipsilateral SCDH with intramuscular injection of Ad-MOCK or Ad-GDNF (A). The expression levels of GDNF and GDNFRa-1 with respect to each tested group were shown as bar charts of relative ratio (B–C). Immunohistochemical (D–K) staining was used to confirm GDNF expression. (D–G: 200X magnification, H–K: 400X magnification) $^*P<0.05$ $^{**}P<0.01$ compared with control group.

Results

GDNF attenuates CCI-induced allodynia and hyperalgesia

To measure the seriousness of neuropathic pain, the Von Frey filament and hot-plantar test were used to establish the animal model. The result showed that CCI induced allodynia and thermal hyperagia at day 1 after surgery (Fig. 1A & 1B). Allodynia was maintained 28 days in CCI group (Fig.1A), whereas thermal hyperalgesia was maintained 14 days but returned to the same level as the control group at day 28 (Fig. 1B). At day 28, rats in the CCI group showed a significantly lower weight for the left hind paw corresponding to the sites where the stimuli were applied (at site of sciatic nerve constriction) compared to controls. Allodynia and thermal hyperalgesia did not differ significantly between the CCI and Ad-MOCK group. Ad-GDNF started to significantly alleviate both allodynia and thermal hyperalgesia associated with CCI at day 5 after surgery, but showed no effect at day 1 and 3 (Fig. 1A & 1B). Therefore, we further investigated the molecular changes underlying the beneficial effect of Ad-GDNF at day 5 in our study.

GDNF inhibits matrix metalloproteinase expression on SCDH

To check GDNF and GDNFRa1 protein expression on the SCDH after adenovirus-mediated GDNF was delivered by intramuscular injection, samples prepared from the ipsilateral SCDH at day 5 after surgery were immunoblotted. GDNF and GDNFRa1 expression in both the CCI and Ad-MOCK group was significantly lower than control. After delivery of Ad-GDNF at day 1 after surgery, GDNF and GDNFRa1 expression returned to control levels at day 5 (Fig. 2A–C). Immunohistochemical analysis of GDNF expression was consistent with the results from immunoblotting (Fig. 2D–K). Since Kawasaki Y et al. reported that MMP-9 induces neuropathic pain through interleukin-1β cleavage and microglial activation at early onset [20], we also analyzed MMP-2 and MMP-9 expression. We found no significant

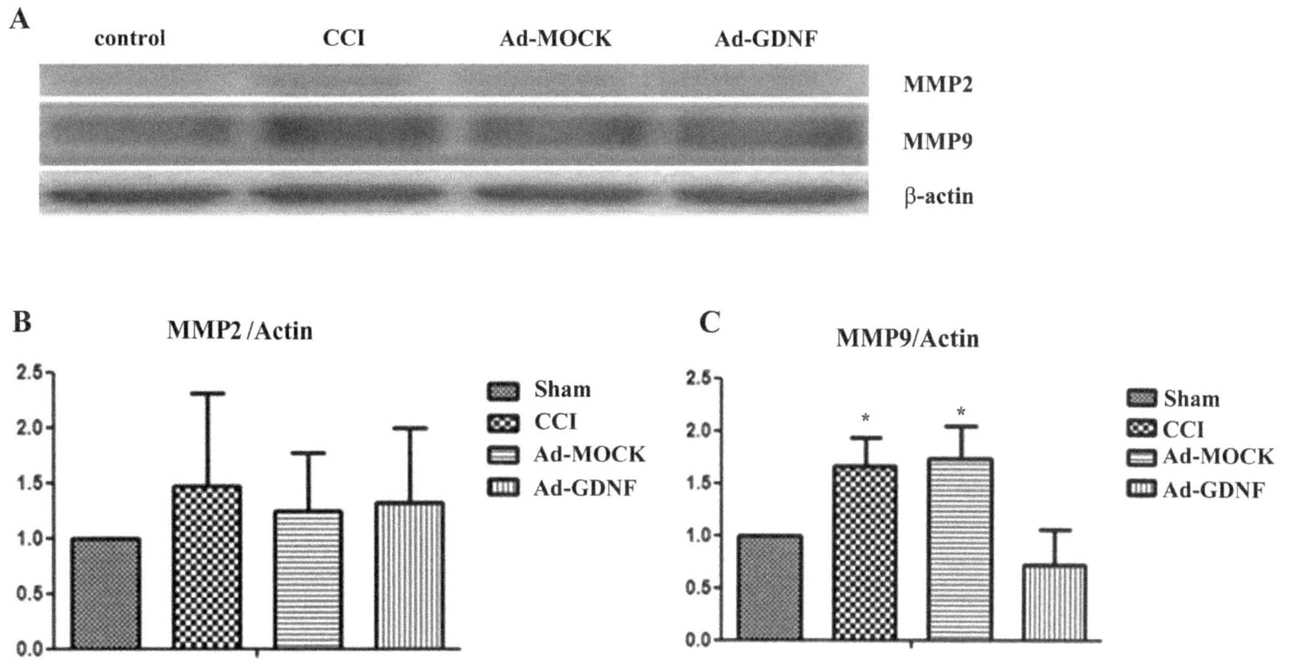

Figure 3. Immunoblotting showing protein expression level with respect to MMP-2 and MMP-9. Western blot analysis showing the expression levels of MMP-2 and MMP-9 in control, CCI, and ipsilateral SCDH with intramuscular injection of Ad-MOCK or Ad-GDNF (A). The expression levels of MMP-2 and MMP-9 with respect to each tested group were shown as bar charts of relative ratio normalized with the expression level of β-actin (B–C). *$P<0.05$ compared with control group.

inter-group difference between any two groups for MMP-2 expression in the SCDH at day 5. In contrast, in the CCI group the MMP-9 expression was significantly higher than that of controls, but no different than the Ad-MOCK group. Administering Ad-GDNF did inhibit MMP-9 expression, which possibly contributed to the attenuation of neuropathic pain (Fig. 3A–C).

GDNF decreases activated microglia and expression of inflammatory factors from CCI on SCDH

A previous study reported that microglia are activated by phosphorylation of p38 and ERK1/2 following peripheral nerve injury including CCI [21]. To confirm this, we detected phosphorylation of p38 and stained for ED-1 expression (microglia marker). Western blot showed that p38 but not ERK1/2 (data not shown) was phosphorylated. In addition, ED-1 expression was elevated in the CCI group. These results may indicate that CCI induced microglia activation and proliferation through the phosphorylation of p38. In contrast, in the Ad-GDNF group the expression of phosphorylated-p38 and ED-1 was significantly lower than in the CCI and Ad-MOCK groups (Fig 4A–C). Double immunofluorescent staining for phosphorylated-p38 and OX42, a microglia marker, showed that expression levels with respect to OX42 and phosphorylated p38 were obviously enhanced after CCI, but phosphorylated p38 was no longer highly expressed after administration of Ad-GDNF (Fig 4D–N). These results revealed CCI-induced phosphorylation of p38 on microglia at SCDH, which returned to normal after GDNF delivery. In CNS, microglia is not only a support cell but is also involved in immune regulation. Microglia activation releases pro-inflammatory cytokines such as TNF-α, IL-1β and IL-6. We examined expression with respect to IL-6 and IL-1β in the different tested groups. Immunoblotting showed that CCI up-regulated IL-6 and IL-1β in the SCDH. After treatment with Ad-GDNF, IL-6 and IL-1β protein expression in the Ad-GDNF group was significantly lower than in the CCI and Ad-MOCK groups, but not the control group (Fig. 5A–C).

GDNF prevents CCI-induced programmed cell death on SCDH

It had been reported that inflammatory factors induced wallerian degeneration at the lesion site following peripheral nerve injury [22].We also observed SCDH tissue loss by H&E staining after CCI and this hallmark was not recovered by Ad-MOCK administration (Fig. 6F&G). We hypothesized that the tissue loss is possibly due to neuronal reduction caused by programmed cell death. To address this question, we used terminal deoxynucleotidyl transferase dUTP nick end labeling (TUNEL) and immunofluorescent microscopy (Fig.7A–H). We found a significant difference between the CCI, Ad-MOCK and Ad-GDNF group by TUNEL staining (Fig.7 F–H&M), as well as double labeling of TUNEL and NeuN (Fig. 7J–L&N). These results may indicate that SCDH neuron cells underwent apoptosis after CCI and that this phenomenon was reversed by Ad-GDNF. To confirm this finding, we also detected the expressions of several apoptotic proteins. Based on our data, the expressions of apoptosis inducing factor (AIF), cleaved caspase-9, cleaved caspase-3, cleaved Poly (ADP-ribose) polymerase (PARP), cleaved SPECTRIN and Beclin-1 were enhanced in the CCI group (Fig. 8A–G). Interestingly, expression levels of these proteins were attenuated to control group levels after administration of Ad-GDNF. These results suggested that adenoviral-mediated delivery of GDNF successfully inhibited CCI-induced apoptosis in the SCDH (Fig. 8A–G).

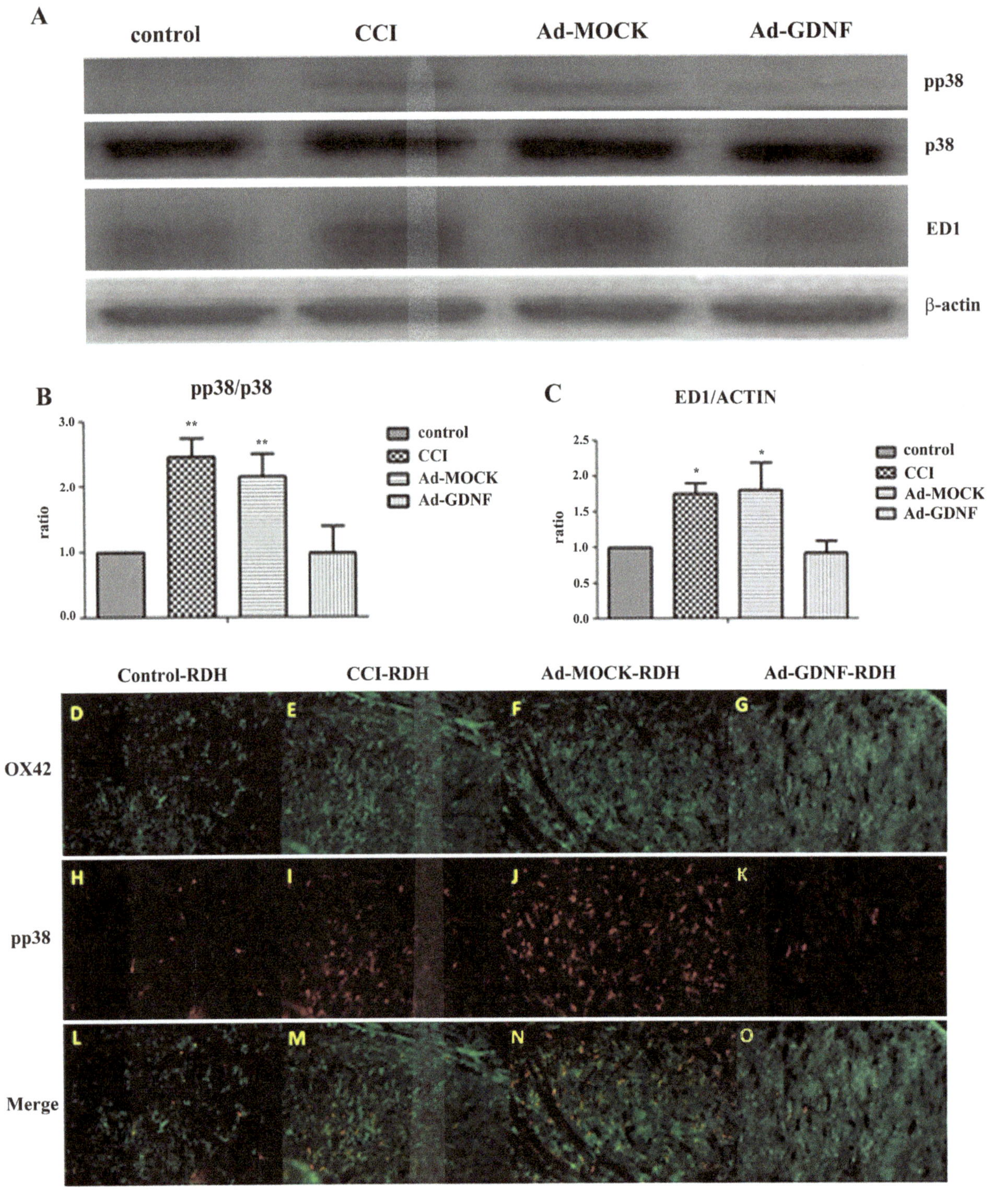

Figure 4. Immunoblotting showing protein expression level with respect to phosphor-p38, p38 and ED-1. Western blot analysis showing the expression levels of phospho-p38, p38 and ED-1 in control, CCI, and ipsilateral SCDH with intramuscular injection of Ad-MOCK or Ad-GDNF (A). The expression levels of phospho-p38 and ED-1 with respect to each tested group were shown as bar charts of relative ratio normalized with expression levels of p38 and β-actin, respectively (B-C). *$P<0.05$, **$P<0.01$ compared with the Ad-GDNF group. Double immunofluorescence staining of OX42 (D–G), a microglia marker, and phosphor-p38 (H–K) in different tested groups. The expression levels with respect to OX42 and phospho-p38 were obviously enhanced after CCI, but phospho-p38 was no longer highly expressed after administration of Ad-GDNF as shown in merged images (L–O).

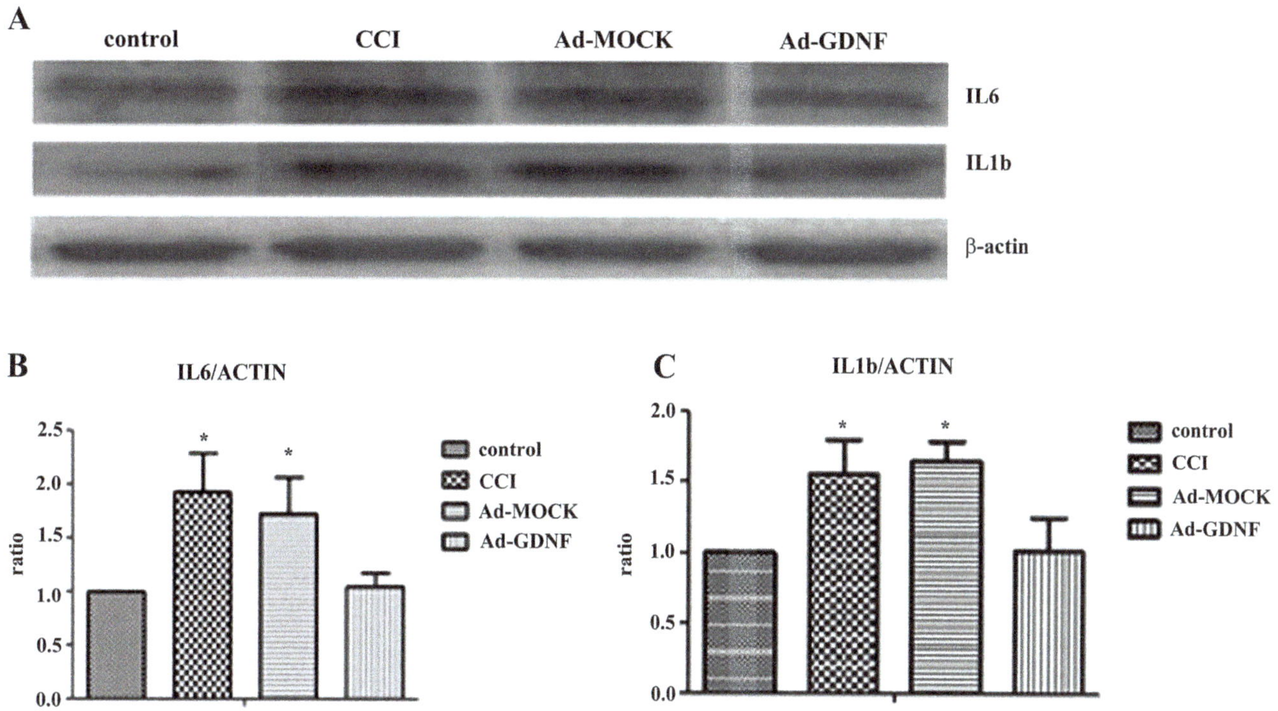

Figure 5. Immunoblotting showing protein expression level with respect to IL-6 and IL-1β. Western blot analysis showing the expression levels of IL-6 and IL-1β in control, CCI, and ipsilateral SCDH with intramuscular injections of Ad-MOCK or Ad-GDNF (A). The expression levels of IL-6 and IL-1β with respect to each tested group were shown as bar charts of relative ratio normalized with the expression levels of β-actin (B–C). *P<0.05, **P<0.01 compared with control group.

GDNF blocks CCI-induced cellular signaling in SCDH

Mao J et al. reported that PKCγ was increased after CCI [23]. In our results, consistent with previous reports, CCI increased both PKCδ and PKCγ protein expression, but in the Ad-GDNF group expression with respect to PKCδ and PKCγ was significant lower than the Ad-MOCK and CCI group, respectively (Fig. 9A–C). These data clearly indicated that GDNF modulated both PKCδ and PKCγ protein expression on the SCDH after CCI. In addition to examining PKC signaling, we also detected the expressions of NOS family proteins including iNOS, nNOS, and eNOS, since NMDA/PKC signaling was associated with NOS expression. Among these three NOS, only iNOS was increased following CCI and this effect was reversed by Ad-GDNF (Fig. 10B). These data suggested that GDNF may have a role in attenuating CCI-induced PKC/iNOS signaling associated with its neuroprotective effect in the SCDH.

Discussion

In the CCI-induced nerve injury animal model, microglia activation and abnormal pro-inflammatory cytokine profiling are

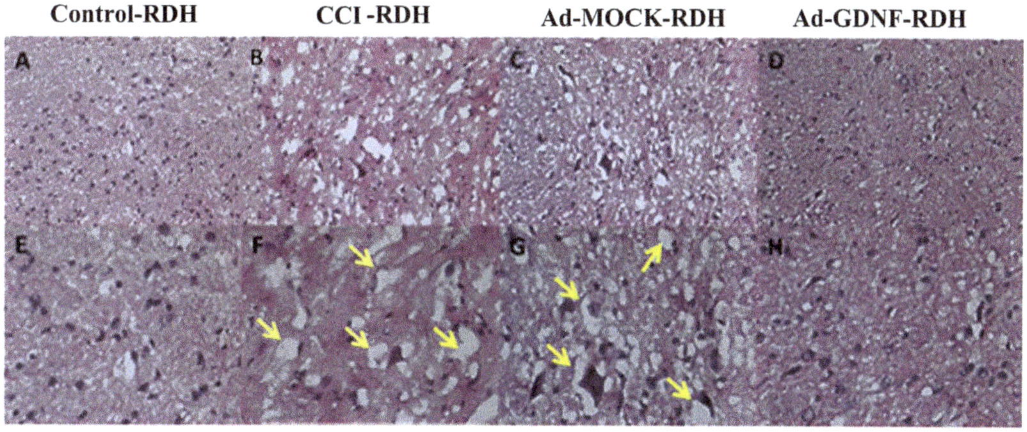

Figure 6. The result of Hematoxylin-Eosin staining (H&E staining) in detecting the morphological changes after administrated with Ad-GDNF. The morphological charges in tight junctions of ipsilateral SCDH among the different tested groups (A–D: 200X, E–G: 400X). Yellow arrows represent possible wallerian degeneration, which was no longer observed after administration of Ad-GDNF.

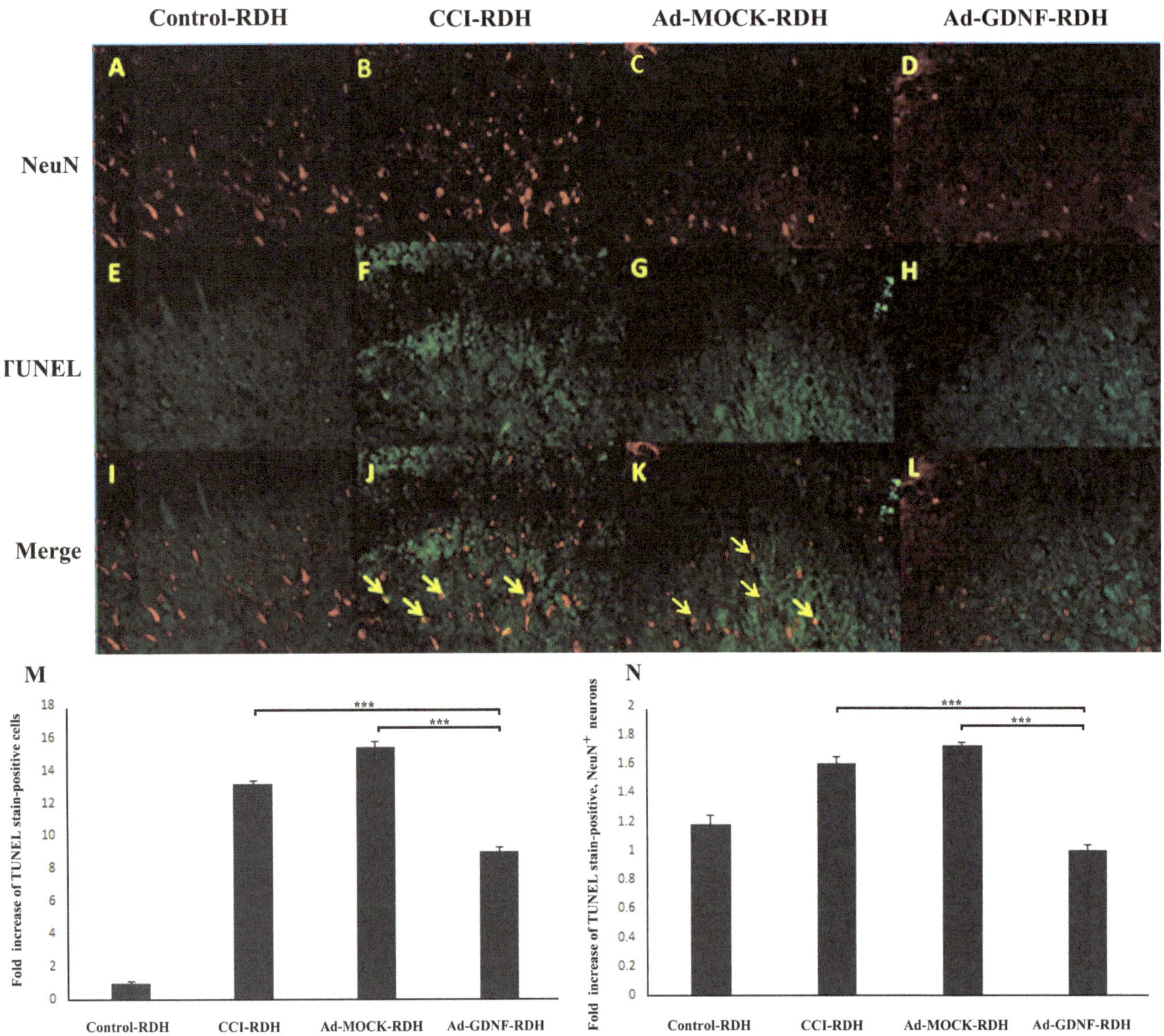

Figure 7. Double immunofluorescent staining of TUNEL and a neuronal cell marker, NeuN, in the rat ipsilateral SCDH in different treatment groups. Tissue samples were detected using antibodies against NeuN (A–D) and TUNEL staining for apoptosis (E–H). The merged images show neuron apoptosis in the ipsilateral SCDH (I–L). Yellow arrows indicate TUNEL-positive neurons. The bar chart with respect to fold increase of TUNEL staining positivity (M) and double labeling (TUNEL and NeuN, N) revealed that apoptotic events triggered by CCI were attenuated by Ad-GDNF.

suggested to be crucial in maintaining neuropathic pain. In fact, microglia are derived from myeloid precursor cells in the periphery and penetrate the CNS during embryogenesis. Microglia are the resident macrophages in the CNS, and mediate signaling crosstalk between peripheral and CNS nerves. Moreover, microglia are also important in CNS neuroinflammation. Mechanical or biochemical stressor insults affecting CNS homeostasis usually induce rapid responses in microglia morphology, gene expression profile and functional behavior and these events are collectively termed 'microgliosis'. Interestingly, damage to the nervous system outside the CNS, such as axotomy of a peripheral nerve, can lead to microgliosis in the spinal cord. In addition, it is also reported that peripheral nerve injury nociceptive inputs from sensory neurons appear to be critical for triggering the development of spinal microgliosis. CCI-induced neuropathic pain is also associated with microgliosis in the SCDH [24]. However, the physiological role of microglia in spinal cord circuitry development and pain transmission remains to be investigated.

Increasing evidence suggests the important role of spinal cord microglia in the genesis of persistent pain, by releasing the proinflammatory cytokines tumor necrosis factor-alpha (TNFα), Interleukine-1beta (IL-1β), and brain derived neurotrophic factor (BDNF). Nerve injury-induced microglial activation occurs by phosphorylation of MAP kinases such as p38 MAPK kinase and extracellular signal-related kinase (ERK) isoforms 1 and 2, and Src-family kinases [21,25–27]. The morphological changes associated with microgliosis may also be mediated by the activation of ERK/MAPK [28]. A number of signaling pathways such as neuregulin-1, matrix metalloproteases (e.g. MMP-9) and multiple chemokines enable direct communication between injured prima-

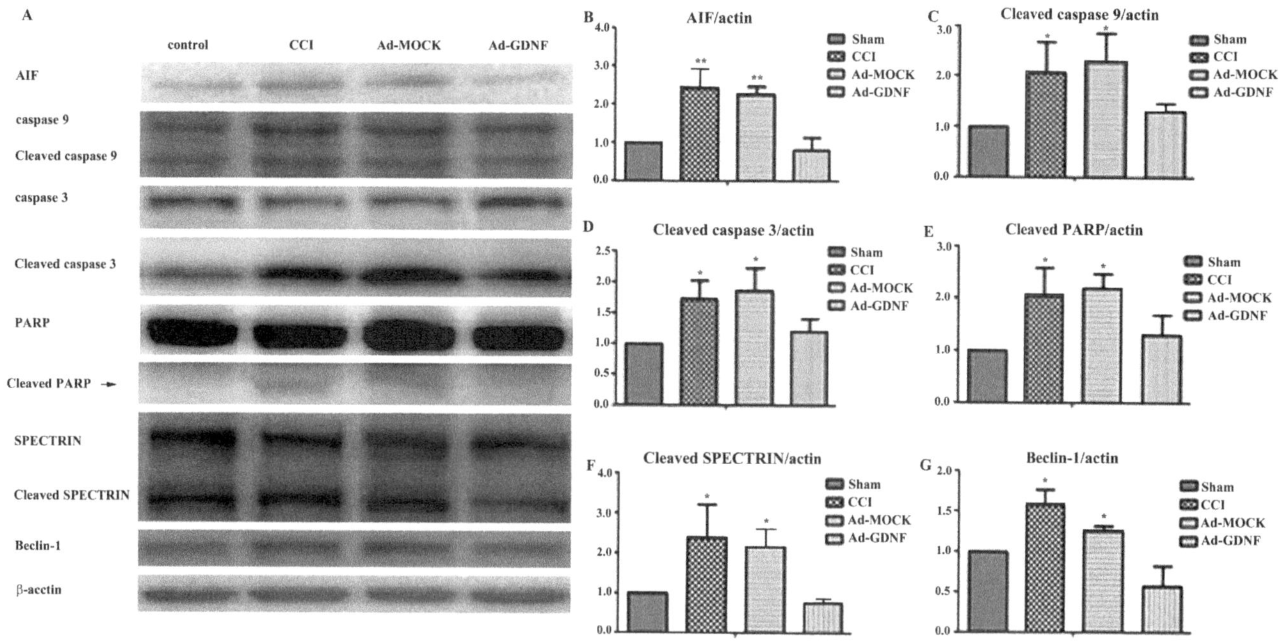

Figure 8. Immunoblotting showing protein expression level with respect to apoptotic and autophagic marker. Western blot analysis of the effect of CCI on the expression of AIF, caspase-9, cleaved caspase-9, caspase-3, cleaved caspase-3, PARP, cleaved PARP, SPECTRIN, cleaved SPECTRIN, and Beclin-1 on ipsilateral SCDH by intramuscular injection with adenovirus plus GDNF gene (A). Ratios of AIF, cleaved caspase-9, cleaved caspase-3, cleaved PARP, cleaved SPECTRIN, Beclin-1 with β-actin on ipsilateral SCDH were measured using western blot analysis (B–G). $^*P<0.05$, $^{**}P<0.01$ compared with the CCI group.

ry afferents and microglia. According to current knowledge regarding p38 MAPK signaling and increased the pain sensitivity, several molecules have been reported to activate p38, such as TNFα [29], IL-1β[30], CCL2[31], MCP-1, CX3CL1[32], iNOS[33], MMP-9[20], P2X4 and P2X7. Some of these microglial activators, such as ATP, CCL2, fractalkine, and MMP-9, are suggested to be released from primary afferent neurons [34,35]. When microglia are activated, the p38 pathway induces expression of molecules such as NFκB, COX2, iNOS, BDNF, TNFα, IL-1β, and IL-6 [30,36,37]. p38 activation in microglia also results in increased release of BDNF and TNFα [38]. Microglial production of proinflammatory cytokines can further recruit additional microglia, activate surrounding astrocytes, and promote the sensitization of central nervous system nociceptive circuits.

We observed CCI induced activation of microglia by phosphorylation of p38 rather than ERK. Spinal microglial activation in both dorsal and ventral horns peaked 1 week after injury and returned after several weeks. Our results support the idea that that microglia affect inflammatory reactions at an early stage. Yasuhiko Kawasaki et al. reported that after spinal nerve ligation (SNL), MMP-9 induced neuropathic pain through interleukin-1 cleavage and microglial activation at early times, whereas MMP-2 maintained neuropathic pain through interleukin-1 cleavage and astrocyte activation at later times [20]. In our study, MMP-9 was induced at day 5 after CCI, and MMP-2 showed no effect. Microglial activation might be just the first step in a cascade of immune responses in the CNS. Zhuang et al. showed the activation of ERK in neurons, then microglia, and then astrocytes in a neuropathic pain model [27]. Microglia may initiate neuropathic pain, and astrocytes probably respond to maintain neuropathic pain. Microglial MAP kinases can be activated by IL-1β and TNF-α, inducing, via transcription factors such as NFκB, additional production of IL-1β, TNF-α, IL-6, IL-10, TGF-β, PGE2, BDNF, and cathepsin S and promoting the deleterious effects of microglial infiltration and phagocytosis in neuropathic pain. Blocking the signaling pathways mediated by IL-1β or IL-6 diminishes behaviors related to neuropathic pain [39]. In this study, GDNF inhibited the activation of microglia and IL-1βand IL-6 release. This can be one of reasons for the decline in pain behaviors after Ad-GDNF administration.

The present study explored how CCI-induced peripheral nerve injury can cause type I (apoptosis) and II (autophagy) programmed cell death. These molecular events can also be attenuated by adenoviral-mediated GDNF delivery. Consistent with other studies, the present data revealed that pro-inflammatory cytokine signaling, such as TNFα, p38, and MMP-9, may contribute to apoptosis induction in the SCDH after CCI. Previous studies suggested that either apoptosis or inflammation plays an important role in neuropathic pain. Peripheral nerve injury produces neuron apoptosis in the dorsal horn of the spinal cord [40–42] and DRG [43,44]. Specifically, apoptosis in satellite glial cells (SGC) (not in neurons) of CCI rat ipsilateral dorsal root ganglia (DRG) at day 30 after injury was revealed [45].

Cleaved caspase-3 and caspase-9 expression is the effector with respect to apoptosis and post-mitochondrial apoptosis. Our results showed that GDNF can reduce CCI-induced caspase expression and activation, which may be associated with relief of pain behavior. This data suggests that caspase signaling pathways are involved in pain development. Apoptosis inducing factor (AIF) is used as a marker of mitochondrial apoptosis. Both caspases and AIF can trigger SPECTRIN cleavage by activating cleaved Poly (ADP-ribose) polymerase (PARP). All of them are apoptosis markers. In our results, CCI induced the expression and activation of chosen markers involved in either mitochondrial or non-

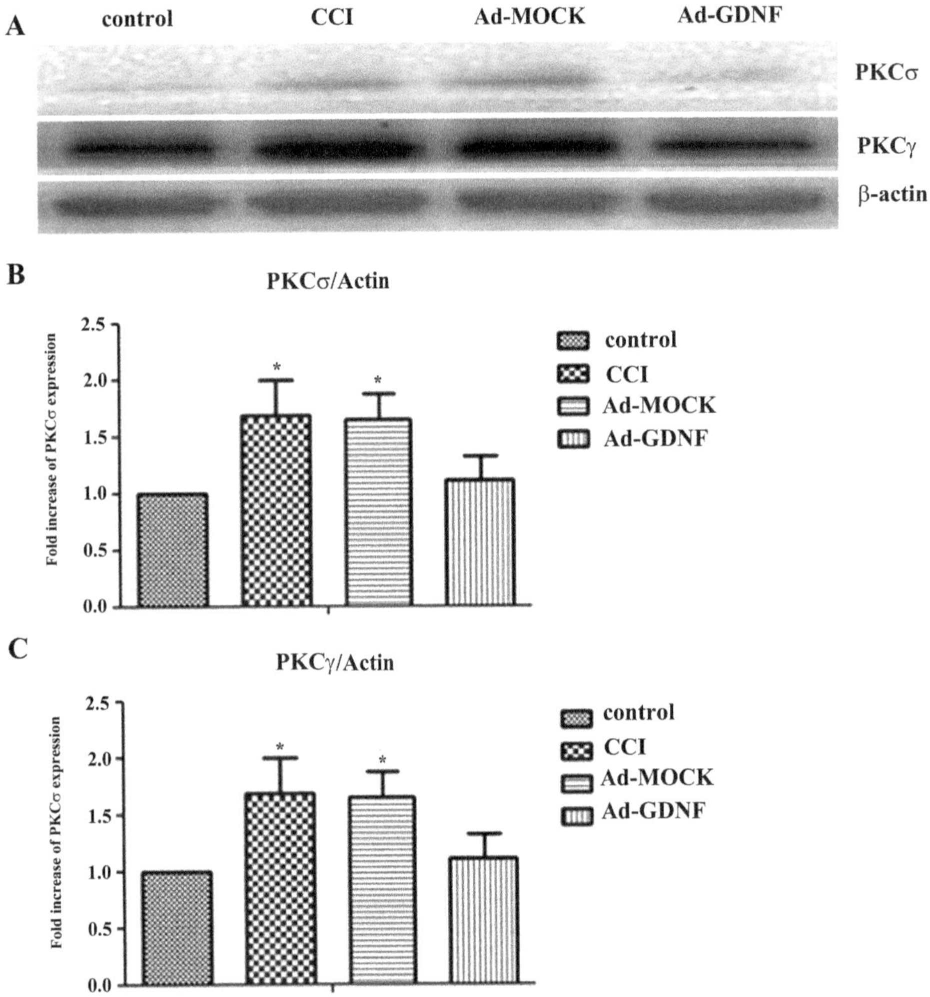

Figure 9. Immunoblotting showing protein expression level with respect to PKCδ and PKCγ. Western blot analysis showing the expression levels of PKCδ and PKCγ in control, CCI, and ipsilateal SCDH with intramuscular injection with Ad-MOCK or Ad-GDNF (A). The expression levels of PKCδ and PKCγ with respect to each tested group were shown as bar charts of relative ratio normalized with the expression levels of β-actin (B–C). *P<0.05, **P<0.01 compared with the Ad-GDNF group.

mitochondrial apoptosis. Moreover, using adenovirally delivered GDNF successfully attenuated apoptotic protein expression.

Autophagy is an intracellular membrane trafficking pathway controlling the delivery of cytoplasmic material to the lysosomes for degradation. It plays an important role in cell homeostasis in both normal settings and abnormal or stressful conditions[46]. LC3B and Beclin-1 are autophagy markers involved in different stages of autophagy. Previous studies reported that L5 spinal nerve ligation induced autophagy in the SCDH. Both LC3 and Beclin-1 are observed to be significantly elevated in the ipsilateral L5 spinal dorsal horn on day 14 following spinal nerve ligation. These two proteins are mainly located at GABAergic interneurons of the spinal dorsal horn after SNL, indicating that autophagic disruption in GABAergic interneurons and astrocytes following peripheral nerve injury might be involved in the induction and maintenance of neuropathic pain [47]. Besides, the mTOR pathway (autophagy-associated) is also reported to be activated in the SCDH in CCI-induced neuropathic pain, and the intrathecal injection of rapamycin can reduce mechanical allodynia [48]. In this study, CCI-induced peripheral nerve injury did lead to autophagy induction on the SCDH and GDNF prevented the elevated expression of Beclin-1 due to CCI-induced nerve injury.

In conclusion, intramuscular injection with Ad-GDNF not only attenuates neuropathic pain but also protects cells from neuropathic pain-associated programmed cell death (microglia inactivation through down-regulating IL-6, IL-1β, p38 and MMP-9). In addition, administration of GDNF also enhanced expression of inducible nitric oxide synthases by modulating the PKC pathway in the SCDH following chronic constriction injury. Adenoviral GDNF-based gene therapy may be an alternative therapeutic approach for treating neuropathic pain in patients.

Although our results provide evidence that GDNF can be applied to attenuate CCI-induced neuropathic pain, the experimental limitations should be noted. First, CCI-induced nerve injury was recently associated with autophagy induction. Many proteins are used as hallmarks of autophagy, such as ATG family proteins, p62, Beclin 1 and LC3B. In this study, we only measured Beclin 1 and LC3B to compare the results with the SNL model. Second, for evaluating apoptotic events after CCI-induced nerve injury on the SCDH, we only used TUNEL staining, NeuN staining and immunostaining of apoptotic proteins. This may not

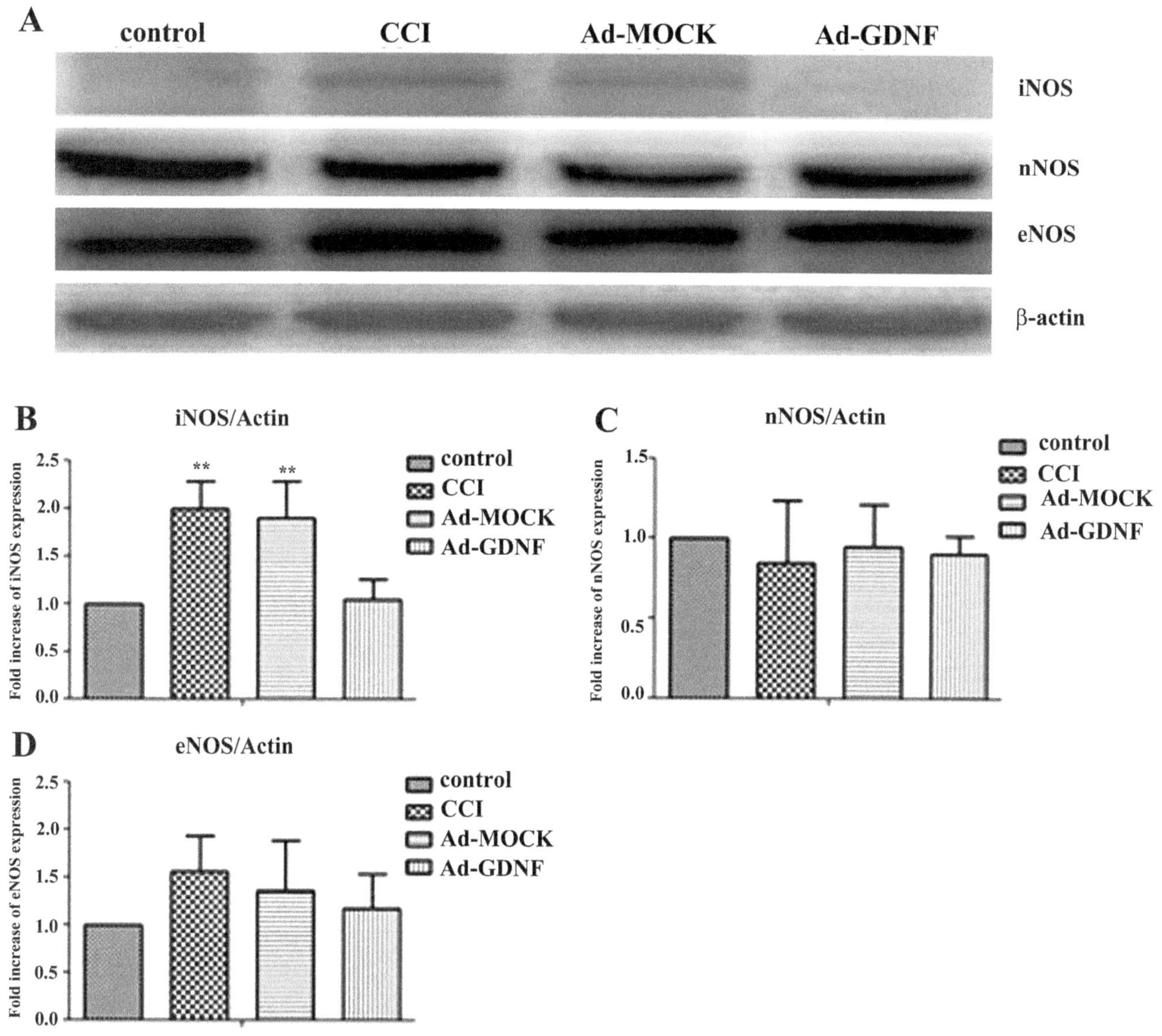

Figure 10. Immunoblotting showing protein expression level with respect to different NOS isoform. Western blot analysis showing the expression levels of iNOS, nNOS and eNOS in control, CCI, and ipsilateral SCDH with intramuscular injection with Ad-MOCK or Ad-GDNF (A). The expression levels of iNOS, nNOS and eNOS with respect to each tested group were shown as bar charts of relative ratio normalized with the expression levels of β-actin (B–D). **$P<0.01$ compared with Ad-GDNF group.

fully characterize the apoptosis. Information regarding DNA content and cell-cycle distribution consequent to CCI and Ad-GDNF treatment was not obtained. Third, the lack of another neurotrophic factor such as BDNF, NGF and NT3 as control to compare with results of GDNF limited our conclusions about the therapeutic value of Ad-GDNF. Finally, to discriminate the signaling pathways associated with the beneficial effects attributed to GDNF in attenuating CCI-induced nerve injury, we only directly observed the modulating role of GDNF on target protein expressions rather than introducing any pathway inhibitors.

Our major finding was that adenovirally mediated delivery of GDNF successfully decreased neuropathic pain behaviors and their associated protein expressions. GDNF appears to inhibit microglia activation, pro-inflammatory cytokine production, and at least two types of programmed cell death (apoptosis and autophagy). Future work on signaling pathways and cross-talk consequent to GDNF administration will provide further insights into its therapeutic action in terms of CCI-induced neuropathic pain attenuation, and provide a starting point for developing new strategies for pain control.

Acknowledgments

We thank Gary Mawyer for English editing. Authors also grateful for technical assistance provided from graduated students and technicians in laboratory owned by Dr. Ming-Hong Tai in NSYSU.

Author Contributions

Conceived and designed the experiments: AKC MHT ALK YRH. Performed the experiments: AKC MHT. Analyzed the data: MCY. Contributed reagents/materials/analysis tools: MCY HPT CYC MHT YRH. Wrote the paper: MCY.

References

1. Lekan HA, Carlton SM, Coggeshall RE (1996) Sprouting of A beta fibers into lamina II of the rat dorsal horn in peripheral neuropathy. Neurosci Lett 208: 147–150.
2. Woolf CJ, Shortland P, Coggeshall RE (1992) Peripheral nerve injury triggers central sprouting of myelinated afferents. Nature 355: 75–78.
3. Shortland P, Wang HF, Molander C (1999) Distribution of transganglionically labelled soybean agglutinin primary afferent fibres after nerve injury. Brain Res 815: 206–212.
4. Bridges D, Thompson SW, Rice AS (2001) Mechanisms of neuropathic pain. Br J Anaesth 87: 12–26.
5. Airaksinen MS, Saarma M (2002) The GDNF family: signalling, biological functions and therapeutic value. Nat Rev Neurosci 3: 383–394.
6. Bennett DL, Michael GJ, Ramachandran N, Munson JB, Averill S, et al. (1998) A distinct subgroup of small DRG cells express GDNF receptor components and GDNF is protective for these neurons after nerve injury. J Neurosci 18: 3059–3072.
7. Boucher TJ, Okuse K, Bennett DL, Munson JB, Wood JN, et al. (2000) Potent analgesic effects of GDNF in neuropathic pain states. Science 290: 124–127.
8. Hao S, Mata M, Wolfe D, Huang S, Glorioso JC, et al. (2003) HSV-mediated gene transfer of the glial cell-derived neurotrophic factor provides an antiallodynic effect on neuropathic pain. Mol Ther 8: 367–375.
9. Ramer MS, Priestley JV, McMahon SB (2000) Functional regeneration of sensory axons into the adult spinal cord. Nature 403: 312–316.
10. Eslamboli A (2005) Assessment of GDNF in primate models of Parkinson's disease: comparison with human studies. Rev Neurosci 16: 303–310.
11. Gill SS, Patel NK, Hotton GR, O'Sullivan K, McCarter R, et al. (2003) Direct brain infusion of glial cell line-derived neurotrophic factor in Parkinson disease. Nat Med 9: 589–595.
12. Manabe Y, Nagano I, Gazi MS, Murakami T, Shiote M, et al. (2002) Adenovirus-mediated gene transfer of glial cell line-derived neurotrophic factor prevents motor neuron loss of transgenic model mice for amyotrophic lateral sclerosis. Apoptosis 7: 329–334.
13. Wang LJ, Lu YY, Muramatsu S, Ikeguchi K, Fujimoto K, et al. (2002) Neuroprotective effects of glial cell line-derived neurotrophic factor mediated by an adeno-associated virus vector in a transgenic animal model of amyotrophic lateral sclerosis. J Neurosci 22: 6920–6928.
14. Bennett GJ, Xie YK (1988) A peripheral mononeuropathy in rat that produces disorders of pain sensation like those seen in man. Pain 33: 87–107.
15. Tai MH, Cheng H, Wu JP, Liu YL, Lin PR, et al. (2003) Gene transfer of glial cell line-derived neurotrophic factor promotes functional recovery following spinal cord contusion. Exp Neurol 183: 508–515.
16. Giraud C, Winocour E, Berns KI (1995) Recombinant junctions formed by site-specific integration of adeno-associated virus into an episome. J Virol 69: 6917–6924.
17. Hargreaves K, Dubner R, Brown F, Flores C, Joris J (1988) A new and sensitive method for measuring thermal nociception in cutaneous hyperalgesia. Pain 32: 77–88.
18. Eftekhari S, Edvinsson L (2011) Calcitonin gene-related peptide (CGRP) and its receptor components in human and rat spinal trigeminal nucleus and spinal cord at C1-level. BMC Neurosci 12: 112.
19. Yamazaki K, Wakasugi N, Tomita T, Kikuchi T, Mukoyama M, et al. (1988) Gracile axonal dystrophy (GAD), a new neurological mutant in the mouse. Proc Soc Exp Biol Med 187: 209–215.
20. Kawasaki Y, Xu ZZ, Wang X, Park JY, Zhuang ZY, et al. (2008) Distinct roles of matrix metalloproteases in the early- and late-phase development of neuropathic pain. Nat Med 14: 331–336.
21. Jin SX, Zhuang ZY, Woolf CJ, Ji RR (2003) p38 mitogen-activated protein kinase is activated after a spinal nerve ligation in spinal cord microglia and dorsal root ganglion neurons and contributes to the generation of neuropathic pain. J Neurosci 23: 4017–4022.
22. George A, Buehl A, Sommer C (2004) Wallerian degeneration after crush injury of rat sciatic nerve increases endo- and epineurial tumor necrosis factor-alpha protein. Neurosci Lett 372: 215–219.
23. Mao J, Price DD, Phillips LL, Lu J, Mayer DJ (1995) Increases in protein kinase C gamma immunoreactivity in the spinal cord dorsal horn of rats with painful mononeuropathy. Neurosci Lett 198: 75–78.
24. Tsuda M, Inoue K, Salter MW (2005) Neuropathic pain and spinal microglia: a big problem from molecules in "small" glia. Trends Neurosci 28: 101–107.
25. Katsura H, Obata K, Mizushima T, Sakurai J, Kobayashi K, et al. (2006) Activation of Src-family kinases in spinal microglia contributes to mechanical hypersensitivity after nerve injury. J Neurosci 26: 8680–8690.
26. Svensson CI, Fitzsimmons B, Azizi S, Powell HC, Hua XY, et al. (2005) Spinal p38beta isoform mediates tissue injury-induced hyperalgesia and spinal sensitization. J Neurochem 92: 1508–1520.
27. Zhuang ZY, Gerner P, Woolf CJ, Ji RR (2005) ERK is sequentially activated in neurons, microglia, and astrocytes by spinal nerve ligation and contributes to mechanical allodynia in this neuropathic pain model. Pain 114: 149–159.
28. Calvo M, Zhu N, Grist J, Ma Z, Loeb JA, et al. (2011) Following nerve injury neuregulin-1 drives microglial proliferation and neuropathic pain via the MEK/ERK pathway. Glia.
29. Svensson CI, Schafers M, Jones TL, Powell H, Sorkin LS (2005) Spinal blockade of TNF blocks spinal nerve ligation-induced increases in spinal P-p38. Neurosci Lett 379: 209–213.
30. Sung CS, Wen ZH, Chang WK, Chan KH, Ho ST, et al. (2005) Inhibition of p38 mitogen-activated protein kinase attenuates interleukin-1beta-induced thermal hyperalgesia and inducible nitric oxide synthase expression in the spinal cord. J Neurochem 94: 742–752.
31. Abbadie C, Lindia JA, Cumiskey AM, Peterson LB, Mudgett JS, et al. (2003) Impaired neuropathic pain responses in mice lacking the chemokine receptor CCR2. Proc Natl Acad Sci U S A 100: 7947–7952.
32. Zhuang ZY, Kawasaki Y, Tan PH, Wen YR, Huang J, et al. (2007) Role of the CX3CR1/p38 MAPK pathway in spinal microglia for the development of neuropathic pain following nerve injury-induced cleavage of fractalkine. Brain Behav Immun 21: 642–651.
33. Tang Q, Svensson CI, Fitzsimmons B, Webb M, Yaksh TL, et al. (2007) Inhibition of spinal constitutive NOS-2 by 1400W attenuates tissue injury and inflammation-induced hyperalgesia and spinal p38 activation. Eur J Neurosci 25: 2964–2972.
34. Clark AK, Malcangio M (2012) Microglial signalling mechanisms: Cathepsin S and Fractalkine. Exp Neurol 234: 283–292.
35. Ji RR, Xu ZZ, Wang X, Lo EH (2009) Matrix metalloprotease regulation of neuropathic pain. Trends Pharmacol Sci 30: 336–340.
36. Svensson CI, Marsala M, Westerlund A, Calcutt NA, Campana WM, et al. (2003) Activation of p38 mitogen-activated protein kinase in spinal microglia is a critical link in inflammation-induced spinal pain processing. J Neurochem 86: 1534–1544.
37. Ji RR, Suter MR (2007) p38 MAPK, microglial signaling, and neuropathic pain. Mol Pain 3: 33.
38. Wen YR, Tan PH, Cheng JK, Liu YC, Ji RR (2011) Microglia: a promising target for treating neuropathic and postoperative pain, and morphine tolerance. J Formos Med Assoc 110: 487–494.
39. Wolf G, Gabay E, Tal M, Yirmiya R, Shavit Y (2006) Genetic impairment of interleukin-1 signaling attenuates neuropathic pain, autotomy, and spontaneous ectopic neuronal activity, following nerve injury in mice. Pain 120: 315–324.
40. Maione S, Siniscalco D, Galderisi U, de Novellis V, Uliano R, et al. (2002) Apoptotic genes expression in the lumbar dorsal horn in a model neuropathic pain in rat. Neuroreport 13: 101–106.
41. Moore KA, Kohno T, Karchewski LA, Scholz J, Baba H, et al. (2002) Partial peripheral nerve injury promotes a selective loss of GABAergic inhibition in the superficial dorsal horn of the spinal cord. J Neurosci 22: 6724–6731.
42. Whiteside GT, Munglani R (2001) Cell death in the superficial dorsal horn in a model of neuropathic pain. J Neurosci Res 64: 168–173.
43. Campana WM, Myers RR (2003) Exogenous erythropoietin protects against dorsal root ganglion apoptosis and pain following peripheral nerve injury. Eur J Neurosci 18: 1497–1506.
44. Sekiguchi M, Kobayashi H, Sekiguchi Y, Konno S, Kikuchi S (2008) Sympathectomy reduces mechanical allodynia, tumor necrosis factor-alpha expression, and dorsal root ganglion apoptosis following nerve root crush injury. Spine (Phila Pa 1976) 33: 1163–1169.
45. Schaeffer V, Meyer L, Patte-Mensah C, Eckert A, Mensah-Nyagan AG (2010) Sciatic nerve injury induces apoptosis of dorsal root ganglion satellite glial cells and selectively modifies neurosteroidogenesis in sensory neurons. Glia 58: 169–180.
46. Mizushima N, Levine B, Cuervo AM, Klionsky DJ (2008) Autophagy fights disease through cellular self-digestion. Nature 451: 1069–1075.
47. Zhang E, Yi MH, Ko Y, Kim HW, Seo JH, et al. (2013) Expression of LC3 and Beclin 1 in the spinal dorsal horn following spinal nerve ligation-induced neuropathic pain. Brain Res 1519: 31–39.
48. Zhang W, Sun XF, Bo JH, Zhang J, Liu XJ, et al. (2013) Activation of mTOR in the spinal cord is required for pain hypersensitivity induced by chronic constriction injury in mice. Pharmacol Biochem Behav 111C: 64–70.

3

Involvement of ERK Phosphorylation of Trigeminal Spinal Subnucleus Caudalis Neurons in Thermal Hypersensitivity in Rats with Infraorbital Nerve Injury

Ikuko Suzuki[1], Yoshiyuki Tsuboi[1], Masamichi Shinoda[1], Kazuo Shibuta[1], Kuniya Honda[1,2], Ayano Katagiri[1], Masaaki Kiyomoto[1], Barry J. Sessle[3], Shingo Matsuura[4], Kinuyo Ohara[4], Kentaro Urata[5], Koichi Iwata[1,6,7]*

1 Department of Physiology, Nihon University School of Dentistry, Chiyoda-ku Tokyo, Japan, **2** Department of Oral and Maxillofacial Surgery, Nihon University School of Dentistry, Chiyoda-ku Tokyo, Japan, **3** Department of Oral Physiology, Faculty of Dentistry, University of Toronto, Toronto, Ontario, Canada, **4** Department of Endodontics, Nihon University School of Dentistry, Chiyoda-ku Tokyo, Japan, **5** Department of Prosthodontics, Nihon University School of Dentistry, Chiyoda-ku Tokyo, Japan, **6** Division of Functional Morphology, Dental Research Center, Nihon University School of Dentistry, Tokyo, Japan, **7** Division of Applied System Neuroscience Advanced Medical Research Center, Nihon University Graduate School of Medical Science, Tokyo, Japan

Abstract

To evaluate the involvement of the mitogen-activated protein kinase (MAPK) cascade in orofacial neuropathic pain mechanisms, this study assessed nocifensive behavior evoked by mechanical or thermal stimulation of the whisker pad skin, phosphorylation of extracellular signal-regulated kinase (ERK) in trigeminal spinal subnucleus caudalis (Vc) neurons, and Vc neuronal responses to mechanical or thermal stimulation of the whisker pad skin in rats with the chronic constriction nerve injury of the infraorbital nerve (ION-CCI). The mechanical and thermal nocifensive behavior was significantly enhanced on the side ipsilateral to the ION-CCI compared to the contralateral whisker pad or sham rats. ION-CCI rats had an increased number of phosphorylated ERK immunoreactive (pERK-IR) cells which also manifested NeuN-IR but not GFAP-IR and Iba1-IR, and were significantly more in ION-CCI rats compared with sham rats following noxious but not non-noxious mechanical stimulation. After intrathecal administration of the MEK1 inhibitor PD98059 in ION-CCI rats, the number of pERK-IR cells after noxious stimulation and the enhanced thermal nocifensive behavior but not the mechanical nocifensive behavior were significantly reduced in ION-CCI rats. The enhanced background activities, afterdischarges and responses of wide dynamic range neurons to noxious mechanical and thermal stimulation in ION-CCI rats were significantly depressed following i.t. administration of PD98059, whereas responses to non-noxious mechanical and thermal stimulation were not altered. The present findings suggest that pERK-IR neurons in the Vc play a pivotal role in the development of thermal hypersensitivity in the face following trigeminal nerve injury.

Editor: Renping Zhou, Rutgers University, United States of America

Funding: This study was supported in part by Research grants from Sato and Uemura Funds from Nihon University School of Dentistry, and Grant from Dental Research Center, Nihon University School of Dentistry; Nihon University multidisciplinary research grant and Individual Research Grant; a Grant from the Ministry of Education, Culture, Sports, Science and Technology to promote multi-disciplinary research Projects (KAKENHI (Grant-in-Aid for Young Scientist (B)) # 22792021 to MS); grants from the Ministry of Education, Culture, Sports, Science, Technology to promote multidisciplinary research projects "Brain Mechanisms for Cognition, Memory and Behavior" and "Translational Research Network on Orofacial Neurological Disorders" at Nihon University, and Japan-Canada (CIHR) Joint Health Research Program, and National Institutes of Health grant DE015420. The funders had no role in study design, data collection and analysis, decision to publish, or preparation of the manuscript.

Competing Interests: The authors have declared that no competing interests exist.

* E-mail: iwata-k@dent.nihon-u.ac.jp

Introduction

Peripheral nerve injury may result in neuropathic pain which is characterized by severe persistent pain in the areas innervated by the injured nerve [1,2,3,4,5]. Following orofacial surgical treatment such as third molar tooth extraction, dental pulpectomy or dental implantation, neuropathic pain sometimes occurs in the orofacial region and is difficult to diagnose and treat, and its underlying mechanisms are unclear [6,7,8,9,10,11].

A variety of animal models with trigeminal nerve injury have been developed to evaluate mechanisms underlying orofacial neuropathic pain, and include chronic constriction injury of the infraorbital nerve (ION-CCI) and inferior alveolar nerve (IAN) transection [6,11,12,13,14]. Molecular changes and enhancement of neuronal excitability can be observed in trigeminal ganglion (TG) neurons [15,16,17] and trigeminal spinal subnucleus caudalis (Vc) neurons after infraorbital or cervical nerve injury [18,19,20]. Mitogen-activated protein (MAP) kinase is one of the important molecules involved in the intracellular transduction cascade resulting in neuronal excitability changes [21,22,23,24]. Extracellular signal-regulated kinase (ERK), p38 and c-Jun N-terminal kinases in sensory neurons are known to have different functions in sensory processing [25,26,27]. In the trigeminal nociceptive system, ERK is phosphorylated in Vc and upper cervical spinal cord (C1/C2) neurons within 5 min after strong noxious stimulation of the orofacial region, and the number of phosphorylated ERK (pERK)-immunoreactive (IR) Vc neurons increases as noxious stimulus intensity is increased [28,29,30].

It has also been reported that pERK-IR neurons are somatotopically organized in the Vc and C1/C2 following capsaicin injection into restricted areas of the orofacial region [31]. These findings strongly suggest that the ERK phosphorylation in Vc neurons is involved in modulation of neuronal excitability following various noxious stimuli. However, the functional involvement of ERK phosphorylation in Vc neurons in trigeminal neuropathic pain states is not fully understood, but it is very important to clarify mechanisms underlying ERK phosphorylation following trigeminal nerve injury in order to understand orofacial neuropathic pain mechanisms. Therefore, the aim of the present study was to assess nocifensive behavior evoked by mechanical or thermal stimulation of the whisker pad skin, phosphorylation of ERK in Vc neurons, and Vc neuronal responses to mechanical or thermal stimulation of the whisker pad skin in ION-CCI rats.

Materials and Methods

Animals

One hundred fifty nine male Sprague Dawley rats weighing 300–400 g (ION-CCI: n = 120, sham operation: n = 39) were used in this study. The rats were housed under 12 h light/dark cycle conditions and had free access to food and water except during the test period. To minimize animal suffering, the number of animals used was based on the minimum required for statistically valid results. Behavioral and electrophysiological analysis were carried out in a blind manner. This study was approved by the Animal Experimentation Committee at the Nihon University. All surgery and animal care were conducted in accordance with the National Institutes of Health Guide for the Care and Use of Laboratory Animals and the guidelines for Institutional Animal Care, and the guidelines of the International Association for the Study of Pain.

Infraorbital nerve constriction

Rats were initially anesthetized with pentobarbital sodium (50 mg/kg, i.p.). For ION ligation, rats were placed on a warm mat and a small incision was made on the buccal mucous membrane at buccal side of the upper molar and ION was exposed. The ION was loosely ligated with 4-0 chromic guts (Myco Medical Supplies Unc., NC) at two points of the nerve trunk and the wound was sutured after ION ligation. For sham-operated rats, the mucous membrane was cut and ION was exposed but not ligated, and the wound was sutured.

Behavioral testing

As previously described in detail, rats were trained daily to stay in a plastic cage for 20 min, to protrude their perioral region including the whisker pad skin through a hole on the wall of the plastic cage for 5 min and to keep their snout protruding through a hole while mechanical, heat and cold stimulation were applied to whisker pad skin [11,32]. Rats could escape freely from stimulation under this condition. The experimenter was kept blind to the experimental conditions.

Previously described approaches were also used to test mechanical or thermal sensitivity in these rats [11]. Mechanical sensitivity of the whisker pad skin was assessed by the use of von Frey filaments (North Coast Medical, Morgan Hill, Calif). The mechanical stimulation was applied to the whisker pad skin ipsilateral or contralaterally in ION-CCI rats or ipsilaterally in sham rats with von Frey filaments before and on days 1, 3, 7, 14 and 21 after ION-CCI. The head-withdrawal threshold to mechanical stimulation of the whisker pad skin was defined as the minimum pressure needed to evoke an escape more than 3 times of 5 stimuli. A cutoff of 60 g was established to prevent tissue damage. Heat sensitivity of the whisker pad skin was assessed using a radiant heat stimulator (Intercross-2000, Intercross, Tokyo, Japan) applied ipsilaterally or contralaterally in ION-CCI rats or ipsilaterally in sham rats. Animals were restrained in the plastic cage, and the head-withdrawal latency to radiant heat stimulation was manually recorded with a chronometer before and on days 1, 3, 7, 14 and 21 after ION-CCI or sham operation. A cutoff of 10 s was established to prevent tissue damage. Cold sensitivity of the whisker pad skin was assessed using 50 μl acetone applied ipsilaterally or contralaterally in ION-CCI rats or ipsilaterally in sham rats. The number of face scratches was counted for 1 min before and on days 1, 3, 7, 14 and 21 after ION-CCI or sham operation.

Immunohistochemistries

Since neuropathic pain behavior to mechanical, heat and cold stimuli was obvious at 7 days after ION-CCI, immunohistochemical studies were conducted in the rats on day 7 after the ION-CCI, sham operation or naïve rats. pERK immunohistochemistry was conducted in ION-CCI or sham rats or in ION-CCI rats with i.t. infusion of MEK1 inhibitor PD98059 (EMD Biosciences, La Jolla, CA) or isotonic saline (as vehicle control) that had received low-intensity (6 g) or high-intensity (60 g) mechanical stimulation to the maxillary whisker pad skin (1 Hz, duration for 15 min) with von Frey filaments. Five min after cessation of the stimulation, the rats were perfused with isotonic saline followed by 4% paraformaldehyde (PFA) in 0.1 M phosphate buffer (pH 7.4, 1 L/kg). Labeling of astroglial and microglial cells was also conducted by using glial fibrillary acid protein (GFAP) and ionized calcium binding adaptor molecule 1 (Iba1) immunohistochemistries in ION-CCI rats with i.t. infusion of PD98059 or isotonic saline; rats were anesthetized with pentobarbital sodium (50 mg/kg, i.p.) and perfused with the same solution as used for pERK immunohistochemistry.

The medulla and upper cervical spinal cord were removed and post-fixed in 4% PFA for 3 days at 4°C. The tissues were then transferred to 20% sucrose (w/v) in 0.01 M phosphate-buffered saline (PBS) for several days for cryoprotection. Thirty-micron-thick sections were cut with a freezing microtome and every fourth section was collected in 0.01 M PBS. Free-floating tissue sections were rinsed in 0.01 M PBS, 3% normal goat serum in PBS for 1.5 h, and then incubated in rabbit anti-phospho-p44/42 MAP kinase (Thr202/Tyr204) antibody (1:1000, Cell signaling Technology, Beverly, MA) or rabbit anti-GFAP polyclonal antibody (1:1000, Dako, Glostrup Denmark) or rabbit anti-Iba1 antibody (1:1000, Wako, Tokyo, Japan) for 3 days at 4°C. Next, the sections were incubated in biotinylated goat anti-rabbit IgG (1:600; Vector Labs, Burlingame, CA, USA) for 2 h at room temperature. After washing, the sections were incubated in peroxidase-conjugated avidin-biotin complex (1:100; ABC, Vector Labs) for 1 h at room temperature. They were then washed in 0.05 M tris buffer (TB), and next incubated in 0.035% 3,3′-diaminobenzidine-tetra HCl (DAB, Tokyo Chemical Industry, Tokyo, Japan), 0.2% nickel ammonium sulfate, and 0.009% peroxide in 0.05 M TB (pH 7.4). The sections were then washed in 0.01 M PBS, serially mounted on gelatin-coated slides, dehydrated in a series of alcohols (from 50 to 100%) and cover slipped.

The pERK- immunoreactive (pERK-IR) cells were drawn under a light microscope with an attached camera lucida drawing tube (Neurolucida 2000 MicroBrightField, Colchester. UT, U.S.A). The number of all pERK-IR cells in Vc was counted from 3 sections of every 6th section and the mean number of pERK-IR cells (/3 sections /rat) was calculated from each animal, in order to reduce the variability of the number of immunoreactive neurons in each section. For GFAP and Iba1 immunohistochemical analyses, the square grid area ($26.67 \times 26.67\ \mu m^2$) occupied by the GFAP- and Iba1-immunoproducts in Vc was measured by using a computer-assisted imaging analysis system (Image J 1.37v, NIH, Bethesda, Maryland).

Double immunofluorescence histochemistry was also used to determine if the pERK-IR cells expressed a neuronal label (NeuN), GFAP or Iba1. ION-CCI rats received high-intensity mechanical stimulation (60 g) of the maxillary whisker pad skin (1 Hz, duration for 15 min) and 5 min later were perfused. Thirty-micron-thick sections of the caudal medulla and upper cervical spinal cord were cut with a freezing microtome and processed for double-labeling immunohistochemistry for pERK and NeuN, pERK and GFAP or pERK and Iba1 in the Vc area receiving afferent input from the 2nd branch of the trigeminal nerve [33]. Free-floating tissue sections were rinsed in 0.01 M PBS, 3% normal goat serum in 0.01 M PBS for 1.5 h, and then incubated in rabbit anti-phospho-p44/42 MAPK antibody (1:300) and mouse anti-NeuN antibody (1:1000; Chemicon, Temecula, CA), or mouse anti-phospho-p44/42 MAP kinase antibody (1:200, Cell signaling Technology, Beverly, MA) and rabbit anti-Iba1 antibody (1:1000) or rabbit anti-GFAP polyclonal antibody (1:5000) 3 days at 4°C and secondary antibodies (anti-rabbit Arexa Fluor 488 IgG and anti-mouse Arexa Fluor 568, 1:1000; Invitrogen, Eugene, OR) conjugated for 2 h at room temperature in a dark room. Then the sections were washed in 0.01 M PBS 3 times for 5 min. Sections were mounted on slides and cover-slipped in PermaFluor (Thermo scientific, Fremont, CA).

PD98059 administration

We used PD98059 as the MEK1 inhibitor to test its effect on the nocifensive behavior, pERK-IR, GFAP-IR or Iba1-IR cells, and Vc neuronal activities in ION-CCI or naïve rats; the solution with 10% DMSO and isotonic saline was used as the vehicle control. PD98059 was dissolved with 10% DMSO and isotonic saline (0.05 μg/ml or 0.1 μg/μl of PD98059) for i.t. administration for 8 days. One day before the ION-CCI rats were anesthetized with pentobarbital Na (50 mg/kg, i.p.) and the C7 spinal process was removed. The silicone tube was inserted into the subdural space from the C7 spinal cord level, and the tip of the silicone tube was placed at the C1/C2 level. The silicone tube was connected with the osmotic pressure pump embedded under the dorsal skin for continuous administration of PD98059. The location of the tip of the tube was determined at the end of the experiment.

Single neuron recording from Vc

Mechanical head-withdrawal threshold was measured in each rat on day 7 after ION-CCI or sham operation, and the ION-CCI rats showing neuropathic pain behavior and sham rats without neuropathic pain behavior were used for recordings of activity from the Vc (ION-CCI: n = 13, sham: n = 14, ION-CCI+PD98059: n = 8, ION-CCI+vehicle: n = 8). Each group of rats was anesthetized with pentobarbital sodium (50 mg/kg, i.p.) and the trachea and left jugular veins were cannulated to allow artificial respiration and intravenous administration of drugs. Anesthesia was maintained with isoflurane (1–2%) mixed with oxygen during surgery. The rats were mounted in a stereotaxic frame, the medulla was exposed, and a mineral oil pool was made with the skin flaps surrounding the laminectomy. A head holder was rigidly secured to the skull by stainless-steel screws and dental acrylic resin, and the ear bars and nose holder were removed to access to the orofacial region conveniently.

After surgery, anesthesia was maintained throughout the experiment by continuous inhalation of isoflurane (1–2%) mixed with oxygen. During recording sessions, the rats were immobilized with pancuronium bromide (1 mg/kg/h, i.v.) and ventilated artificially. The expired CO_2 concentration was monitored and maintained between 3.0–4.0%. Rectal temperature was maintained at 37–38°C by a thermostatically-controlled heating pad (Nihon kohden, Tokyo, Japan) and the electrocardiogram was monitored. When the heart beat rate increased more than 300/min, the isoflurane concentration increased appropriately.

Electrophysiological recording procedures were similar to those previously described in detail [11]. Briefly, enamel-coated tungsten microelectrodes (impedance = 10–12 Megohms, 1000 Hz) were advanced into the Vc about 2 mm caudal to the obex in 1 μm steps. Vc neurons were searched by applying mechanical stimulation (pressure or brush) to the craniofacial region. When a single neuron was isolated, its response to mechanical stimulation of the facial skin was carefully examined and its cutaneous receptive field (RF) was mapped. Graded mechanical stimuli were applied to the most sensitive area of the RF. Mechanical stimuli consisted of brushing with a camel hair brush, graded pressure produced by von Frey filaments (1, 6, 15, 26 and 60 g) and pinch produced by a small arterial clip. In order to avoid sensitization due to repeated stimulation, noxious mechanical stimuli were applied to only small area of the RF of each neuron. If the non-noxious RF of the first and second encountered nociceptive neurons overlapped with each other, the second neuron was not included in the analysis. Each neuron was classified either as 1) a low-threshold mechanoreceptive (LTM) neuron; 2) a wide dynamic range (WDR) neuron; or 3) a nociceptive-specific (NS) neuron. In this study only WDR neurons were further studied and their data analyzed. When a WDR neuron was identified, heat and cold stimuli were applied to the most sensitive area of the mechanical RF by a contact thermal probe (5 mm in diameter, adapting temperature: 35°C, Intercross Tokyo Japan). If the neuron responded to cooling of the RF, it was then tested with heat stimulation. The tip of the thermal probe was 5 mm in diameter, and the rate of temperature change was set at 10°C/s. Before application of the thermal stimulus to the RF, the surface temperature was adapted to 35°C for 180 s. Skin heating ranged from 44 to 50°C and lasted for 10 s. Cold stimuli consisted of cooling of the skin from 10 to 30°C. The thermal stimuli were applied to the RF at 190-s intervals (adaptation time: 180 s, stimulus time: 10 s) to avoid sensitization of peripheral nociceptors.

Neuronal responses were fed into a hard disc for subsequent analysis of signals. After recording of the response properties of Vc neurons, lesions were made at the recording site by passing direct current of 20 μA for 15 s. The waveform of single or multiple neuronal activities was analyzed off-line. The waveform of each neuron was identified using Spike 2 software (CED, Cambridge, UK). Peristimulus time histograms (bin width = 1 s) were generated in response to each stimulus. Background activity was first recorded for 10 s before application of mechanical or thermal stimulus and then subtracted from the evoked neuronal responses during the subsequent analysis. Afterdischarges were recorded for 10 s after pinching the RF, and expressed as mean spike frequency. The mean firing frequency was calculated during mechanical or thermal stimulation, and stimulus-response (S-R) functions of each Vc neuron were obtained in response to the mechanical or thermal stimuli. The mechanical or thermal stimulation of the RF was considered to have induced an effect

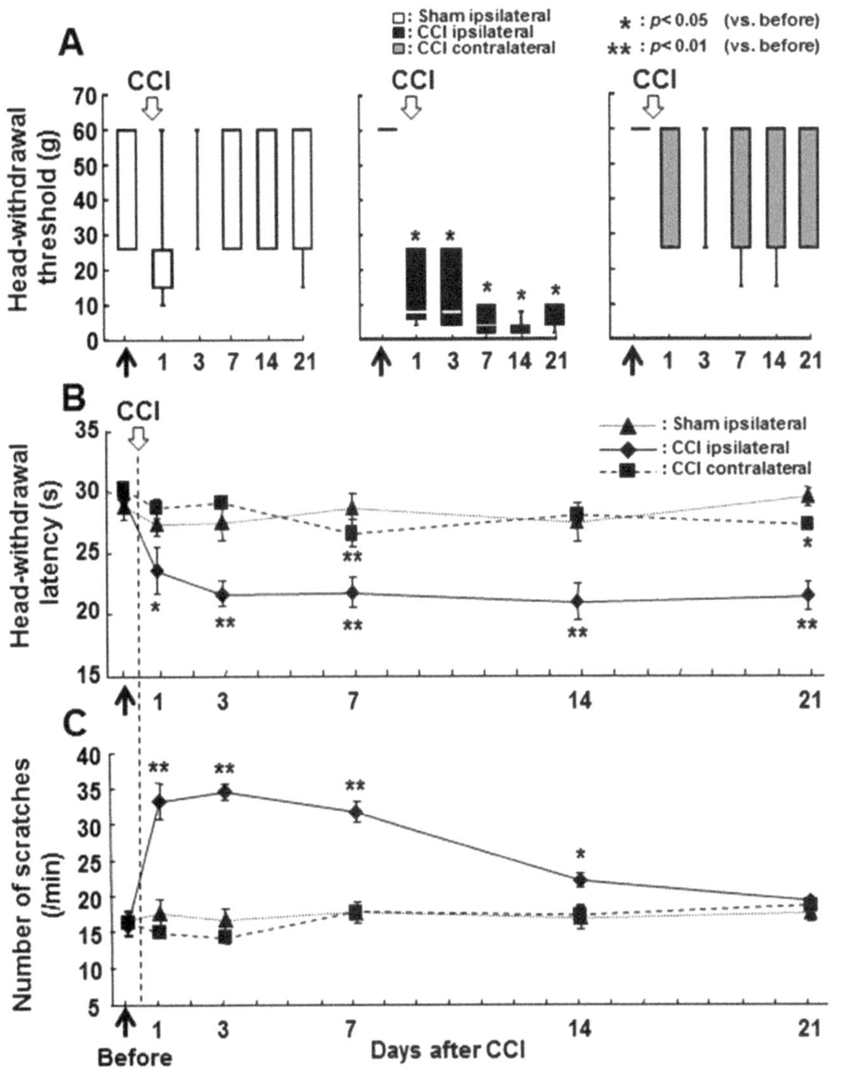

Figure 1. Nocifensive behavior to mechanical, heat or cold stimulation of the whisker pad skin in sham and ION-CCI rats. Time-course change in the head-withdrawal threshold to mechanical stimulation of the whisker pad skin (A), head-withdrawal latency to heat stimulation of the whisker pad skin (B) and face scratching frequency following acetone application to the whisker pad skin (C). Ipsi. to CCI: ipsilateral side to CCI, Contra. to CCI: contralateral side to CCI, Ipsi. to sham: ipsilateral side to sham operation, before: before ION-CCI or sham operation. *: $p<0.05$ (vs. before), **: $p<0.01$ (vs. before).

when the peak firing frequency at 5 s after mechanical and 30 s (one trial for each neuron with 180 s intervals) after thermal stimulation differed from the mean background discharge rate by ±2 S.D. The RF of each neuron was drawn to scale on a standard diagram of the rat head. RF area was calculated using image analysis software (Image J 1.37v).

At the end of the experiment, the rats were overdosed with pentobarbital sodium (80 mg/kg, i.p.) and sacrificed. The brains were removed and placed in cold fixative (4% PFA in 0.01 M PBS) for a few days, then transferred to cold phosphate-buffered 20% sucrose for 48 h. Serial sections (50 µm-thick) were cut along the path of the electrode penetration. The sections were counter-stained with Thionin for identification of recording sites. Recording sites were drawn using Camera lucida drawing tube (Neurolucida 2000).

Statistical analysis

Mechanical head-withdrawal thresholds are presented as median values and other data are shown as mean ± SEM. The one-way ANOVA followed by Bonferroni test was performed on the behavioral test at each time point after the operation. Student t-test was used to compare the number of pERK-IR cells between ION-CCI and sham rats, to compare the number of pERK-IR cells between PD98059-injected and vehicle-injected ION-CCI rats, and to compare the heat and cold nocifensive behavior between PD98059-injected and vehicle-injected ION-CCI rats. Student t-test was also used to compare the background activity, afterdischarge, brush and pinch evoked responses between ION-CCI and sham rats, and to compare between PD98059-injected and vehicle-injected ION-CCI rats. For comparison of mechanical nocifensive behavior between PD98059-injected and vehicle-injected ION-CCI rats, Mann Whitney U-test was used. Two-way repeated measures ANOVA followed by Turky test was used to compare the firing frequency following graded mechanical, heat or cold stimuli between ION-CCI rats and sham rats, and to compare between PD98059-injected ION-CCI rats and vehicle-injected ION-CCI rats. Differences were considered significant at $p<0.05$.

Results

Behavioral responses to mechanical and thermal stimulation of the whisker pad skin

After completion of the training, in which the rats accepted the mechanical stimulation applied to the whisker pad skin, rats underwent the ION-CCI or sham operation. During mechanical or thermal stimulation of the whisker pad skin, vocalization and autotomy were never observed in ION-CCI and sham rats. Figure 1 illustrates the head-withdrawal threshold to mechanical stimulation of the whisker pad skin (A), head-withdrawal latency to heat stimulation of the whisker pad skin (B), and the number of face scratches following cold (acetone) stimulation of the whisker pad skin (C). The head-withdrawal threshold to mechanical stimulation and head-withdrawal latency to heat stimulation of the whisker pad skin were significantly reduced at 1 day after ION-CCI and lasted for 21 days after the CCI compared to that before CCI operation (Fig. 1A and B). The number of face scratches after acetone application to the whisker pad skin was also significantly larger in ION-CCI rats for 14 days after CCI compared to that before the operation. There were no significant changes in head-withdrawal threshold to mechanical stimulation of the whisker pad skin, head-withdrawal latency to heat stimulation, and the number of face scratches after acetone application to the whisker pad skin on the side contralateral to the ION-CCI. In sham rats, the head-withdrawal threshold to mechanical stimulation of the whisker pad skin, the head-withdrawal latency to heat and the number of face scratches after acetone application were also not changed after the operation.

pERK-IR, GFAP-IR and Iba1-IR cells in Vc

All pERK-IR cells following noxious mechanical stimulation of the whisker pad skin also showed NeuN immunoreactivity in ION-CCI rats, indicating that pERK-IR cells observed were neurons (Fig. 2 A, B and C). To test if ERK phosphorylation occurs in astroglial or microglial cells in Vc, we studied pERK, GFAP and Iba1 immunohistochemistries in the Vc of ION-CCI rats. No pERK-IR cells showed GFAP-IR (Fig. 2D, E and F) or Iba1-IR (Fig. 2G, H and I) in Vc.

A large number of pERK-IR cells were observed in the superficial laminae of the Vc on the side ipsilateral to the operation 5 min after non-noxious (6 g) and especially noxious (60 g) mechanical stimulation of the whisker pad skin in sham rats (Figs. 2 J, L and 3 A, B, E) and ION-CCI rats (Figs. 2 N, P and 3 C, D, E) on day 7 after the operation, with the largest number at 1.4 mm caudal to the obex (Fig. 3 A–D). No pERK-IR cells were observed in the contralateral Vc of sham rats (Fig. 2 K and M) and ION-CCI rats (Fig. 2 O and Q). The mean number of pERK-IR cells after noxious stimulation (60 g) of the whisker pad skin was significantly larger in ION-CCI rats compared to sham rats on the side ipsilateral to the operation, whereas no significant difference in the number of pERK-IR cells between sham and ION-CCI rats was observed after non-noxious mechanical stimulation (6 g) of the whisker pad skin (Fig. 3 E). The number of pERK-IR cells following heat (50°C) or cold (acetone administration) stimulation was also significantly larger in ION-CCI rats compared to sham rats (Fig. 3 F and G).

Responses of Vc nociceptive neurons

A total of 27 nociceptive neurons was recorded from Vc in sham and ION-CCI rats (sham: 14, ION-CCI: 13), and electrophysiological properties of functionally identified Vc nociceptive neurons were analyzed. Most of these nociceptive neurons in sham and ION-CCI rats were located in the superficial laminae of the lateral portion of the Vc (Fig. 4 A and B). The nociceptive neurons were defined as WDR neurons based on their responses to mechanical stimulation of their RFs. The RF of each WDR neuron was located on the whisker pad skin, and the mean RF size was not different between sham and ION-CCI rats (Fig. 4 C). Mean background activity and afterdischarge of WDR neurons were significantly larger in ION-CCI rats compared to sham rats (Fig. 5 A and B). WDR neurons showed graded responses to graded stimulation of the RF in sham and ION-CCI rats (Fig. 5 C), and the mean graded pressure responses and brush- and pinch-evoked responses were significantly larger in ION-CCI rats compared to sham rats (Fig. 5 D and E). Heat and cold-evoked responses were also significantly larger in ION-CCI rats compared to sham rats (Fig. 5 F and G).

Effect of i.t. PD98059 administration on ERK phosphorylation in Vc neurons, nocifensive behavior, Vc WDR neuronal activities, GFAP-IR cells and Iba1-IR cells

Many pERK-IR cells after noxious mechanical stimulation (60 g) of the whisker pad skin were apparent in the superficial laminae of the Vc in ION-CCI rats after i.t. vehicle injection (Fig. 6 A), but the mean number of pERK-IR cells was significantly smaller in 0.1 μg/μl concentration of PD98059-injected ION-CCI rats compared to vehicle-injected ION-CCI rats after 60 g stimulation of the whisker pad skin (Fig. 6 C). We also tested the effect of 0.05 μg/μl concentration of PD98059 on ERK phosphorylation in Vc neurons. The number of pERK-IR cells was slightly smaller than saline-injected rats but not reached to the significant level (Fig. 6C). In naïve rats, we could not observe significant effect of PD98059 administration on pERK expression and nocifensive behaviors. The mean head-withdrawal threshold to mechanical stimulation of the whisker pad skin was not different between PD98059-injected and vehicle-injected ION-CCI rats (Fig. 6 D). On the other hand, mean head-withdrawal latency to heat stimulation of the whisker pad skin was significantly longer in PD98059-injected ION-CCI rats compared to vehicle-injected ION-CCI rats (Fig. 6 E), and the mean number of face scratches after acetone administration to the whisker pad skin was also significantly smaller in PD98059-injected ION-CCI rats compared to vehicle-injected ION-CCI rats (Fig. 6 F).

We also studied the effect of i.t. administration of PD98059 on Vc WDR neuronal activities in ION-CCI rats. A total of 16 WDR neurons was tested with i.t. administration of vehicle or PD98059 in ION-CCI rats (PD98059: $n=8$, vehicle: $n=8$). Mean background activity and afterdischarge in Vc WDR neurons were significantly smaller in PD98059-administered ION-CCI rats compared to vehicle-administered ION-CCI rats (Fig. 7 A and B). Evoked responses of Vc WDR neurons following noxious (60 g) but not non-noxious mechanical stimulation (less than 15 g) of the whisker pad skin were significantly smaller in PD98059-administered ION-CCI rats compared to vehicle-administered ION-CCI rats (Fig. 7 C). Responses to brushing of the RF were not affected by PD98059 administration in ION-CCI rats (Fig. 7 D), whereas responses to pinching of the RF were significantly depressed after PD98059 administration (Fig. 7 E). Noxious heat (50°C) or cold (10°C)-evoked responses of Vc WDR neurons were also signifi-

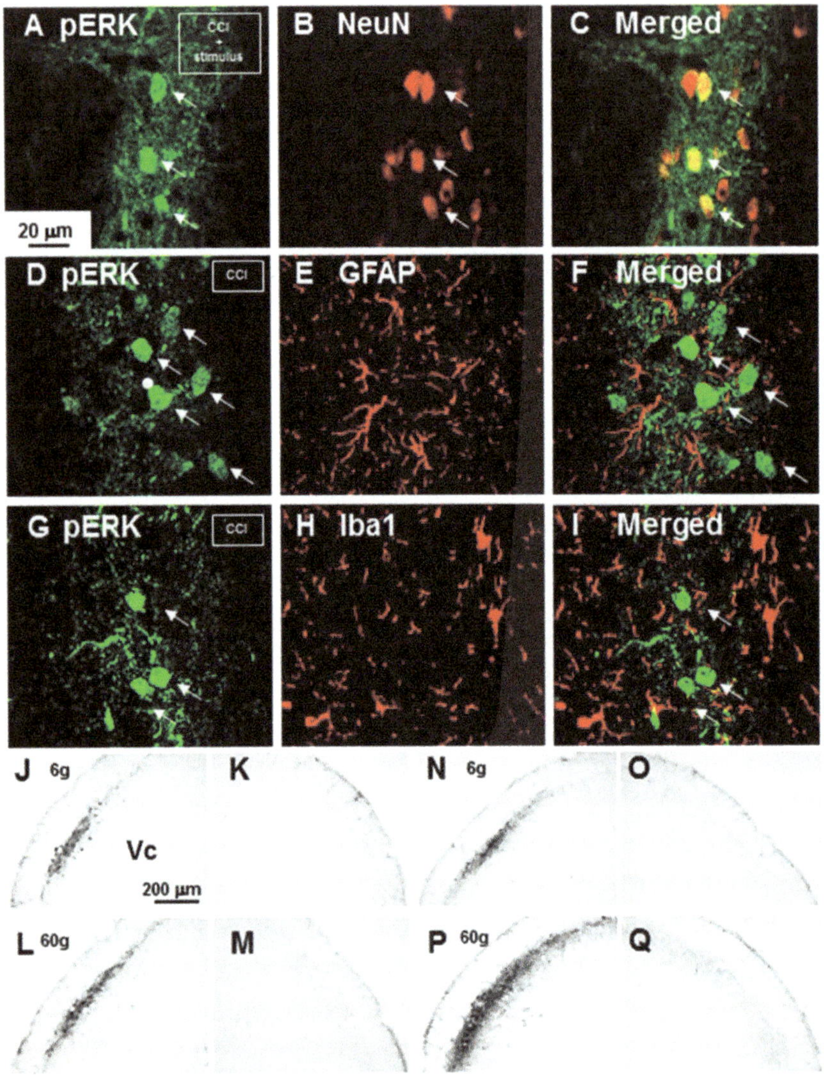

Figure 2. Photomicrographs of pERK-IR, NeuN-IR, GFAP-IR and Iba1-IR cells in Vc. A–C: Fluorescent photomicrographs of pERK-IR cells (A), NeuN-IR cells (B) and merged photomicrograph of A and B (C) ION-CCI rats. D–F: Fluorescent photomicrographs of pERK-IR cells (D), GFAP-IR cells (E) and merged photomicrograph of D and E (F) in ION-CCI rats. G–I: Fluorescent photomicrographs of pERK-IR cells (G), Iba1-IR cells (H) and merged photomicrograph of G and H (I) in ION-CCI rats. J–M: pERK-IR cells following 6 g stimulation of the whisker pad skin on the side ipsilateral to the sham operation (J), those in the contralateral side (K), those following 60 g stimulation on the ipsilateral side (L) and those in the contralateral side (M), N–Q: pERK-IR cells following 6 g stimulation of the whisker pad skin on the side ipsilateral to the ION-CCI (N), those in the contralateral side (O), those following 60 g stimulation in the ipsilateral side (P) and those in the contralateral side (Q).

cantly suppressed in ION-CCI rats after i.t. administration of PD98059 (Fig. 7 F and G).

To evaluate the effect of i.t. administration of PD98059 on glial cell hyperactivation in Vc of ION-CCI rats (PD98059: n = 5, vehicle: n = 5), GFAP and Iba1 immunoreactive cells were studied in ION-CCI rats following i.t. administration of PD98059 or vehicle. Many GFAP-IR (Fig. 8 A and B) or Iba1-IR cells (Fig. 8 C and D) were observed in Vc of ION-CCI rats with PD98059 or vehicle administration, and the areas occupied by GFAP-IR and Iba1-IR immuno-products in Vc were not significantly different between PD98059-administered and vehicle-administered ION-CCI rats (Fig. 8 E and F).

Discussion

The present study has provided novel findings of the effects of ION-CCI on the rat, documenting mechanical or thermal behavioral hypersensitivity of the whisker pad skin innervated by the injured ION, significant increases in the number of pERK-IR cells in the Vc following noxious but not non-noxious stimulation of the whisker pad skin, and changes in the response properties of Vc WDR neurons that are indicative of Vc central sensitization. Further novel findings were that the thermal but not mechanical behavioral hypersensitivity, the number of pERK-IR cells and responses of Vc WDR neurons to noxious mechanical or thermal stimuli but not non-noxious stimuli could be significantly suppressed after i.t. injection of MEK1 inhibitor in ION-CCI rats, suggesting that ERK phosphorylation in Vc WDR neurons

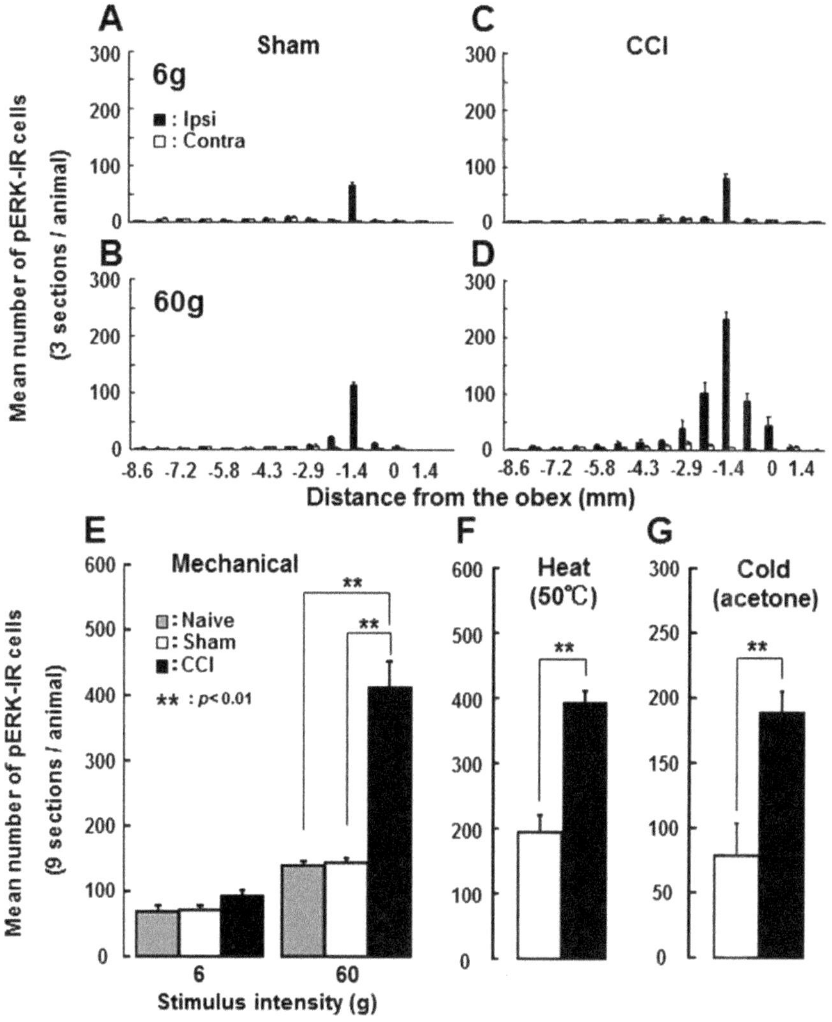

Figure 3. Rostro-caudal distribution and mean number of pERK-IR cells. A and B: rostro-caudal distribution of pERK-IR cells following 6 g (A) and 60 g (B) mechanical stimulation of the whisker pad skin in sham rats. C and D: rostro-caudal distribution of pERK-IR cells following 6 g (C) and 60 g (D) mechanical stimulation of the whisker pad skin in ION-CCI rats. E: Mean number of pERK-IR cells following 6 or 60 g stimulation of the whisker pad skin in naïve, sham and ION-CCI rats. **: $p<0.001$ (sham vs. ION-CCI).

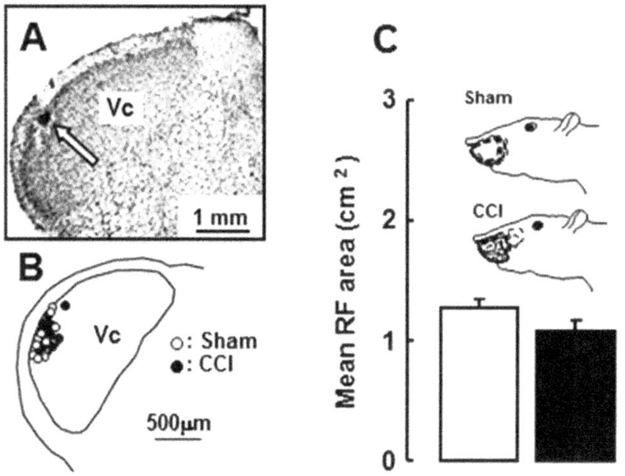

Figure 4. Recording sites and receptive field size. A and B: location of recording sites in Vc. C: Drawings of RFs and mean RF area in ION-CCI and sham rats.

may contribute to thermal but not mechanical hypersensitivity in the face following trigeminal nerve injury.

Mechanical and thermal hypersensitivity following ION-CCI

ION-CCI produced sustained modifications in sensory processing, resulting in long-lasting mechanical and heat hypersensitivity and transient hypersensitivity to cold stimulation in the area innervated by the injured ION. In our ION-CCI rats, mechanical and heat hypersensitivity was obvious at 1 day after ION ligation and lasted for at least 21 days, whereas cold hypersensitivity lasted only 14 days although it also had an early onset. The hypersensitivity to mechanical and heat stimulation to the hind paw in rats with sciatic nerve ligation has been reported to be apparent at 2 days post-injury and to last for more than 30 days [34,35], and cold hypersensitivity of the hind paw has also been reported in rats following sciatic nerve ligation to last for more than 21 days at the early onset (1 day after the ligation) [36]. Thus, sciatic or trigeminal nerve injury induces hind paw or face mechanical and heat hypersensitivity with an early onset that

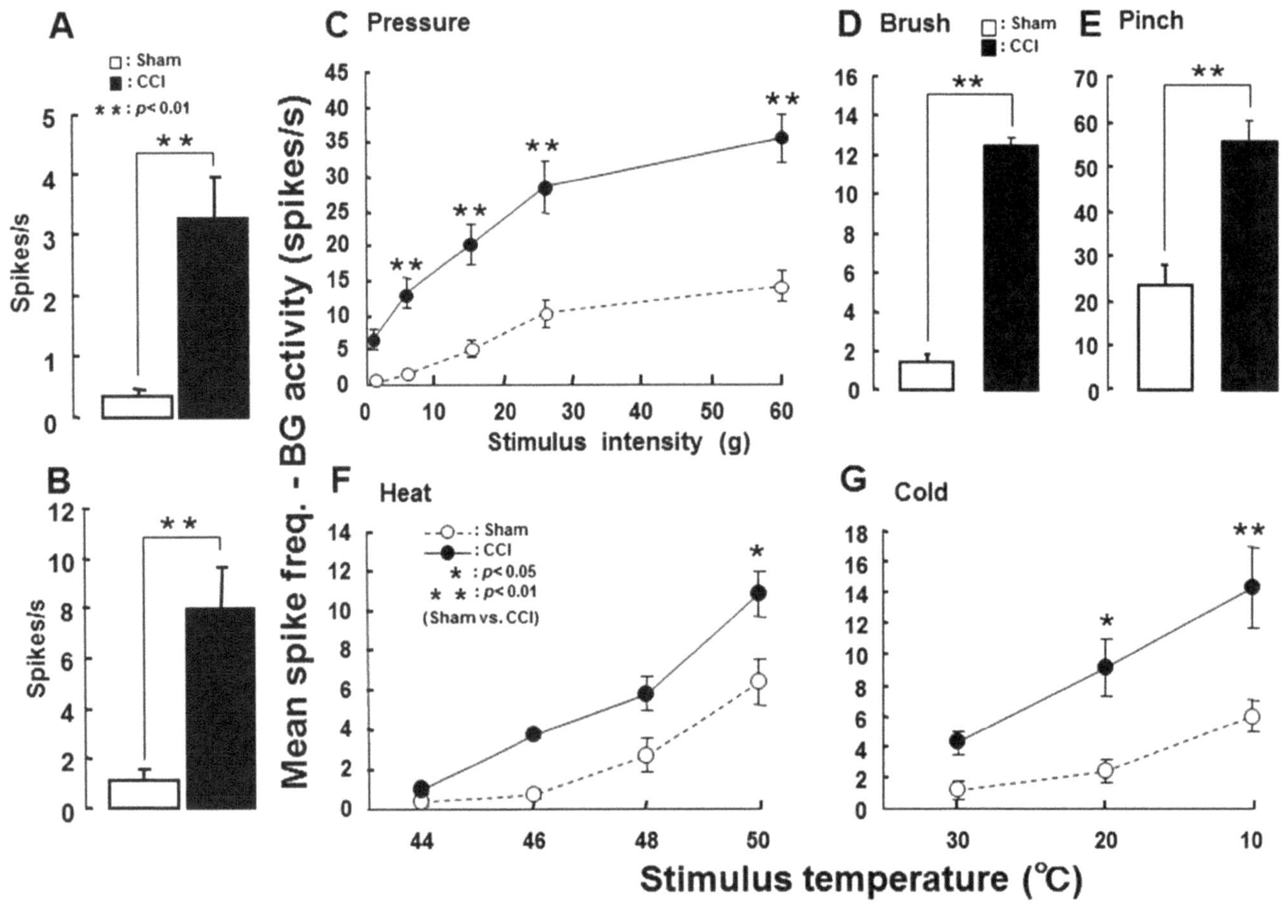

Figure 5. Single neuronal activity of Vc WDR neurons in ION-CCI and sham rats. A: Mean background activities. B: Mean afterdischarges. C: Mean spike frequency following graded mechanical stimuli. D: Mean spikes following brushing to the RF. E: Mean spikes following pinching to the RF. F: Mean spike frequency following graded heat stimuli. G: Mean spike frequency following graded cold stimuli. *: p<0.05 (sham vs. ION-CCI), **: p<0.01 (sham vs. ION-CCI).

persists for a long period, whereas cold hypersensitivity lasts for short period following trigeminal nerve injury and persists for a long period after sciatic nerve injury.

Changes in Vc neuronal activity associated with mechanical and thermal hypersensitivity

It has been reported that the behavioral hypersensitivity to innocuous mechanical or thermal stimulation following spinal nerve injury originates from increased neuronal excitability in the peripheral and central nervous system [37,38,39]. In the case of peripheral changes, numerous studies have shown that primary afferent fibers have significantly higher spontaneous activity following spinal nerve injury [40,41,42], and sensitization of the injured primary afferent fibers may occur [17,41,43]. A number of papers have also described altered electrophysiological properties and protein production in myelinated and unmyelinated fibers in sciatic nerve-ligated rats [43,44,45,46] and that TRPM8 and TRPV1 channel expression is significantly enhanced in DRG neurons after sciatic nerve injury [47]. In the orofacial region, ION-CCI and IAN-transection models have been developed to evaluate mechanisms underlying orofacial neuropathic pain [6,11,12,13,14]. Molecular changes and enhancement of neuronal excitability can be observed in TG neurons [15,16,17] and Vc neurons after infraorbital or cervical nerve injury [18,19,20]. These findings suggest that the mechanical and thermal hypersensitivity that we documented after ION-CCI may be associated with hyperexcitability of injured myelinated or unmyelinated ION primary afferent fibers. It is noteworthy that the heat and mechanical hypersensitivity lasted for at least 21 days after the ION-CCI, whereas cold hypersensitivity lasted for 14 days after ION-CCI. It is possible that the different time-courses in nocifensive behaviors between mechanical or heat hypersensitivity and cold hypersensitivity in the ION-CCI rats may be due, at least in part, to different effects of ION-CCI on mechanical or heat sensitive primary afferent fibers versus cold-sensitive fibers, such as channel or receptor expression in each type of primary afferent neurons after the CCI [17].

The possibility of central nervous mechanisms contributing to the above differences also cannot be ruled out. Spinal dorsal horn (DH) and thalamic nociceptive neurons have high background activity and enhancement of mechanical and/or thermal evoked responses following peripheral nerve injury [4,37,48]. Moreover, both non-noxious and noxious responses may be enhanced after spinal nerve injury, indicating that these CNS neuronal changes may contribute to the mechanical and thermal hypersensitivity is produced by peripheral nerve injury [34,37]. In the trigeminal system, it has also been reported that non-noxious and noxious responses of Vc neurons as well as IAN fibers are enhanced following IAN injury [6,32,49]. The ION-CCI-induced increase in

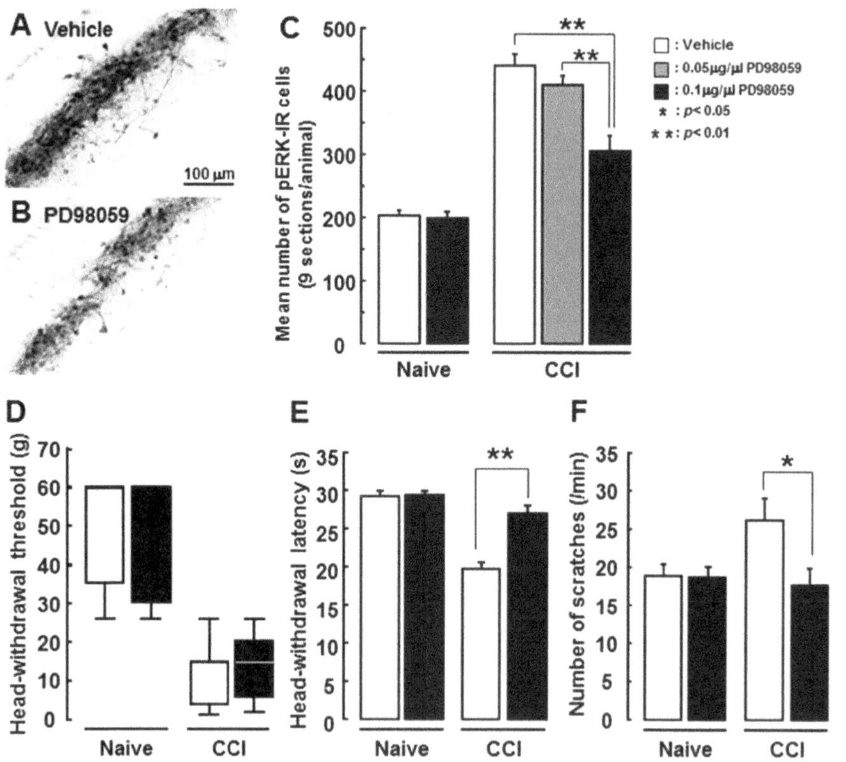

Figure 6. Effect of i.t. administration of PD98059 on ERK phosphorylation in Vc neurons and nocifensive behavior. A and B: photomicrographs of pERK-IR cells in Vc following 60 g stimulation of the whisker pad skin in ION-CCI rats with i.t. vehicle (A) or PD98059 (B) administration. C: Mean number of pERK-IR cells in naïve and ION-CCI rats with vehicle or PD98059 administration. D–F: Mean head-withdrawal threshold to mechanical stimulation of the whisker pad skin (D), mean head-withdrawal latency to heat stimulation of the whisker pad skin (E) and mean number of face scratches after acetone application to the whisker pad skin (F) in naïve and ION-CCI rats with vehicle or PD98059 administration. *: $p<0.05$, **: $p<0.01$ (vehicle vs. PD98059).

Vc neuronal excitability documented in this study reflected changes in Vc neuronal properties indicative of central sensitization of Vc nociceptive neurons and were similar to those reported in these previous studies, in that background activity, afterdischarges and mechanical and thermal-evoked responses were significantly enhanced in IAN-injured rats compared to sham rats. These findings suggest that these Vc neuronal changes likely contributed to the mechanical, heat and cold hypersensitivity in the face following ION-CCI. We also observed a significant increase in the number of pERK-IR cells double-labeled with NeuN following noxious but not non-noxious mechanical stimulation of the whisker pad skin in ION-CCI rats compared to sham rats. This observation suggests that the hyperexcitability of Vc nociceptive neurons is associated with an enhancement of ERK phosphorylation in Vc nociceptive neurons following noxious but not non-noxious mechanical stimulation of the whisker pad skin in ION-CCI rats.

Functional implications of ERK phosphorylation in trigeminal neuropathic pain

We also studied the effect of the MEK1 inhibitor PD98095 on the head-withdrawal behavior to mechanical or heat stimulation of the whisker pad skin and on face scratching behavior evoked by acetone application to the whisker pad skin in ION-CCI rats. The head-withdrawal latency to heat stimulation and face scratching frequency to acetone application were significantly reduced in the ION-CCI rats following i.t. administration of PD98059, whereas the head-withdrawal threshold to mechanical stimulation of the whisker pad skin was not affected by the PD98059 administration. We also demonstrated that Vc neuronal responses evoked by noxious heat, cold and noxious mechanical stimulation but not by non-noxious mechanical stimulation were significantly suppressed following i.t. PD98059 administration compared to vehicle administration in the ION-CCI rats. Non-noxious stimulus which was almost same intensity as mechanical head-withdrawal threshold causes ERK phosphorylation in the small number of Vc and C1–C2 neurons in ION-CCI rats. Furthermore, the number of pERK-IR cells following non-noxious mechanical stimulation in ION-CCI rats was not significantly larger than that of sham rats, and we could not observe significant effect of PD98059 on the excitability of WDR neurons in IN-CCI rats. These results suggest that pERK-IR cells are involved in noxious thermal and/or noxious mechanical responses of Vc and C1–C2 neurons but not non-noxious mechanical responses. Furthermore, the number of pERK-IR cells ION-CCI rats was not significantly larger in sham rats following non-noxious mechanical stimulation of the lateral facial skin. The head-withdrawal threshold and non-noxious responses of WDR neurons were not affected by PD98059 administration. These data are consistent with our behavioral data, in which head-withdrawal responses to non-noxious mechanical stimulation of the whisker pad skin was not affected by PD98059 administration in ION-CCI and sham rats. In addition, the increased number of pERK-IR cells following noxious stimuli in ION-CCI rats could be significantly reduced by PD98059 administration. There is evidence that ERK phosphorylation is involved in the enhanced neuronal activity in

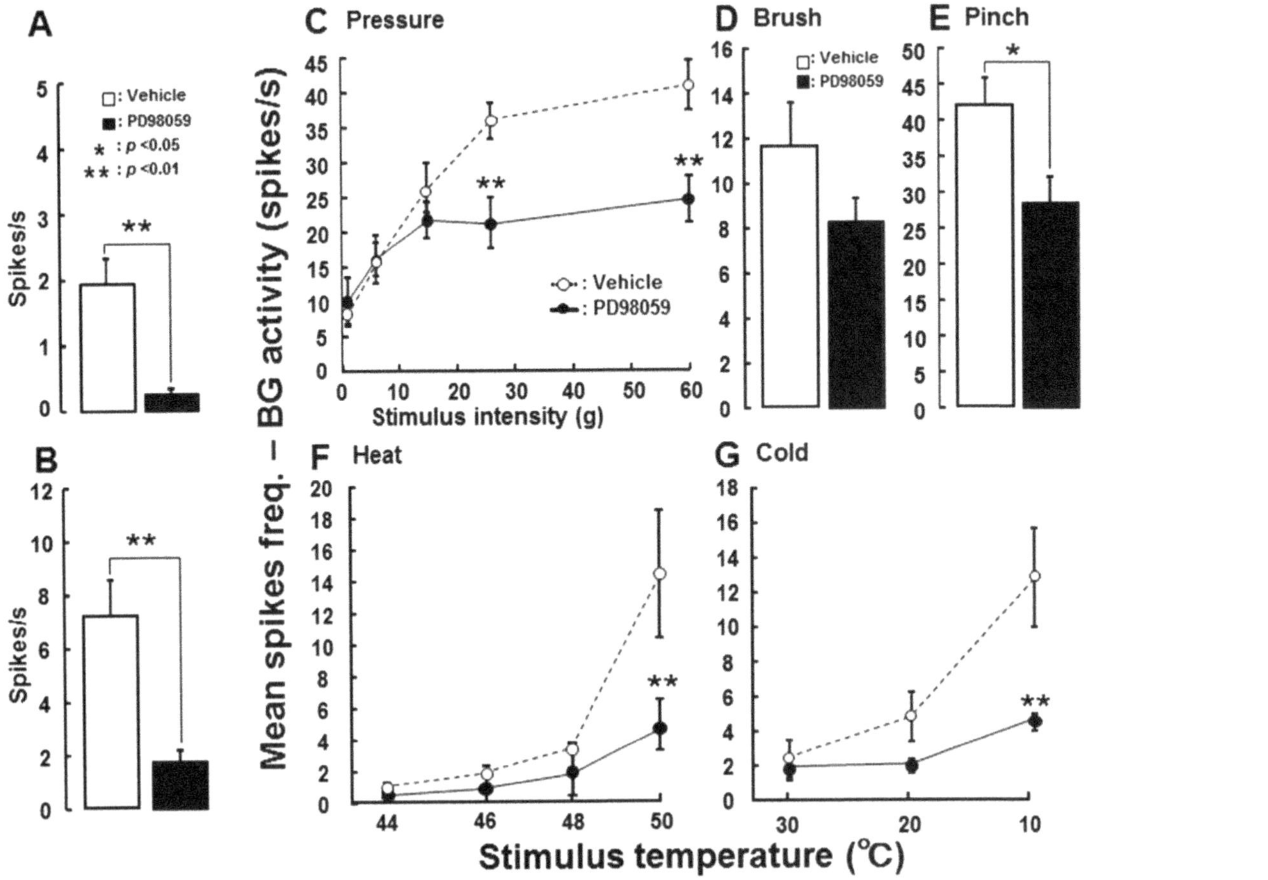

Figure 7. Effect of i.t. administration of PD98059 on Vc WDR neuronal activities in ION-CCI rats. A: Mean background activities. B: Mean afterdischarges. C: Mean spike frequency following graded mechanical stimuli. D: Mean spikes following brushing the RF. E: Mean spikes following pinching the RF. F: Mean spike frequency following graded heat stimuli. G: Mean spike frequency following graded cold stimuli. *: $p<0.05$, **: $p<0.01$ (vehicle vs. PD98059).

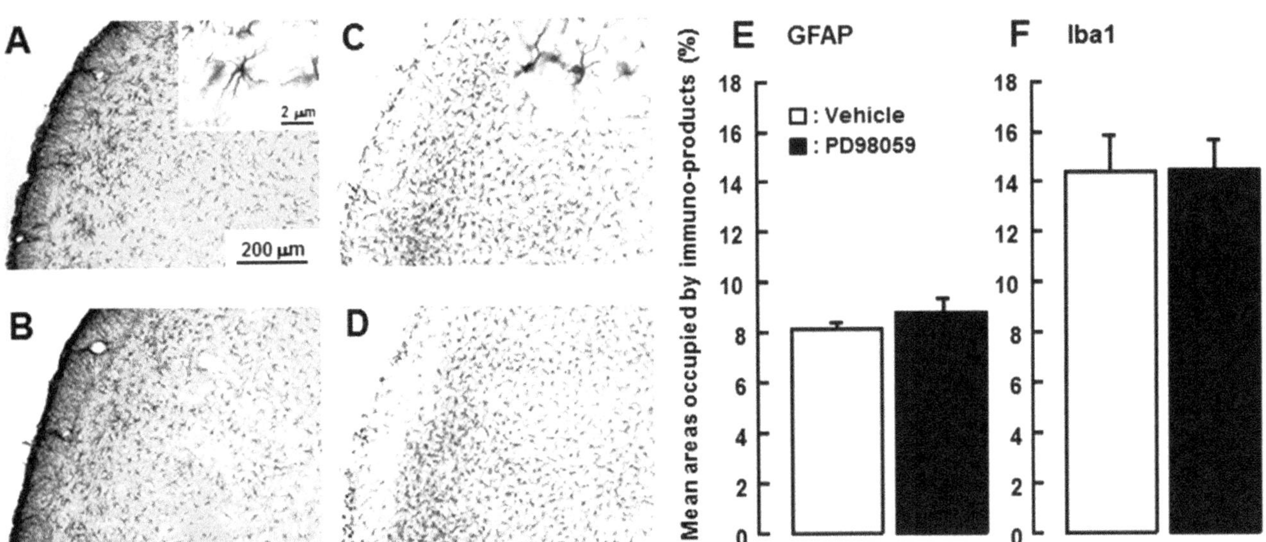

Figure 8. Effect of PD98059 administration on GFAP and Iba1 immunoreactivities in ION-CCI rats. A and B: Photomicrographs of GFAP-IR cells in Vc in ION-CCI rats with i.t. PD98059 (A) or vehicle (B) administration. C and D: Photomicrographs of Iba1-IR cells in Vc in ION-CCI rats with i.t. PD98059(C) or vehicle (D) administration. E and F: Mean areas occupied by GFAP-IR (E) and Iba1-IR (F) immuno-products in ION-CCI rats with i.t. vehicle or PD98059 administration.

the spinal DH following strong noxious stimuli, injury or inflammation since the increased firing of DH neurons induced by repetitive electrical stimulation of the sciatic nerve at C-fiber intensity can be significantly suppressed following i.t. administration of the MEK1 inhibitor U0126 [50,51,52,53,54,55], and significant enhancement of pERK expression occurs in DH nociceptive neurons following peripheral nerve injury or inflammation that also can be suppressed by MEK1 inhibitor administration [27,56,57,58]. We have also documented increased pERK-IR cells in Vc following other types of noxious stimuli [18,28,30,31]. Together with these previous data, the findings suggest that ERK phosphorylation is involved in the enhancement of the Vc nociceptive neuronal activity in ION-CCI rats that results from activation of small-diameter primary afferent fibers by strong noxious mechanical or thermal stimulation.

Since some previous studies have documented that ERK phosphorylation occurs in glial cells in rats with sciatic nerve injury or spinal nerve ligation [59,60], we also tested if i.t. administration of PD98059 in ION-CCI rats affects expression of GFAP and Iba1 that are markers for astroglial and microglial cells, respectively. We did not observe any differences in the areas occupied by GFAP and Iba1 immuno-products between PD98059- and vehicle-administered ION-CCI rats. There was also no evidence of any pERK-IR cells showing GFAP and Iba1 immunoreactivities in ION-CCI rats, but all pERK-IR cells showed NeuN immunoreactivity. These findings suggest that ERK may be phosphorylated in neurons but not in astroglial or microglial cells in Vc in this neuropathic pain model.

Taken together with previous results, the present findings suggest that ERK phosphorylation in Vc neurons is involved in central sensitization of Vc nociceptive neurons following trigeminal nerve injury, resulting in orofacial thermal hypersensitivity associated with trigeminal neuropathic pain.

Author Contributions

Conceived and designed the experiments: KI. Performed the experiments: IS YT MS KS KH AK MK BJS SM KO KU KI. Analyzed the data: IS YT MS KS KH AK MK BJS SM KO KU KI. Contributed reagents/materials/analysis tools: MS BJS. Wrote the paper: KI MS BJS. Read and approved the final manuscript: IS YT MS KS KH AK MK BJS SM KO KU KI. Provided data interpretation: IS YT MS KS KH AK MK BJS SM KO KU KI. Helped finalize the manuscript: IS YT MS KS KH AK MK BJS SM KO KU KI. Conceptualized the hypothesis: KI. Supervised the experiments: KI. Directed the data analysis: KI. Finalized the manuscript: KI.

References

1. Gautron M, Jazat F, Ratinahirana H, Hauw JJ, Guilbaud G (1990) Alterations in myelinated fibres in the sciatic nerve of rats after constriction: possible relationships between the presence of abnormal small myelinated fibres and pain-related behaviour. Neurosci Lett 111: 28–33.
2. Guilbaud G, Benoist JM, Jazat F, Gautron M (1990) Neuronal responsiveness in the ventrobasal thalamic complex of rats with an experimental peripheral mononeuropathy. J Neurophysiol 64: 1537–1554.
3. Carlton SM, Dougherty PM, Pover CM, Coggeshall RE (1991) Neuroma formation and numbers of axons in a rat model of experimental peripheral neuropathy. Neurosci Lett 131: 88–92.
4. Laird JM, Bennett GJ (1993) An electrophysiological study of dorsal horn neurons in the spinal cord of rats with an experimental peripheral neuropathy. J Neurophysiol 69: 2072–2085.
5. Woolf CJ, Max MB (2001) Mechanism-based pain diagnosis: issues for analgesic drug development. Anesthesiology 95: 241–249.
6. Robinson PP, Boissonade FM, Loescher AR, Smith KG, Yates JM, et al. (2004) Peripheral mechanisms for the initiation of pain following trigeminal nerve injury. J Orofac Pain 18: 287–292.
7. Vickers ER, Cousins MJ, Walker S, Chisholm K (1998) Analysis of 50 patients with atypical odontalgia. A preliminary report on pharmacological procedures for diagnosis and treatment. Oral Surg Oral Med Oral Pathol Oral Radiol Endod 85: 24–32.
8. Truelove E (2004) Management issues of neuropathic trigeminal pain from a dental perspective. J Orofac Pain 18: 374–380.
9. Jaaskelainen SK (2004) The utility of clinical neurophysiological and quantitative sensory testing for trigeminal neuropathy. J Orofac Pain 18: 355–359.
10. Forssell H, Tenovuo O, Silvoniemi P, Jaaskelainen SK (2007) Differences and similarities between atypical facial pain and trigeminal neuropathic pain. Neurology 69: 1451–1459.
11. Iwata K, Imai T, Tsuboi Y, Tashiro A, Ogawa A, et al. (2001) Alteration of medullary dorsal horn neuronal activity following inferior alveolar nerve transection in rats. J Neurophysiol 86: 2868–2877.
12. Imamura Y, Kawamoto H, Nakanishi O (1997) Characterization of heat-hyperalgesia in an experimental trigeminal neuropathy in rats. Exp Brain Res 116: 97–103.
13. Vos BP, Strassman AM, Maciewicz RJ (1994) Behavioral evidence of trigeminal neuropathic pain following chronic constriction injury to the rat's infraorbital nerve. J Neurosci 14: 2708–2723.
14. Nomura H, Ogawa A, Tashiro A, Morimoto T, Hu JW, et al. (2002) Induction of Fos protein-like immunoreactivity in the trigeminal spinal nucleus caudalis and upper cervical cord following noxious and non-noxious mechanical stimulation of the whisker pad of the rat with an inferior alveolar nerve transection. Pain 95: 225–238.
15. Tsuboi Y, Takeda M, Tanimoto T, Ikeda M, Matsumoto S, et al. (2004) Alteration of the second branch of the trigeminal nerve activity following inferior alveolar nerve transection in rats. Pain 111: 323–334.
16. Takeda M, Tsuboi Y, Kitagawa J, Nakagawa K, Iwata K, et al. (2011) Potassium channels as a potential therapeutic target for trigeminal neuropathic and inflammatory pain. Mol Pain 7: 5.
17. Kitagawa J, Takeda M, Suzuki I, Kadoi J, Tsuboi Y, et al. (2006) Mechanisms involved in modulation of trigeminal primary afferent activity in rats with peripheral mononeuropathy. Eur J Neurosci 24: 1976–1986.
18. Kobayashi A, Shinoda M, Sessle BJ, Honda K, Imamura Y, et al. (2011) Mechanisms involved in extraterritorial facial pain following cervical spinal nerve injury in rats. Mol Pain 7: 12.
19. Nakajima A, Tsuboi Y, Suzuki I, Honda K, Shinoda M, et al. (2011) PKCgamma in Vc and C1/C2 is involved in trigeminal neuropathic pain. J Dent Res 90: 777–781.
20. Xu M, Aita M, Chavkin C (2008) Partial infraorbital nerve ligation as a model of trigeminal nerve injury in the mouse: behavioral, neural, and glial reactions. J Pain 9: 1036–1048.
21. Fields RD, Eshete F, Stevens B, Itoh K (1997) Action potential-dependent regulation of gene expression: temporal specificity in ca2+, cAMP-responsive element binding proteins, and mitogen-activated protein kinase signaling. J Neurosci 17: 7252–7266.
22. Martin KC, Michael D, Rose JC, Barad M, Casadio A, et al. (1997) MAP kinase translocates into the nucleus of the presynaptic cell and is required for long-term facilitation in Aplysia. Neuron 18: 899–912.
23. Fields RD (1998) Effects of ion channel activity on development of dorsal root ganglion neurons. J Neurobiol 37: 158–170.
24. Impey S, Obrietan K, Storm DR (1999) Making new connections: role of ERK/MAP kinase signaling in neuronal plasticity. Neuron 23: 11–14.
25. Ji RR, Gereau RWt, Malcangio M, Strichartz GR (2009) MAP kinase and pain. Brain Res Rev 60: 135–148.
26. Dai Y, Iwata K, Fukuoka T, Kondo E, Tokunaga A, et al. (2002) Phosphorylation of extracellular signal-regulated kinase in primary afferent neurons by noxious stimuli and its involvement in peripheral sensitization. J Neurosci 22: 7737–7745.
27. Ji RR, Befort K, Brenner GJ, Woolf CJ (2002) ERK MAP kinase activation in superficial spinal cord neurons induces prodynorphin and NK-1 upregulation and contributes to persistent inflammatory pain hypersensitivity. J Neurosci 22: 478–485.
28. Shimizu K, Asano M, Kitagawa J, Ogiso B, Ren K, et al. (2006) Phosphorylation of Extracellular Signal-Regulated Kinase in medullary and upper cervical cord neurons following noxious tooth pulp stimulation. Brain Res 1072: 99–109.
29. Suzuki I, Kitagawa J, Noma N, Tsuboi Y, Kondo M, et al. (2008) Attenuation of naloxone-induced Vc pERK hyper-expression following capsaicin stimulation of the face in aged rat. Neurosci Lett 442: 39–43.
30. Honda K, Kitagawa J, Sessle BJ, Kondo M, Tsuboi Y, et al. (2008) Mechanisms involved in an increment of multimodal excitability of medullary and upper cervical dorsal horn neurons following cutaneous capsaicin treatment. Mol Pain 4: 59.
31. Noma N, Tsuboi Y, Kondo M, Matsumoto M, Sessle BJ, et al. (2008) Organization of pERK-immunoreactive cells in trigeminal spinal nucleus caudalis and upper cervical cord following capsaicin injection into oral and craniofacial regions in rats. J Comp Neurol 507: 1428–1440.
32. Saito K, Hitomi S, Suzuki I, Masuda Y, Kitagawa J, et al. (2008) Modulation of trigeminal spinal subnucleus caudalis neuronal activity following regeneration of transected inferior alveolar nerve in rats. J Neurophysiol 99: 2251–2263.

33. Shibuta K, Suzuki I, Shinoda M, Tsuboi Y, Honda K, et al. (2012) Organization of hyperactive microglial cells in trigeminal spinal subnucleus caudalis and upper cervical spinal cord associated with orofacial neuropathic pain. Brain Res 1451: 74–86.
34. Bennett GJ, Xie YK (1988) A peripheral mononeuropathy in rat that produces disorders of pain sensation like those seen in man. Pain 33: 87–107.
35. Xing H, Chen M, Ling J, Tan W, Gu JG (2007) TRPM8 mechanism of cold allodynia after chronic nerve injury. J Neurosci 27: 13680–13690.
36. Allchorne AJ, Broom DC, Woolf CJ (2005) Detection of cold pain, cold allodynia and cold hyperalgesia in freely behaving rats. Mol Pain 1: 36.
37. Palecek J, Dougherty PM, Kim SH, Paleckova V, Lekan H, et al. (1992) Responses of spinothalamic tract neurons to mechanical and thermal stimuli in an experimental model of peripheral neuropathy in primates. J Neurophysiol 68: 1951–1966.
38. Scholz J, Woolf CJ (2002) Can we conquer pain? Nat Neurosci 5 Suppl: 1062–1067.
39. Aita M, Byers MR, Chavkin C, Xu M (2010) Trigeminal injury causes kappa opioid-dependent allodynic, glial and immune cell responses in mice. Mol Pain 6: 8.
40. Lisney SJ, Devor M (1987) Afterdischarge and interactions among fibers in damaged peripheral nerve in the rat. Brain Res 415: 122–136.
41. Tal M, Eliav E (1996) Abnormal discharge originates at the site of nerve injury in experimental constriction neuropathy (CCI) in the rat. Pain 64: 511–518.
42. Kajander KC, Bennett GJ (1992) Onset of a painful peripheral neuropathy in rat: a partial and differential deafferentation and spontaneous discharge in A beta and A delta primary afferent neurons. J Neurophysiol 68: 734–744.
43. Shir Y, Seltzer Z (1990) A-fibers mediate mechanical hyperesthesia and allodynia and C-fibers mediate thermal hyperalgesia in a new model of causalgiform pain disorders in rats. Neurosci Lett 115: 62–67.
44. Molander C, Hongpaisan J, Grant G (1992) Changing pattern of c-FOS expression in spinal cord neurons after electrical stimulation of the chronically injured sciatic nerve in the rat. Neuroscience 50: 223–236.
45. Noguchi K, Kawai Y, Fukuoka T, Senba E, Miki K (1995) Substance P induced by peripheral nerve injury in primary afferent sensory neurons and its effect on dorsal column nucleus neurons. J Neurosci 15: 7633–7643.
46. Noguchi K, Dubner R, De Leon M, Senba E, Ruda MA (1994) Axotomy induces preprotachykinin gene expression in a subpopulation of dorsal root ganglion neurons. J Neurosci Res 37: 596–603.
47. Kobayashi K, Fukuoka T, Obata K, Yamanaka H, Dai Y, et al. (2005) Distinct expression of TRPM8, TRPA1, and TRPV1 mRNAs in rat primary afferent neurons with adelta/c-fibers and colocalization with trk receptors. J Comp Neurol 493: 596–606.
48. Palecek J, Paleckova V, Dougherty PM, Carlton SM, Willis WD (1992) Responses of spinothalamic tract cells to mechanical and thermal stimulation of skin in rats with experimental peripheral neuropathy. J Neurophysiol 67: 1562–1573.
49. Nakagawa K, Takeda M, Tsuboi Y, Kondo M, Kitagawa J, et al. (2010) Alteration of primary afferent activity following inferior alveolar nerve transection in rats. Mol Pain 6: 9.
50. Fukui T, Dai Y, Iwata K, Kamo H, Yamanaka H, et al. (2007) Frequency-dependent ERK phosphorylation in spinal neurons by electric stimulation of the sciatic nerve and the role in electrophysiological activity. Mol Pain 3: 18.
51. Liu XG, Sandkuhler J (1995) Long-term potentiation of C-fiber-evoked potentials in the rat spinal dorsal horn is prevented by spinal N-methyl-D-aspartic acid receptor blockage. Neurosci Lett 191: 43–46.
52. Liu X, Sandkuhler J (1997) Characterization of long-term potentiation of C-fiber-evoked potentials in spinal dorsal horn of adult rat: essential role of NK1 and NK2 receptors. J Neurophysiol 78: 1973–1982.
53. Sandkuhler J, Liu X (1998) Induction of long-term potentiation at spinal synapses by noxious stimulation or nerve injury. Eur J Neurosci 10: 2476–2480.
54. Svendsen F, Tjolsen A, Hole K (1998) AMPA and NMDA receptor-dependent spinal LTP after nociceptive tetanic stimulation. Neuroreport 9: 1185–1190.
55. Vikman KS, Siddall PJ, Duggan AW (2005) Increased responsiveness of rat dorsal horn neurons in vivo following prolonged intrathecal exposure to interferon-gamma. Neuroscience 135: 969–977.
56. Ji RR, Baba H, Brenner GJ, Woolf CJ (1999) Nociceptive-specific activation of ERK in spinal neurons contributes to pain hypersensitivity. Nat Neurosci 2: 1114–1119.
57. Song XS, Cao JL, Xu YB, He JH, Zhang LC, et al. (2005) Activation of ERK/CREB pathway in spinal cord contributes to chronic constrictive injury-induced neuropathic pain in rats. Acta Pharmacol Sin 26: 789–798.
58. Peng G, Han M, Du Y, Lin A, Yu L, et al. (2009) SIP30 is regulated by ERK in peripheral nerve injury-induced neuropathic pain. J Biol Chem 284: 30138–30147.
59. Ma W, Quirion R (2002) Partial sciatic nerve ligation induces increase in the phosphorylation of extracellular signal-regulated kinase (ERK) and c-Jun N-terminal kinase (JNK) in astrocytes in the lumbar spinal dorsal horn and the gracile nucleus. Pain 99: 175–184.
60. Zhuang ZY, Gerner P, Woolf CJ, Ji RR (2005) ERK is sequentially activated in neurons, microglia, and astrocytes by spinal nerve ligation and contributes to mechanical allodynia in this neuropathic pain model. Pain 114: 149–159.

4

Spinal Changes of a Newly Isolated Neuropeptide Endomorphin-2 Concomitant with Vincristine-Induced Allodynia

Yang Yang[1]ⁿ, Yong-Gang Zhang[2], Guo-An Lin[3], He-Qiu Xie[4], Hai-Tao Pan[5], Ben-Qing Huang[6], Ji-Dong Liu[1], Hui Liu[1], Nan Zhang[7], Li Li[1]*, Jian-Hua Chen[1]*

1 Department of Neurosurgery, The Zhumadian City Center Hospital, Zhumadian, P.R. China, **2** Department of ICU, The Zhumadian City Center Hospital, Zhumadian, P.R. China, **3** Department of Burn, The 159th Hospital of PLA, Zhumadian, P.R. China, **4** Department of Pain, The Zhumadian City Center Hospital, Zhumadian, P.R. China, **5** School of Statistics, Xi'an University of Finance and Economics, Xi'an, P.R. China, **6** Department of Oncology, The 159th Hospital of PLA, Zhumadian, P.R. China, **7** Department of student affairs, Xinxiang Medical University, Xinxiang, P.R. China

Abstract

Chemotherapy-induced neuropathic pain (CNP) is the major dose-limiting factor in cancer chemotherapy. However, the neural mechanisms underlying CNP remain unclear. There is increasing evidence implicating the involvement of spinal endomorphin-2 (EM2) in neuropathic pain. In this study, we used a vincristine-evoked rat CNP model displaying mechanical allodynia and central sensitization, and observed a significant decrease in the expression of spinal EM2 in CNP. Also, while intrathecal administration of exogenous EM2 attenuated allodynia and central sensitization, the mu-opioid receptor antagonist β-funaltrexamine facilitated these events. We found that the reduction in spinal EM2 was mediated by increased activity of dipeptidylpeptidase IV, possibly as a consequence of chemotherapy-induced oxidative stress. Taken together, our findings suggest that a decrease in spinal EM2 expression causes the loss of endogenous analgesia and leads to enhanced pain sensation in CNP.

Editor: Shao-Jun Tang, University of Texas Medical Branch, United States of America

Funding: This study was supported by the Natural Science Foundation of Zhumadian City (2013m5218) and the National Natural Science Foundation of China (Nos. 81172095, 81171135, 81200324). The funders had no role in study design, data collection and analysis, decision to publish, or preparation of the manuscript.

Competing Interests: The authors have declared that no competing interests exist.

* E-mail: LLiZhumadian@163.com (LL); JHChenZhumadian@163.com (JHC)

These authors contributed equally to this work.

Introduction

Chemotherapy-induced neuropathic pain (CNP) is a common, dose-limiting side effect of cancer treatment using chemotherapeutic drugs. CNP limits the maximum dose of drug that can be safely administered as well as the duration of treatment, and hence impairs the quality of life [1]. Unlike neuropathic pain induced by trauma and diabetes, CNP occurs in the absence of axonal degeneration in peripheral nerves, suggesting that the mechanisms underlying CNP are elusive and complex [2,3]. CNP is often resistant to standard analgesics. Hence, it is crucial to investigate the mechanisms causing CNP and subsequently devise effective treatment strategies [4].

Opioid receptors in the spinal cord play a critical role in modulating nociceptive transmission. Approximately 70% of opiate ligand-mediated signaling in the spinal cord occurs through the mu-opioid receptor (MOR); the most potent opiate drugs are known to act as ligands of MOR [5]. Endomorphin-1 (EM1) and endomorphin-2 (EM2) were newly isolated endogenous opioid peptides and identified as the endogenous ligands of MOR [6–8]. While EM1-like immunoreactivity (-LI) is primarily restricted to the brain, EM2-LI is found mainly in the spinal cord and suspected to modulate pain signaling at that level [9,10]. In rat models of neuropathic pain, administration of exogenous EM2 at the spinal level results in a much stronger analgesic effect than morphine [11–13]. Following partial ligation of the sciatic nerve, EM2-LI in the spinal dorsal horn ipsilateral to the nerve injury was shown to be greatly reduced, suggesting that the loss of endogenous inhibitory signals might be responsible for the subsequent chronic pain [14].

One study reported that paclitaxel- and vincristine-induced CNP seems relatively resistant to opioid therapy, and that large doses of morphine alone did not have a significant analgesic effect [15]. While studying the relationship between the spinal opioid system and CNP, two recent studies demonstrated the involvement of spinal opioid receptors in electroacupuncture or magnetic stimulation induced analgesia in CNP. They showed that administration of opioid receptor antagonists could successfully block electroacupuncture or magnetic stimulation mediated inhibition of allodynia and hyperalgesia in rat CNP models [16,17]. To further understand the pathophysiology of CNP, it is essential to determine whether the expression of endogenous inhibitory peptides such as EM1 and EM2 is modified in CNP. No studies thus far have investigated the relationship between spinal EM2 and CNP.

In this study, we examined the role of spinal EM2 in the pathophysiology of CNP. We used a rat model of CNP implanted with a mini-osmotic pump to continuously deliver vincristine sulfate, and analyzed changes in the expression of EM2 in the spinal cord during the development and progression of CNP. Further, we examined the threshold of pain tolerance following intrathecal administration of β-funaltrexamine (β-FNA) and exogenous EM2. In addition, to determine whether the reduction in spinal EM2 expression is a consequence of increased activity of dipeptidylpeptidase IV (DPP IV), we treated our CNP models systemically with diprotin A, an inhibitor of DPP IV. We also investigated the role of chemotherapy- induced oxidative stress in modulating the activity of DPP IV.

Materials and Methods

Animals

Adult male Sprague–Dawley rats, weighing 200 g, were used. Rats were housed under standard conditions. All procedures of our experiments were approved by the Committee of Animal Use for Research and Education of Zhumadian City Center Hospital (Zhumadian, Henan Province, P.R. China), and all efforts were made to minimize the number of animals used and their suffering [18]. (Permit Number: zmd-13-6688).

Mini-osmotic Pump Implantation

As described previously [19,20], rats were anesthetized with halothane (5% to induce, 2–3% to maintain), and their right external jugular vein was catheterized with a vincristine-filled miniosmotic pump (0.5 μl/h, 14 days; Alzet Model 2002, Durect Corporation, Cupertino, CA, USA) that had been primed overnight to deliver 30 mg/kg/day vincristine sulfate (Sigma-Aldrich, St Louis, MO, USA) (Vincristine group). Control rats were implanted with primed mini-osmotic pump containing 0.9% saline (Sham group).

Drugs

Endomorphin-2, Endomorphin-1, β-funaltrexamine (β-FNA, antagonist for mu-opioid receptor), phenyl N-tert-butylnitrone (PBN, scavenger for reactive oxygen species) and diprotin A (inhibitor of dipeptidylpeptidase IV) were purchased from Sigma-Aldrich.

Experimental Design

In the first series of experiments, rats were divided into Naive group, Sham group, Vincristine group. The baseline values of pain behavior were recorded before osmotic pump implantation. Then, from 1 day post osmotic pump implantation (1d) to 28 days post osmotic pump implantation (28d), pain behavioral tests were performed once a day in each group (n = 10/group). Body weight and motor function were detected once a week to monitor the toxicity of vincristine (n = 10/group).

In the second series of experiments, rats in these three groups were sacrificed on 3d, 5d, 7d, 10d, 14d and 21d, and the spinal cords and dorsal root ganglia were harvested and preserved (n = 5/d in Naive and Sham groups, n = 10/d in Vincristine group). The spinal cords were used for immunostaining of EM2, EM1 or MOR, Western blot analysis of MOR, the detection of spinal content of EM2 or EM1, spinal activity of dipeptidylpeptidase IV and spinal reactive oxygen species; the dorsal root ganglia were used for immunostaining of EM2 and the detection of the content of EM2.

In the third series of experiments, rats of Vincristine group were injected intraperitoneally with PBN (1.5 mg/kg/d) [21,22] from 1d to 7d. The spinal cords of rats were harvested for detection of activity of DPP IV after pain behavioral test on 3d, 5d, 7d, 10d, 14d and 21d (n = 10/d).

In the fourth series of experiments, rats of Vincristine group were injected intraperitoneally with diprotin A (3.5 mg/kg/d) [23,24] from 1d to 7d. The spinal cords of rats were harvested for detection of content of EM2 after pain behavioral test on 3d, 5d, 7d, 10d, 14d and 21d (n = 10/d).

In the fifth series of experiments, saline, EM2, EM1 or β-FNA was injected intrathecally in Vincristine group at 2 weeks post osmotic pump implantation (2w). After injection, pain behavior was immediately measured (n = 10).

In the sixth series of experiments, saline, EM2 or β-FNA was injected intrathecally in Vincristine group at 2w, and a total of 30 wide dynamic range (WDR) neurons were immediately recorded in each group (Sham group, Vincristine+Saline group, Vincristine+EM2 group and Vincristine+β-FNA group; n = 30/group).

Rotarod Test

In order to assess whether the dosage of vincristine used in the present experiment could impair motor function, which might influence the pain behavioral results, the motor function of Vincristine group was assessed by the rotarod test [25]. Rats were placed on the 7650 Rotarod accelerator treadmill (Ugo Basile, Varese, Italy) set at a constant speed of 25 RPM. As the animal took a grip of the drum, the accelerator mode was selected on the treadmill, the rotation rate of the drum was increased linearly. Thereafter, the time was measured from the start of the acceleration period until the rat fell off the drum. The cut-off time was 30 s.

EM Content Assay

EM2 or EM1 content was measured from spinal cord or dorsal root ganglion using a commercially available enzyme-linked immunosorbent assay kit (S12460001, Bachem, King of Prussia, PA, USA) [26]. The rats were euthanized and the L4-5 spinal cords or dorsal root ganglia were removed and immediately frozen in liquid nitrogen. Tissue samples were sonicated in 200 μl of lysis buffer, centrifuged at 17,000 *g* for 15 min, and the supernatant collected. In the assay, tissue EM2 or EM1 competed with exogenously added biotinylated EM2 or EM1 for a limited amount of immobilized antibody binding sites and the amount of biotinylated EM2 or EM1 was determined by colorimetric analysis. The amount of EM2 or EM1 present in the tissue samples was calculated from standard curve of known EM2 or EM1 concentration and was expressed in ng/mg protein. A portion of the tissue supernatant was used to measure total protein using a standard Bradford assay (BioRad, Hercules, CA, USA).

Spinal Reactive Oxygen Species (ROS) Assay

The rats were euthanized and the spinal cord was dissected and homogenized. The supernatants were collected for ROS assay. The production of ROS was measured by 2′,7′-Dichlorodihydrofluorescein (DCFH) oxidation as described previously [27]. DCFH reacts with ROS to form 2′,7′-dichlorofluorescein (DCF), the fluorescent product. The fluorescence was read at 485 nm excitation and 530 nm emission on a fluorescence plate reader. The results were calculated as percentage of Vincristine 14d group.

Measurement of Spinal Dipeptidylpeptidase IV (DPP IV) Activity

The rats were euthanized and the spinal cord was dissected and homogenized. The supernatants were collected for DPP IV activity assay. DPP IV activity of the spinal cord was measured by using the chromogenic substrate Gly-Pro-p-nitroanilide (Gly-

Pro-pNA; Sigma) as previously reported [24]. 100 μl of supernatant was incubated at 37°C with 1.5 mM Gly-Pro-pNA in 100 μl of phosphate-buffered saline containing 10 mg/ml bovine serum albumin. Absorbance was measured at 405 nm on a microplate reader at 3-min intervals for a total of 60 min, and the number of picomoles of pNA formed was calculated by comparison to a pNA standard curve. The results were plotted as picomoles of pNA versus time, giving a measure of DPP IV activity expressed as picomoles per minute. The peak pNA production rate was used for analysis between groups.

Intrathecal Catheter Insertion and Drug Administration

A polyethylene-10 catheter (Becton-Dickinson, Sparks, MD, USA) was intrathecally inserted according to a previous method [28]. The rats were allowed to recover for 1 day. Only the rats judged as neurologically normal were used for the subsequent drug administration. The dosage of each drug used in the present study was according to the previous reports. Treatment group received intrathecal injection of EM2 (0.3, 1, 3 μg) [13] or EM1 (3 μg) [13] or β-FNA (3, 10 μg) [29], while the same volume of normal saline was injected in control group. Each drug was dissolved in 10 μl of saline and injected intrathecally by the way of a single acute administration.

Pain Behavioral Test

For the pain behavioral tests, the same room in which the rats were routinely housed was used. The rats were placed under inverted plastic boxes ($30\times30\times50$ cm^3) on an elevated mesh floor and allowed to habituate for at least 15 min before the threshold testing. The observers of the behaviors were blinded to the treatment of the rats. To observe how different drug treatments affected the pain threshold, behavioral tests were performed 6 h before the drugs administration to provide baseline scores. After intrathecal drug injection, pain threshold was measured for every 10 min.

Von frey monofilaments. As previously described [30], a set of von Frey monofilaments (Stoelting, Chicago, IL, USA) was used to test the mechanical withdrawal threshold of the hindpaws. The monofilaments were applied with increasing force until the rat withdrew the paw. Lifting of the paw due to normal locomotory behavior was ignored. Each monofilament was applied five times. The threshold was taken as the lowest force that evoked a brisk withdrawal response to one of the five repetitive stimuli. The withdrawal thresholds were measured three or four times in order to obtain two consecutive values that differed not more than 10%.

Hargreaves' method. Thermal nociceptive threshold to radiant heat was quantified using the paw withdrawal test [31]. Briefly, rats were placed in a Perspex enclosure, without restraint and a movable infrared radiant heat source placed directly under the plantar surface of the hind paw (Ugo Basile, Italy). The paw withdrawal latency to radiant heat was defined as the time from onset of the radiant heat to the withdrawal of the rat hind paw. The average of three estimations was taken to yield a mean paw withdrawal latency.

Electrophysiological Testing

The rats were anesthetized and artificially ventilated. Core body temperature was monitored and maintained at 37.5±0.5°C. A laminectomy was performed from the T13 to L2 vertebrae to expose the lumbosacral enlargement of the spinal cord. Extracellular single unit recordings were made from L4-5 spinal dorsal horn with glass capillary microelectrodes (10–15 MΩ filled with 0.5 M sodium acetate). According to previous reports [32,33], the dorsal horn neurons were identified as WDR units on the basis of their characteristic responses: (1) having a receptive field consisting of a small low threshold center and a large high threshold surround ipsilateral to the recording site; (2) responding with an increasing firing rate to brush, pressure and noxious pinch applied to the low threshold center; (3) showing no apparent accommodation when continuous noxious stimulation was applied. After successful identification of a single WDR unit, the unit responsiveness to 10 s mechanical stimuli was recorded. The spike trains were monitored with a memory oscilloscope and the numbers of neuronal firing were simultaneously recorded and saved on a computer via an A/D converter following spike discriminator and counter.

Immunohistochemical Staining

Tissue preparation. Rats were anesthetized and perfused transcardially with paraformaldehyde. The L4-5 spinal cords and dorsal root ganglia were removed and transferred into 30% sucrose in 0.1 M phosphate buffer (PB, pH 7.4) for cryoprotection. The spinal cords were cut into 30 μm thick sections and collected in 0.01 M phosphate-buffered saline (PBS, pH 7.4). The dorsal root ganglia were cut into longitudinal sections measuring 10 μm thick and mounted onto gelatin-coated glass slides.

Immunofluorescence. After washed in PBS, the spinal cord sections were incubated at room temperature with rabbit antiserum against EM2 (AB5104, 1:200; Chemicon, Temecula, CA, USA), rabbit antiserum against EM1 (AB5102, 1:200; Chemicon) or guinea pig antiserum against MOR (AB1774, 1:3000; Chemicon) in 0.01 M PBS containing 5% (v/v) normal donkey serum (NDS), 0.3% (v/v) Triton X-100, 0.05% (w/v) NaN3 and 0.25% (w/v) carrageenan (PBS-NDS, pH 7.4) for 24 h, followed by biotinylated goat anti-rabbit IgG (BA-1000, 1:200; Vector Laboratories, Burlingame, CA, USA) or biotinylated goat anti-guinea pig IgG (BA-7000, 1:200; Vector) diluted with PBS-NDS for another 4 h, and then with avidin-biotin-peroxidase complex Elite Kit (1:100 dilution; Vector) in PBS for 1 h. Finally, the sections were reacted with 0.05 M Tris–HCl buffer (pH 7.6) containing 0.04% diaminobenzidine tetrahydrochloride (Dojin, Kumamoto, Japan) and 0.0003% H_2O_2 for visualizing EM2-LI, EM1-LI or MOR-LI. After staining, all the sections were observed with a bright-field microscope (Olympus AH2 VANOX, Tokyo, Japan). The dorsal root ganglion sections were incubated sequentially with: (1) rabbit antiserum against EM2 (1:200) in PBS-NDS for 48 h at 4°C; (2) Cy3-labeled donkey anti-rabbit IgG (AP184F, 1:200; Chemicon) in PBS-NDS for 12 h at 4°C. After staining, all the sections were observed with Olympus FV1000 confocal laser scanning microscope.

Western Blot Analysis

Rats were anesthetized and the lumbar segments of spinal cord innervated by the L4-5 dorsal roots were rapidly removed. The collected tissue was mechanically homogenized and centrifuged. The supernatant was collected and stored at −80°C. Protein concentrations of the supernatant were determined using the BCA Protein Assay Kit (Pierce, Rockford, IL, USA). Proteins of interest were separated by SDS-PAGE electrophoresis (20 μg of total protein per well), and transferred onto nitrocellulose membranes. The membranes were placed in a blocking solution (Tris-buffered saline with 0.02% Tween and 5% non-fat dry milk powder) for 1 h, and incubated overnight with guinea pig antiserum against MOR (AB1774, 1:1000; Chemicon). After washing, the membranes were incubated in peroxidase-conjugated secondary antibody (1:1000; Santa Cruz Biotechnology, Santa Cruz, CA, USA) for 1 h, and then the membranes were detected by the enhanced chemiluminescence detection method (Amersham

Pharmacia Biotech Inc., Piscataway, NJ, USA). The densities of protein blots were analyzed by using Labworks Software (Ultra-Violet Products Ltd., Cambridge, UK) and normalized to β-actin levels.

Data Analysis

All data were collected by experimenters blinded to the surgery and reagents treatments and statistical analyses were done by using SPSS software (version 12). Data were expressed as mean ±standard error mean (mean±SEM). Statistical analysis of the data was carried out with a one-way analysis of variance (ANOVA) followed by Bonferroni post hoc analysis. A Pearson correlation was used to determine the correlation between the content of EM2 and pain behavioral performance. Comparisons between two means were performed by a Student's T-test. Significance level was set at $P<0.05$.

Results

Mechanical Allodynia Occurred in Vincristine Treated Rats

No difference in body weight was observed between Sham group (341±25.1 g; 4w) and Vincristine group (351±17.1 g; 4w), and the body weight of these two groups was persistently elevated through the period tested (Fig. 1A). Also, no difference in motor function was observed between Sham group (21.4±3.7 s; 4w) and Vincristine group (22±2.2 s; 4w), and these values were maintained at normal levels at all time points tested (Fig. 1B). These data indicated that vincristine treatment exerted no significant toxicity.

Compared to Sham group (25.9±1.6 g; 5d), the paw withdrawal threshold of Vincristine group was significantly decreased at 5d (14.9±2.1 g), reached the lowest value at 14d (5.3±1.4 g), and thereafter was at persistent low level (n = 10/group; $P<0.05$) (Fig. 1C). In contrast with the severe mechanical allodynia, no significant changes in thermal withdrawal thresholds were observed between Sham group (13.5±1.2 s; 4w) and Vincristine group (13.2±1.4 s; 4w) (Fig. 1D). These data indicated that vincristine treatment induced mechanical allodynia.

Spinal EM2 was Significantly Decreased after Chemotherapy

Immunohistochemistry indicated that compared to Naive group and Sham group, EM2-LI was significantly decreased in the spinal dorsal horn of Vincristine group (Fig. 2A). Using ELISA, we detected that compared to Naive group (80±5.1 ng/mg protein; 5d) and Sham group (83±4.2 ng/mg protein; 5d), spinal EM2 content was significantly decreased in Vincristine group at 5d (53±7.6 ng/mg protein). EM2 downregulation peaked at 2w (24±3.8 ng/mg protein) and thereafter persisted at low level (n = 10/group; $P<0.05$) (Fig. 2B). Thus, the time course change of spinal EM2 content was similar to that of mechanical allodynia. Furthermore, the content of EM2 was found to be significantly correlated to the paw withdrawal threshold in Vincristine group ($P<0.001$, $r = 0.939$) (Fig. 2C).

With regard to MOR expression in spinal cord, immunostaining (Fig. 2D) and Western blot (Fig. 2E) showed that there was no difference among Naive group, Sham group and Vincristine group at any time points tested. In all the rats, MOR expression was unchanged through the period tested.

Immunohistochemistry indicated that compared to Sham group, EM2-immunopositive neurons was significantly decreased in the dorsal root ganglion of Vincristine group (Fig. 3A). Using ELISA, we detected that compared to Naive group (39±7.1 ng/mg protein; 14d) and Sham group (41±5.9 ng/mg protein; 14d), the EM2 content of dorsal root ganglion was significantly decreased in Vincristine group (13±3.6 ng/mg protein; 14d) (Fig. 3B).

Immunohistochemistry indicated that there was no detectable EM1-immunopositive structures in spinal cord in the three groups (Fig. 3C). Using ELISA, we detected that the spinal cords of the three groups contained almost no EM1 (Fig. 3D). Furthermore, pain behavior test showed that EM2 exerted more effective antinociception compared with corresponding dose of EM1 (Fig. 3E).

Decreased Spinal EM2 Contributed to Allodynia and Central Sensitization

We injected EM2 or β-FNA intrathecally and observed their effects on mechanical allodynia in Vincristine group (2w). While the exogenous EM2 dose-dependently attenuated the allodynia (Fig. 4A), the mu-opioid receptor antagonist β-FNA facilitated the mechanical allodynia (Fig. 4B).

The responsiveness of WDR neurons was gradually increased with the increase in mechanical intensity (brush, pressure and pinch) (Fig. 5A–D). The stimulus-response functional curves for mechanical sensitivity of the spinal dorsal horn WDR neurons are shown in each group (Fig. 5E). Compared to Sham group, the responsiveness of WDR neurons was significantly enhanced with a distinct leftward shift of the stimulus-response functional curve in Vincristine group (2w), which indicated that spinal central sensitization occurred in Vincristine group rats (Fig. 5E). We injected EM2 or β-FNA intrathecally and observed their effects on increased responsiveness of WDR neurons in Vincristine group (2w). The increased responsiveness was significantly attenuated by EM2, whereas it was significantly facilitated by β-FNA (Fig. 5E).

Spinal Decreased EM2 was Induced by Increased Activity of DPP IV, and Chemotherapy-induced Oxidative Stress might be the Causative Factor for Increased Activity of DPP IV

Compared to Naive group (150±20.2 pmol/min) and Sham group (145±19.3 pmol/min), the activity of DPP IV was significantly increased in Vincristine group (373±50.2 pmol/min) at 7d ($P<0.05$). The activity of DPP IV peaked at 2W (680±60.4 pmol/min) and persisted thereafter, which correlated with the changing course of spinal EM2 content (Fig. 6A). On the other hand, some Vincristine group rats were treated with diprotin A (inhibitor of dipeptidylpeptidase IV), which produced a significant inhibition of the decrement of spinal EM2 (Fig. 6B). These data indicated that increased activity of DPP IV contributed to decreased spinal EM2 after chemotherapy.

We observed that spinal reactive oxygen species was significantly increased in Vincristine group (Fig. 6C), and a systemic treatment with PBN (reactive oxygen species scavenger) significantly reduced the increased activity of DPP IV (Fig. 6D), which indicated that Vincristine-induced oxidative stress may mediate the development of increased activity of DPP IV in Vincristine group.

In addition, the treatment with PBN and diprotin A prevented the occurrence of mechanical allodynia in Vincristine group rats (Fig. 6E and F). On the other hand, neither PBN nor diprotin A treatment affected the motor performance of Vincristine group rats, the motor function of all the rats maintained at normal level from 1d to 28d (data not shown).

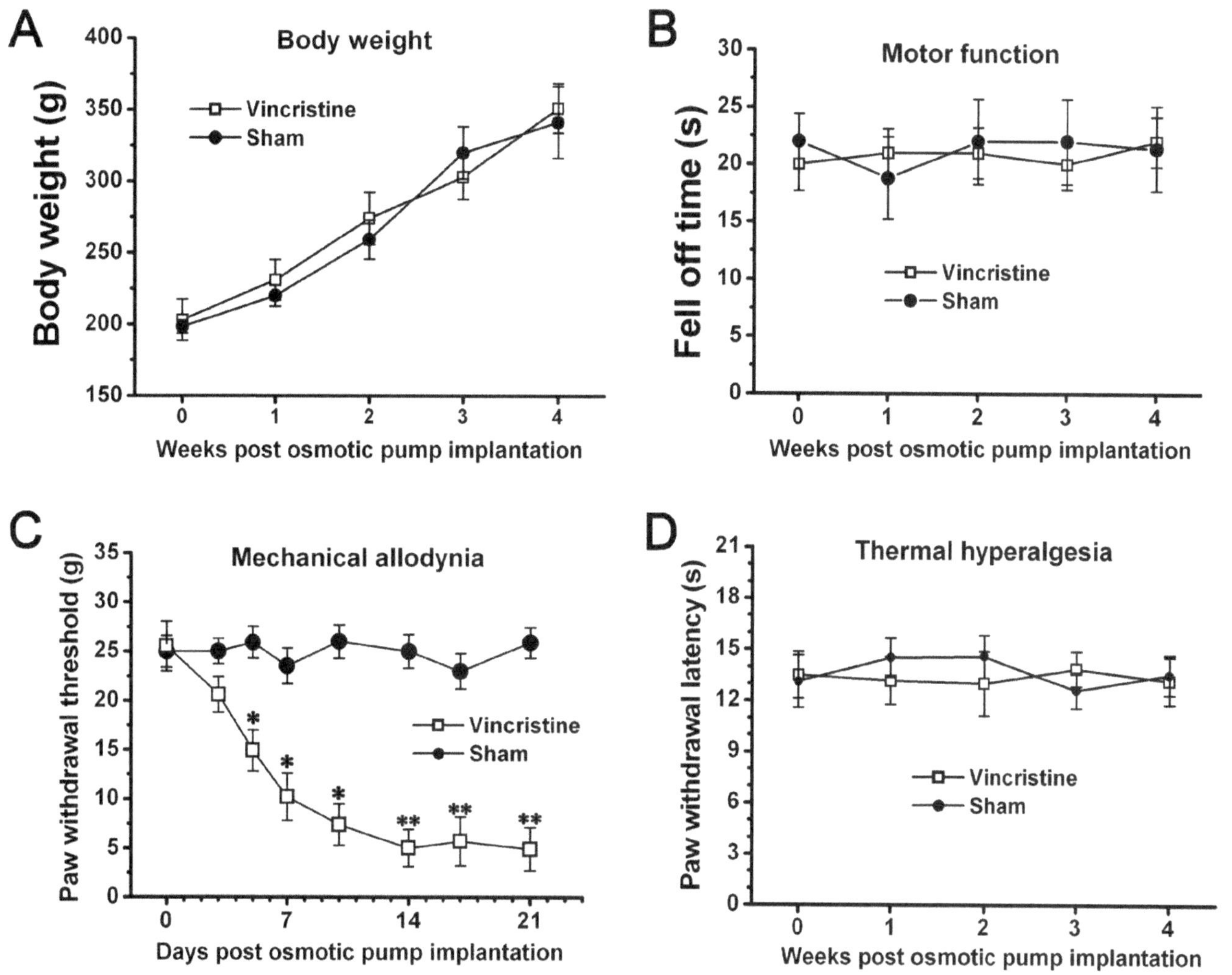

Figure 1. Mechanical allodynia occurred in vincristine treated rats. With regard to (A) body weight and (B) motor function, there was no difference between Vincristine group and Sham group. (C) Compared to Sham group, the paw withdrawal threshold of Vincristine group was significantly decreased. (D) No significant changes in thermal withdrawal thresholds were observed between Vincristine group and Sham group. All data were calculated as mean ± SEM (n = 10/group). *P<0.05, **P<0.01 vs. Sham group in C.

Discussion

The mechanisms underlying CNP are unclear and need to be investigated further [28]. To our knowledge, there are no analgesic drugs that could be labeled both safe and effective in treating CNP [20,34–38]. To identify such therapeutic strategies, it is necessary and crucial to elucidate the molecular mechanisms resulting in CNP following chemotherapy. This study is the first to provide conclusive evidence that decreased levels of EM2 in the spinal cord contribute to allodynia and central sensitization in CNP. We also show that this decrease is likely due to increased activity of dipeptidylpeptidase IV (DPP IV), caused by chemotherapy-induced oxidative stress.

Technical Considerations

In this study, we modeled CNP in rats by implanting a mini-osmotic pump to provide continuous infusion of vincristine for 2 weeks, such that its concentration in blood is maintained at a consistent level [19,20]. Compared to other previously established methods such as consecutive intraperitoneal injections, our method has several advantages: the procedure needs to be performed only once, is quick, ensures reliable intravenous drug delivery, and animals show good tolerance [19].

Although endogenously expressed endomorphins have been isolated from tissue, the identity of the gene encoding the precursor protein from which the endomorphin peptides are derived has not been identified. Due to the small molecular weight of EMs (<1 kDa), PCR and Western blotting methods could not be used to perform quantitative analyses. However, researchers have successfully used ELISA to precisely determine the content of spinal EM2 [26].

Decreased Spinal EM2 Expression after Chemotherapy Contributes to Allodynia in CNP Rat

CNP is characterized by allodynia, hyperalgesia and spontaneous pain, features that are also found in other forms of neuropathic pain. Although it is still unclear how chemotherapeutics interact with the nervous system to induce changes in pain sensation and behavior, the neural mechanisms underlying CNP may be similar to other forms of neuropathic pain [4]. Like neuropathic pain (and inflammatory pain) induced by trauma and diabetes, hypersensi-

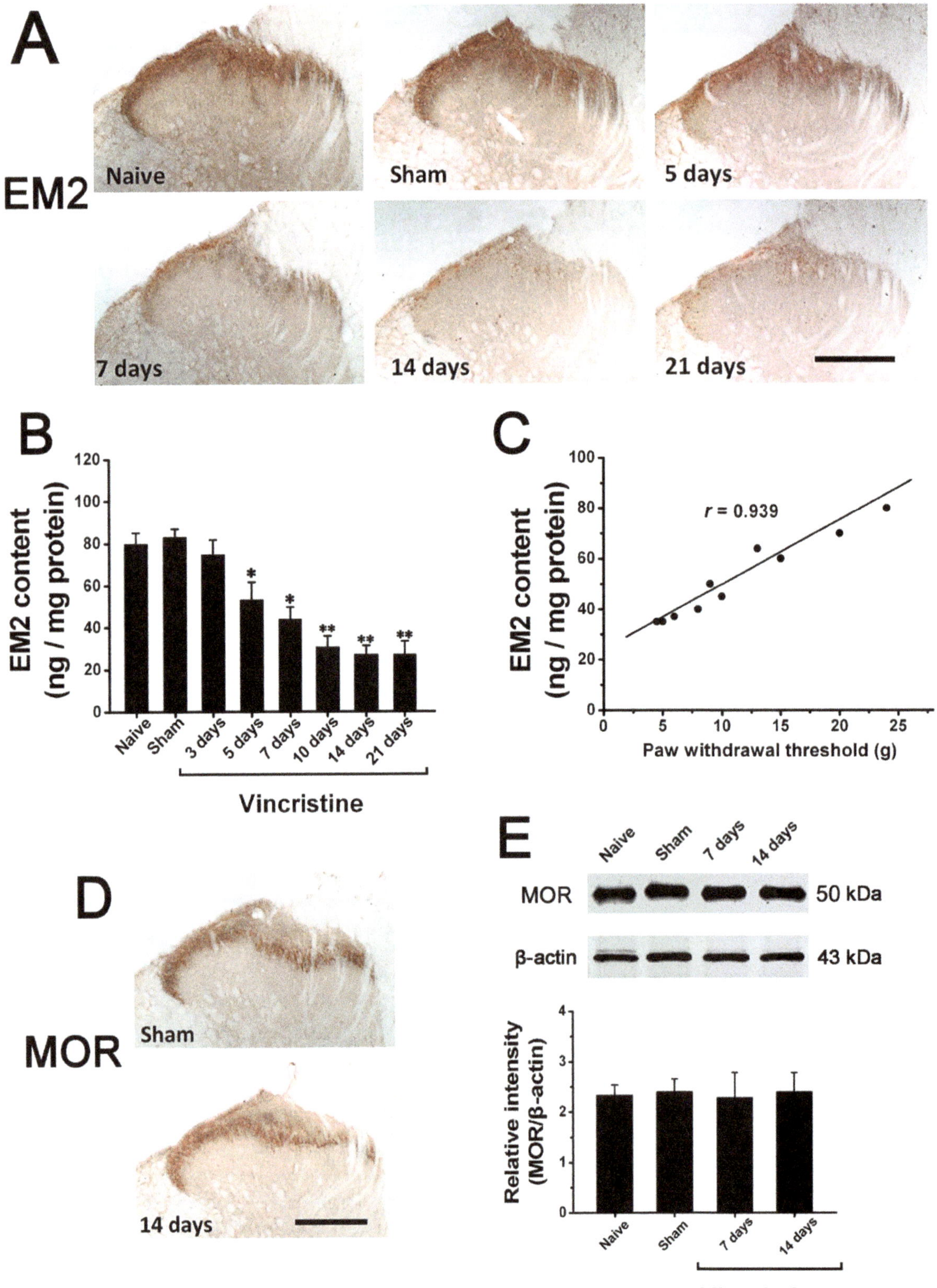

Figure 2. Spinal EM2 was significantly decreased in vincristine treated rats. (A) Compared to Sham group, EM2-like immunoreactivity in spinal dorsal horn of Vincristine group was significantly decreased. Bar = 200 μm. (B) Compared to Naive group and Sham group, ELISA showed that spinal EM2 content was significantly decreased in Vincristine group. (C) The content level of EM2 was found to be significantly correlated to the paw withdrawal threshold in Vincristine group ($P<0.001$, $r=0.939$). (C) With regard to MOR-like immunoreactivity in spinal dorsal horn, there was no difference between Sham group and Vincristine group. Bar = 200 μm. (D) With regard to MOR expression in spinal cord, Western blot analysis showed that there was no difference between Sham group and Vincristine group. In vincristine treated rats, MOR expression was unchanged through the

period tested. All data were calculated as mean ± SEM (n = 10/group). *P<0.05, **P<0.01 vs. Naive group and Sham group in (B). EM2: endomorphin2; MOR: mu-opioid receptor.

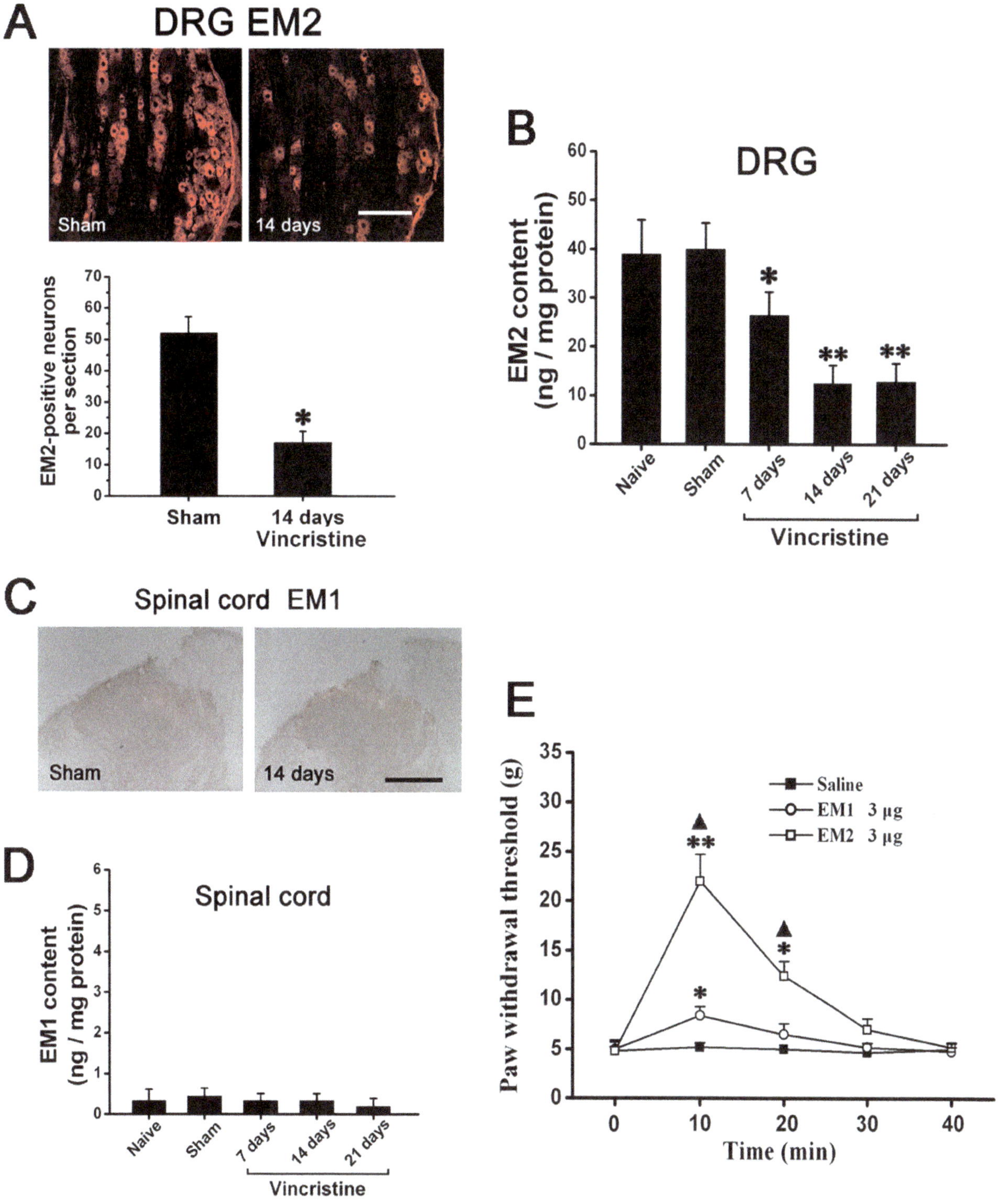

Figure 3. EM2 in dorsal root ganglion was significantly decreased, and there was almost no spinal EM1 in vincristine treated rats. (A) The number of EM2-immunopositive dorsal root ganglion neurons in Vincristine group was significantly decreased compared to Sham group. Bar = 100 μm. (B) Compared to Naive group and Sham group, ELISA showed that the EM2 content of dorsal root ganglion was significantly decreased in Vincristine group. (C) There was almost no EM1-immunopositive structures in spinal cord in Sham group and Vincristine group. (D) ELISA showed that the spinal cords of all the rats contained almost no EM1. (E) EM2 showed more effective antinociception than EM1. *P<0.05, **P<0.01 vs. Naive group and Sham group in (A) and (B). *P<0.05, **P<0.01 vs. Saline group; ▲ P<0.05 vs. EM1 group in (E).

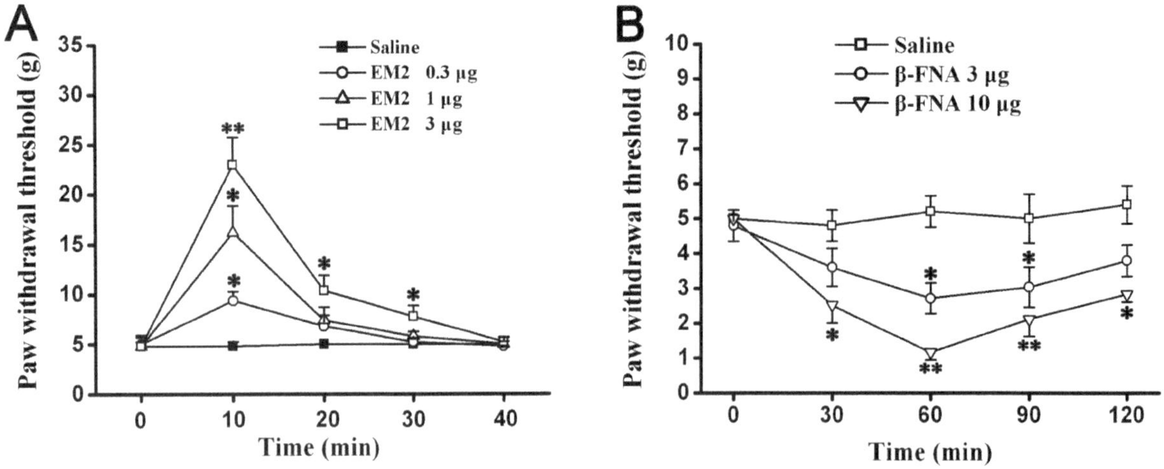

Figure 4. Decreased spinal EM2 contributed to mechanical allodynia in vincristine treated rats. (A) In Vincristine group, intrathecal injection of EM2 significantly attenuated the allodynia in a dose-dependent manner. (B) In Vincristine group, intrathecal administration of the mu-opioid receptor antagonist β-FNA made the mechanical allodynia more serious. *$P<0.05$, **$P<0.01$ vs. Saline group.

tivity of C-fiber nociceptors following treatment with the antitumor agent vincristine, has been noted in some neurophysiological studies [39]. Also reported is central sensitization of the wide dynamic range neurons of the spinal cord in response to vincristine treatment [40]. Studies investigating the mechanisms causing CNP have hypothesized that the fundamental pathology of CNP is a toxic effect on axonal mitochondria. The subsequent impairment in mitochondrial function may lead to membrane depolarization

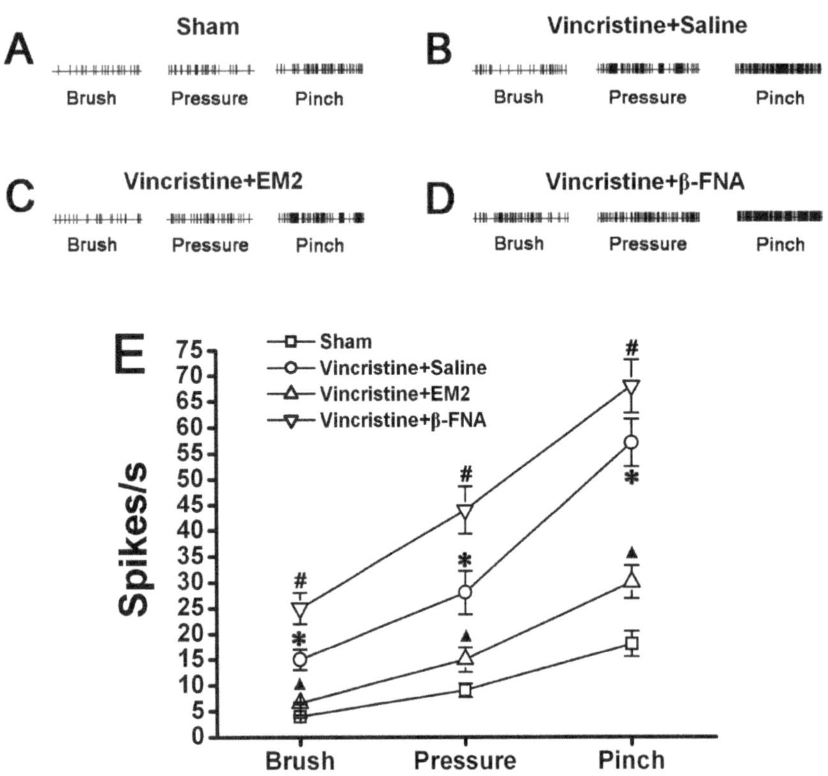

Figure 5. Decreased spinal EM2 contributed to spinal central sensitization in vincristine treated rats. Comparative recordings of responsiveness of spinal dorsal horn wide dynamic range (WDR) neurons to mechanical (brush, pressure and pinch) stimuli in Sham group (A), Vincristine +Saline group (B), Vincristine+EM2 group (C) and Vincristine+β-FNA group (D). (A–D) The responsiveness of WDR neurons was gradedly increased with the increase in mechanical intensity (brush, pressure and pinch). (E) Compared to Sham rats, the responsiveness of WDR neurons was significantly enhanced with a distinct leftward shift of the stimulus-response functional curve in vincristine treated rats. While the exogenous EM2 significantly attenuated the increased responsiveness, the mu-opioid receptor β-FNA aggratated the increased responsiveness. *$P<0.05$ vs. Sham group; ▲ or # $P<0.05$ vs. Vincristine+Saline group.

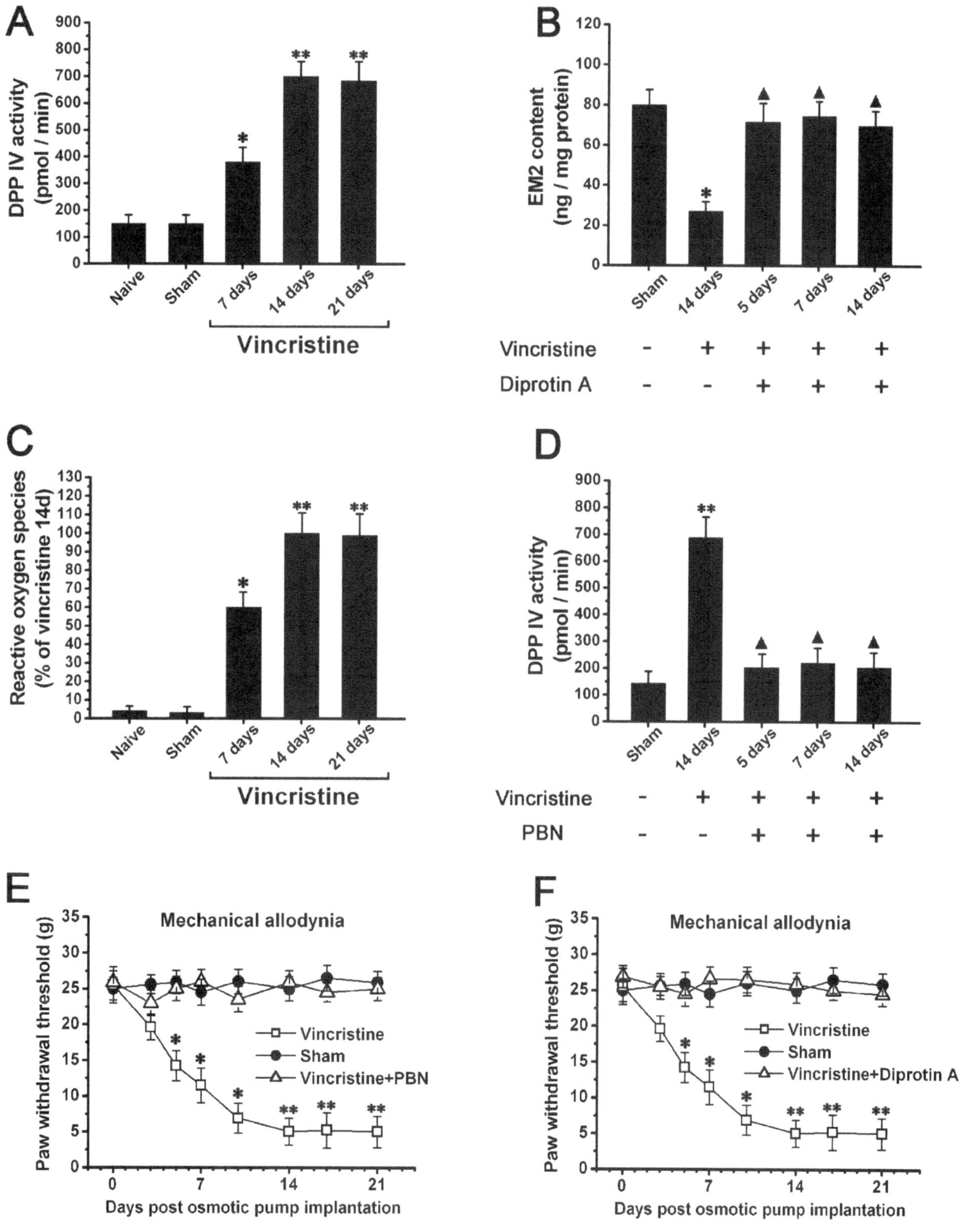

Figure 6. Spinal decreased EM2 was induced by oxidative stress mediated increased activity of dipeptidylpeptidase IV (DPP IV). (A) Compared to Naive group and Sham group, the activity of spinal DPP IV was significantly increased in Vincristine group. (B) A systemic treatment with diprotin A (inhibitor of DPP IV) blocked the decrement of spinal EM2 in Vincristine group. (C) Compared to Naive group and Sham group, the spinal reactive oxygen species was significantly increased in Vincristine group. (D) A systemic treatment with PBN (a scavenger for reactive oxygen species) significantly attenuated the increased activity of DPP IV in Vincristine group. (E) The treatment with PBN prevented the forming of mechanical allodynia in Vincristine group. (F) The treatment with diprotin A prevented the forming of mechanical allodynia in Vincristine group rats. *$P<0.05$, **$P<0.01$ vs. Naive group and Sham group; ▲ $P<0.05$ vs. Vincristine group at 14 days.

and action potentials [41]. More research is needed to corroborate this hypothesis and further dissect the pathways contributing to CNP.

It has been shown that after partial ligation of the sciatic nerve, EM2-LI is significantly decreased in the spinal dorsal horn ipsilateral to the nerve injury based on immunohistochemical analysis. Smith et al first reported the decrease in endogenous EM2 levels in chronic pain [14]. We made similar findings in this study, and showed, using immunohistochemistry and ELISA, a significant reduction in EM2 in the spinal dorsal horn and dorsal root ganglion in a rat CNP rat model. Since measurement of the concentration of neuropeptides by immunohistochemistry is only semiquantitative, we used ELISA to determine more accurately the change in spinal EM2 levels.

Changes in the opioidergic systems have been studied in other neuropathic pain models. Several reports have shown an upregulation of dynorphin using immunocytochemistry [42], radioimmunoassay [43] and mRNA [44] measurements after nerve injury. Although the predominant cellular effect of opioids is inhibition of neuronal excitability, dynorphin has been shown to enhance dorsal horn neuronal hyperexcitability in nerve injury models of chronic pain [43]. Administration of dynorphin can induce allodynia that in turn can be attenuated by endomorphins [45]. Metenkephalin, another naturally occurring opioid peptide, has been shown not to change significantly after nerve injury [44,46]. Our results provide the first evidence that reduction in the levels of an endogenous opioid in primary afferents is significantly associated with CNP. This indicates that the chronic pain associated with CNP might be due to the loss of an inhibitory effect on pain signal transmission.

Examination of several pain models revealed significant alterations in the expression of MOR in the spinal dorsal horn and dorsal root ganglion. For example, MOR expression is decreased in the spinal dorsal horn and the inhibitory effect of MOR agonists is reduced in neuropathic pain and bone cancer pain [47,48]. Peripheral inflammation increases MOR expression in the dorsal horn and dorsal root ganglion [49,50], with an increase in the inhibitory effect of MOR agonists [51]. Interestingly, this study found that MOR expression in the spinal cord remains unchanged after vincristine treatment. It therefore seems that the reduction in spinal EM2 level does not induce a compensatory increase in MOR expression, suggesting that spinal MOR may not be involved in the initiation and maintenance of chronic pain in CNP rats.

Although Smith et al provided the first evidence of a decrease in endogenous EM2 levels in the spinal cord following partial ligation of the sciatic nerve, they did not perform behavioral tests to assess pain and to evaluate the effect of intrathecal administration of exogenous EM2 or the mu-opioid receptor antagonist β-FNA [14]. Therefore, the causal relationship between decreased spinal EM2 and pain behavior could not be established. In this study, we demonstrated that the mechanical allodynia in CNP rats is attenuated by intrathecal administration of EM2, while administration of β-FNA further decreased the von Frey threshold for mechanical sensitivity. These behavioral results further elucidated the contribution of decreased spinal EM2 levels to decreased endogenous inhibitory influence on pain transmission. The loss of endogenous pain inhibition may be one of the most important mechanisms underlying the chronic pain associated with CNP.

EM1 and EM2 are structurally different by only one amino acid residue; hence, some comparative studies were performed to reveal the functional difference between EM1 and EM2. EM1-immunopositive structures are predominantly located in the brain while EM2-immunopositive structures are mainly found in the lower brainstem and spinal cord. While EM2-immunopositive structures exist at high density in the spinal dorsal horn, almost no EM1-immunopositive structures could be detected at the spinal level [52,53]. Similar to previous reports, our immunohistochemistry and ELISA assays showed there is almost no expression of EM1 in the spinal cord of both control and vincristine-treated rats. Although there is enough evidence indicating both EM1 and EM2 play pivotal roles in inhibiting nociceptive transmission at the spinal cord level, it has also been shown that EM2 is a more potent analgesic in the spinal cord than EM1 when administered intrathecally [54,55]. Similarly, our pain behavior test showed that EM2 has a more effective antinociceptive function than similar doses of EM1. An electrophysiological study suggested that the difference in behaviorally examined antinociceptive functions of EM1 and EM2 may be due to differences in their enzymatic degradation [56].

The Decrease in Spinal EM2 Levels Contribute to Central Sensitization of Spinal Neurons in CNP Rats

Emerging reports have suggested that EM2 expression in the spinal dorsal horn might functionally affect nociception by binding to pre-synaptically localized mu-opioid receptors causing inhibition of neurotransmitter release, and by binding to post-synaptic mu-opioid receptors causing hyperpolarization of spinal dorsal horn neurons [9,10]. Therefore, a reduction in EM2 in the spinal cord could lead to a loss of inhibition and may contribute to central sensitization. Spinal dorsal horn wide dynamic range (WDR) neurons are more plastic following tissue injury and are believed to be responsible for the spinally-organized central sensitization [57]. In this study, we found that WDR neurons show significantly increased responsiveness to stimuli during CNP. This suggests that spinal central sensitization does occur in CNP rats. Our findings corroborate previous reports of central sensitization following vincristine treatment [40]. Most importantly, intrathecal administration of exogenous EM2 significantly attenuated the central sensitization, and administration of β-FNA exerted opposite effects. Our findings demonstrate that the decrease in spinal EM2 plays an important role in causing the excessively increased activity of dorsal horn neurons.

Decreased Spinal EM2 Expression is Caused by Increased Activity of DPP IV

DPP IV is a membrane-bound serine proteinase that removes dipeptides from the amino terminus of peptides containing proline as the penultimate amino acid [58]. Endomorphins satisfy this substrate requirement, and were shown to be excellent substrates for DPP IV, which can liberate the N-terminal Tyr-Pro with high activity [59]. The use of DPP IV inhibitor enhanced and prolonged EM2-induced analgesia, and established the function of this enzyme in endomorphin degradation [60]. In the current study, we detected a significant increase in the activity of spinal DPP IV following vincristine treatment. We therefore hypothesize that the decrease in spinal EM2 levels is caused by chemotherapy-induced increase in the activity of DPP IV. We confirmed this by demonstrating that systemic treatment with diprotin A (an inhibitor of DPP IV) can block the downregulation of spinal EM2.

Chemotherapy-induced Oxidative Stress Might Cause Increased DPP IV Activity

Primary afferent sensory terminals and spinal dorsal horn are regions of high metabolic demand. The terminals of sensory afferents contain an unusually high concentration of mitochondria [61,62]. It has been shown that chemotherapy-evoked neuropathy is caused by a toxic effect on axonal mitochondria [41]. Impaired mitochondrial function in turn produces an excessive amount of reactive oxygen species (ROS), which induces significant oxidative stress [63]. In this study, we examined the level of reactive oxygen species in the spinal cord of CNP rats, and found them to be significantly increased following vincristine treatment.

Oxidative stress has been shown to influence the activity of DPP IV [24]. Based on our observations, we hypothesized that chemotherapy-induced oxidative stress may be a key mechanism causing increased activity of DPP IV. We confirmed this by treating CNP rats with PBN (a scavenger of reactive oxygen species) and showing a significant reduction in the increased activity of DPP IV. Hence, oxidative stress seems to induce the increase in DPP IV activity in vincristine treated rats.

In summary, our study of a rat CNP model provides the first evidence that spinal EM2 levels, but not MOR, are significantly decreased in CNP. We have shown that the allodynia and central sensitization associated with CNP is induced by a loss of endogenous inhibitory influence on pain transmission. Finally, our data suggest that chemotherapy-induced oxidative stress induces an increase in the activity of DPP IV, which in turn contributes to the reduction in spinal EM2 expression.

Acknowledgments

We are grateful to Prof. Uel Jack McMahan from Stanford University, USA for his critical reading and suggestions on the manuscript.

Author Contributions

Conceived and designed the experiments: YY LL JHC. Performed the experiments: YY YGZ GAL HQX HTP. Analyzed the data: YY HTP. Contributed reagents/materials/analysis tools: BQH JDL HL NZ. Wrote the paper: LL JHC.

References

1. Kautio AL, Haanpää M, Kautiainen H, Kalso E, Saarto T (2011) Burden of chemotherapy-induced neuropathy–a cross-sectional study. Support Care Cancer 19: 1991–1996.
2. Topp KS, Tanner KD, Levine JD (2000) Damage to the cytoskeleton of large diameter sensory neurons and myelinated axons in vincristine induced painful peripheral neuropathy in the rat. J Comp Neurol 424: 563–576.
3. Polomano RC, Mannes AJ, Clark US, Bennett GJ (2001) A painful peripheral neuropathy in the rat produced by the chemotherapeutic drug, paclitaxel. Pain 94: 293–304.
4. Farquhar-Smith P (2011) Chemotherapy-induced neuropathic pain. Curr Opin Support Palliat Care 5: 1–7.
5. Besse D, Lombard MC, Zajac JM, Roques BP, Besson JM (1990) Pre- and postsynaptic location of mu, delta and kappa opioid receptors in the superficial layers of the dorsal horn of the rat spinal cord. Prog Clin Biol Res 328: 183.
6. Zadina JE, Hackler L, Ge LJ, Kastin AJ (1997) A potent and selective endogenous agonist for the μ-opiate receptor. Nature 386: 499–502.
7. Zadina JE, Martin-Schild S, Gwerall AA, Kastin AJ, Hackler L, et al. (1999) Endomorphins: novel endogenous μ-opiate receptor agonist in regions of high μ-opiate receptor density. Ann N Y Acad Sci 897: 136–144.
8. Zadina JE (2002) Isolation and distribution of endomorphins in the central nervous system. Jpn J Pharmacol 89: 203–208.
9. Aicher SA, Mitchell JL, Swanson KC, Zadina JE (2003) Endomorphin-2 axon terminals contact mu-opioid receptor-containing dendrites in trigeminal dorsal horn. Brain Res 977: 190–198.
10. Sanderson Nydahl K, Skinner K, Julius D, Basbaum AI (2004) Colocalization of endomorphin-2 and substance P in primary afferent nociceptors and effects of injury: a light and electron microscopic study in the rat. Eur J Neurosci 19: 1789–1799.
11. Przewlocka B, Mika J, Labuz D, Toth G, Przewlocki R (1999) Spinal analgesic action of endomorphins in acute, inflammatory and neuropathic pain in rats. Eur J Pharmacol 367: 189–196.
12. Przewlocki R, Labuz D, Mika J, Przewlocka B, Tomboly C, et al. (1999) Pain inhibition by endomorphins. Ann NY Acad Sci 897: 154–164.
13. Grass S, Wiesenfeld-Hallin Z, Xu XJ (2000) The effect of intrathecal endomorphin-2 on the flexor reflex in normal, inflamed and axotomized rats: reduced effect in rats with autotomy. Neuroscience 98: 339–344.
14. Smith RR, Martin-Schild S, Kastin AJ, Zadina JE (2001) Decreases in endomorphin-2-like immunoreactivity concomitant with chronic pain after nerve injury. Neuroscience 105: 773–778.
15. Flatters SJ, Bennett GJ (2004) Ethosuximide reverses paclitaxel- and vincristine-induced painful peripheral neuropathy. Pain 109: 150–161.
16. Meng X, Zhang Y, Li A, Xin J, Lao L, et al. (2011) The effects of opioid receptor antagonists on electroacupuncture-produced anti-allodynia/hyperalgesia in rats with paclitaxel-evoked peripheral neuropathy. Brain Res 1414: 58–65.
17. Ami N, Okamoto K, Oshima H (2012) Analgesic effect of magnetic stimulation on paclitaxel-induced peripheral neuropathic pain in mice. Brain Res 1461: 24–29.
18. Zimmermann M (1983) Ethical guidelines for investigations of experimental pain in conscious animals. Pain 16: 109–110.
19. Nozaki-Taguchi N, Chaplan SR, Higuera ES, Ajakwe RC, Yaksh TL (2001) Vincristine-induced allodynia in the rat. Pain 93: 69–76.
20. Lynch 3rd JJ, Wade CL, Zhong CM, Mikusa JP, Honore P (2004) Attenuation of mechanical allodynia by clinically utilized drugs in a rat chemotherapy induced neuropathic pain model. Pain 110: 56–63.
21. Liao YH, Zhang GH, Jia D, Wang P, Qian NS, et al. (2011) Spinal astrocytic activation contributes to mechanical allodynia in a mouse model of type 2 diabetes. Brain Res 1368: 324–335.
22. Schwartz ES, Lee I, Chung K, Chung JM (2008) Oxidative stress in the spinal cord is an important contributor in capsaicin-induced mechanical secondary hyperalgesia in mice. Pain 138: 514–524.
23. Janecka A, Staniszewska R, Gach K, Fichna J (2008) Enzymatic degradation of endomorphins. Peptides 29: 2066–2073.
24. Wang CH, Cherng WJ, Yang NI, Hsu CM, Yeh CH, et al. (2008) Cyclosporine increases ischemia-induced endothelial progenitor cell mobilization through manipulation of the CD26 system. Am J Physiol Regul Integr Comp Physiol 294: 811–818.
25. Nadeson R, Tucker A, Bajunaki E, Goodchild CS (2002) Potentiation by ketamine of fentanyl antinociception. I. An experimental study in rats showing that ketamine administered by non-spinal routes targets spinal cord antinociceptive systems. Br J Anaesth 88: 685–691.
26. Wolfe D, Hao S, Hu J, Srinivasan R, Goss J, et al. (2007) Engineering an endomorphin-2 gene for use in neuropathic pain therapy. Pain 133: 29.
27. Yang S, Zhang D, Yang Z, Hu X, Qian S, et al. (2008) Curcumin protects dopaminergic neuron against LPS induced neurotoxicity in primary rat neuron/glia culture. Neurochem Res 33: 2044–2053.
28. Storkson RV, Kjorsvik A, Tjolsen A, Hole K (1996) Lumbar catheterization of the spinal subarachnoid space in the rat. J Neurosci Methods 65: 167–172.
29. Zhao M, Wang JY, Jia H, Tang JS (2007) Roles of different subtypes of opioid receptors in mediating the ventrolateral orbital cortex opioid-induced inhibition of mirror-neuropathic pain in the rat. Neuroscience 144: 1486–1494.
30. Hao JX, Xu IS, Xu XJ, Wiesenfeld-Hallin Z (1999) Effects of intrathecal morphine, clonidine and baclofen on allodynia after partial sciatic nerve injury in the rat. Acta Anaesthesiol Scand 43: 1027–1034.
31. Hargreaves K, Dubner R, Brown F, Flores C, Joris J (1988) A new and sensitive method for measuring thermal nociception in cutaneous hyperalgesia. Pain 32: 77–88.
32. Li KC, Chen J (2004) Altered pain-related behaviors and spinal neuronal responses produced by s.c. injection of melittin in rats. Neuroscience 126: 753–762.
33. Sun YY, Li KC, Chen J (2005) Evidence for peripherally antinociceptive action of propofol in rats: behavioral and spinal neuronal responses to subcutaneous bee venom. Brain Res 1043: 231–235.
34. Uhm JH, Yung WKA (1999) Neurologic complications of cancer therapy. Curr Treat Options Neurol 1: 428–437.
35. Bosnjak S, Jelic S, Susnjar S, Luki V (2002) Gabapentin for relief of neuropathic pain related to anticancer treatment: a preliminary study. J Chemother 14: 214–219.
36. Hempenstall K, Rice ASC (2002) Current treatment options in neuropathic pain. Curr Opin Investig Drugs 3: 441–448.
37. Meuser T, Pietruck C, Radbruch L, Stute P, Lehmann KA, et al. (2001) Symptoms during cancer pain treatment following WHO-guidelines: a longitudinal follow-up study of symptom prevalence, severity and etiology. Pain 93: 247–257.
38. Dahl JL (2002) Working with regulators to improve the standard of care in pain management: the U.S. experience. J Pain Symptom Manage 24: 136–147.
39. Tanner KD, Reichling DB, Gear RW, Paul SM, Levine JD (2003) Altered temporal pattern of evoked afferent activity in a rat model of vincristine-induced painful peripheral neuropathy. Neuroscience 118: 809–817.
40. Weng HR, Cordella JV, Dougherty PM (2003) Changes in sensory processing in the spinal dorsal horn accompany vincristine-induced hyperalgesia and allodynia. Pain 103: 131–138.
41. Flatters SJL, Bennett GJ (2006) Studies of peripheral sensory nerves in paclitaxel-induced painful peripheral neuropathy: Evidence for mitochondrial dysfunction. Pain 122: 245–257.

42. Kajander K, Sahara Y, Iadarola M, Bennett G (1990) Dynorphin increases in the dorsal spinal cord in rats with a painful peripheral neuropathy. Peptides 11: 719–728.
43. Malan TP, Ossipov M, Gardell L, Ibrahim M, Bian D, et al. (2000) Extraterritorial neuropathic pain correlates with multisegmental elevation of spinal dynorphin in nerve-injured rats. Pain 86: 185–194.
44. Draisci G, Kajander K, Dubner R, Bennett G, Iadarola M (1991) Up-regulation of opioid gene expression in spinal cord evoked by experimental nerve injuries and in£ammation. Brain Res 560: 186–192.
45. Stone L, Fairbanks C, Laughlin T, Nguyen HO, Bushy T, et al. (1997) Spinal analgesic actions of the new endogenous opioid peptides endomorphin-1 and -2. NeuroReport 8: 3131–3135.
46. Delander GE, Schott E, Brodin E, Fredholm BB (1997) Temporal changes in spinal cord expression of mRNA for substance P, dynorphin and enkephalin in a model of chronic pain. Acta Physiol Scand 161: 509–516.
47. Kohno T, Ji RR, Ito N, Allchorne AJ, Befort K, et al. (2005) Peripheral axonal injury results in reduced mu opioid receptor pre- and post-synaptic action in the spinal cord. Pain 117: 77–87.
48. Yamamoto J, Kawamata T, Niiyama Y, Omote K, Namiki A (2008) Down-regulation of mu opioid receptor expression within distinct subpopulations of dorsal root ganglion neurons in a murine model of bone cancer pain. Neuroscience 151: 843–853.
49. Ji RR, Zhang Q, Law PY, Low HH, Elde R, et al. (1995) Expression of mu-, delta-, and kappa-opioid receptor-like immunoreactivities in rat dorsal root ganglia after carrageenan-induced inflammation. J Neurosci 15: 8156–8166.
50. Maekawa K, Minami M, Masuda T, Satoh M (1996) Expression of mu and kappa-, but not delta-, opioid receptor mRNAs is enhanced in the spinal dorsal horn of the arthritic rats. Pain 64: 365–371.
51. Stanfa LC, Dickenson AH (1993) Cholecystokinin as a factor in the enhanced potency of spinal morphine following carrageenin inflammation. Br J Pharmacol 108: 967–973.
52. Martin-Schild S, Gerall AA, Kastin AJ, Zadina JE (1999) Differential distribution of endomorphin 1- and endomorphin 2-like immunoreactivities in the CNS of the rodent. J Comp Neurol 405: 450–471.
53. Pierce TL, Wessendorf MW (2000) Immunocytochemical mapping of endomorphin-2 immunoreactivity in rat brain. J Chem Neuroanat 18: 181–207.
54. Tseng LF, Narita M, Suganuma C, Mizoguchi H, Ohsawa M, et al. (2000) Differential antinociceptive effects of endomorphin-1 and endomorphin-2 in the mouse. J Pharmacol Exp Ther 292: 576–583.
55. Grass S, Xu IS, Wiesenfeld-Hallin Z, Xu X-J (2002) Comparison of the effect of intrathecal endomorphin-1 and endomorphin-2 on spinal cord excitability in rats. Neurosci Lett 324: 197–200.
56. Fujita T, Kumamoto E (2006) Inhibition by endomorphin-1 and endomorphin-2 of excitatory transmission in adult rat substantia gelatinosa neurons. Neuroscience 139: 1095–1105.
57. Basbaum AI, Bautista DM, Scherrer G, Julius D (2009) Cellular and Molecular Mechanisms of Pain. Cell 139: 267–284.
58. Cunningham DF, O'Connor B (1997) Proline specific peptidases. Biochim Biophys Acta 1343: 160–186.
59. Janecka A, Staniszewska R, Gach K, Fichna J (2008) Enzymatic degradation of endomorphins. Peptides 29: 2066–2073.
60. Shane R, Wilk S, Bodnar RJ (1999) Modulation of endomorphin-2- induced analgesia by dipeptidyl peptidase IV. Brain Res 815: 278–286.
61. Heppelmann B, Messlinger K, Neiss WF, Schmidt RF (1994) Mitochondria in fine afferent nerve fibres of the knee joint in the cat: a quantitative electron-microscopical examination. Cell Tissue Res 275: 493–501.
62. Chang DT, Honick AS, Reynolds IJ (2006) Mitochondrial trafficking to synapses in cultured primary cortical neurons. J Neurosci 26: 7035–7045.
63. Virmani A, Gaetani F, Binienda Z (2005) Effects of metabolic modifiers such as carnitines, coenzyme Q10, and PUFAs against different forms of neurotoxic insults: metabolic inhibitors, MPTP, and methamphetamine. Ann NY Acad Sci 21053: 183–191.

5

Molecular Mechanisms Underlying the Enhanced Analgesic Effect of Oxycodone Compared to Morphine in Chemotherapy-Induced Neuropathic Pain

Karine Thibault[1,2,3*¤], Bernard Calvino[1,2], Isabelle Rivals[4], Fabien Marchand[5,6], Sophie Dubacq[1,2], Stephen B. McMahon[3], Sophie Pezet[1,2]

1 Brain Plasticity Unit, ESPCI-ParisTech, Paris, France, **2** Centre National de la Recherche Scientifique, UMR 8249, Paris, France, **3** Neurorestoration Group, The Wolfson Centre for Age-Related Diseases, King's College London, London, United Kingdom, **4** Equipe de Statistique Appliquée, ESPCI-ParisTech, Paris, France, **5** Institut National de la Santé et de la Recherche Médicale, Unité 1107, NEURO-DOL, Clermont-Ferrand, France, **6** Clermont Université, Université d'Auvergne, Pharmacologie Fondamentale et Clinique de la Douleur, Clermont-Ferrand, France

Abstract

Oxycodone is a μ-opioid receptor agonist, used for the treatment of a large variety of painful disorders. Several studies have reported that oxycodone is a more potent pain reliever than morphine, and that it improves the quality of life of patients. However, the neurobiological mechanisms underlying the therapeutic action of these two opioids are only partially understood. The aim of this study was to define the molecular changes underlying the long-lasting analgesic effects of oxycodone and morphine in an animal model of peripheral neuropathy induced by a chemotherapic agent, vincristine. Using a behavioural approach, we show that oxycodone maintains an optimal analgesic effect after chronic treatment, whereas the effect of morphine dies down. In addition, using DNA microarray technology on dorsal root ganglia, we provide evidence that the long-term analgesic effect of oxycodone is due to an up-regulation in $GABA_B$ receptor expression in sensory neurons. These receptors are transported to their central terminals within the dorsal horn, and subsequently reinforce a presynaptic inhibition, since only the long-lasting (and not acute) anti-hyperalgesic effect of oxycodone was abolished by intrathecal administration of a $GABA_B$ receptor antagonist; in contrast, the morphine effect was unaffected. Our study demonstrates that the $GABA_B$ receptor is functionally required for the alleviating effect of oxycodone in neuropathic pain condition, thus providing new insight into the molecular mechanisms underlying the sustained analgesic action of oxycodone.

Editor: Michael Costigan, Boston Children's Hospital and Harvard Medical School, United States of America

Funding: This work was supported by the "Institut UPSA de la douleur" and the "Centre National de la Recherche Scientifique", CNRS. KT received a two year doctoral fellowship from Mundipharma laboratory (ML). KT received one year of post-doctoral fellowship from "Fondation pour la Recherche Medicale". The funders had no role in study design, data collection and analysis, decision to publish, or preparation of the manuscript.

Competing Interests: The authors have declared that no competing interests exist.

* E-mail: karine.thibault@parisdescartes.fr

¤ Current address: Glia-Glia & Glia-Neuron Interactions in Neurophysiopathology Group, CNRS FR3636, Paris Descartes University, Paris, France

Introduction

Approximately 7–8% of the European population suffers from neuropathic pain, and 5% of these cases may be severe [1]. Unfortunately, the pharmacotherapy of neuropathic pain is frequently unsatisfactory for patients. One reason for their poor efficacy is the lack of a clear understanding of the neurobiological mechanisms that underlie neuropathic pain. Morphine is the most commonly used opioid analgesic in the past 30 years. However, repeated use of opioids induces a tolerance phenomenon, which significantly reduces their analgesic effects. Among clinically used opioids, oxycodone shows excellent anti-hyperalgesic and anti-allodynic effects against neuropathic pain [2,3]. Oxycodone is a semi-synthetic opioid analgesic, and has been used in clinics since 1917 [4]. Like other opioids, including morphine, the analgesic effect of oxycodone is mainly mediated through the activation of the μ-opioid receptor. Interestingly, the analgesic effect of oxycodone seems to be as potent as morphine on different types of pain, including visceral pain [5], post-operative pain [6] and cancer pain [7,8]. Moreover, the oxycodone-paracetamol combination was shown to be effective against chronic lower back pain [9], whereas morphine treatment did not show any beneficial effect [10]. In patients with neuropathic pain, oxycodone treatment (mostly in combination with anticonvulsants) improves health-related quality of life and diminishes the impact of pain on physical activity and sleep [11]. However, the neurobiological mechanisms underlying the therapeutic action of these two opioids are currently only partially understood. The aim of this study was to identify the molecular changes that produce the different analgesic effects of morphine and oxycodone.

Vincristine is an anti-neoplasic drug used to treat a wide variety of cancers. Nonetheless, it induces a peripheral neurotoxicity and subsequent neuropathic pain in both patients [12,13] and animal models [14–17]. Here, we observed in an animal model of vincristine-induced neuropathic pain that oxycodone has a longer lasting analgesic effect than morphine. Based on DNA microarray technology in dorsal root ganglia, we report an important list of genes that are differentially expressed in oxycodone-treated rats, as compared to morphine-treated subjects. This provides clues on the mechanisms underlying their different long-term actions. Furthermore, we provide direct evidence for an involvement of $GABA_B$ receptors in the long-lasting effect of oxycodone on neuropathic pain.

Materials and Methods

All experiments were performed in agreement with the European Community Council Directive of 24 November 1986 (86/609/EEC) and with guidelines on ethical standards for the investigation of experimental pain in animals, published in a Guest Editorial in the journal 'Pain' (Committee for Research and Ethical issues of the I.A.S.P., 1980). This study was approved by the ethics committee C2EA-59: 'Comité d'éthique en matière d'expérimentation animale Paris Centre et Sud'. Accordingly to the rule of the '3R' of the European regulation for the use of laboratory animals, the number of animals was kept to the minimum possible. Experiments were performed on 123 male Sprague Dawley rats (Janvier, Le Genest St Isle, France) weighing 150–175 g at the beginning of the experiments. Great care was taken, particularly with regard to housing conditions, to avoid or minimize discomfort of the animals: rats were housed four in a cage to minimize the possibility of painful interactions. The animals were kept on solid floor cages with a deep layer of sawdust to accommodate the excess of urination and cages were changed three times a week. They were kept at a constant temperature of 22°C, with a 12 h alternative light/dark cycle. Food and water were available *ad libitum.*

Induction of peripheral neuropathy by vincristine and analgesic treatment

Animals were randomly chosen and tested by an experimenter blinded to the animal's treatment. Fifty-seven rats received intraperitoneal (i.p.) injections of vincristine (0.1 mg/kg/day; Oncovin-1 mg, EG LABO, Boulogne-Billancourt, France) for two 5-day cycles with a 2-day pause between cycles, as previously described [17]. Thirty control rats received i.p. injections of the vehicle (saline: 9‰ NaCl) according to the same protocol. At the end of vincristine treatment (D15), each group was divided into 3 sub-groups that received chronic injections of morphine (3.33 mg/kg diluted in saline, i.p. injection; laboratoire Cooper, France), oxycodone (3.33 mg/kg diluted in saline, i.p. injection; OxyNorm, Napp Pharmaceuticals Ltd, Cambridge, UK) or saline during 5 days (D19). These doses were chosen according to a previous report [18], as well as unpublished preliminary data showing an equipotent analgesic effect of morphine and oxycodone on mechanical hyperalgesia (pinch test) in naive animals, when used at 3.33 mg/kg.

Influence of the $GABA_B$ receptor on the long-lasting analgesic effect of repeated oxycodone injections: intrathecal administration of saclofen

This experiment was performed to evaluate the involvement of $GABA_B$ receptors in the analgesic effect of oxycodone. Intrathecal injections were performed by lumbar puncture, as previously described [19,20]. Briefly, a rat was slightly anesthetized with isoflurane gas (Baxter, Maurepas, France) and held in one hand by the pelvic girdle; a 25-gauge x1-inch needle connected to a 10-µl Hamilton syringe was then inserted into the subarachnoidal space between the spinous processes of L5 and L6, until a tail-flick was elicited. The syringe was held in position for several seconds after the injection of saclofen (10 µl; Ref S166, Sigma-Aldrich, St. Louis, MO) or saline. Saclofen was diluted to a concentration of 1 µg/µl in saline. This dose was chosen according to [21,22]. Twenty-four rats received i.p. injections of vincristine. At D15, rats were subdivided into two groups: 12 rats received chronic injections of oxycodone, and the other 12 received chronic injections of saline (over a 5 day-treatment). At D19, each group was further divided into 2 sub-groups that received an i.t. injection of saclofen or saline (n = 6 vincristine-oxycodone-saclofen treated rats; n = 6 vincristine-oxycodone-saline treated rats; n = 6 vincristine-saline-saclofen treated rats; n = 6 vincristine-saline-saline treated rats).

Influence of the $GABA_B$ receptor on the analgesic effect of acute injection of morphine and oxycodone and repeated injections of morphine: intrathecal administration of saclofen

Thirty-six rats received i.p. vincristine injections. The role of the $GABA_B$ receptor on the analgesic effect of acute injection of opioids was tested at D15 (n = 6 vincristine-oxycodone-saclofen treated rats; n = 6 vincristine-oxycodone-saline treated rats; n = 6 vincristine-morphine-saclofen treated rats; n = 6 vincristine-morphine-saline treated rats; n = 6 vincristine-saline-saclofen treated rats; n = 6 vincristine-saline-saline treated rats). The role of the $GABA_B$ receptor on the analgesic effect of chronic injections of morphine was tested at D19, as with oxycodone (see above).

Behavioural tests

The animals received a two-week habituation period prior to the start of the peripheral neuropathy-inducing vincristine injections, as previously described [23].

Chronic effects of analgesic treatment. Behavioural tests were performed on D1 and D15 of vincristine treatment in 21 vincristine-treated rats and 18 control rats. The time-course study on the effects of oxycodone and morphine was performed at D15 and D19, in which behavioural tests were repeated 30, 60 and 90 minutes following morphine (n = 7 vincristine-morphine treated rats; n = 6 saline-morphine treated rats), oxycodone (n = 7 vincristine-oxycodone treated rats; n = 6 saline-oxycodone treated rats), or saline injections (n = 7 vincristine-saline treated rats; n = 6 saline-saline treated rats).

$GABA_B$ receptor antagonist study on the long-lasting analgesic effect of repeated injections of oxycodone. Behavioural tests were performed on D1 and D15 of vincristine treatment in 24 vincristine-treated rats. Behavioural tests were performed on D15 as a control for the development of neuropathic pain state; the animals were then repeatedly treated with oxycodone. The rats received one injection of oxycodone or saline at D19, and were then tested 30 minutes later as a control for the long-lasting analgesic effect of oxycodone (D19). Four hours after this first injection, rats were injected again with oxycodone or saline (D19′). Fifteen minutes after this second injection, rats were anesthetized with isoflurane (Baxter, Maurepas, France) and injected intrathecally with saclofen (10 µg; Ref S166, Sigma-Aldrich, St. Louis, MO) diluted in saline. Rats were behaviourally tested once again, 15 minutes after the saclofen injection (n = 6 vincristine-oxycodone-saclofen treated rats; n = 6 vincristine-oxycodone-saline treated rats; n = 6 vincristine-saline-saclofen treated rats; n = 6 vincristine-saline-saline treated rats).

$GABA_B$ receptor antagonist study on the analgesic effect of acute injection of oxycodone or morphine and chronic injections of morphine. Behavioural tests were performed on D1 of vincristine treatment in 36 vincristine-treated rats. The rats received one injection of oxycodone, morphine or saline at D15. Fifteen minutes later, rats were anesthetized with isoflurane and injected intrathecally with saclofen (10 μg; Ref S166, Sigma-Aldrich, St. Louis, MO) diluted in saline. Rats were tested again 15 minutes after the saclofen injection (n = 6 vincristine-oxycodone-saclofen treated rats; n = 6 vincristine-oxycodone-saline treated rats; n = 6 vincristine-morphine-saclofen treated rats; n = 6 vincristine-morphine-saline treated rats; n = 6 vincristine-saline-saclofen treated rats; n = 6 vincristine-saline-saline treated rats). At D19 (*i.e.* 5 days after the start of opioids treatment), the same experiment was performed following chronic injections of morphine (n = 6 vincristine-morphine-saclofen treated rats; n = 6 vincristine-morphine-saline treated rats; n = 6 vincristine-saline-saclofen treated rats; n = 6 vincristine-saline-saline treated rats). For ease of reading, we have presented the results in two separate figures: the effect of saclofen after acute injection of oxycodone, and the effect of saclofen after morphine treatment.

Assessment of static mechanical sensitivity. The static mechanical allodynia was measured using the electronic Von Frey test, as previously described [23]. Briefly, an Electronic Von Frey hair unit (EVF-3, Bioseb, Chaville, France) was used to measure the sensitivity threshold in one test; measurements ranged from 0 to 500 grams with a 0.2 gram accuracy. Paw sensitivity threshold was defined as the minimal pressure required to elicit a robust and immediate withdrawal reflex of the paw. The stimulus was applied to each hind paw five times within a five-second interval; by convention, the threshold for each rat was the average of ten measured values. Static mechanical allodynia was defined as a significant decrease in withdrawal thresholds to Von Frey application.

The results for each group in the $GABA_B$ receptor antagonist study were expressed as follows: δ-paw withdrawal threshold (% ± S.E.M.), calculated from individual paw withdrawal thresholds: $\left[\frac{(T30-T0)}{T0}\right]\times 100$ at D19 and $\left[\frac{(T30'-T0)}{T0}\right]\times 100$ at D19′. The effect of saclofen on mechanical allodynia was defined as a significant decrease in δ-paw withdrawal threshold to Von Frey application.

Assessment of static mechanical hyperalgesia. Static mechanical hyperalgesia was measured using the 'Pinch' test, as previously described [23]. Rats were individually taken by the experimenter and held without restraint on the experimenter's lap for 5 min. The threshold of static mechanical sensitivity was determined using a 'Pincher' unit (Bioseb, Chaville, France). Briefly, pressure was applied with a calibrated forceps (ranging from 0–800 g) to the mid-plantar area of each hind paw, to elicit a robust and immediate withdrawal reflex of the stimulated paw. The stimulus was applied to each hind paw three times within a 2 minute-interval; by convention, the threshold for a rat was the average of the six measured values. Static mechanical hyperalgesia was defined as a significant decrease in withdrawal thresholds to pincher application.

The results for each group in the $GABA_B$ receptor antagonist study were expressed as follows: δ-paw withdrawal threshold (% ± S.E.M.), calculated from individual paw withdrawal thresholds: $\left[\frac{(T30-T0)}{T0}\right]\times 100$ at D19 and $\left[\frac{(T30'-T0)}{T0}\right]\times 100$ at D19′. The effect of saclofen on mechanical allodynia was defined as a significant decrease in the δ-paw withdrawal threshold to pincher application.

Assessment of dynamic mechanical allodynia and hyperaesthesia: the "Paint-brush test". The dynamic mechanical allodynia observed in neuropathic patients was measured as previously developed in our laboratory and described in Thibault *et al.* [24]. First, a stimulus was applied with a smooth (marten hair) paint-brush to each hind paw, five times within a five-second interval. Each stimulus that resulted in a response was scored as '1', and the absence of a response was scored as '0'. The 10 stimulation scores were added, giving a total score between 0 and 10 for each rat. Next, the stimulation was applied with a rough (pig bristle) paint-brush, using the same protocol. Dynamic mechanical allodynia or hyperesthesia were defined as a significant increase in the total score using the smooth or the rough brush, respectively.

Statistical analysis of the behavioural data. Behavioural data from electronic Von Frey and Pinch tests were examined using two-way analysis of variance (ANOVA) followed by a Student Newman–Keuls test for two-by-two comparisons. Behavioural data from paint-brush tests were examined with a Kruskal–Wallis test followed by a Wilcoxon matches pairs test and a Mann–Whitney U test for two-by-two comparisons. Data were expressed as means ± SEM, and the levels of significance were set at: *$p<0.05$; **$p<0.01$; ***$p<0.001$.

DNA microarray analysis

RNA preparation for microarray analysis and microarray hybridisation. Two hours after the end of the behavioural study (D19), rats were deeply anaesthetized with pentobarbital (60 mg/kg i.p; Ceva Santé Animale, Libourne, France) and decapitated (n = 4 vincristine-morphine, n = 4 vincristine-oxycodone, n = 4 vincristine-saline treated rats; and n = 4 saline-morphine, n = 4 saline-oxycodone, n = 4 saline-saline rats). Lumbar dorsal root ganglia (DRGs) L2 through L5 were dissected and immediately frozen on dry ice. Tissues were kept at −80°C until homogenisation. Total RNA from individually dissected frozen DRGs was extracted and treated with DNAse using the RNeasy® Lipid Tissue Mini kit (Qiagen, Courtaboeuf, France), according to the manufacturer's protocol. The quality and quantity of each RNA sample was checked using an Agilent 2100 Bioanalyzer with RNA 6000 NanoChips (Agilent Technologies, Massy, France). Five hundred ng of RNA were sent to the Integragen Illumina microarray facility (Integragen, Evry, France, www.integragen.com) for sample processing. Illumina pangenomic rat microarrays (RatRef-12 Expression BeadChips), including 22,517 probes, were also performed at the Integragen Illumina microarray facility (Evry, France), according to the Illumina procedures.

DNA microarray statistical analysis. All manipulations and statistical analyses were performed with the R freeware. For Illumina beadchip data, all spots with a detection p-value greater than 0.05% were excluded. A two-way ANOVA was performed, using vincristine treatment as the first factor and analgesic treatment as the second factor. Student t-tests were performed to find differentially expressed genes between morphine and oxycodone treatment, in vincristine-treated rats or controls. The reported p-values correspond to the control of the type I error risk of each individual gene (no adjustment for multiple testing). The data have been deposited in NCBIs Gene Expression Omnibus (http://www.ncbi.nlm.nih.gov/geo/) and assigned Series accession number GSE53897.

Real-time quantitative PCR. Quantitative real-time PCR was performed using the fluorescent binding-dye SYBR Green (Absolute Blue SYBR Green Rox mix, ABgene, Thermo Scientific) on a real-time PCR machine (LightCycler Technology, Roche) with primer sets designed at the Roche website (www.roche-applied-science.com). Each qPCR assay was conducted in triplicate, using cDNA derived from 50 ng total RNA from each animal. Each sample well contained 4 μl of cDNA (5 ng/μl), with a primer concentration of 0.5 μM plus 5 μl of SYBR Green. Each qPCR assay was conducted with one candidate housekeeping gene for normalisation (actin, beta: Actb). The following primers were used: Gabbr2, 5′-AAGACCTTTGAAACACTCTGCAC-3′ (forward) and 5′-CCAAAGGCAGTTGTGTAGCC-3′ (reverse); Actb, 5′-CCCGCGAGTACAACCTTCT-3′ (forward) and 5′-CGTCATCCATGGCGAACT-3′ (reverse). qPCR was performed on all samples (saline-saline; saline-oxycodone; saline-morphine; vincristine-saline; vincristine-oxycodone; vincristine-morphine). All fluorescence data were processed using a post-PCR data analysis software program (LightCycler relative Quantification Software version 1.0; Roche), providing an automatic calculation of a normalized ratio. Saline samples were used for normalisation. The ratios of each gene of interest were compared among samples, using an unpaired t-test.

Immunohistochemistry

Tissue preparation. Twelve rats receiving vincristine treatment and 12 others receiving saline treatment were used for the immunohistochemistry experiment. At D15, each group was divided into 3 sub-groups that received chronic injections of morphine ($n = 4$ vincristine-morphine, $n = 4$ saline-morphine treated rats), oxycodone ($n = 4$ vincristine-oxycodone, $n = 4$ saline-oxycodone treated rats) or saline ($n = 4$ vincristine-saline, $n = 4$, saline-saline treated rats). Rats were deeply anaesthetized at the end of analgesic treatment (D19) with a 25 mg/ml urethane injection (1.5 g/kg i.p), and perfused transcardially with 200 ml of 0.9% NaCl, followed by 500 ml of 4% paraformaldehyde (PFA) in 0.1 M phosphate buffer (PB), pH 7.4. Tissues were dissected out and post-fixed at 4°C in the same fixative, either overnight (spinal cord) or for 2 hours (DRGs). All tissues were further cryoprotected in 30% sucrose (in 0.1 M PB, pH 7.4) overnight at 4°C. DRG sections (14 μm thick) were serially cut using a cryostat (HM550, Microm Microtech). Sections were mounted directly onto a Superfrost slide such that two series of six slides corresponding to the whole ganglion could be obtained. Two slides per animal were used for each labelling. Spinal cord sections (30 μm thick) were cut using a cryostat and collected in phosphate buffer saline (PBS; 0.02 M) containing 0.02% sodium azide.

Characterisation of the rabbit anti-GABAB2 antibody

Western Blot. The anti-$GABA_{B2}$ antibody was tested using the western blot method. Briefly, a rat was deeply anaesthetized with pentobarbital (60 mg/kg i.p.; Ceva Santé Animale, Libourne, France) and then euthanised by decapitation. The cortex of a control animal was homogenised in RIPA (radioimmunoprecipitation assay buffer; 50 mM Tris, pH 8, 150 mM NaCl, 1% NP-40, 0.5% deoxycholate, 0.1% SDS, 1 mM sodium orthovanadate) containing Complete protease inhibitor mixture (Complete, Roche, Neuilly-sur-seine, France). The protein concentrations were determined using a Biorad DC Protein Assay kit (Bio-Rad Laboratories, California, USA). Spinal cord samples (30 μg of proteins) were separated by 10% SDS-PAGE, and transferred to nitrocellulose membranes. The membrane was then incubated with the primary antibody rabbit anti-$GABA_{B2}$ (ref. 52248, Abcam, Cambridge, UK), diluted 1:1000 in 20 mM Tris, pH 7.5, 500 mM NaCl, 0.1% Tween 20 (TBS-T). After several washes in TBS-T, the membrane was incubated in an anti-rabbit IgG HRP secondary antibody (1:10000) for 1 h at room temperature. Following several washes in TBS-T, the membrane was treated with the ECL-plus reagent (10 min) for detection by autoradiography. A specific band was observed at 106-110 kDa, corresponding to the GABAB2 receptor (Figure S1A).

Immunohistochemistry. Immunostainings performed with this antibody on spinal cord revealed characteristic $GABA_{B2}$ receptor staining. As previously reported [25,26], we observed staining in the superficial laminae (Figure S1B) and in deeper laminae (Figure S1B). Spinal cord sections incubated without primary antibody did not display any staining (data not shown).

GABAB2 receptor labelling in dorsal root ganglia

Immunostainings were performed on tissues from 4 animals per group. Double immunofluorescent stainings for $GABA_{B2}$ receptor and βIII tubulin (a marker of all neuronal cells) were performed to determine the percentage of neurons expressing $GABA_{B2}$ receptors. Sections were incubated overnight at room temperature with a rabbit anti-$GABA_{B2}$ receptor antibody (1:300, ref. 52248, Abcam, Cambridge, UK) and mouse anti-βIII Tubulin antibody (1:2000, ref. G7121, Promega, San Luis Obispo, CA USA); antibodies were diluted in PBS-T-azide (PBS 0.02 M containing 0.3% Triton X-100 and 0.02% sodium azide). Following several washes in PBS, sections were incubated for 2 h at room temperature in Alexa Fluor® 488 anti-rabbit IgG and Alexa Fluor® 350 anti-mouse IgG (Invitrogen, California, USA), diluted 1:1000 in PBS-T. Following several washes in PBS, sections were mounted in Vectashield medium (Vector Laboratories, Burlingame, USA). A similar procedure was performed for $GABA_{B2}$ receptor-$GABA_{B1}$ receptor double immunostaining, using the anti-$GABA_{B1}$ receptor antibody (1:500; mouse anti-$GABA_{B1}$ receptor, ref. 55051, Abcam, Cambridge, UK) and Alexa Fluor® 546 anti-mouse IgG.

Quantification of βIII tubulin- and GABAB2 receptor-positive neurons. Black and white 256 grey level images were acquired using a 40X objective on a Zeiss microscope equipped with a Zeiss Axiocam MRm camera. All acquisitions were performed using the same acquisition setup. Quantification of the percentage of $GABA_{B2}$ receptor-positive cells was performed by counting both the number of $GABA_{B2}$ and βIII tubulin immunopositive cells in DRG. At least 200 cells were counted per DRG (more than four or five sections per rat). An analysis of staining intensity and size diameter distribution was performed using Image J software (http://rsb.info.nih.gov/ij/). The background staining intensity was subtracted from each image, and results were expressed as the mean intensity of immunoreactivity ± SEM. The mean diameter, percentage of positively stained cells, and mean intensity of $GABA_{B2}$ staining in DRG neurons were compared between all groups by one-way ANOVA using SigmaStat software, followed by the Student Newman–Keuls test to detect differences between different groups.

GABAB2 receptor labelling in the spinal dorsal horn. Free floating serial sections from the lumbar segment L4-L5 were incubated in rabbit anti-$GABA_{B2}$ receptor antibody (1:300; ref. 52248, Abcam, Cambridge, UK). This was either performed alone for quantification, or in combination with the following antibodies for double or triple staining: 1) IB4, a FITC-conjugated isolectine (1:700; Isolectin B4 FITC conjugate, ref. L 2895, Sigma-Aldrich, St. Louis, MO); 2) mouse anti-CGRP (1:500; ref. C 9487, Sigma-Aldrich, St. Louis, MO); 3) guinea pig anti-vGlut2 (1:5000; ref. AB2251, Chemicon, Temecula, CA USA); or 4) mouse anti-$GABA_{B1}$ receptor (1:500; ref. 55051, Abcam, Cambridge, UK, [27]). Tissues were finally washed in PBS, and mounted in Vectashield medium (Vector, Burlingame, USA).

Quantification of GABAB2 receptor labelling in the spinal dorsal horn. To quantify $GABA_{B2}$ receptor staining in the dorsal horn of all subject groups, black and white 256 grey level images were acquired using a 40X objective on a Zeiss microscope equipped with a Zeiss Axiocam MRm camera. All acquisitions were performed using the same acquisition setup. A 100 μm ×

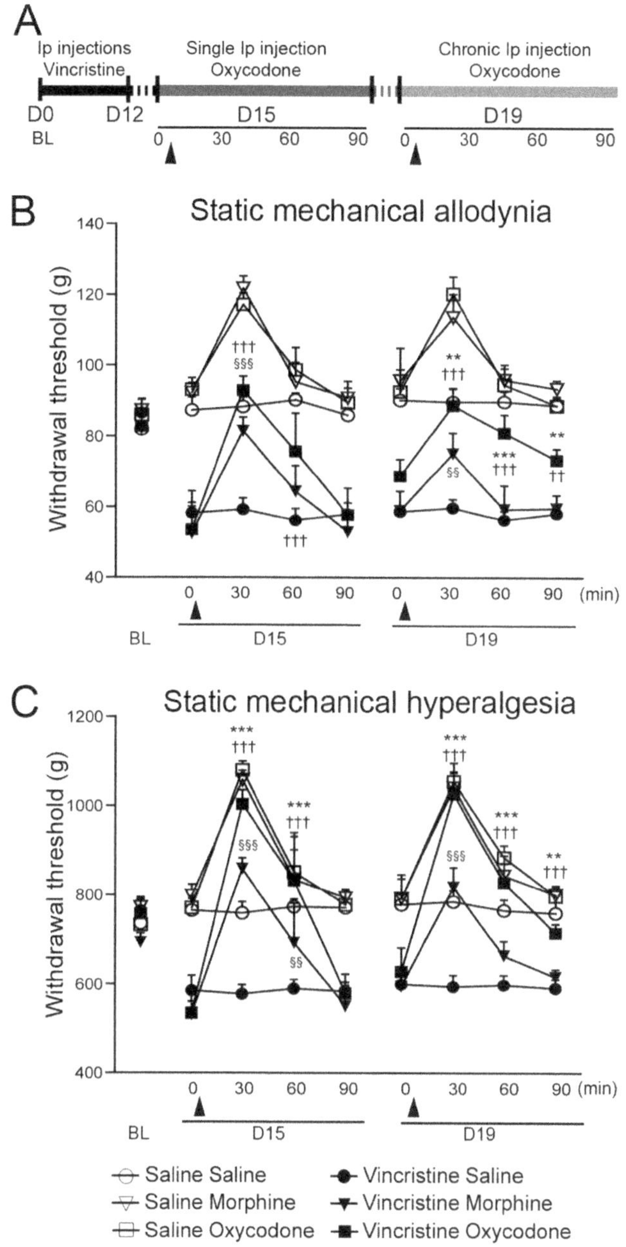

Figure 1. Time-course of static mechanical sensitivity. A: Schematic representation of the experimental paradigm. Rats received i.p. injections of vincristine (0.1 mg/kg/day) during 2 cycles of 5 days. Analgesic treatment started at D15, and was performed for 5 days until D19. The analgesic effect of oxycodone or morphine was tested on D15 and D19, with a time-course of 30, 60 and 90 minutes after injection. These injections are illustrated by black triangles. At D15, all groups of vincristine-treated rats presented static mechanical allodynia (B) and hyperalgesia (C), as compared to control rats and the baseline (BL). B: Static mechanical allodynia measured using the electronic Von Frey test. The measured static mechanical allodynia was totally reversed after a single injection of morphine or oxycodone, although only oxycodone maintained a strong analgesic effect at D19. C: Static mechanical hyperalgesia measured by the "Pinch Test". Oxycodone induced an analgesic effect in vincristine-oxycodone treated rats after a single injection, and maintained its analgesic effect at D19. All data are expressed as mean ± SEM. (n = 7 vincristine-morphine treated rats; n = 6 saline-morphine treated rats), (n = 7 vincristine-oxycodone treated rats; n = 6 saline-oxycodone treated rats), and (n = 7 vincristine-saline treated rats; n = 6 saline-saline treated rats). $^{*}p<0.05$, $^{**}p<0.01$, $^{***}p<0.001$: vincristine-oxycodone treated rats vs. vincristine-morphine treated rats; † $p<0.05$, †† $p<0.01$, ††† $p<0.001$: vincristine-oxycodone treated rats vs. vincristine-saline treated rats; §§ $p<0.01$, §§§ $p<0.001$: vincristine-morphine treated rats vs. vincristine-saline treated rats. For figure clarity, the statistical significance symbols for the vincristine vs. saline groups are not shown.

500 µm region of interest was placed on the dorsal horn to measure fluorescence intensity (FI) plot profiles (gray levels, in arbitrary units, with respect to the distance from the surface, in micrometers). Statistical significance was determined with a Student's unpaired t test for specific depth point, or one way ANOVA followed by a Student Newman–Keuls test for mean fluorescent intensity analysed per lamina (for all statistical tests: $^{**}p<0.01$;$^{*}p<0.05$).

As a final note, each type of immunostaining in the DRG or dorsal horn was simultaneously performed for all animals, in order to maintain consistency and allow a statistical analysis of all results. Omission of the primary antibody, or any other stage in the protocol, did not result in any labelling.

Results

Oxycodone maintained a strong analgesic effect after chronic treatment as compared to morphine in vincristine-treated rats

As previously observed [28], at the end of vincristine treatment (D15), vincristine-treated rats displayed a significant increased static (Figure 1B-C) and dynamic (Figure S2A–B) mechanical sensitivity, as compared to the baseline (BL, *i.e.* beginning of the treatment) and saline-treated rats. A single injection of morphine or oxycodone was capable of totally reversing static mechanical allodynia, hyperalgesia (D15 T30, Figures 1B and C, respectively) and dynamic mechanical allodynia (D15 T30, Figure S2A). The analgesic effect of oxycodone (measured by the Pinch test) was more potent than the analgesic effect of morphine on static mechanical hyperalgesia (D15 T30, Figure 1C). Moreover, dynamic mechanical hyperesthesia (measured with the rough paintbrush test) was only attenuated by morphine, whereas it was totally reversed by oxycodone (D15 T30, Figure S2B). At the end of the analgesic chronic treatment on day 19 (D19), only oxycodone was able to maintain the analgesic effect observed at D15 on mechanical sensitivity (D19 T30, Figure 1B-C and Figure S2A–B). By this point, morphine had completely lost its analgesic effect on dynamic mechanical sensitivity (Figure S2A–B).

Extensive analysis of gene expression modified by chronic analgesic treatment

We conducted a large-scale DNA microarray study based on pan-genomic chips, using Illumina technology on the dorsal root ganglion (DRG). This was aimed at systematically detecting genes whose expression was altered by chronic morphine or oxycodone treatment in either saline- or vincristine-treated rats. Among the 22,517 probes included in the microarray, 757 were differentially expressed by the end of analgesic treatment (D19), corresponding to 316 genes (Table S1). The complete list of dysregulated genes is catalogued in Table S1. Among these results, we report 145 genes that are differentially expressed after analgesic treatment in control rats (Table S1). This list could be applied to improve our understanding of the molecular mechanisms underlying chronic opioid treatment in steady state, and in particular the mechanisms of tolerance observed after chronic morphine treatment.

In this study, we chose to investigate the molecular mechanisms controlling the sustained analgesic effect of oxycodone in

Table 1. List of genes differentially regulated between vincristine-morphine vs. vincristine-oxycodone treated animals.

								Variance analysis Vin vs Control	Mor vs Oxy Vincritsine animals		Mor vs Oxy Control animals	
ACCESSION	**SYMBOL**	**V-Mor**	**V-Oxy**	**V-NaCl**	**S-Mor**	**S-Oxy**	**S-NaCl**	**p**	**p**	**diff**	**p**	**diff**
NM_144737	Fmo2	7,19	7,67	7,27	7,01	7,03	7,01	0,01	0,04	−0,48	0,92	−0,02
NM_145670	Bcas1	8,88	9,22	8,95	9,16	8,81	9,15	0,77	0,01	−0,34	0,01	0,35
NM_031345	Dsipi	11,74	12,02	11,78	11,86	11,83	11,71	0,52	0,04	−0,28	0,82	0,03
NM_012829	Cck	6,26	6,53	6,29	6,34	6,31	6,31	0,48	0,01	−0,27	0,79	0,03
NM_134398	P34	6,06	6,28	6,22	6,24	6,16	6,24	0,57	0,01	−0,22	0,26	0,08
NM_053349	Sox11	6,02	6,24	6,09	6,12	6,12	6,05	0,8	0,02	−0,22	0,98	0
NM_013066	Mtap2	6,16	6,39	6,33	6,29	6,18	6,35	0,73	0,03	−0,22	0,27	0,11
NM_001004132	Pctk1	8,5	8,71	8,54	8,84	8,73	8,7	0,01	0,04	−0,21	0,28	0,1
NM_203367	Zmynd11	6,2	6,4	6,48	6,43	6,34	6,41	0,5	0,02	−0,2	0,28	0,09
NM_001006985	Mrpl13	10,81	11,01	10,97	10,97	10,92	10,92	0,95	0,02	−0,2	0,46	0,06
NM_053555	Vamp5	8,05	8,25	8,18	8,15	8,13	8,12	0,62	0,03	−0,2	0,85	0,02
NM_031613	Tmod2	7,74	7,94	7,82	7,81	7,82	7,93	0,68	0,04	−0,19	0,93	−0,01
NM_031802	**Gabbr2**	**11,15**	**11,34**	**11,17**	**11,19**	**11,19**	**11,22**	**0,64**	**0,04**	**−0,19**	**0,99**	**0**
NM_012839	Cycs	12,27	12,44	12,4	12,33	12,22	12,33	0,11	0,04	−0,18	0,2	0,11
NM_134351	Mat2a	6,27	6,45	6,4	6,36	6,19	6,39	0,11	0,01	−0,18	0,01	0,17
XM_343564	Col5a2	9,93	10,1	10,12	10,14	9,93	10,18	0,45	0,04	−0,17	0,02	0,21
NM_001005884	Letm1	8,99	9,14	9,12	9,05	9,15	9,04	1	0,04	−0,15	0,15	−0,1
NM_080577	Nploc4	6,09	6,24	6,18	6,18	6,12	6,11	0,35	0,03	−0,14	0,38	0,05
NM_053527	Cdc5l	9,2	9,34	9,34	9,38	9,18	9,32	0,98	0,03	−0,14	0	0,2
NM_080586	**Gabrg1**	**6,16**	**6,29**	**6,33**	**6,26**	**6,2**	**6,24**	**0,43**	**0,04**	**−0,13**	**0,31**	**0,06**
NM_017065	**Gabrb3**	**5,95**	**6,07**	**6,01**	**6,07**	**6,05**	**6,06**	**0,08**	**0,01**	**−0,12**	**0,59**	**0,02**
NM_053483	Kpna2	9,33	9,45	9,41	9,4	9,49	9,41	0,28	0,04	−0,12	0,1	−0,1
NM_001004206	Pa2g4	6,03	5,92	5,98	6	5,99	5,96	0,8	0,01	0,1	NaN	NaN
NM_171993	Cdc20	6,43	6,32	6,35	6,38	6,55	6,44	0,01	0,04	0,11	0,01	−0,17
NM_053854	Nat2	6,04	5,92	6,03	6,01	6,12	6,04	0,05	0,02	0,11	0,02	−0,11
NM_031129	Tceb2	11,07	10,95	11	11,02	11,02	10,93	0,54	0,04	0,12	0,99	0
NM_021657	Phlpp	8,19	8,07	8,09	8,21	8,21	8,2	0,01	0,03	0,12	0,96	0
NM_133553	B3galt4	6,42	6,26	6,42	6,41	6,39	6,41	0,3	0,02	0,16	0,67	0,03
NM_058208	Socs2	6,33	6,13	6,1	6,12	6,19	6,23	0,85	0	0,2	0,24	−0,07
NM_017030	Pccb	6,7	6,5	6,6	6,66	6,57	6,66	0,48	0,01	0,2	0,25	0,09
NM_001004259	Pnkp	6,6	6,39	6,51	6,52	6,55	6,46	0,78	0,01	0,21	0,63	−0,03
NM_053719	Emb	8,22	8	8,16	8,03	8,11	8	0,15	0,03	0,22	0,38	−0,09
NM_001007626	Ggps1	7,43	7,18	7,26	7,2	7,34	7,24	0,61	0,02	0,24	0,16	−0,14

Table 1. Cont.

ACCESSION	SYMBOL	V-Mor	V-Oxy	V-NaCl	S-Mor	S-Oxy	S-NaCl	Variance analysis Vin vs Control	Mor vs Oxy Vincritsine animals		Mor vs Oxy Control animals	
								p	p	diff	p	diff
NM_030834	Slc16a3	6,94	6,66	6,76	6,73	6,72	6,6	0,19	0,04	0,28	0,92	0,01
NM_001007612	Ccl7	6,51	6,21	6,57	6,5	6,51	6,45	0,44	0,03	0,3	0,91	−0,01
NM_012947	Eef2k	8,77	7,65	8,67	7,65	8,92	9,18	0,48	0,04	1,12	0,03	−1,27
NM_031010	Alox15	10,66	9,43	10,22	6,43	6,29	6,38	0	0,01	1,22	0,74	0,13

Data are illustrated as follows: 1) Gene accession number; 2) Gene symbol; 3) Mean expression of the genes for the six different groups; 4) results of variance analysis between vincristine and control: p-value; 5) results of Student's t-test between morphine and oxycodone in vincristine-treated rats: p-value and expression difference (morphine – oxycodone); 6) results of Student's t-test between morphine and oxycodone in control rats: p-value and expression difference (morphine – oxycodone).

neuropathic pain, as compared to morphine. Our analysis was focused on genes differentially expressed after analgesic treatment in vincristine-treated rats; we thus identified 37 genes (Table S1). The difference in gene expression between vincristine-morphine and vincristine-oxycodone conditions was calculated (Table 1), revealing 15 genes whose expression was up-regulated after morphine treatment; this can also be expressed as (vincristine-morphine gene expression) - (vincristine-oxycodone gene expression) >0. Furthermore, we identified 22 genes whose expression was up-regulated after oxycodone treatment; this can also be expressed as (vincristine-morphine gene expression) - (vincristine-oxycodone gene expression) <0 (Table 1). Among the genes up-regulated after oxycodone treatment, we observed 3 genes that regulate receptor activity, classified in the 'Receptor' subcategory. Interestingly, these genes were: i) Gabbr2, coding for the $GABA_{B2}$ receptor; and ii) Gabrb3 and Gabrg1, coding respectively for the $GABA_A$ R subunit β3 and $GABA_A$ R subunit γ1 (Table 2). The differential expression of these three genes was significant between morphine- and oxycodone-treated rats after vincristine treatment.

Although we could not exclude a role of the $GABA_A$ receptor in chronic opioid treatment, as reported in previous studies [29,30], we chose to concentrate the second part of this study on $GABA_{B2}$ receptor expression, and their potential role in the long-lasting analgesic effect of oxycodone on neuropathic pain.

Chronic oxycodone treatment induced an increase in $GABA_{B2}$ receptor expression in small diameter DRG neurons, as well as their terminals in superficial laminae of the dorsal horn

In order to validate our results, we verified the differential expression of the $GABA_{B2}$ receptor (Gabbr2) in the DRG of vincristine-treated and control animals at the RNA and protein levels. Using qPCR, we observed an up-regulation of Gabbr2 expression in vincristine-oxycodone treated animals as compared to vincristine-morphine treated animals (1.91 ± 0.48 *vs.* 0.47 ± 0.24; $p<0.05$) (Figure 2D). At the protein level, $GABA_{B2}$ receptors were exclusively expressed in small and medium diameter neurons in DRGs (size ≤34 µm, Figures 2A-C and E). The size distribution histogram of $GABA_{B2}$ receptor immunoreactivity in DRG cells was similar in all animal groups, with a peak at 24 µm (Figure 2E). However, we observed an increase in the percentage of neurons positive for $GABA_{B2}$ staining in oxycodone-treated animals as compared to morphine-treated animals, following vincristine treatment (Figure 2F). Moreover, quantification of the mean intensity of $GABA_{B2}$ receptor staining showed a 53% increase in vincristine-oxycodone treated rats as compared to vincristine-morphine treated rats, and an 84% increase compared to vincristine-saline treated rats (Figure 2G).

In the spinal dorsal horn, the intensity of $GABA_{B2}$ staining exhibited a significant increase in both lamina I and the outer part of lamina II (Figure 3A–D), with a 70% increase in lamina I only in the vincristine-oxycodone treated group (Figure 3E). In contrast, there was no significant change in the other groups, or in deep laminae (Figure 3D).

Functionality and localisation of $GABA_{B2}$ receptors

To be functional, $GABA_B$ receptors must be organised as heterodimers comprising one $GABA_{B1}$ and one $GABA_{B2}$ subunit (for review see [31]). Using double immunostaining, we effectively observed their colocalisation in small and medium sized DRG neurons (Figure S3A–C) and in superficial layers of the dorsal horn (Figure S3D–F), suggesting that functional $GABA_B$ receptors are expressed at these levels. In addition, we observed that

Table 2. Modification of genes regulating GABA receptor activity expression after oxycodone treatment.

	$GABA_A$ R subunit β3	$GABA_A$ R subunit γ1	$GABA_{B2}$ R
Mean Expression			
Vincristine-morphine	5.95±0.05	6.16±0.10	11.15±0.08
Vincristine-oxycodone	6.07±0.09	6.29±0.04	11.34±0.12
Vincristine-saline	6.01±0.02	6.33±0.10	11.17±0.13
Control-morphine	6.07±0.03	6.26±0.07	11.19±0.12
Control-oxycodone	6.05±0.02	6.20±0.11	11.19±0.14
Control-saline	6.06±0.09	6.24±0.03	11.22±0.16
Statistics			
p-value vincristine vs. control	0.081	0.429	0.644
Difference of expression	−0.048	0.027	0.024
p-value morphine vs. oxycodone in vincristine animals	**0.012**	**0.038**	**0.047**
Difference of expression	**−0.118**	**−0.129**	**−0.192**
p-value morphine vs. oxycodone in control animals	0.591	0.312	0.992
Difference of expression	0.023	0.060	−0.001

Data are illustrated as follows: 1) Mean expression value for all groups; 2) Statistical analysis: results of variance analysis between vincristine and control: p-value and expression difference (vincristine – control); results of Student's t test between morphine and oxycodone in vincristine-treated rats: p-value and expression difference (morphine – oxycodone); results of Student's t test between morphine and oxycodone in control rats: p-value and expression difference (morphine – oxycodone). The three genes regulating GABA receptor activity expression were exclusively modified after analgesic treatment in vincristine-treated animals.

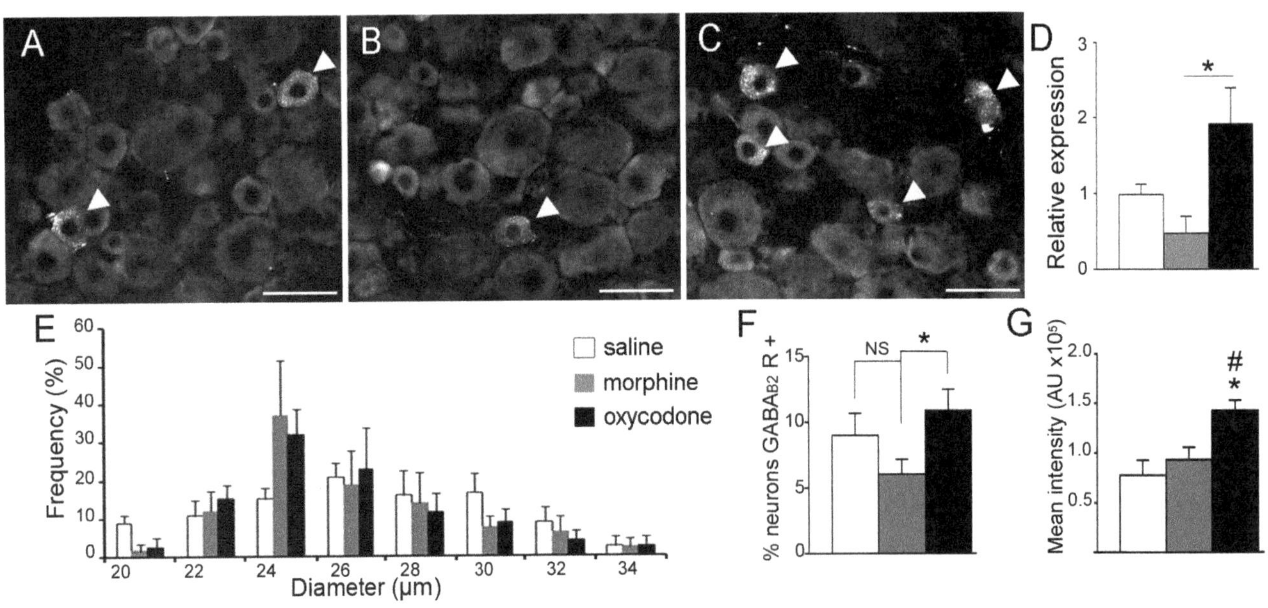

Figure 2. Up-regulation of $GABA_{B2}$ receptor expression in small diameter DRG neurons after chronic oxycodone treatment. A–C: Immunofluorescent staining showing $GABA_{B2}$ receptor immunoreactive neurons (arrowheads) in representative vincristine-saline (A), vincristine-morphine, (B) and vincristine-oxycodone (C) treated animals. Scale bars = 50 μm. D: Relative expression of Gabbr2 in the DRG of vincristine-treated rats determined by qPCR. The results validate the up-regulation of the Gabbr2 gene observed by DNA microarray in the vincristine-oxycodone treated rat, as compared to a vincristine-morphine treated rat. Data obtained from vincristine-treated rats were normalized to control rat data (n = 4 per group; *$p<0.05$ between vincristine-oxycodone treated rats and vincristine-morphine treated rats). Data were expressed as mean ± SEM. E: Histogram showing the size distribution frequency of $GABA_{B2}$ receptor expression in the DRG for all vincristine groups. Note that the size distribution frequency was identical in the three groups studied. F: Percentage of $GABA_{B2}$ receptor-positive neurons in the three animal groups. Oxycodone induced an increased percentage of $GABA_{B2}$ receptor-positive neurons as compared to morphine treatment. G: Analysis of the mean intensity of $GABA_{B2}$ receptor staining in the three vincristine-treated animals. Oxycodone induced a 53% increase in $GABA_{B2}$ receptor staining in vincristine-oxycodone treated rats as compared to vincristine-morphine treated rats, and an 84% increase as compared to vincristine-saline treated rats. (n = 4 vincristine-morphine treated rats, n = 4 vincristine-oxycodone treated rats, and n = 4 vincristine-saline treated rats) *$p<0.05$ between vincristine-oxycodone treated rats and vincristine-morphine treated rats; #$p<0.05$ between vincristine-oxycodone treated rats and vincristine-saline treated rats. Data are expressed as mean ± SEM.

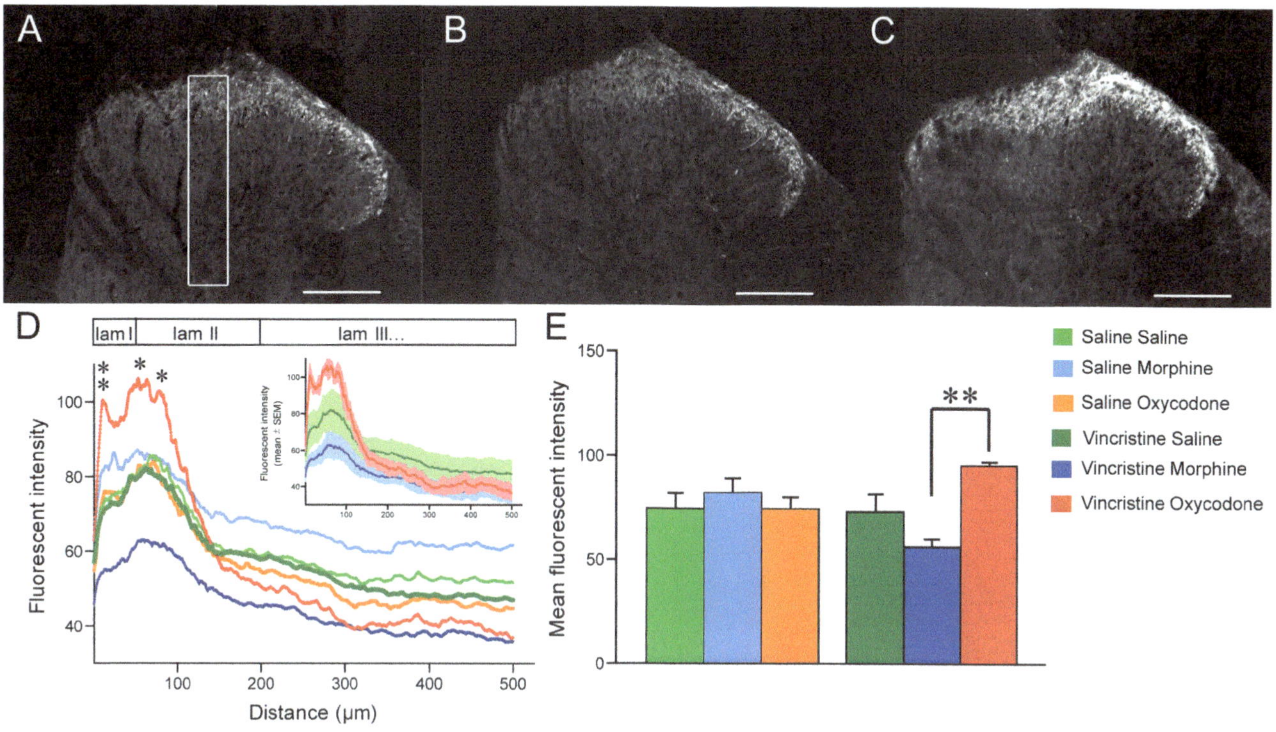

Figure 3. Up-regulation of $GABA_{B2}$ receptor expression in superficial laminae of the spinal cord after chronic oxycodone treatment. A–C: Immunofluorescent staining showing $GABA_{B2}$ receptor labelling in the dorsal horn in (A) vincristine-saline, (B) vincristine-morphine, and (C) vincristine-oxycodone treated animals. D: Analysis of the fluorescence intensity profiles of $GABA_{B2}$ receptor immunoreactivity from superficial to deeper layers in control/vincristine treated animals chronically treated with saline, morphine or oxycodone. The selected zone was a vertical area in laminae I through IV (white selection in A). The insert shows the mean fluorescent intensity ± SEM in the three groups of vincristine-treated rats as mean ± SEM. For ease of reading, it was not possible to show the SEM of all groups. E: Mean fluorescent intensity of $GABA_{B2}$ receptor immonoreactivity at the level of the first 50 µm of the spinal cord dorsal horn. Vincristine treatment did not alter the intensity of $GABA_{B2}$ receptor staining as compared to saline-treated animals. However, oxycodone (but not morphine) significantly increased the intensity of $GABA_{B2}$ receptor staining in the superficial lamina. (n = 4 vincristine-morphine treated rats; n = 4 saline-morphine treated rats), (n = 4 vincristine-oxycodone treated rats; n = 4 saline-oxycodone treated rats), and (n = 4 vincristine-saline treated rats; n = 4 saline-saline treated rats) $^*p<0.05$ and $^{**}p<0.01$ vincristine-oxycodone vs. vincristine-morphine. Data are expressed as mean ± SEM.

$GABA_{B2}$ receptors mainly colocalised within peptidergic CGRP-positive fibres (Figure S4A–C; Figure 4B–C–D, crossed arrows), and not in non-peptidergic IB4-positive terminals (Figure S4D–F). Notably, we observed that $GABA_{B2}$ receptors were present in glutamatergic presynaptic terminals (vGlut2 positive) containing CGRP (Figure 4A–D, arrows).

We directly examined the role of $GABA_B$ receptors in the long-lasting analgesic effect of oxycodone by assessing the effect of intrathecal administration of saclofen (10 µg), a selective $GABA_B$ receptor antagonist [21,22] (Figure 5A). The relieving effect of oxycodone on static mechanical allodynia was totally blocked by the antagonist (Figure 5B), whereas its analgesic effect on mechanical hyperalgesia was only partially blocked (Figure 5C). Interestingly, intrathecal administration of saclofen had no effect on the analgesic action of oxycodone after a single injection at D15 (Figure S5A–B). Moreover, in order to demonstrate the specific involvement of up-regulated $GABA_B$ receptor function in the long-lasting analgesic effect of chronic oxycodone injection, we assessed the effect of an intrathecal administration of saclofen after a single injection (D15) and after chronic administration of morphine (D19). These results indicate that saclofen does not inhibit the effect of acute or chronic treatment of morphine on mechanical sensitivity in vincristine-treated rats (Figure S6A–B).

Discussion

The aim of this study was two-fold: to better understand the mechanisms underlying the analgesic effect of both oxycodone and morphine; and to compare these mechanisms of action in a model of neuropathic pain induced by vincristine. Our results demonstrate that a large number of genes are dysregulated after opioid analgesic treatment in vincristine-treated animals. These findings also suggest an increased GABAergic tone in the superficial dorsal horn induced by oxycodone treatment that is mediated by $GABA_{B2}$ receptor; this would explain the enhanced alleviation of chronic neuropathic pain that we observed.

Attenuation of the analgesic effect of morphine

Vincristine-treated rats displayed all of the behavioural characteristics of peripheral sensory neuropathy observed in this model, *i.e.* static and dynamic mechanical allodynia and hyperalgesia [15,17,24,32]. As previously described in both patients and animal models [2,3,5,8,33–35], we observed that administration of oxycodone or morphine alleviated symptoms of chronic neuropathic pain. However, repeated morphine injections lead to an attenuation of its analgesic effect, while oxycodone maintained a strong analgesic effect even after multiple injections. These observations are consistent with previous reports demonstrating morphine's inefficacy in the symptomatic relief of neuropathic

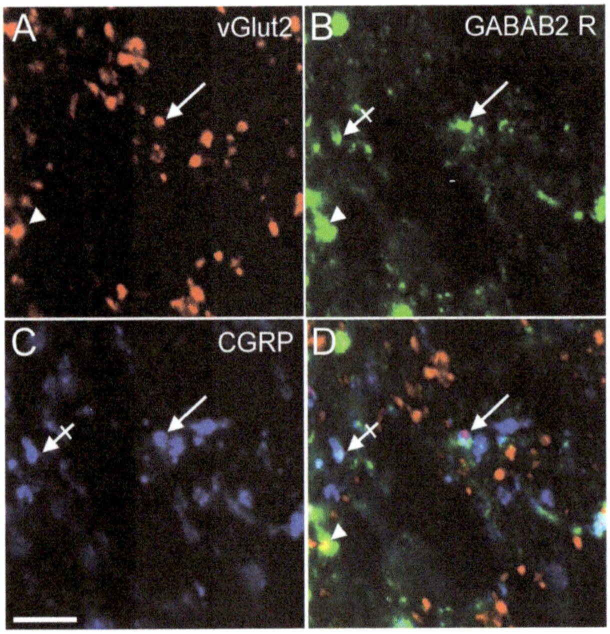

Figure 4. The $GABA_{B2}$ receptor is located in CGRP-positive glutamatergic presynaptic terminals. Confocal images of triple immunostainings, comprised of vGlut2 (A, red), $GABA_{B2}$ receptor (B, green) and CGRP (C, blue), in a vincristine-oxycodone treated animal. D is a merge of images A–C. We observed $GABA_{B2}$ receptor expression in CGRP-immunoreactive glutamatergic presynaptic terminals (arrow). Glutamatergic presynaptic terminals immunoreactive for $GABA_{B2}$ receptor were also observed (arrowhead), as well as CGRP-positive $GABA_{B2}$ terminals (crossed arrow). Scale bar A-D = 5 μm.

pain in STZ-induced diabetes models [36,37], as well as an observed slower rate of tolerance to oxycodone-6-oxyme (an oxycodone derivative compound) as compared to morphine in naive animals [18]. While morphine and oxycodone are both μ-opioid receptor agonists, previous studies have shown that these two opioids exhibit different efficiencies and distinct analgesic profiles in various pain models, such as the bone cancer pain model and the SNL model [33]. A more recent study from that same group has shown that modification of the μ-opioid receptor is responsible for the distinct analgesic effect of oxycodone and morphine, and that μ-opioid receptor activation is less attenuated by oxycodone than by morphine [38]. Although the authors of that study dismiss the hypothesis that, in the bone cancer pain model, a change in the number of μ-opioid receptors or a change in the μ-opioid receptor binding affinity might be the underlying mechanisms, these hypotheses remain valid in our model. Finally, as proposed by Nakamura *et al.*, the differential activation of the μ-opioid receptor by oxycodone or morphine might be due to the mechanism that regulates GTP binding onto G proteins in the μ-receptor [38]. These changes in μ-opioid receptor activation might produce subtle but functionally important variations in intracellular cascade signalling, possibly leading to a modified gene expression that is observed after oxycodone treatment, but not after morphine treatment.

Previous studies have reported that repeated opiate administration alters gene expression in different regions of the nervous system in rodents [29,30,39], which may contribute to plastic changes associated with tolerance. It has also been shown that morphine treatment alters the expression of several receptors in the amygdala, including the $GABA_A$ receptor [29]. Moreover, chronic treatment of morphine leads to a decrease in GABAergic tonus [40,41]. Our DNA microarray analysis confirms this down-regulation of $GABA_A$ receptor subunits (β3 and γ1) in DRG neurons induced by chronic morphine treatment. The functional consequence of this decreased $GABA_A$ receptor synthesis in DRG neurons could be a reduction in the spinal pre-synaptic GABAergic tone, ultimately resulting in a persistent alteration of synaptic signalling.

DNA microarray analysis as a tool to dissect molecular mechanisms involved in opioid treatment

Our DNA microarray experiment was designed to address distinct yet complementary questions. First, which genes are differentially expressed by vincristine treatment at the end of the chronic analgesic treatment? This analysis is important to comprehending the mechanisms underlying the maintenance of neuropathic pain symptoms associated with vincristine treatment. Since our DNA microarray experiment was performed days after the end of the treatment and several weeks after the development of neuropathic pain [17,28], these genes are likely to be involved in the maintenance (and not development) of neuropathic pain symptoms. Second, which genes are differentially expressed in control animals when they are chronically treated with oxycodone or morphine? As stated above, chronic morphine treatment leads to an attenuation of its analgesic effect and the development of tolerance. Understanding the different targets of gene alteration induced by morphine at a steady state is important to clarifying the molecular mechanisms involved in the drug action and the development of this tolerance. As a final point, analysing the genes differentially expressed by oxycodone or morphine treatment in vincristine-treated animals provides us with further insight into the molecular mechanisms controlling the sustained analgesic effect of opioids in the neuropathic pain state.

Although these points are all important to address, their thorough pursuit was beyond the scope of this study. Future studies that aim to inquire into these different questions should greatly benefit from the complete database of dysregulated genes that we report here.

The $GABA_B$ receptor is involved in the long-lasting analgesic effect of oxycodone

The spinal cord is the site of both pro- and anti-nociceptive modulations. Released from primary afferent fibres, Substance P (SP), CGRP and glutamate exacerbate neuronal activity and have a pro-nociceptive action. Conversely, activation of $GABA_B$ receptors inhibits voltage-dependent calcium channels via G-protein-coupled adenylate cyclase [42,43] and reduces the release of excitatory amino acids and SP from primary afferent terminals in the spinal cord [44,45]. Therefore, an increase in the GABAergic tonus decreases neuronal excitation and has an anti-nociceptive property.

In vincristine-treated animals (but not in naive animals), chronic treatment with oxycodone specifically induced an up-regulation of $GABA_{B2}$ receptor expression as compared to vincristine-morphine treated rats. We also found that $GABA_{B2}$ receptors were expressed in superficial layers of the dorsal horn, particularly in glutamatergic presynaptic terminals containing CGRP. As previously reported, the up-regulation of $GABA_B$ receptors in DRG neurons leads to an increase in inhibitory transmission tonus and a decrease in excitatory transmission tonus, which could explain the long-lasting analgesic effect observed during chronic oxycodone administration in neuropathic pain conditions. Our hypothesis is that the up-regulation of $GABA_{B2}$ receptor expression in CGRP

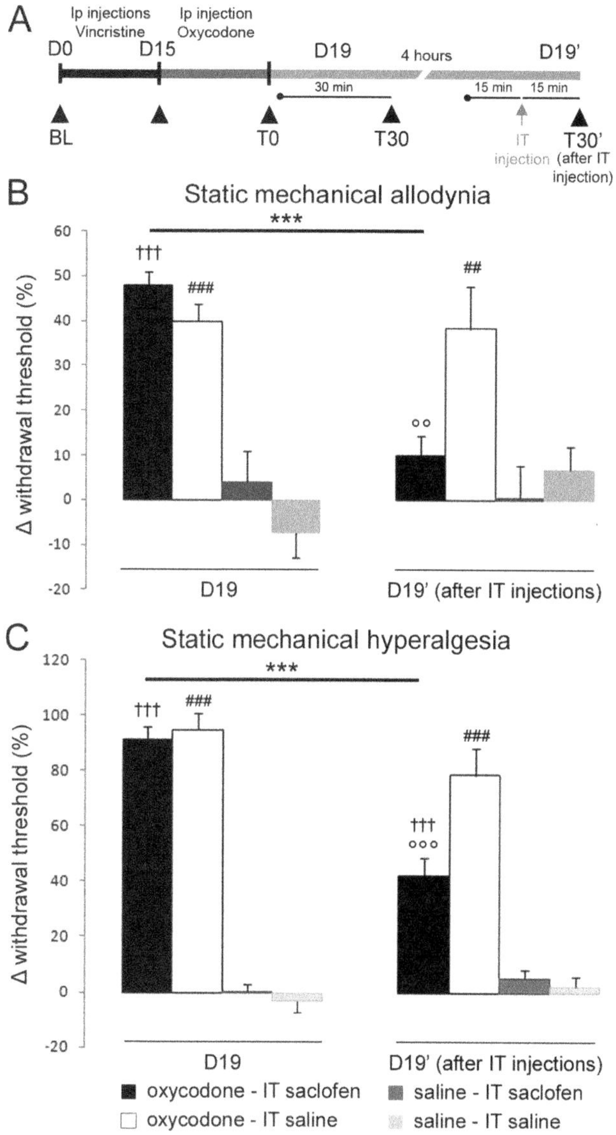

Figure 5. The long-lasting analgesic effect of oxycodone is reversed by i.t. injection of a GABA$_B$ antagonist. A: Schematic representation of the experimental paradigm. Rats received i.p. injection of vincristine (black horizontal bar). The oxycodone treatment started at D15, while animals presented mechanical hyperalgesia (dark grey horizontal bar). Behavioural tests, illustrated by black triangles, were performed at D0 (BL), D15 and D19, before (T0) and 30 min after (T30) oxycodone injection, to control for the analgesic effect of oxycodone. The functional involvement of GABA$_B$ receptors in this long-asting analgesic effect of oxycodone was tested by intrathecal (i.t.) injection of saclofen (10 μg) versus saline injection (grey arrow), 4 hours after the previous test (D19). Rats were injected again with oxycodone or saline (D19'). Fifteen minutes after this second injection, rats were injected intrathecally with saclofen or saline and tested 15 minutes after the i.t. injection (T30'). B, C: Effect of saclofen intrathecal injection on oxycodone's long-lasting effect on static mechanical allodynia (B) and static mechanical hyperalgesia (C). Results are expressed as mean δ withdrawal threshold ± SEM. The δ-withdrawal threshold was calculated using individual values as follows: $\left[\frac{(T30-T0)}{T0}\right] \times 100$ at D19 and $\left[\frac{(T30'-T0)}{T0}\right] \times 100$ at D19'. The results confirm the analgesic action of oxycodone (left panel, D19), and show that saclofen completely reversed the analgesic action on mechanical allodynia (B), while only partially reversing the effect on static mechanical hyperalgesia (C). (n = 6, vincristine-oxycodone-saclofen treated rats; n = 6, vincristine-oxycodone-saline treated rats; n = 6 vincristine-saline-saclofen treated rats; n = 6, vincristine-saline-saline treated rats). ***$p < 0.001$: vincristine-oxycodone treated rats compared at different time points; ## $P < 0.01$, ### $p < 0.001$: vincristine-oxycodone treated rats vs. vincristine-saline treated rats; °°$p < 0.01$, °°°$p < 0.001$: vincristine-oxycodone-saclofen treated rats vs. vincristine-oxycodone-saline treated rats; ††† $p < 0.001$: vincristine-oxycodone-saclofen treated rats vs. vincristine-saline-saclofen treated rats.

sensory afferents observed after chronic oxycodone treatment may counteract the increased neuronal excitability induced by vincristine treatment. The inhibition of oxycodone's analgesic effect following an intrathecal injection of a selective GABAB receptor antagonist confirms this hypothesis. Therefore, the alleviating effect of oxycodone in neuropathic pain condition seems to involve the spinal GABAergic tonus though GABAB receptors.

Although functional GABA$_B$ receptors must be comprised of a heterodimer of GABA$_{B1}$ and GABA$_{B2}$ receptor subtypes to be active [31], some studies report tissues in which the expression of GABA$_{B1}$ and GABA$_{B2}$ receptors do not overlap. For example, some tissues only express GABA$_{B1}$ receptor subtypes (and not GABA$_{B2}$), suggesting a distinct role for GABA$_{B1}$ in the absence of GABA$_{B2}$ [25]. In addition, independent maturation of GABA$_{B1}$ and GABA$_{B2}$ receptor subtypes has been observed during postnatal development in the brain [46]. It has been demonstrated that no biochemical or functional responses from the GABA$_B$ receptor (or homomeric GBR1 or GBR2) are detectable in the brain or retina of a GABA$_{B1}$ -/- mouse mutant. [47–51]. There is a partial preservation of the GABA$_{B2}$ receptor subtype staining in the brain of GABA$_{B1}$ -/- juvenile mice, suggesting a functional role for GABA$_{B2}$ receptor subtype proteins in the immature brain, in addition to its contribution as a dimer in GABA$_B$ receptor complexes[46]. Together, these data suggest that the GABA$_{B1}$ and GABA$_{B2}$ receptor subtypes may play other roles, independent of the presence of their partner. We could not exclude a different role for the up-regulation of the GABA$_{B2}$ receptor subtype in our model.

In conclusion, this study provides evidence that treatment with oxycodone produces a profound anti-nociceptive effect under a neuropathic pain-like state. Furthermore, our results reveal a thorough list of genes that are dysregulated in DRGs at the end of chronic analgesic treatment. These findings will be indispensable to future studies that aim to understand the analgesic effects of oxycodone as compared to morphine in chemotherapy-induced neuropathic pain.

Supporting Information

Figure S1 Anti-GABA$_{B2}$ receptor antibody specificity. A: Representative western blotting of one spinal cord lysate, using the anti-GABA$_{B2}$ receptor antibody. A single band was observed at 106–110 kDa, corresponding to the expected weight of the GABA$_{B2}$ receptor protein. B: Anti-GABA$_{B2}$ immunostaining on a spinal cord section. Representative example of GABA$_{B2}$ staining in the dorsal horn, located primarily in the superficial laminae (arrowheads). Some staining was observed in deep laminae as well (arrows). Spinal cord sections incubated without primary antibody showed no staining (data not shown).

Figure S2 Time-course of dynamic mechanical sensitivity. At D15, rats in all vincristine-treated groups suffered from dynamic mechanical allodynia (A) and hyperesthesia (B). A: Mean number of positive responses to the smooth paint-brush test. The measured dynamic mechanical allodynia was totally reversed after a single injection of morphine or oxycodone, although only oxycodone maintained an analgesic effect at the end of the chronic analgesic treatment (D19). B: Mean number of positive responses to the rough paint-brush test. Only oxycodone maintained an analgesic effect at the end of the chronic analgesic treatment (D19). All data are expressed as mean ± SEM. (n = 7 vincristine-morphine treated rats; n = 6 saline-morphine treated rats), (n = 7 vincristine-oxycodone treated rats; n = 6 saline-oxycodone treated rats), and (n = 7 vincristine-saline treated rats; n = 6 saline-saline treated rats). *$p<0.05$: vincristine-oxycodone treated rats vs. vincristine-morphine treated rats; † $p<0.05$, †† $p<0.01$: vincristine-oxycodone treated rats vs. vincristine-saline treated rats; § $p<0.05$: vincristine-morphine treated rats vs. vincristine-saline treated rats. For figure clarity, the statistical significance symbols for the vincristine vs. saline groups are not shown.

Figure S3 Colocalisation between $GABA_{B1}$ and $GABA_{B2}$ receptors in sensory neurons. A–F: Double immunostaining showing the colocalisation of $GABA_{B1}$ receptor (A, D) with $GABA_{B2}$ receptor (D, E) in the DRG (A–C) and in the spinal dorsal horn (D–F) of a representative vincristine-oxycodone treated animal. C and F are merged images of A and B, and D and E, respectively. The results indicate colocalisation of both $GABA_{B1}$ and $GABA_{B2}$ in small DRG neurons (arrow in A, B and C) and in the superficial spinal dorsal horn (arrowheads in the magnification of D, E and F). A–C, scale bar = 30 μm; D–F, scale bar = 150 μm.

Figure S4 The $GABA_{B2}$ receptor and CGRP colocalise in superficial laminae of the dorsal horn. A–C: Double immunostaining showing CGRP (A, C, red)/$GABA_{B2}$ receptor (B, C, green) positive fibres in a vincristine-oxycodone treated animal. C is a merged image of A and B, showing colocalisation in laminae I and II. D–F: Double immunostaining of IB4 (D, F, green)/ $GABA_{B2}$ receptor (E, F, red) indicates little colocalisation in a vincristine-oxycodone treated animal. Colocalisation was observed principally in laminae II 'out'. F is a merge of D and E. Scale bar = 100 μm.

Figure S5 The acute analgesic effect of oxycodone is not reversed by i.t. injection of a $GABA_B$ antagonist. A, B: Effect of intrathecal saclofen (10 μg) injection on the acute analgesic effect of oxycodone on static mechanical allodynia (A) and static mechanical hyperalgesia (B). After i.t. injection of saclofen, the analgesic effect of a single injection of oxycodone at D15 was not modified (ns: vincristine-oxycodone-saclofen treated rats vs. vincristine-oxycodone-saline treated rats). All data are expressed as mean ± SEM. ††† $p<0.001$: vincristine-oxycodone-saclofen treated rats vs. vincristine-saline-saclofen treated rats; ### $p<0.001$: vincristine-oxycodone-saline treated rats vs. vincristine-saline-saline treated rats.

Figure S6 The analgesic effect of morphine is not modified by i.t. injection of a GABA $_B$ antagonist. A, B: Effect of intrathecal saclofen (10 μg) injection on the acute (D15) and chronic (D19) analgesic effect of morphine on static mechanical allodynia (A) and static mechanical hyperalgesia (B). After i.t. injection of saclofen, the analgesic effect of a single injection of morphine at D15 was not modified (ns: vincristine-morphine-saclofen treated rats vs. vincristine-morphine-saline treated rats). The analgesic effect of morphine was decreased at D19 as compared to D15 (as expected), and was not modified by the i.t. injection of saclofen (ns). All data are expressed as mean ± SEM. § $p<0.05$, §§§ $p<0.001$: vincristine-morphine-saclofen treated rats vs. vincristine-saline-saclofen treated rats; # $p<0.05$, ### $p<0.001$: vincristine-morphine-saline treated rats vs. vincristine-saline-saline treated rats.

Table S1 Complete list of genes dysregulated at the end of analgesic treatment. Data are illustrated as follows: 1) Gene accession number; 2) Gene symbol; 3) Mean expression of the genes for the six different groups; 4) ident: an identifying z-z-z for the statistical analysis significance (z corresponding to the three tests; z = 1 if the null hypothesis is rejected with a risk of 5% or z = 0); 5) results of variance analysis between vincristine and control: p-value; 6) results of Student's t test between morphine and oxycodone in vincristine-treated rats: p-value and expression difference (morphine – oxycodone); 7) results of Student's t test between morphine and oxycodone in control rats: p-value and expression difference (morphine – oxycodone). Peach highlight corresponds to an identifying number of 1_1_1 *i.e.* with a statistically significant difference between vincristine and control, and morphine and oxycodone in vincristine-treated rats, and between morphine and oxycodone in control rats. Yellow highlight corresponds to an identifying number of 1_0_1 *i.e.* with a statistically significant difference between vincristine and control, and between morphine and oxycodone in control rats. Green highlight corresponds to an identifying number of 1_0_0 *i.e.* with a statistically significant difference between vincristine and control, only. Purple highlight corresponds to an identifying number of 0_1_1 *i.e.* with a statistically significant difference between morphine and oxycodone in vincristine-treated rats, and between morphine and oxycodone in control rats. Blue highlight corresponds to an identifying number of 0_1_0 *i.e.* with a statistically significant difference between morphine and oxycodone in vincristine-treated rats, only. In this group, there was significant differential expression of several genes corresponding to the $GABA_A$ R subunit β3 (Gabrb3), the $GABA_A$ R subunit γ1 (Gabrg1), and the $GABA_{B2}$ receptor (Gabbr2). Dark blue highlight corresponds to an identifying number of 0_0_1 *i.e.* with a statistically significant difference between morphine and oxycodone in control rats, only.

Acknowledgments

The authors thank Mundipharma laboratory for kindly providing oxycodone for this study. We also thank Brandon Loveall of 'Improvence' for English proofreading of the manuscript.

Author Contributions

Conceived and designed the experiments: KT BC SBM SP. Performed the experiments: KT FM SD. Analyzed the data: KT IR. Wrote the paper: KT SP.

References

1. Bouhassira D, Lanteri-Minet M, Attal N, Laurent B, Touboul C (2008) Prevalence of chronic pain with neuropathic characteristics in the general population. Pain 136: 380–387.
2. Watson CP and Babul N (1998) Efficacy of oxycodone in neuropathic pain: a randomized trial in postherpetic neuralgia. Neurology 50: 1837–1841.

3. Watson CP, Moulin D, Watt-Watson J, Gordon A, Eisenhoffer J (2003) Controlled-release oxycodone relieves neuropathic pain: a randomized controlled trial in painful diabetic neuropathy. Pain 105: 71–78.
4. Falk E (1917) Eukodal, ein neues Narkotikum. Munchener Medizinische Wochenschrift 20: 381–384.
5. Lenz H, Sandvik L, Qvigstad E, Bjerkelund CE, Raeder J (2009) A comparison of intravenous oxycodone and intravenous morphine in patient-controlled postoperative analgesia after laparoscopic hysterectomy. Anesth Analg 109: 1279–1283.
6. Curtis GB, Johnson GH, Clark P, Taylor R, Brown J, et al. (1999) Relative potency of controlled-release oxycodone and controlled-release morphine in a postoperative pain model. Eur J Clin Pharmacol 55: 425–429.
7. Bruera E, Belzile M, Pituskin E, Fainsinger R, Darke A, et al. (1998) Randomized, double-blind, cross-over trial comparing safety and efficacy of oral controlled-release oxycodone with controlled-release morphine in patients with cancer pain. J Clin Oncol 16: 3222–3229.
8. Mucci-LoRusso P, Berman BS, Silberstein PT, Citron ML, Bressler L, et al. (1998) Controlled-release oxycodone compared with controlled-release morphine in the treatment of cancer pain: a randomized, double-blind, parallel-group study. Eur J Pain 2: 239–249.
9. Gatti A, Sabato AF, Carucci A, Bertini L, Mammucari M, et al. (2009) Adequacy assessment of oxycodone/paracetamol (acetaminophen) in multimodal chronic pain: a prospective observational study. Clin Drug Investig 29 Suppl 1: 31–40.
10. Khoromi S, Cui L, Nackers L, Max MB (2007) Morphine, nortriptyline and their combination vs. placebo in patients with chronic lumbar root pain. Pain 130: 66–75.
11. Barrera-Chacon JM, Mendez-Suarez JL, Jauregui-Abrisqueta ML, Palazon R, Barbara-Bataller E, et al. (2011) Oxycodone improves pain control and quality of life in anticonvulsant-pretreated spinal cord-injured patients with neuropathic pain. Spinal Cord 49: 36–42.
12. Casey EB, Jellife AM, Le Quesne PM, Millett YL (1973) Vincristine neuropathy. Clinical and electrophysiological observations. Brain 96: 69–86.
13. Sandler SG, Tobin W, Henderson ES (1969) Vincristine-induced neuropathy. A clinical study of fifty leukemic patients. Neurology 19: 367–374.
14. Aley KO, Reichling DB, Levine JD (1996) Vincristine hyperalgesia in the rat: a model of painful vincristine neuropathy in humans. Neuroscience 73: 259–265.
15. Authier N, Gillet JP, Fialip J, Eschalier A, Coudore F (2003) A new animal model of vincristine-induced nociceptive peripheral neuropathy. Neurotoxicology 24: 797–805.
16. Nozaki-Taguchi N, Chaplan SR, Higuera ES, Ajakwe RC, Yaksh TL (2001) Vincristine-induced allodynia in the rat. Pain 93: 69–76.
17. Weng HR, Cordella JV, Dougherty PM (2003) Changes in sensory processing in the spinal dorsal horn accompany vincristine-induced hyperalgesia and allodynia. Pain 103: 131–138.
18. Kiraly KP, Riba P, D'Addario C, Di BM, Landuzzi D, et al. (2006) Alterations in prodynorphin gene expression and dynorphin levels in different brain regions after chronic administration of 14-methoxymetopon and oxycodone-6-oxime. Brain Res Bull 70: 233–239.
19. Mestre C, Pelissier T, Fialip J, Wilcox G, Eschalier A (1994) A method to perform direct transcutaneous intrathecal injection in rats. J Pharmacol Toxicol Methods 32: 197–200.
20. Marchand F, Ardid D, Chapuy E, Alloui A, Jourdan D, et al. (2003) Evidence for an involvement of supraspinal delta- and spinal mu-opioid receptors in the antihyperalgesic effect of chronically administered clomipramine in mononeuropathic rats. J Pharmacol Exp Ther 307: 268–274.
21. Malan TP, Mata HP, Porreca F (2002) Spinal GABA(A) and GABA(B) receptor pharmacology in a rat model of neuropathic pain. Anesthesiology 96: 1161–1167.
22. Park JH, Han JB, Kim SK, Park JH, Go DH, et al. (2010) Spinal GABA receptors mediate the suppressive effect of electroacupuncture on cold allodynia in rats. Brain Res 1322: 24–29.
23. Thibault K, Calvino B, Pezet S (2011) Characterisation of sensory abnormalities observed in an animal model of multiple sclerosis: a behavioural and pharmacological study. Eur J Pain 15: 231–16.
24. Thibault K, Bonnard E, Dubacq S, Fournié-Zaluski MC, Roques B, et al. (2008) Antinociceptive and anti-allodynic effects of oral PL37, a complete inhibitor of enkephalin-catabolizing enzymes, in a rat model of peripheral neuropathic pain induced by vincristine. Eur J Pharmacol 600: 71–77.
25. Calver AR, Medhurst AD, Robbins MJ, Charles KJ, Evans ML, et al. (2000) The expression of GABA(B1) and GABA(B2) receptor subunits in the cNS differs from that in peripheral tissues. Neuroscience 100: 155–170.
26. Charles KJ, Evans ML, Robbins MJ, Calver AR, Leslie RA, et al. (2001) Comparative immunohistochemical localisation of GABA(B1a), GABA(B1b) and GABA(B2) subunits in rat brain, spinal cord and dorsal root ganglion. Neuroscience 106: 447–467.
27. Bartoi T, Rigbolt KT, Du D, Kohr G, Blagoev B, et al. (2010) GABAB receptor constituents revealed by tandem affinity purification from transgenic mice. J Biol Chem 285: 20625–20633.
28. Thibault K, Van Steenwinckel J, Brisorgueil MJ, Fischer J, Hamon M, et al. (2008) Serotonin 5-HT2A receptor involvement and Fos expression at the spinal level in vincristine-induced neuropathy in the rat. Pain 140: 305–322.
29. Rodriguez Parkitna JM, Bilecki W, Mierzejewski P, Stefanski R, Ligeza A, et al. (2004) Effects of morphine on gene expression in the rat amygdala. J Neurochem 91: 38–48.
30. Ammon-Treiber S and Hollt V (2005) Morphine-induced changes of gene expression in the brain. Addict Biol 10: 81–89.
31. Goudet C, Magnaghi V, Landry M, Nagy F, Gereau RW, et al. (2009) Metabotropic receptors for glutamate and GABA in pain. Brain Res Rev 60: 43–56.
32. Authier N, Coudore F, Eschalier A, Fialip J (1999) Pain related behaviour during vincristine-induced neuropathy in rats. Neuroreport 10: 965–968.
33. Minami K, Hasegawa M, Ito H, Nakamura A, Tomii T, et al. (2009) Morphine, oxycodone, and fentanyl exhibit different analgesic profiles in mouse pain models. J Pharmacol Sci 111: 60–72.
34. Kato A, Minami K, Ito H, Tomii T, Matsumoto M, et al. (2008) Oxycodone-induced analgesic effects in a bone cancer pain model in mice. Oncology 74 Suppl 1: 55–60.
35. Kaplan R, Parris WC, Citron ML, Zhukovsky D, Reder RF, et al. (1998) Comparison of controlled-release and immediate-release oxycodone tablets in patients with cancer pain. J Clin Oncol 16: 3230–3237.
36. Courteix C, Bourget P, Caussade F, Bardin M, Coudore F, et al. (1998) Is the reduced efficacy of morphine in diabetic rats caused by alterations of opiate receptors or of morphine pharmacokinetics? J Pharmacol Exp Ther 285: 63–70.
37. Malcangio M and Tomlinson DR (1998) A pharmacologic analysis of mechanical hyperalgesia in streptozotocin/diabetic rats. Pain 76: 151–157.
38. Nakamura A, Hasegawa M, Minami K, Kanbara T, Tomii T, et al. (2013) Differential activation of the mu-opioid receptor by oxycodone and morphine in pain-related brain regions in a bone cancer pain model. Br J Pharmacol 168: 375–388.
39. Tapocik JD, Letwin N, Mayo CL, Frank B, Luu T, et al. (2009) Identification of candidate genes and gene networks specifically associated with analgesic tolerance to morphine. J Neurosci 29: 5295–5307.
40. Chen YP, Chen SR, Pan HL (2005) Effect of morphine on deep dorsal horn projection neurons depends on spinal GABAergic and glycinergic tone: implications for reduced opioid effect in neuropathic pain. J Pharmacol Exp Ther 315: 696–703.
41. Dunbar SA, Karamian I, Yeatman A, Zhang J (2006) Effects of recurrent withdrawal on spinal GABA release during chronic morphine infusion in the rat. Eur J Pharmacol 535: 152–156.
42. Holz GG, Kream RM, Spiegel A, Dunlap K (1989) G proteins couple alpha-adrenergic and GABAb receptors to inhibition of peptide secretion from peripheral sensory neurons. J Neurosci 9: 657–666.
43. Holz GG, Rane SG, Dunlap K (1986) GTP-binding proteins mediate transmitter inhibition of voltage-dependent calcium channels. Nature 319: 670–672.
44. Fox S, Krnjevic K, Morris ME, Puil E, Werman R (1978) Action of baclofen on mammalian synaptic transmission. Neuroscience 3: 495–515.
45. Malcangio M and Bowery NG (1993) Gamma-aminobutyric acidB, but not gamma-aminobutyric acidA receptor activation, inhibits electrically evoked substance P-like immunoreactivity release from the rat spinal cord in vitro. J Pharmacol Exp Ther 266: 1490–1496.
46. Fritschy JM, Sidler C, Parpan F, Gassmann M, Kaupmann K, et al. (2004) Independent maturation of the GABA(B) receptor subunits GABA(B1) and GABA(B2) during postnatal development in rodent brain. J Comp Neurol 477: 235–252.
47. Benke D, Honer M, Michel C, Bettler B, Mohler H (1999) gamma-aminobutyric acid type B receptor splice variant proteins GBR1a and GBR1b are both associated with GBR2 in situ and display differential regional and subcellular distribution. J Biol Chem 274: 27323–27330.
48. Benke D, Michel C, Mohler H (2002) Structure of GABAB receptors in rat retina. J Recept Signal Transduct Res 22: 253–266.
49. Prosser HM, Gill CH, Hirst WD, Grau E, Robbins M, et al. (2001) Epileptogenesis and enhanced prepulse inhibition in GABA(B1)-deficient mice. Mol Cell Neurosci 17: 1059–1070.
50. Schuler V, Luscher C, Blanchet C, Klix N, Sansig G, et al. (2001) Epilepsy, hyperalgesia, impaired memory, and loss of pre- and postsynaptic GABA(B) responses in mice lacking GABA(B(1)). Neuron 31: 47–58.
51. Queva C, Bremner-Danielsen M, Edlund A, Ekstrand AJ, Elg S, et al. (2003) Effects of GABA agonists on body temperature regulation in GABA(B(1))-/- mice. Br J Pharmacol 140: 315–322.

6

Molecular Hydrogen Attenuates Neuropathic Pain in Mice

Masanori Kawaguchi, Yasushi Satoh*, Yukiko Otsubo, Tomiei Kazama

Department of Anesthesiology, National Defense Medical College, Tokorozawa, Saitama, Japan

Abstract

Neuropathic pain remains intractable and the development of new therapeutic strategies are urgently required. Accumulating evidence indicates that overproduction of oxidative stress is a key event in the pathogenesis of neuropathic pain. However, repeated intra-peritoneal or intrathecal injections of antioxidants are unsuitable for continuous use in therapy. Here we show a novel therapeutic method against neuropathic pain: drinking water containing molecular hydrogen (H_2) as antioxidant. The effect of hydrogen on neuropathic pain was investigated using a partial sciatic nerve ligation model in mice. As indicators of neuropathic pain, temporal aspects of mechanical allodynia and thermal hyperalgesia were analysed for 3 weeks after ligation. Mechanical allodynia and thermal hyperalgesia were measured using the von Frey test and the plantar test, respectively. When mice were allowed to drink water containing hydrogen at a saturated level *ad libitum* after ligation, both allodynia and hyperalgesia were alleviated. These symptoms were also alleviated when hydrogen was administered only for the induction phase (from day 0 to 4 after ligation). When hydrogen was administered only for the maintenance phase (from day 4 to 21 after ligation), hyperalgesia but not allodynia was alleviated. Immunohistochemical staining for the oxidative stress marker, 4-hydroxy-2-nonenal and 8-hydroxydeoxyguanosine, showed that hydrogen administration suppressed oxidative stress induced by ligation in the spinal cord and the dorsal root ganglion. In conclusion, oral administration of hydrogen water may be useful for alleviating neuropathic pain in a clinical setting.

Editor: Shao-Jun Tang, University of Texas Medical Branch, United States of America

Funding: This work was supported by JSPS (Japan Society for the Promotion of Science, Tokyo, Japan; Grant number 25293331). The funders had no role in study design, data collection and analysis, decision to publish, or preparation of the manuscript.

Competing Interests: The authors have declared that no competing interests exist.

* Email: wndlt3@gmail.com

Introduction

Neuropathic pain is one of abnormal chronic pain that is produced after trauma or disease of the peripheral or the central nervous system. The common symptoms of neuropathic pain are mechanical allodynia, a painful response to innocuous tactile stimuli, and hyperalgesia, a decrease in nociceptive thresholds to the stimuli. Neuropathic pain remains intractable and many patients suffering from this disease exact a tremendous cost to the economy. Anti-inflammatories including non-steroidal anti-inflammatory drug and some narcotic analgesics are not effective for managing neuropathic pain and the need for higher dosages of these drugs leads to unsatisfactory side effects. Therefore, the development of new therapeutic strategies is urgently required.

Reactive oxygen species (ROS) are reported to be involved in the pathomechanism of neuropathic pain [1–4]. Although the mechanism by which excessive ROS produce pain is largely unclear, antioxidants have received attention as novel analgesics against neuropathic pain [3]. It was reported that systemic administration of antioxidants produced an analgesic effect in animal models of neuropathic pain. For instance, phenyl-*N-tert*-butylnitrone (PBN), 5,5-dimethylpyrroline-N-oxide, vitamin E, and 4-hydroxy-2,2,6,6-tetramethylpiperidine-1-oxyl (TEMPOL) could ameliorate the behavioral signs of neuropathic pain [5–8]. In these reports, analgesia was extended by repeated injections of drugs at short intervals. Thus, if these agents are to be useful in therapy, they will have to be given continuously or at relatively short interval, which is unsuitable for clinical medication.

Molecular hydrogen has recently received attention as a novel antioxidant with high efficacy and no currently known side effect [9]. Because of its small size and electrically neutral properties, molecular hydrogen can reach target organs easily. Drinking water with dissolved hydrogen has been reported to be effective in preventing oxidative stress in some animal models of other diseases [10–12]. In addition, hydrogen does not accumulate in living cells nor produce noxious metabolites, which sometimes cause distress in other antioxidants.

ROS include hydroxyl radical, hydrogen peroxide, superoxide, nitric oxide, and nitroperoxide. Among them, hydroxyl radical is extremely toxic and has no currently known beneficial role. Furthermore, no defense system against hydroxyl radical has been found in mammalian cells. On the other hand, hydrogen peroxide, superoxide, and nitric oxide have important roles in various biological processes at low concentrations [13–15]. Thus, there is a concern about continuous use of antioxidant that might cause serious side effect. Hydrogen is a more attractive antioxidant, in that unlike other antioxidants it can selectively neutralize the hydroxyl radical, while having minimal effect on beneficial ROS [9].

In the present study, we show that molecular hydrogen can ameliorate mechanical allodynia and thermal hyperalgesia. Our results indicate that hydrogen administration by the oral pathway may have potential for the management of neuropathic pain.

Materials and Methods

Ethics Statement

The care and use of all mice in this study was carried out in accordance with institutional ethical guidelines for animal experiments of the National Defense Medical College (Tokorozawa, Saitama, Japan), and were approved by the Committee for Animal Research at the National Defense Medical College. Guidelines of the Committee for Research and Ethical Issues of the International Association for the Study of Pain [16] was strictly adhered to in this study.

Animals

We used C57BL/6 mice at 8-weeks old when subjected to nerve ligation. These mice were maintained on a 12-h light–dark cycle (lights on from 07:00 to 19:00) with room temperature at 21±1°C. They had access to water and food *ad libitum.*

Hydrogen Water

Hydrogen water was produced by Blue Mercury Inc. (Tokyo, Japan), which contained more than 0.6 mM hydrogen. Hydrogen water was put in an aluminium bottle (60 ml) to maintain the concentration of hydrogen. Mice were allowed to drink hydrogen water *ad libitum* for indicated time. Hydrogen water was exchanged every day to keep the hydrogen concentration constant. Control groups were supplied with distilled water. There was no significant difference in the amounts of water consumed between hydrogen group and control group (3.87±0.13 vs. 3.91±0.15 ml, mean ± SEM, n = 12 mice for each). Amount of water consumed was monitored by recording the volume of water in the bottle.

Mouse Study Design

Siblings from the same litter were randomly allocated into one of the following groups so that each group was balanced on littermate. Ligation group: n = 12, Ligation+hydrogen (day 0–21) group: n = 12, Ligation+hydrogen (day 0–4) group: n = 12, Ligation+hydrogen (day 4–21) group: n = 12, Sham group: n = 12, Sham+hydrogen (day 0–21) group: n = 12.

Nerve Injury Pain Model

Throughout the experiment, we used a partial sciatic nerve ligation (PSNL) model as a neuropathic pain model (Seltzer model) as described previously [17]. Briefly, the sciatic nerve located in the right hind paw was exposed via a small incision and approximately 1/3–1/2 the diameter of the nerve was tightly ligated with an 8–0 silk suture. PSNL caused a fast and pronounced development of mechanical allodynia and thermal hyperalgesia in mice. In the sham-operated groups, sciatic nerves were exposed without ligation. The pain behaviors were assessed by the von Frey test and the plantar test for mechanical allodynia and thermal hyperalgesia, respectively. These behaviors were tested before (Pre) and after PSNL operation (day 1, 4, 7, 14, and 21). Measurement was carried out by an investigator blinded to the hydrogen treatment.

Measurement of Mechanical Allodynia

To quantify mechanical allodynia, paw withdrawal responses to mechanical stimulation were assessed with von Frey filaments as previously described [17]. Briefly, mice were habituated for at least 1 h prior to testing in a clear acrylic cylinder (20 cm in height and 10 cm in diameter) on an elevated mesh floor. Calibrated von Frey filaments (North Coast Medical, Gilroy, CA) were then applied through the mesh to the plantar surface on hind paw. Filaments were applied for 1 s and this was repeated 5 times at a frequency of 0.5 Hz. Filaments were pressed until the filament bent. Paw movements associated with locomotion or weight shifting were not counted as responses. The lightest filament of 0.008 g bending force was initially applied with progressively increasing force (0.02, 0.04, 0.07, 0.16, 0.4, 0.6, 1.0, 1.4, and 2.0 g). Measurement was finished when paw withdrawals were evoked at least three withdrawals out of five applications, and the calibrated bending force of the filament was defined as the paw withdrawal threshold.

Measurement of Thermal (Heat) Hyperalgesia

Response to thermal stimulation were measured as previously described [18] with some modifications using a plantar test apparatus (ANESTHESIA RESEARCH Lab, University of California, San Diego, CA). The intensity of the thermal stimulus was adjusted to achieve a baseline paw-withdrawal latency of approximately 7–9 sec on average in naive mice. Paw withdrawal latency was determined as the average of three scores per paw.

Immunohistochemical Studies

Immunohistochemical study on the dorsal root ganglion (DRG) and the spinal cord of at the lumbar level was performed as previously described [19]. Briefly, paraffin sections (5 μm thick) were deparaffinized and immersed in unmasking solution (Vector H3300; Vector Laboratories, Burlingame, CA) for antigenic retrieval and heated in an autoclave (121°C) for 5 min. The sections were then incubated in a nonspecific blocking reagent (Dako, Glostrup, Denmark) for 30 min to reduce background staining. Sections were then incubated with primary antibodies overnight in a humidified chamber at 4°C. Primary antibodies used in this study were anti-4-hydroxy-2-nonenal (4-HNE) (mouse monoclonal, Japan Institute for the Control of Aging, Shizuoka, Japan), anti-8-hydroxydeoxyguanosine (8-OHdG) (mouse monoclonal, Japan Institute for the Control of Aging), anti-neuronal nuclear antigen (NeuN) (rabbit polyclonal, Millipore, Billerica, MA), anti-glial fibrillary acidic protein (GFAP) (rabbit polyclonal, Thermo Fisher Scientific, Waltham, MA), anti-NG2 (rabbit polyclonal, Abcam, Cambridge, UK), anti-Olig2 (rabbit polyclonal, Abcam), and anti-Iba1 (rabbit polyclonal, Wako, Osaka, Japan) antibodies.

For fluorescent staining, sections were incubated with Alexa-Fluor 488-conjugated goat anti-rabbit IgG (1:200; Molecular Probes, Eugene, OR) for primary antibodies derived from mouse. For primary antibody derived from rabbit, Alexa-Fluor 546-conjugated goat anti-mouse IgG (1:200; Molecular Probes) was used. Sections were examined using a Nikon fluorescence microscopy system (Nikon, Tokyo, Japan) with electron-multiplying (EM) CCD digital camera (ImagEM, Hamamatsu Photonics, Hamamatsu, Japan).

Samples from six slides (from six mice) per experimental conditions were examined. For quantification of the spinal cord sections, total number of positive cells for 4-HNE or 8OHdG was counted. For quantification of the DRG sections, the proportion of positive cells was determined by positive neuron profile divided by the total neuronal profiles on each section. Counting of immunostaining was performed by an investigator blinded to the treatment conditions.

Statistics

Statistical analysis was performed using GraphPad Prism 5 (GraphPad Software Inc.). Comparisons of the means of each group were performed using a Student's *t* test or two-way repeated measures analysis of variance (two-way RM ANOVA) with a Bonferroni post-hoc test. Details regarding specific statistical tests are included in the results. Values are presented as the mean ± SEM.

Results

Mechanical Allodynia and Hyperalgesia Induced by PSNL was Alleviated by Hydrogen Water

To examine the effect of hydrogen water against neuropathic pain, we tested whether *ad libitum* drinking of hydrogen water modified mechanical allodynia and hyperalgesia in PSNL model mice. In control mice (without hydrogen), PSNL caused a significant and long-lasting decrease in their mechanical threshold measured with von Frey hairs (Figure 1A). A two-way RM ANOVA confirmed this, indicating a significant difference between the ipsilateral and the contralateral sides to ligation ($F = 91.46$, $P < 0.0001$). On the other hand, in the sham operated group, there was no significant difference in mechanical thresholds between the ipsilateral and the contralateral sides to operation (Figure 1B; two-way RM ANOVA, ipsilateral vs. contralateral, $P > 0.05$).

When mice were supplied with hydrogen water for the whole experimental period (from day 0 (right after PSNL operation) to 21), they exhibited a significant and long-lasting decrease in their mechanical threshold on the ipsilateral side to ligation compared with the contralateral side (Figure 1A; two-way RM ANOVA, ipsilateral vs. contralateral, $F = 16.21$, $P < 0.001$), similar to mice without hydrogen treatment. However, the hydrogen-treated mice exhibited higher threshold on the ipsilateral side to ligation when compared with mice without hydrogen treatment (Figure 1A). A two-way RM ANOVA indicated a significant difference between hydrogen-treated mice and controls (ipsilateral H_2 (+) vs. ipsilateral H_2 (−), $F = 9.43$, $P < 0.0046$). In the sham-operated group with hydrogen treatment, there was no significant difference in mechanical thresholds between the ipsilateral and the contralateral sides to operation (Figure 1B; two-way RM ANOVA, ipsilateral vs. contralateral, $P > 0.05$). These results indicate that hydrogen treatment significantly alleviated mechanical allodynia caused by PSNL.

In the plantar test, control mice exhibited significant reduction of paw withdrawal latency only on the ipsilateral side to the ligation compared with the contralateral side (Figure 2A). A two-way RM ANOVA conformed this, indicating a significant difference between the ipsilateral and the contralateral sides to ligation (ipsilateral vs. contralateral, $F = 13.36$, $P = 0.0014$). On the other hand, in the sham operated group, there was no significant difference in paw withdrawal latency between the ipsilateral and the contralateral sides to operation (Figure 2B; two-way RM ANOVA, ipsilateral vs. contralateral, $P > 0.05$).

When mice were supplied with hydrogen water for the whole experimental period, they did not exhibit significant reduction in paw withdrawal latency on the ipsilateral side to ligation compared with the contralateral side (Figure 2A; two-way RM ANOVA, ipsilateral vs. contralateral, $P > 0.05$). Furthermore, paw withdrawal latency on the ipsilateral side of mice with hydrogen treatment was significantly longer than that of mice without hydrogen treatment (Figure 2A). A two-way RM ANOVA indicated a significant difference between them (ipsilateral H_2 (+) vs. ipsilateral H_2 (−), $F = 11.42$, $P = 0.0027$). In the sham-operated group with hydrogen treatment, there was no significant difference in paw withdrawal latency between the ipsilateral and the contralateral sides to operation (Figure 2B; two-way RM ANOVA, ipsilateral H_2 (+) vs. contralateral H_2 (+), $P > 0.05$). These results indicate that both mechanical allodynia and thermal hyperalgesia induced by PSNL can be alleviated by drinking hydrogen water.

Hydrogen Treatment was Effective against the Development Phase but not against the Maintenance Phase of Mechanical Allodynia

In the Seltzer model, the time course of the pain responses consists of two-phases. The pain responses in the von Frey and the

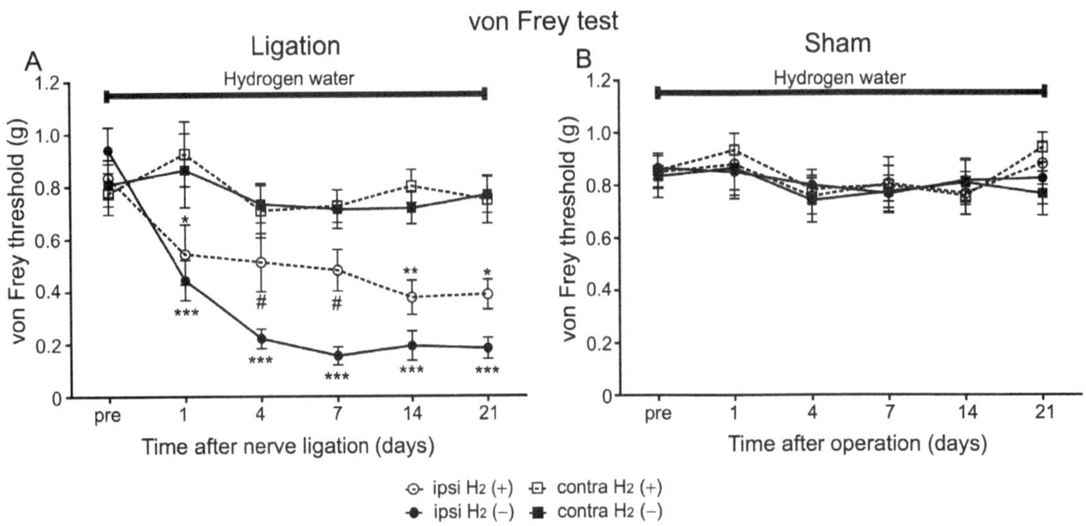

Figure 1. Hydrogen treatment suppressed mechanical allodynia in the PSNL model. Neuropathic mechanical allodynia was analysed by the von Frey test. Hydrogen was supplied for the whole experimental period right after PSNL or sham operation. The control group received distilled water from day 0 to 21. (A) The hydrogen-treated mice exhibited higher threshold on the ipsilateral side to ligation than controls (n = 12 mice for each group). (B) Sham operation did not caused mechanical allodynia regardless of hydrogen treatment (n = 12 mice for each group). We used a two-way RM ANOVA with a Bonferroni post-hoc test; *$P < 0.05$, **$P < 0.01$, ***$P < 0.001$ vs. contralateral side of control mice, #$P < 0.05$ vs. ipsilateral side of control mice.

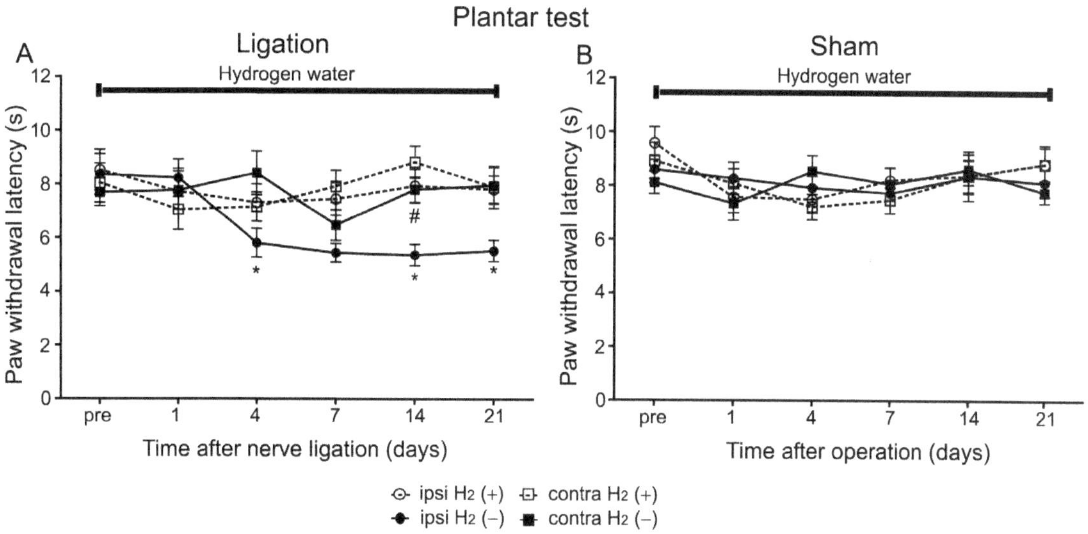

Figure 2. Hydrogen treatment suppressed thermal hyperalgesia in the PSNL model. Thermal hyperalgesia was analysed by the plantar test. The same sets of mice used for the von Frey test were used in the plantar test. (A) The reduction of paw withdrawal latency was attenuated in mice with hydrogen compared with those without hydrogen (n = 12 mice for each group). (B) Sham operation did not cause hyperalgesia regardless of hydrogen treatment (n = 12 mice for each group). We used a two-way RM ANOVA with a Bonferroni post-hoc test; $*P<0.05$ vs. contralateral side of control mice, $^{\#}P<0.05$ vs. ipsilateral side of control mice.

plantar test were gradually increased till 4 days after PSNL and then followed by sustained pain behaviors as observed in figures 1 and 2. To examine the effect of hydrogen on the induction phase, hydrogen was administered from day 0 to 4. The von Frey test revealed that mice with hydrogen treatment exhibited a higher threshold on the ipsilateral side when compared with that of mice without hydrogen (Figure 3A). A two-way RM ANOVA indicated a significant difference between hydrogen-treated mice and controls (ipsilateral H_2 (+) vs. ipsilateral H_2 (−), $F=9.06$, $P=0.0064$). These results indicate that hydrogen treatment was effective on the development of mechanical allodynia. It is worth noting that an analgesic effect lasted for the whole experiment period even after the termination of hydrogen treatment (Figure 3A).

When hydrogen was administered from day 4 to 21 (maintenance phase), the von Frey test indicated that there was no significant difference in mechanical thresholds on the ipsilateral side to ligation between mice with hydrogen treatment and controls (Figure 3B; two-way RM ANOVA, ipsilateral H_2 (+) vs. ipsilateral H_2 (−), $P>0.05$). These results indicate that hydrogen treatment is effective against the induction phase, but not against the maintenance phase in mechanical allodynia.

Hydrogen Treatment was Effective against both Induction and Maintenance Phases in Thermal Hyperalgesia

The plantar test also revealed that hydrogen treatment attenuated the induction of hyperalgesia. When hydrogen was administered from day 0 to 4, these mice exhibited significantly longer paw withdrawal latency on the ipsilateral side compared with mice without hydrogen (Figure 4A; two-way RM ANOVA, ipsilateral H_2 (+) vs. ipsilateral H_2 (−), $F=6.66$, $P=0.017$).

When mice were administered hydrogen water from day 4 to 21, they also exhibited significantly longer paw withdrawal latency on the ipsilateral side compared with that in mice without hydrogen (Figure 4B; two-way RM ANOVA, ipsilateral H_2 (+) vs. ipsilateral H_2 (−), $F=4.64$, $P=0.04$). These results indicate that hydrogen treatment is effective against both induction and maintenance phases in thermal hyperalgesia.

Hydrogen Suppressed the Increase of Oxidative Stress in the Spinal Cord Dorsal Horn and the DRG 4 days after PSNL

To examine the effect of hydrogen water against oxidative stress, we conducted immunohistochemical analysis using antibodies against oxidative stress markers. We evaluated the numbers of 4-HNE or 8-OHdG positive cells in the spinal cord (at the level of L5) at the end of 4 days period after PSNL or sham operation. The number of 4-HNE positive cells was increased in the spinal cord dorsal horn from mice with PSNL (Figure 5A) compared with the sham-operated controls (Figures 5C). However, the number of positive cells was decreased in mice that received hydrogen water from day 0 (right after PSNL operation) to 4 (Figures 5B) compared with mice without hydrogen (Figures 5A). The quantification confirmed this, indicating a significant difference between them (Figure 5G; *t* test, H_2 (−) vs. H_2 (+), $t=2.33$, $P=0.021$). Similarly, the number of 8-OHdG positive cells was increased in the spinal cord dorsal horn from mice with PSNL (Figure 5D) compared with the sham-operated controls (Figures 5F). The number of positive cells was decreased in mice treated with hydrogen (Figures 5E) compared with mice without hydrogen (Figures 5D). The quantification indicated a significant difference between them (Figure 5H; *t* test, H_2 (−) vs. H_2 (+), $t=1.83$, $P=0.049$). These results indicate that drinking of hydrogen water suppress the increase of oxidative stress induced by PSNL in the spinal cord dorsal horn.

We also evaluated staining for 4-HNE and 8-OHdG in the DRG (at the level of L5) at the end of 4 days period after PSNL. Weak staining for 4-HNE was detected in mice with PSNL (Figures 6A), but not from the sham-operated controls (Figures 6C). Judging from the morphological appearance, 4-HNE was mainly located in the membrane region of neuronal cells (Figures 6A).

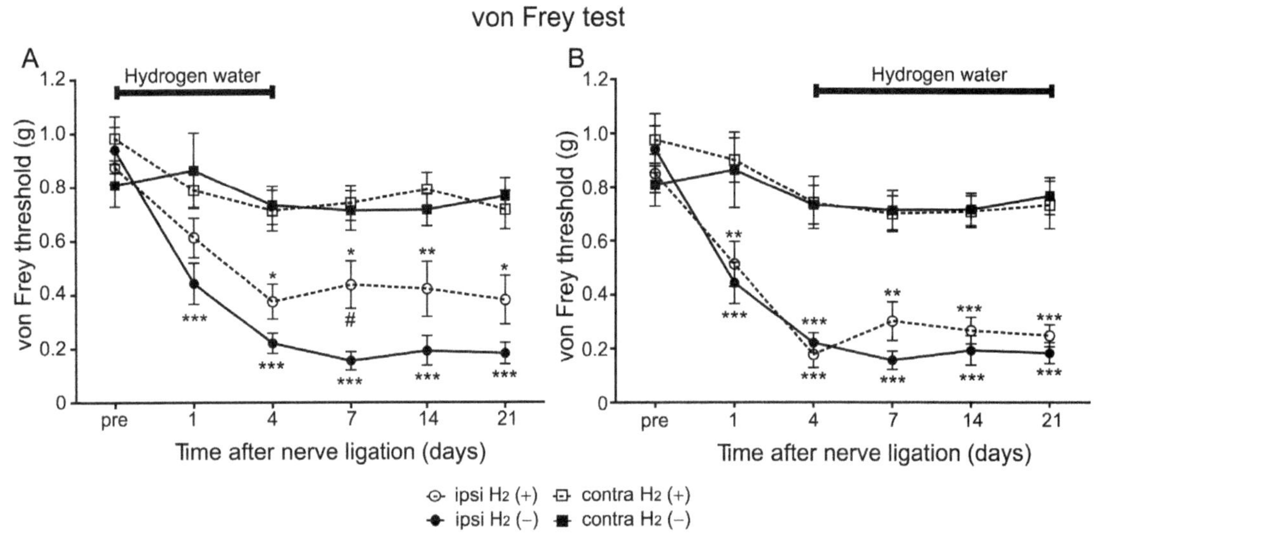

Figure 3. Hydrogen treatment was effective against the induction phase but not against the maintenance phase of mechanical allodynia. (A) Hydrogen water was supplied from day 0 to 4, and after then changed to distilled water. Paw withdrawal threshold was significantly lower in the H_2 (+) group when compared with the H_2 (–) group (n = 12 mice for each group). Note that the lower threshold in the H_2 (+) group lasted beyond the termination of hydrogen treatment. (B) Hydrogen water was supplied from day 4 to 21. There was no significant difference in paw withdrawal threshold between the H_2 (+) and the H_2 (–) groups (n = 12 mice for each group). These experiments were performed concurrently with those in Figure 1. We used a two-way RM ANOVA with a Bonferroni post-hoc test; *$P<0.05$, **$P<0.01$, ***$P<0.001$ vs. contralateral side of same mice. #$P<0.05$ vs. ipsilateral side of H_2 (–) mice.

Staining for 4-HNE was reduced in mice treated with hydrogen (Figures 6B) compared with mice without hydrogen (Figures 6A). The quantification indicated a significant difference between them (Figure 6D; 4-HNE, *t* test, H_2 (–) vs. H_2 (+), $t = 2.08$, $P = 0.032$). These data indicate that drinking of hydrogen water suppress the increase of 4-HNE induced by PSNL in the DRG. On the contrary, the 8-OHdG positive cells were hardly detected in the DRG from mice with PSNL as well as in those from the sham-operated controls.

We further analyzed the properties of 4-HNE expression in the spinal cord dorsal horn from mice with PSNL at the end of 4 days period after ligation. 4-HNE was hardly detected in neuronal cells, as indicated by double staining for 4-HNE and the neuronal marker NeuN (Figure 7A). Similarly, double staining for 4-HNE

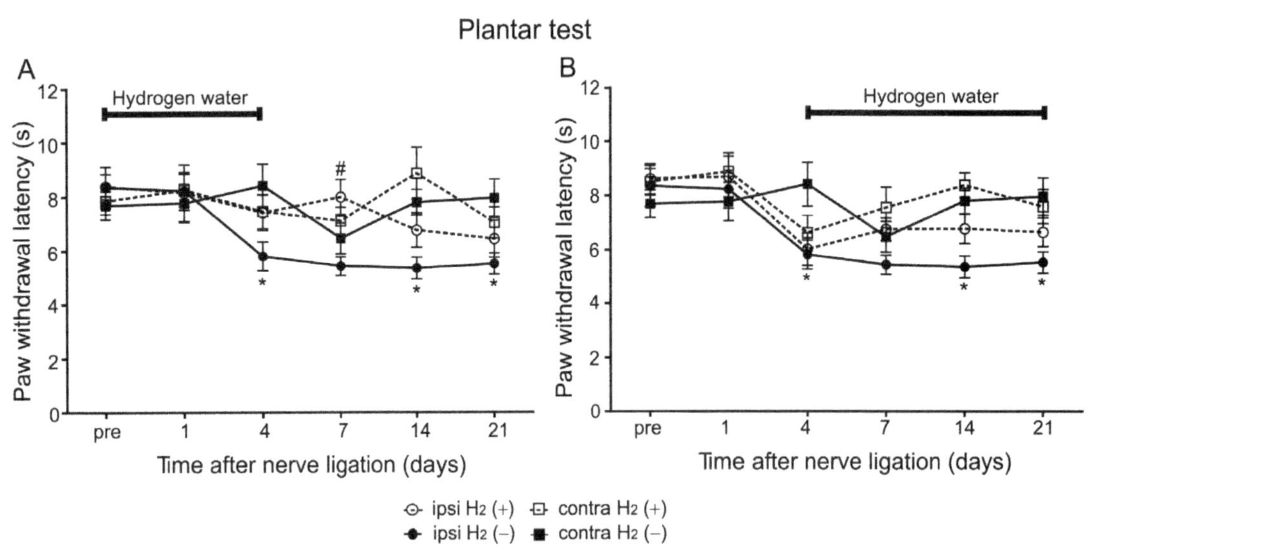

Figure 4. Hydrogen treatment was effective against both induction and maintenance phases of thermal hyperalgesia. (A) When hydrogen water was supplied from day 0 to 4, paw withdrawal latency was longer in the H_2 (+) group when compared with the H_2 (–) group (n = 12 mice for each group). Note that the lower threshold in the H_2 (+) group lasted beyond the termination of hydrogen treatment. (B) When hydrogen water was supplied from day 4 to 21, there was a significant difference in paw withdrawal latency between the H_2 (+) and the H_2 (–) groups (n = 12 mice for each group). These experiments were performed concurrently with those in Figure 2. We used a two-way RM ANOVA with a Bonferroni post-hoc test; *$P<0.05$ vs. contralateral side of same mice. #$P<0.05$ vs. ipsilateral side of H_2 (–) mice.

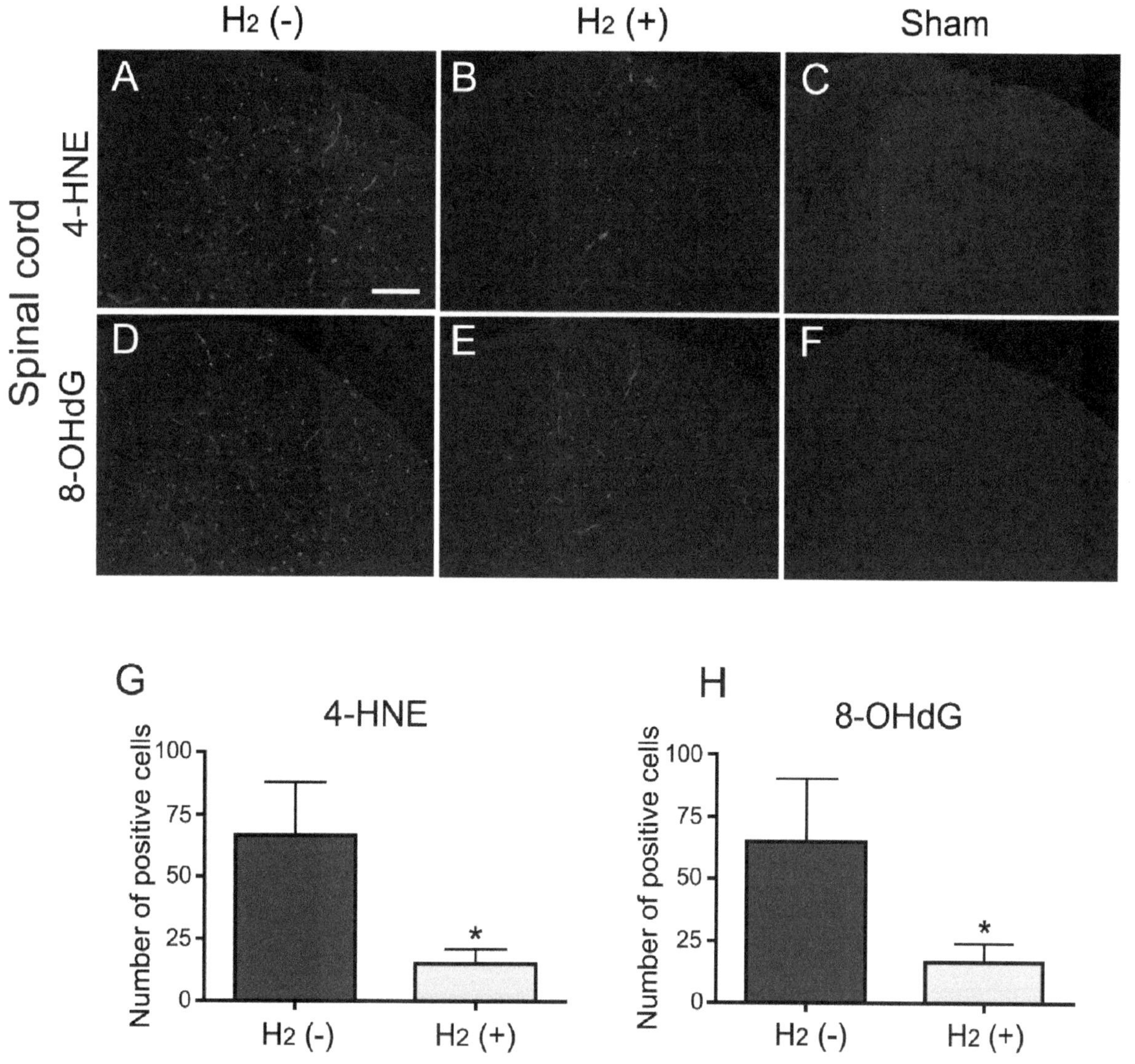

Figure 5. Hydrogen suppressed the development of oxidative stress in the spinal cord dorsal horn. (A–F) Representative images of immunohistochemical staining for the oxidative stress markers 4-HNE (A–C) and 8-OHdG (D-F) in the spinal cord dorsal horn at the level of L5. Staining for 4-HNE was increased in the spinal cord at the end of 4 days period after PSNL (A) compared with sham operation (C). (B) The number of 4-HNE positive cells was decreased in mice with hydrogen when compared with the H_2 (–) group (A). Similarly, staining for 8-OHdG was also increased in the spinal cord from mice with PSNL (D) compared with sham operation (F). (E) The number of 8-OHdG positive cells was decreased in mice with hydrogen at the end of 4 days period after PSNL when compared with the H_2 (–) group (D). (G, H) The numbers of positive cells for both markers were significantly decreased when compared with the H_2 (–) group. $^*P<0.05$ compared with control (t test, n = 6 mice for each). Scale bar: 200 μm.

and the astrocyte marker GFAP indicated that 4-HNE was not expressed in astrocytes (Figure 7B). On the other hand, double staining for 4-HNE and the oligodendrocyte marker NG2 indicated the expression of 4-HNE in oligodendrocyte (Figure 7C). Furthermore, double staining for 4-HNE and another oligodendrocyte marker Olig2 confirmed the expression of 4-HNE in oligodendrocyte (Figure 7D). Double staining for 4-HNE and the specific microglia marker Iba1 showed that 4-HNE was not expressed in microglia (Figure 7E). These data indicate that 4-HNE is expressed mainly in oligodendrocyte at the end of 4 days period after PSNL.

Discussion

In this report, we show that hydrogen has a potent analgesic effect against neuropathic pain. Our result is consistent with other previous studies that reported the analgesic effects of ROS scavengers against neuropathic pain. Systemic injection of PBN, which is a non-specific ROS scavenger that scavenges all types of ROS indiscriminately, relieved mechanical allodynia induced by spinal nerve ligation in the rat [5]. Tal et al. reported that systemic injection of TEMPOL reduced hyperalgesia induced by chronic constriction injury in rats [7]. Kim et al. reported that systemic injection of vitamin E attenuated mechanical allodynia and thermal hyperalgesia caused by spinal nerve ligation in rodents [8]. PBN and vitamin E were also effective in producing analgesia by intrathecal injection, indicating that the spinal mechanism is, at least in part, important in neuropathic pain [5,8]. On the other hand, peripheral ROS also seem to be involved in the generation of pain [1].

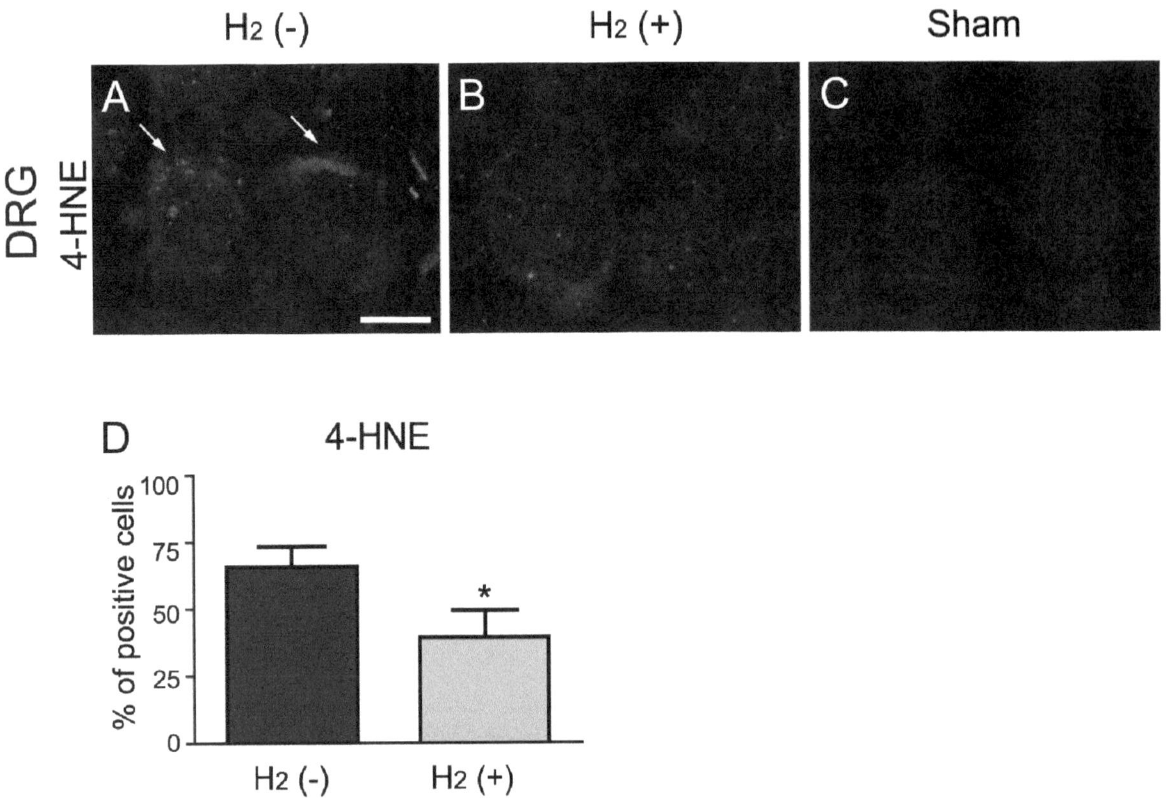

Figure 6. Hydrogen suppressed the development of oxidative stress in the DRG. (A–C) Representative images of immunohistochemical staining for oxidative stress markers 4-HNE in the DRG at the level of L5. Weak staining for 4-HNE (arrows) was observed in the DRG from mice without hydrogen at the end of 4 days period after PSNL (A), whereas staining for 4-HNE was not observed in sham operation mice (C). (B) Staining for 4-HNE was reduced in mice with hydrogen at the end of 4 days period after PSNL. (D) The proportion of 4-HNE positive cells was significantly decreased when compared with the H_2 (–) group (A). Results are expressed as percent of total neurons. *$P<0.05$ compared with control (*t* test, n = 6 mice for each). Scale bar: 20 μm.

We observed that hydrogen reduced oxidative stress caused by PSNL in the spinal cord and the DRG, although little is known about how oxidative stress contribute to neuropathic pain. In this study, we used 4-HNE and 8-OHdG as biomarkers for oxidative stress. 4-HNE is an aldehyde toxic end product of lipid peroxidation and used as a biomarker for membrane lipid peroxidation. 8-OHdG is an oxidized nucleoside accumulated in both mitochondrial and nuclear DNA and used as a biomarker for oxidative DNA damage. 4-HNE and 8-OHdG as well-known biomarkers for oxidative insults caused by hydroxyl radical. Because hydrogen selectively reduces hydroxyl radical [9], 4-HNE and 8-OHdG are suitable for analysing anti-oxidative effect of hydrogen [9–11,20]. In this relation, it was reported that 4-HNE was significantly reduced by drinking hydrogen water in mouse model of Parkinson's disease, whereas intensity of dihydroethidium, which was oxidized by superperoxide, was not significantly reduced by hydrogen water [11].

Our results indicated that, in the spinal cord, 4-HNE was located mainly in oligodendrocyte at the end of 4 days period after PSNL. Oligodendrocyte is responsible for myelinisation in the CNS and myelin ensheathes neuronal axons allowing fast nerve conduction. Although less is known about the possible role of oligodendrocyte in neuropathic pain, recent report suggests the involvement of spinal oligodendrocyte in neuropathic pain. For instance, spinal transportation of oligodendrocyte progenitor cells reduced spinal cord injury-induced chronic neuropathic pain by enhancing remyelination [21]. Further studies will be needed to to understand the role of 4-HNE in oligodendrocyte for neuropathic pain.

We observed the weak staining for 4-HNE in the DRG at the end of 4 days period after PSNL, which was located in neuronal cells. Staining for 8-OHdG was hardly detected in the DRG in contrary to the spinal cord. Currently, we cannot know the reason for the different expression pattern of markers for oxidative stress between in the DRG and in the spinal cord. Further study is required to understand the role of oxidative stress in the spinal cord and the DRG to neuropathic pain.

We must emphasize that hydrogen was given orally in the current study. Generally, administration of agents by oral pathways is less effective than administration by intra-peritoneal or intrathecal methods. Thus, the efficacy of oral administration is very important from a clinical point of view because continuous intra-peritoneal or intrathecal injections are intolerable. Molecular hydrogen is electrically neutral and has a low molecular weight. Thus, hydrogen readily passes through the blood brain barrier and reaches target cells, unlike other antioxidants that have higher molecular weights and/or polarized structures, making it difficult to reach the target. These specific propensities of hydrogen may contribute to its high efficacy in spite of oral administration. Although we do not know the precise mechanism with which oral hydrogen reduce the increase of oxidative stress after PSNL, oral hydrogen may reach the target site very rapidly. For instance, it was reported that hydrogen molecule can be delivered to the blood in minutes in drinking hydrogen water [10]. It was also suggested

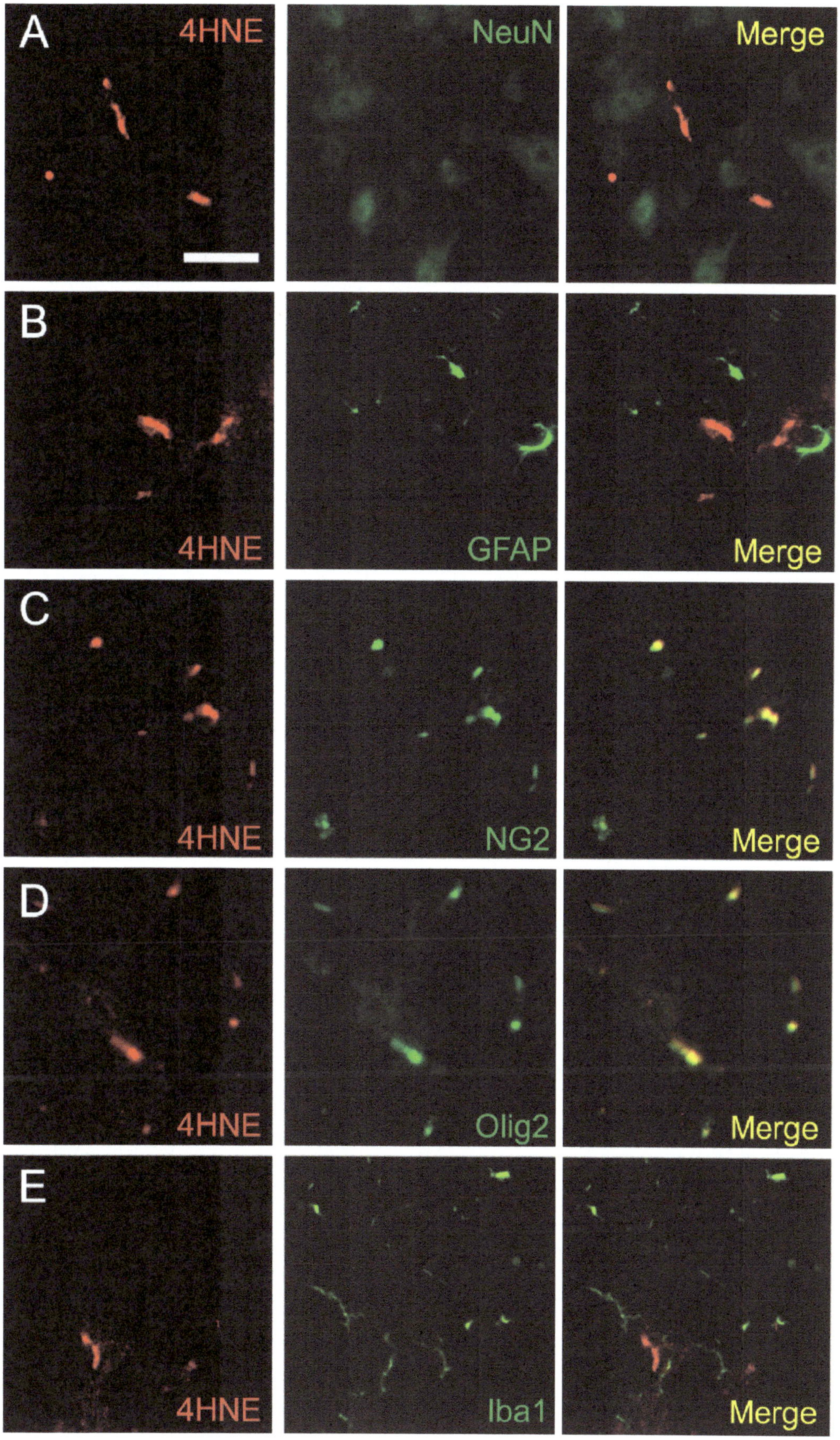
A
4HNE
NeuN
Merge
B
4HNE
GFAP
Merge
C
4HNE
NG2
Merge
D
4HNE
Olig2
Merge
E
4HNE
Iba1
Merge

Figure 7. 4-HNE were mainly produced on oligodendrocyte in the spinal cord 4 days after PSNL. (A–E) Double immunostaining of 4-HNE with cellular markers for neurons (A), astrocyte (B), oligodendrocyte (C, D), and microglia (E). 4-HNE signals were mainly colocalized with the oligodendrocyte marker NG2 and olig2, but not with NeuN, GFAP, and Iba1 in the spinal cord at the end of 4 days period after PSNL. Scale bar: 20 μm.

that hydrogen might reach the target site by gaseous diffusion, which make it highly effective for reducing hydroxyl radicals [9].

Recently, it was reported that intrathecal administration of hydrogen-rich saline relieve neuropathic pain induced by CCI in rats [22]. This accord with our study and further support the possibility of therapeutic use of hydrogen in pain medicine. Based on the result of this report, anti-oxidant effect of hydrogen in the spinal cord is, at least in part, important in alleviating neuropathic pain. It would be helpful for extending hydrogen application if the date from intraperitoneal injection, intravenous injection, and intrathecal injection of hydrogen was collected as a supporting evidence.

Recently, accumulating evidence suggests that hydrogen is a highly effective antioxidant that has therapeutic potencies for some diseases without remarkable side effects. For instance, hydrogen can reportedly ameliorate reperfusion injury [23], atherosclerosis [24], carcinogenesis [25], neurodegenerative disorders [26], hearing disorders [27], and neuroapoptosis induced by neonatal anesthesia [19] without serious harmful side effect. In addition, hydrogen is already used in clinic for the prevention of decompression sickness in divers [9].

It is important to identify which type of ROS is critically involved in neuropathic pain; however, this is difficult because most antioxidants can react with various ROS indiscriminately. Our results indicate that hydroxyl radical has, at least in part, an important role in both induction and maintenance of neuropathic pain because hydrogen acts only with hydroxyl radical. However, our results could not exclude the possibility that other ROS contribute to neuropathic pain. It was reported that the inhibitors of nitric oxide (NO) synthase reduced pain behaviors, indicating that NO is involved in the mechanism of neuropathic pain [28]. In addition, superoxide is also reportedly involved in the mechanism of neuropathic pain since hyperalgesia was reduced by systemic injection of TEMPOL, which removes one type of free radical, the superoxide [7].

Interestingly, in mice that received hydrogen water from day 0 to 4, the analgesic effect continued even after the cessation of drinking hydrogen water. Therefore, it seems likely that the hydroxyl radical in the induction phase may be important to develop neuropathic pain following PSNL. Furthermore, in mice that received hydrogen water from day 4 to 21, thermal hyperalgesia was gradually improved until day 21, although it reached a maximum at day 4, indicating that the analgesic effect of hydrogen water was also effective against established hyperalgesia. Thus, it may be that hydroxyl radical contributes to maintenance as well as induction of thermal hyperalgesia in the PSNL model. In contrast to hyperalgesia, hydrogen did not improve mechanical allodynia when given during day 4 to 21, indicating that the analgesic effect of hydrogen water was not effective for established mechanical allodynia. Although we do not know the reason for the difference between allodynia and hyperalgesia in the maintenance phase, it is intriguing to speculate that the pathomechanism of mechanical allodynia and thermal hyperalgesia may be different with regard to the vulnerability to oxidative stress in the maintenance phase.

In conclusion, oral administration of water containing hydrogen can be an effective and easy strategy for treating neuropathic pain. Another study indicated that removal of excessive ROS could also produce an analgesic effect against acute inflammatory pain [29]. Further studies will be needed to understand the effect of hydrogen on other types of pain.

Acknowledgments

The authors thank Ms. Kiyoko Takamiya and Mrs. Yuko Ogura (Technicians, Department of Anesthesiology, National Defense Medical College, Tokorozawa, Saitama, Japan) for excellent technical help in this study.

Author Contributions

Conceived and designed the experiments: YS. Performed the experiments: MK. Analyzed the data: MK YS. Contributed reagents/materials/analysis tools: MK YO. Wrote the paper: MK YS TK.

References

1. Khalil Z, Liu T, Helme RD (1999) Free radicals contribute to the reduction in peripheral vascular responses and the maintenance of thermal hyperalgesia in rats with chronic constriction injury. Pain 79: 31–37.
2. Twining CM, Sloane EM, Milligan ED, Chacur M, Martin D, et al. (2004) Perisciatic proinflammatory cytokines, reactive oxygen species, and complement induce mirror-image neuropathic pain in rats. Pain 110: 299–309.
3. Janes K, Neumann WL, Salvemini D (2012) Anti-superoxide and anti-peroxynitrite strategies in pain suppression. Biochim Biophys Acta 1822: 815–821.
4. Meeus M, Nijs J, Hermans L, Goubert D, Calders P (2013) The role of mitochondrial dysfunctions due to oxidative and nitrosative stress in the chronic pain or chronic fatigue syndromes and fibromyalgia patients: peripheral and central mechanisms as therapeutic targets? Expert Opin Ther Targets 17: 1081–1089.
5. Kim HK, Park SK, Zhou JL, Taglialatela G, Chung K, et al. (2004) Reactive oxygen species (ROS) play an important role in a rat model of neuropathic pain. Pain 111: 116–124.
6. Lee I, Kim HK, Kim JH, Chung K, Chung JM (2007) The role of reactive oxygen species in capsaicin-induced mechanical hyperalgesia and in the activities of dorsal horn neurons. Pain 133: 9–17.
7. Tal M (1996) A novel antioxidant alleviates heat hyperalgesia in rats with an experimental painful peripheral neuropathy. Neuroreport 7: 1382–1384.
8. Kim HK, Kim JH, Gao X, Zhou JL, Lee I, et al. (2006) Analgesic effect of vitamin E is mediated by reducing central sensitization in neuropathic pain. Pain 122: 53–62.
9. Ohsawa I, Ishikawa M, Takahashi K, Watanabe M, Nishimaki K, et al. (2007) Hydrogen acts as a therapeutic antioxidant by selectively reducing cytotoxic oxygen radicals. Nat Med 13: 688–694.
10. Nagata K, Nakashima-Kamimura N, Mikami T, Ohsawa I, Ohta S (2009) Consumption of molecular hydrogen prevents the stress-induced impairments in hippocampus-dependent learning tasks during chronic physical restraint in mice. Neuropsychopharmacology 34: 501–508.
11. Fujita K, Seike T, Yutsudo N, Ohno M, Yamada H, et al. (2009) Hydrogen in drinking water reduces dopaminergic neuronal loss in the 1-methyl-4-phenyl-1,2,3,6-tetrahydropyridine mouse model of Parkinson's disease. PLoS One 4: e7247.
12. Yanagihara T, Arai K, Miyamae K, Sato B, Shudo T, et al. (2005) Electrolyzed hydrogen-saturated water for drinking use elicits an antioxidative effect: a feeding test with rats. Biosci Biotechnol Biochem 69: 1985–1987.
13. Sauer H, Wartenberg M, Hescheler J (2001) Reactive oxygen species as intracellular messengers during cell growth and differentiation. Cell Physiol Biochem 11: 173–186.
14. Murad F (2004) Discovery of some of the biological effects of nitric oxide and its role in cell signaling. Biosci Rep 24: 452–474.
15. Liu H, Colavitti R, Rovira, II, Finkel T (2005) Redox-dependent transcriptional regulation. Circ Res 97: 967–974.
16. Zimmermann M (1983) Ethical guidelines for investigations of experimental pain in conscious animals. Pain 16: 109–110.
17. Otsubo Y, Satoh Y, Kodama M, Araki Y, Satomoto M, et al. (2012) Mechanical allodynia but not thermal hyperalgesia is impaired in mice deficient for ERK2 in the central nervous system. Pain 153: 2241–2252.

18. Narita M (2005) Protease-Activated Receptor-1 and Platelet-Derived Growth Factor in Spinal Cord Neurons Are Implicated in Neuropathic Pain after Nerve Injury. Journal of Neuroscience 25: 10000–10009.
19. Yonamine R, Satoh Y, Kodama M, Araki Y, Kazama T (2013) Coadministration of hydrogen gas as part of the carrier gas mixture suppresses neuronal apoptosis and subsequent behavioral deficits caused by neonatal exposure to sevoflurane in mice. Anesthesiology 118: 105–113.
20. Ishibashi T, Sato B, Rikitake M, Seo T, Kurokawa R, et al. (2012) Consumption of water containing a high concentration of molecular hydrogen reduces oxidative stress and disease activity in patients with rheumatoid arthritis: an open-label pilot study. Med Gas Res 2: 27.
21. Tao F, Li Q, Liu S, Wu H, Skinner J, et al. (2013) Role of neuregulin-1/ErbB signaling in stem cell therapy for spinal cord injury-induced chronic neuropathic pain. Stem Cells 31: 83–91.
22. Chen Q, Chen P, Zhou S, Yan X, Zhang J, et al. (2013) Hydrogen-rich saline attenuated neuropathic pain by reducing oxidative stress. Can J Neurol Sci 40: 857–863.
23. Hayashida K, Sano M, Ohsawa I, Shinmura K, Tamaki K, et al. (2008) Inhalation of hydrogen gas reduces infarct size in the rat model of myocardial ischemia-reperfusion injury. Biochem Biophys Res Commun 373: 30–35.
24. Ohsawa I, Nishimaki K, Yamagata K, Ishikawa M, Ohta S (2008) Consumption of hydrogen water prevents atherosclerosis in apolipoprotein E knockout mice. Biochem Biophys Res Commun 377: 1195–1198.
25. Nakashima-Kamimura N, Mori T, Ohsawa I, Asoh S, Ohta S (2009) Molecular hydrogen alleviates nephrotoxicity induced by an anti-cancer drug cisplatin without compromising anti-tumor activity in mice. Cancer Chemother Pharmacol 64: 753–761.
26. Fu Y, Ito M, Fujita Y, Ichihara M, Masuda A, et al. (2009) Molecular hydrogen is protective against 6-hydroxydopamine-induced nigrostriatal degeneration in a rat model of Parkinson's disease. Neurosci Lett 453: 81–85.
27. Kikkawa YS, Nakagawa T, Horie RT, Ito J (2009) Hydrogen protects auditory hair cells from free radicals. Neuroreport 20: 689–694.
28. Tedesco LS, Fuseler J, Grisham M, Wolf R, Roerig SC (2002) Therapeutic administration of nitric oxide synthase inhibitors reverses hyperalgesia but not inflammation in a rat model of polyarthritis. Pain 95: 215–223.
29. Ko YK, Youn AM, Hong BH, Kim YH, Shin YS, et al. (2012) Antinociceptive effect of phenyl N-tert-butylnitrone, a free radical scavenger, on the rat formalin test. Korean J Anesthesiol 62: 558–564.

7

Fatty Acid Amide Hydrolase (FAAH) Inhibitors Exert Pharmacological Effects, but Lack Antinociceptive Efficacy in Rats with Neuropathic Spinal Cord Injury Pain

Aldric T. Hama[1]*, Peter Germano[2], Matthew S. Varghese[1], Benjamin F. Cravatt[3], G. Todd Milne[2], James P. Pearson[2], Jacqueline Sagen[1]

1 Miami Project to Cure Paralysis, University of Miami Miller School of Medicine, Miami, Florida, United States of America, 2 Ironwood Pharmaceuticals, Inc., Cambridge, Massachusetts, United States of America, 3 Department of Chemical Physiology, The Skaggs Institute for Chemical Biology, The Scripps Research Institute, La Jolla, California, United States of America

Abstract

Amelioration of neuropathic spinal cord injury (SCI) pain is a clinical challenge. Increasing the endocannabinoid anandamide and other fatty acid amides (FAA) by blocking fatty acid amide hydrolase (FAAH) has been shown to be antinociceptive in a number of animal models of chronic pain. However, an antinociceptive effect of blocking FAAH has yet to be demonstrated in a rat model of neuropathic SCI pain. Four weeks following a SCI, rats developed significantly decreased hind paw withdrawal thresholds, indicative of below-level cutaneous hypersensitivity. A group of SCI rats were systemically treated (i.p.) with either the selective FAAH inhibitor URB597 or vehicle twice daily for seven days. A separate group of SCI rats received a single dose (p.o.) of either the selective FAAH inhibitor PF-3845 or vehicle. Following behavioral testing, levels of the FAA *N*-arachidonoylethanolamide, *N*-oleoyl ethanolamide and *N*-palmitoyl ethanolamide were quantified in brain and spinal cord from SCI rats. Four weeks following SCI, FAA levels were markedly reduced in spinal cord tissue. Although systemic treatment with URB597 significantly increased CNS FAA levels, no antinociceptive effect was observed. A significant elevation of CNS FAA levels was also observed following oral PF-3845 treatment, but only a modest antinociceptive effect was observed. Increasing CNS FAA levels alone does not lead to robust amelioration of below-level neuropathic SCI pain. Perhaps utilizing FAAH inhibition in conjunction with other analgesic mechanisms could be an effective analgesic therapy.

Editor: Vinod K. Yaragudri, Nathan Kline Institute for Psychiatric Research and New York School of Medicine, United States of America

Funding: This work supported in part by Ironwood Pharmaceuticals, Inc. and by the National Institutes of Health Neurological Disorders & Stroke NS61172 (to JS). The funder provided support in the form of salaries for authors PG, GTM and JPP, and research materials but did not have any additional role in the study design, data collection and analysis, decision to publish, or preparation of the manuscript. The specific roles of these authors are articulated in the 'author contributions' section.

Competing Interests: The current work was supported in part by Ironwood Pharmaceuticals, Inc. Co-authors Peter Germano, James P. Pearson and G. Todd Milne are stockholders, Peter Germano and G. Todd Milne are employees, and James P. Pearson is a paid consultant of Ironwood Pharmaceuticals which has a FAAH inhibitor program. The specific roles of these authors are articulated in the 'author contributions' section. Ironwood provided research materials required per the study design. There are no patents, products in development or marketed products to declare that would represent a conflict of interest.

* E-mail: ahama@miami.edu

Introduction

In addition to motor and visceral dysfunction, a serious consequence of spinal cord injury (SCI) is chronic pain. It is estimated that 65% of SCI patients suffer from chronic pain, with about one-third of these patients rating their pain as severe [1]. Although pain can occur above and at the level of the spinal lesion, symptoms with similarity to peripheral neuropathic pain can occur below the spinal lesion [2]. Also, below-level neuropathic pain is particularly challenging to treat in that adverse side effects of commonly prescribed neuropathic pain analgesics may exacerbate existing dysfunctions, such as urinary retention with antidepressants and constipation with opioids. Thus, it is crucial that novel therapeutics be developed for this particular patient population.

A number of studies have shown that activation of the cannabinoid (CB) receptor leads to a robust antinociception in a variety of preclinical pain models [3]. The antinociceptive effects of nonselective CB receptor agonists in rats are blocked with either cannabinoid receptor type-1 (CB_1) or cannabinoid receptor type-2 (CB_2) receptor antagonists. Limited clinical evidence and SCI patient survey suggests that CB receptor activation with CB ligands derived from *Cannabis sativa* reduces SCI pain [4,5]. In humans, the psychological and physiological effects of CB agonists are blocked by treatment with the CB_1 receptor antagonist rimonabant (SR141719A) indicating the importance of CB_1 receptors in mediating the effects of CB [6].

Intrathecal administrations of fatty acid amide (FAA) endocannabinoids, such as *N*-arachidonoylethanolamide (AEA), demonstrate robust antinociception in models of tissue injury-induced cutaneous hypersensitivity [7,8]. One method of enhancing CNS levels of endocannabinoids and other antinociceptive non-cannabinoid FAA, such as *N*-oleoyl ethanolamide (OEA) and *N*-palmitoyl ethanolamide (PEA), is by blocking one of their catabolic enzymes, fatty acid amide hydrolase (FAAH) [9,10]. Systemic as well as intrathecal administration of selective FAAH inhibitors have demonstrated significant antinociception in preclinical models of peripheral neuropathic pain [3,9,11]. The antinociceptive effects positively correlated with increased CNS endocannabinoid levels and were blocked with administration of either CB_1 or CB_2 receptor antagonist [12,13]. Even though the antinociceptive effect is mediated by CB_1 receptors, there is a lack of side effects with FAAH inhibition commonly associated with CB_1 receptor agonists, including hypothermia, catalepsy and decreased locomotor activity [14]. It is possible that a part of the antinociceptive effect of increased CNS FAA is due to a non-CB receptor mediated mechanism, such activity at the transient receptor potential vanilloid receptor (TRPV1) channel [11].

Acute SCI in rats can lead to persistent neuropathic pain-like symptoms [15–17]. Robust cutaneous hypersensitivity of the hind paws to both noxious and innocuous stimuli is obtained following spinal compression [18]. A number of clinical analgesics do not display efficacy in SCI rats despite demonstrating efficacy in other neuropathic pain models [17,18]. However, treatment with a non-subtype selective CB receptor agonist WIN 55,212-2 led to a significant antinociception which was reversed by treatment with rimonabant indicating that therapeutic efficacy was mediated by CB_1 receptors [19]. Furthermore, no tolerance to the antinociceptive effect of WIN 55,212-2 was observed over a seven-day treatment period, whereas morphine efficacy gradually diminished during the same treatment period [20]. While exogenous CB_1 receptor agonists may hold promise as analgesics for neuropathic SCI pain, in addition to target-mediated side effects, their current legal status and difficulty in "blinding" the psychotropic effects of cannabinoids make clinical development controversial [21]. Although antinociceptive efficacy of FAAH inhibitors has been observed in various models of peripheral tissue injury-induced pain, efficacy has yet to be demonstrated in neuropathic SCI pain.

The goal of the current study is to evaluate the effect of blocking FAAH with the inhibitors URB597 and PF-3845 on below-level cutaneous hypersensitivity SCI rats. URB597 is a phenyl carbamate inhibitor and PF-3845 is a piperidine urea FAAH inhibitor [9] which irreversibly bind to FAAH. Most previous studies of URB597 demonstrated antinociception following a single dose, but one study showed that repeated dosing over time was needed to attain significant efficacy [22]. Thus, in the current study, SCI rats were systemically treated with URB597 over a seven-day period. Following the treatment and testing period, brain and spinal cord were collected for measurement of FAA by liquid chromatography-tandem mass spectrometry (LC-MS/MS) analysis. As a comparator, WIN 55,212-2 was tested in parallel with FAAH inhibitors in SCI rats. Whereas treatment with WIN 55,212-2 resulted in marked antinociception, there was a lack of comparable antinociception following FAAH treatment in SCI rats.

Materials and Methods

Animals

All procedures were reviewed and approved by the University of Miami Animal Care and Use Committee (Protocol No. 07-134) and followed the recommendations within the *Guide for the Care and Use of Laboratory Animals* (National Research Council). Every effort was made to use the least possible number of animals and to minimize pain and distress. Male Sprague-Dawley rats (130–150 g at the time of surgery; Harlan, Indianapolis, IN) were housed two per cage and allowed free access to food and water before and after surgery. Lighting was on a 12 hr light/dark cycle. Temperature and humidity were controlled to $22\pm1°C$ and $50\pm10\%$, respectively. Rats were acclimated to the animal facility for at least 5 days prior to use.

General experimental plan

Baseline hind paw withdrawal thresholds and locomotor function were assessed before and 4 weeks following SCI surgery. Spinal cord injured rats were dosed beginning 4 weeks after surgery for seven days. Although SCI rats were dosed daily, withdrawal thresholds were measured only on the first, third and seventh day of dosing (i.e. 28, 30 and 35 days post-SCI surgery). To assess a possible effect of daily compound treatment on locomotor function, locomotor rating scores were obtained from SCI rats 4 weeks after surgery, prior to compound administration, and on the sixth day of compound treatment (i.e. 34 days post-SCI surgery).

Spinal cord injury in the rat

Aseptic surgical technique and sterile instruments were used. The procedure to induce an acute SCI has been previously described [18]. Rats were anesthetized and maintained with isoflurane in O_2 for the duration of the surgery. The back was shaved and the skin cleaned with chlorhexadine. A laminectomy was performed to expose spinal segment T6-T7. A microvascular clip (20 g compressive force, Harvard Apparatus, Hollister, MA) was placed vertically on the exposed thoracic spinal cord, such that clip compressed the entire segment, and then left in place for 60 seconds. Care was taken not to cut the dura or disturb nearby spinal nerve roots. Following spinal compression, the clip was removed, the muscles sutured shut and the skin closed with wound clips. Urinary bladders were expressed twice daily until voiding was regained. Spontaneous voiding returned about 1 or 2 days following spinal compression.

Hind paw withdrawal threshold

Prior to spinal compression surgery, hind paw withdrawal thresholds were measured. The up-down method was used to quantify hind paw responsiveness to innocuous tactile stimulation [23]. Rats were placed in clear Plexiglas containers resting on an elevated wire mesh floor and allowed to acclimate to the chamber for at least 30 min. Eight specific calibrated von Frey filaments were used to determine the withdrawal threshold (0.4, 0.6, 1, 2, 4, 6, 8, 15 grams; Stoelting Co., Woodale, IL). The filament was applied perpendicularly the plantar skin of the hind paw, bowed slightly and held in place for six seconds. A hind paw withdrawal from the filament led to testing with a lower force filament. A lack of response led to the use of the next higher force filament. From the pattern of responses to the filaments, a withdrawal threshold was calculated. Both hind paws were tested and about 5 min separated testing of the opposite paw. An upper withdrawal threshold of 15 g was used. Prior to surgery, rat withdrawal thresholds were 15 g. In order for SCI rats to be included in the study, withdrawal thresholds of one paw needed to be 4 g or less.

Locomotor function: Basso, Beattie, and Bresnahan Score

Following threshold measurement, below-level motor functionality was assessed using a standardized "Locomotor Rating Scale" devised by Basso, Beattie, and Bresnahan (BBB) [24]. The scale ranges from 0, no hind limb function, to 21, normal, coordinated movement of the hind limbs as observed in uninjured rats. Rats were placed in a 1.2 m diameter arena and allowed to continuously move within a four minute observation period. Two observers rated hind limb function, such as movement at joints, hind paw stepping and fore paw-hind paw coordination.

Following the observation period, the scores from both hind limbs were averaged to give a final BBB score. Prior to surgery, BBB scores of naive rats are 21. Spinal cord injured-rats were rated one day prior to the beginning of the treatment period and reassessed on the sixth day of treatment following determination of withdrawal thresholds.

Pharmacological treatments

Following baseline behavioral assessment in SCI rats, rats were divided into four treatment groups. Spinal cord-injured rats were injected with either URB597 (i.p.), WIN 55,212-2 (s.c.) or vehicle (i.p.) twice daily (at approximately 900 and 1700) for 7 days. Withdrawal thresholds were measured following the first daily injection. Following injection, rats were tested once every 30 minutes for up to four hours post-injection. On the sixth day of treatment, following final determination of withdrawal threshold, BBB scores were determined. On the seventh day, immediately following testing at four hours post-injection, rats were deeply anesthetized with isoflurane, decapitated and brain and spinal cord tissues were collected.

In a separate group of SCI rats, either PF-3845 or vehicle was orally administered and rats were tested once every hour up to four hours post-administration. Because of stress associated with p.o. dosing in SCI rats, rats were dosed only once and not treated over a seven-day period. At the last testing time point, rats were deeply anesthetized with isoflurane, decapitated and brain and spinal tissues were collected. Uninjured age-matched rats were also treated with either PF-3845 or vehicle (p.o.) and tissues were collected at the same time as the SCI rats. At the same time, age-matched uninjured rats were treated with either URB597 (i.p.), WIN 55,212-2 (s.c.), or vehicle (i.p.), were deeply anesthetized, decapitated and tissues were collected four hours post-treatment to determine baseline FAA levels and to determine the acute effects of the compounds on FAA levels in uninjured rats. An additional group of uninjured rats were treated with URB597 (i.p.) or vehicle (i.p.), euthanized and brain and spinal cord tissues were collected two hours after treatment.

The spinal cord was divided into four segments: lumbar (L4/L5), a 1 cm segment rostral to the compression epicenter, a 1 cm segment of the epicenter and a 1 cm segment caudal to the epicenter. Tissues were flash frozen on dry ice and stored at −80°C until assay.

Assessment of brain and spinal cord levels of fatty acid amides by liquid chromatography-tandem mass spectrometry

Brain samples were prepared using a method adapted from previously published methods [25]. Briefly, brain samples were removed from −80°C freezer and placed on dry ice. Individual brains were transferred to a clean, tared 50 ml capacity polypropylene conical tube and weights were recorded. A solution of ethyl acetate:hexanes (9:1) was immediately added to each conical tube along with a FAA standard molecule (Palmitoyl Propanolamide, Ironwood Pharmaceuticals, Inc., Cambridge, MA). Samples were homogenized for 15 seconds using an electric-powered mechanical tissue disrupter (Omni Prep Multi-Sample Homogenizer Part Number: 06-021, Omni International, Kennesaw, GA) fitted with stainless steel probe (10 mm×110 mm Stainless Steel Omni Prep/THQ Homogenizer Probe, Omni International, Kennesaw, GA) washed with approximately 30% water, and homogenized for another 15 seconds. Samples were vortexed and centrifuged (2,000×g for 30 minutes at 10°C). After centrifugation, the upper organic layer was recovered and the samples were evaporated to dryness under nitrogen gas. Samples were not subjected to solid phase extraction. After reconstitution in 1 ml chloroform:methanol (1:3), samples were centrifuged (16,000×g for 3 minutes at room temperature) to sediment any particulates. A 100 µl aliquot of each sample supernatant was transferred to individual wells on a 96 well plate. Each sample was diluted 1:1 with methanol containing the internal standard d4-AEA (arachidonoyl-ethanolamide) labeled with 4 deuterium atoms replacing the 4 H's on the methylenes of ethanolamine moiety, Cayman Chemical, Ann Arbor, MI) Waters Acquity/TQD system in positive ion (ES+) mode. Samples were maintained at 6°C.

The procedure for FAA extraction from spinal cord tissue segments was similar to brain FAA extraction procedure listed above with the following change. After evaporation of organic solvents from tissue homogenates the residue from extraction was dissolved in 0.25 ml chloroform:methanol (1:3) instead of 1 ml volume used for brain extracts.

Liquid chromatography-tandem mass spectrometry conditions

Liquid chromatography was conducted using a Higgins Clipeus HPLC column [C8 reverse phase, dimensions 2.1×30 mm, particle size 5 micron (Mountain View, CA)] and samples were eluted using a gradient employing 2 mobile phases A and B from 30%–95% B [HPLC mobile phases A (5 mM ammonium acetate in water) and HPLC mobile phase B (5 mM ammonium acetate in 85:10:5 acetonitrile: isopropanol: water)] using a flow rate of 0.4 ml/min. MS/MS. The following mass transitions were monitored AEA: 348.2>62 m/z, OEA: 326.2>62 m/z, PEA: 300.2>62 m/z, Palmitoyl Propanolamide: 314.2>75.9 m/z, D4-AEA: 352.2>66 m/z (last two are internal standards for fatty acid amides). Chromatograms were integrated and quantified by response to the internal standard peak area using Quanlynx software V4.0 SP4 (Micromass, Ltd).

Compound treatments

URB597 (3 mg/kg, Cayman Chemicals, Ann Arbor, MI) was dissolved in 10% dimethyl sulfoxide (DMSO): 10% Cremophor EL: 80% saline and administered i.p. in a volume of 1.5 ml/kg. URB597 was prepared daily, prior to dosing. WIN 55,212-2 mesylate (3 mg/kg, Sigma-Aldrich Co., St. Louis, MO) was dissolved in 45% (2-Hydroxypropyl)-β-cyclodextrin (Sigma-Aldrich, Co.) in saline and administered s.c. in a volume of 2 ml/kg. PF-3845 (3, 10 mg/kg, synthesized as described by Ahn et al., 2009 b was dissolved in 10% DMSO: 10% Cremophor EL: 80% saline and administered p.o. in a volume of 5 ml/kg.

Statistical analysis

Analyses of LC-MS/MS data were conducted using GraphPad Prism software. For FAA, statistical comparisons between treatment groups were made using an unpaired, two-tailed Student's *t*-test. To determine fold-change in levels of FAA, the levels were normalized to the respective vehicle-treated group. *p* values less than 0.05 were considered significant. To assess the effect of treatment over time on behaviors, a two-way repeated measures analysis of variance (ANOVA) was performed with Student-Newman-Keuls for post hoc analysis. Fatty acid amide levels from each rat were plotted (Fig. 1–5) and the mean ± S.E.M. were calculated. Behavioral data are presented as mean ± S.E.M.

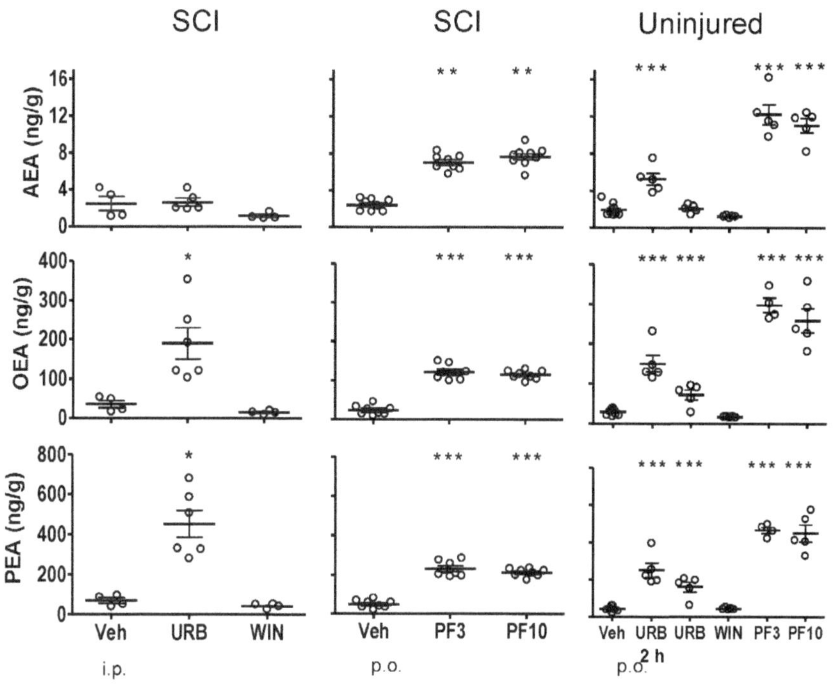

Figure 1. Fatty acid amide concentrations in brain following treatment with FAAH inhibitors, WIN 55,212-2 and vehicle in SCI and uninjured rats. Rats were treated with either URB597 (URB; 3 mg/kg, i.p.), WIN 55,212-2 (WIN; 3 mg/kg, s.c.) or vehicle (Veh; 1.5 ml/kg, i.p.) for seven days and euthanized four hours following the last treatment. One group of URB597 rats were euthanized two hours (2 h) following a single treatment. Rats that received PF-3845 (PF3, PF10; 3, 10 mg/kg, p.o) or vehicle (Veh, p.o.) were treated once and euthanized four hours following dosing. Levels of AEA, OEA and PEA from each rat are shown, the thick horizontal line is the mean and the thin horizontal lines are the S.E.M. n = 4–10/ group. * $p<0.05$, ** $p<0.01$, *** $p<0.001$ vs. vehicle (Student's t-test).

Results

Effect of spinal cord injury on CNS FAA levels

Table 1 summarizes changes in CNS FAA levels four weeks after SCI. The most apparent changes in SCI tissue, compared to uninjured tissues, are of decreased levels of OEA and PEA of thoracic spinal cord at and near the epicenter.

Whole Brain. In untreated, uninjured rats, the mean brain levels of AEA, OEA and PEA were 2.2±0.51, 33.7±3.8 and 67.7±5.0 ng/g tissue, respectively (Fig. 1). In SCI vehicle-treated rats, the mean brain levels of AEA, OEA and PEA were 2.5±0.8, 35.6±9.3 and 69.4±13.6 ng/g tissue, respectively. Brain FAA levels from vehicle-treated SCI rats were not significantly different from brain levels from uninjured rats ($p>0.05$).

Thoracic Spinal Cord. Spinal cord injury led to marked decreases in OEA and PEA content in spinal tissues. The mean level of OEA in thoracic spinal cord from uninjured rats was 652.1±99.1 ng/g tissue. The mean levels of OEA in tissue rostral to the epicenter, the epicenter and caudal to the epicenter from SCI rats were 318.6±44.1, 188.8±17.9 and 275.3±22.3 ng/g tissue, respectively ($p<0.05$, rostral, epicenter and caudal vs. uninjured OEA; Fig. 2–4). The mean level of PEA in thoracic spinal cord from uninjured rats was 1108.0±148.7 ng/g tissue. The mean level of PEA in tissue rostral to the epicenter, the epicenter and caudal to the epicenter from SCI rats were 941.4±122.3, 351.5±56.5 and 740.2±53.2 ng/g tissue (e.g. Fig. 3; $p<0.05$, epicenter and caudal vs. uninjured PEA).

By contrast, mean levels of AEA in spinal tissues from SCI rats were not significantly changed from that of uninjured rats. Levels of AEA in the rostral, epicenter and caudal spinal segments from SCI rats were 5.1±1.1, 4.6±1.3 and 5.4±1.0 ng/g tissue, respectively. Levels of AEA in comparable spinal segments from uninjured rats were 6.0±1.3, 8.0±1.9 and 6.2±0.4 ng/g tissue, respectively. While there was a trend of decreased levels of AEA in spinal tissues from SCI rats, this was not statistically significant from that of uninjured rats ($p>0.05$).

Lumbar Spinal Cord. In lumbar spinal cord from untreated, uninjured rats, the mean levels of AEA, OEA and PEA were 3.8±0.4, 241.0±32.8 and 493.4±61.5 ng/g tissue, respectively. In lumbar spinal cord from SCI rats, the mean levels of AEA, OEA and PEA were 2.6±0.1, 224.1±30.0 and 344.7±53.8 ng/g tissue, respectively. The levels of FAA in lumbar spinal cord from SCI rats, while slightly decreased, were not significantly different from that of uninjured rats ($p>0.05$; Fig. 5).

Effect of FAAH inhibitors and WIN 55,212-2 on CNS FAA levels

URB597. Four hours post-treatment with URB597, levels of AEA, OEA and PEA were significantly increased in spinal segments rostral (Fig. 2) and caudal (Fig. 4) to the injury and lumbar segment (Fig. 5) of spinal cord from SCI rats ($p<0.05$ vs. vehicle treatment). Levels of AEA were unchanged in brains from both uninjured and SCI rats, despite clear increases in OEA and PEA (Fig. 1). To confirm that the dose of URB597 was effective in blocking brain FAAH, uninjured rats were euthanized two hours following URB597 treatment; FAA were significantly increased ($p<0.05$ vs. vehicle; Fig. 1). In contrast to the increases in FAA rostral and caudal to the spinal injury, there was a lack of effect of URB597 treatment at the epicenter four hours after treatment ($p>0.05$ vs. vehicle treatment, Fig. 3).

Table 2 summaries changes in CNS FAA content following URB597 treatment in SCI and uninjured rats. The effects of

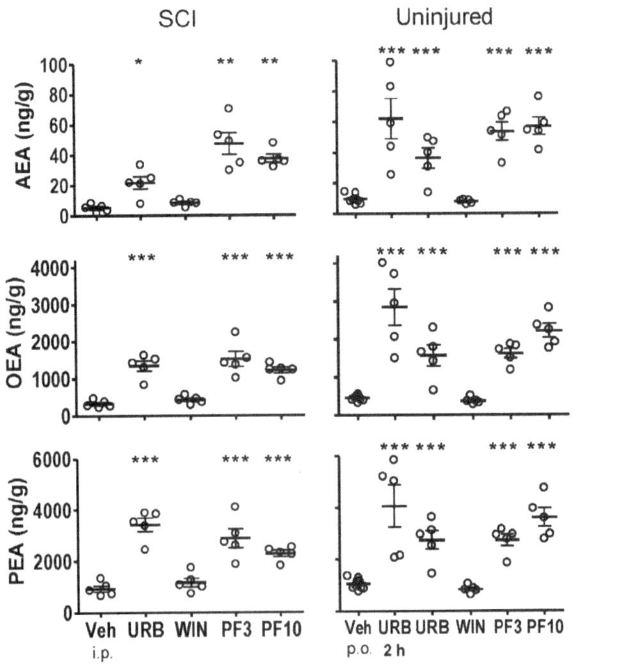

Figure 2. Fatty acid amide concentrations in thoracic spinal cord segments rostral to the spinal injury from SCI rats or comparable thoracic spinal cord segments from uninjured rats following treatment with FAAH inhibitors, WIN 55,212-2 and vehicle. Both SCI and uninjured rats were treated with either URB597 (URB; 3 mg/kg, i.p.), WIN 55,212-2 (WIN; 3 mg/kg, s.c.) or vehicle (Veh; 1.5 ml/kg, i.p.) for seven days and euthanized four hours following the last treatment. Rats that received PF-3845 (PF3, PF10) were treated once (3, 10 mg/kg, p.o.) and euthanized four hours following dosing. One group of uninjured rats was treated once with URB597 and euthanized two hours (2 h) following treatment. The FAA levels of thoracic spinal cord of uninjured rats from this figure are repeated for Figures 3 and 4. Levels of AEA, OEA and PEA from each rat are shown, the thick horizontal line is the mean and the thin horizontal lines are the S.E.M. n = 4–10/group. * $p<0.05$, ** $p<0.01$, *** $p<0.001$ vs. vehicle (Student's t-test).

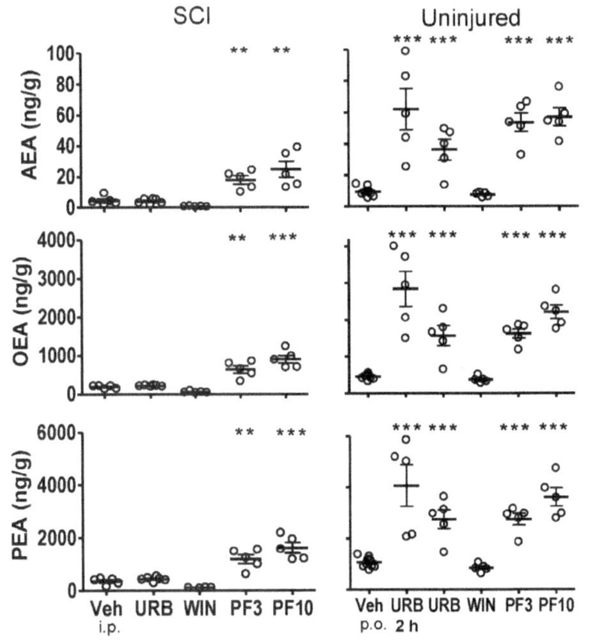

Figure 3. Fatty acid amide concentrations in thoracic spinal cord segments from the epicenter of injury from SCI rats or comparable spinal cord segments from uninjured rats following treatment with FAAH inhibitors, WIN 55,212-2 and vehicle. Both SCI and uninjured rats were treated with either URB597 (URB; 3 mg/kg, i.p.), WIN 55,212-2 (WIN; 3 mg/kg, s.c.) or vehicle (Veh; 1 ml/kg, i.p.) for seven days and euthanized four hours following the last treatment. One group of uninjured rats was treated once with URB597 and euthanized two hours (2 hr) following treatment. Rats that received PF-3845 (PF3, PF10) were treated once (3, 10 mg/kg, p.o.) and euthanized four hours following dosing. Levels of AEA, OEA and PEA from each rat are shown, the thick horizontal line is the mean and the thin horizontal lines are the S.E.M. n = 4–10/group. * $p<0.05$, ** $p<0.01$, *** $p<0.001$ vs. vehicle (Student's t-test).

URB597 treatment, as fold-change over vehicle-treatment, on CNS FAA are summarized following a seven day treatment schedule and following a single treatment.

PF-3845. PF-3845 also consistently increased CNS FAA levels in both uninjured and SCI rats. However, unlike URB597, PF-3845 also elevated FAAs at the epicenter in this experiment, at both doses, four hours after treatment ($p<0.05$ vs. vehicle; Fig. 1–5). Overall, the effect of PF-3845 at 3 mg/kg and 10 mg/kg on tissue FAA appeared to be similar with the potential exception of effects at the epicenter.

Table 3 summaries CNS FAA content, as fold-change over vehicle treatment, following PF-3845 treatment in SCI and uninjured rats.

WIN 55,212-2. Interestingly, there were trends towards changes in FAA concentrations following treatment with the nonselective CB receptor agonist WIN 55,212-2 in both uninjured (single treatment) and SCI rats (seven-day treatment). In brain and thoracic spinal cord from uninjured rats, there were tendencies for reduced FAA (Fig. 1–5; Table 2). However, a trend towards an increase in AEA in lumbar spinal cord in uninjured rats was observed following a single treatment of WIN 55,212-2 ($p>0.05$ vs. vehicle treatment).

In SCI rats, there were trends towards both decreased and increased tissue FAA content following WIN 55,212-2 treatment. A trend towards decreased FAA was observed in brain from SCI rats following seven days WIN 55,212-2 treatment ($p>0.05$ vs. vehicle treatment; Table 2). At the same time, spinal cord rostral and caudal to the epicenter showed increased levels of FAA ($p>0.05$ vs. vehicle treatment; Table 2).

Antinociceptive effect of FAAH inhibitors and WIN 55,212-2 in SCI rats

Prior to seven day dosing, the mean hind paw withdrawal threshold of all SCI rats was 3.9±0.6 g (Fig. 6). The mean baseline withdrawal thresholds, within each treatment group, prior to the morning treatment, did not significantly change over the seven day treatment period ($p>0.05$). Significant increases in withdrawal thresholds were observed 30 min following treatment with WIN 55,212-2 on each day of behavioral testing. In fact, on each day of testing, WIN 55,212-2 fully ameliorated hind paw cutaneous hypersensitivity ($p<0.05$ vs. vehicle treatment and vs. baseline; two-way repeated measures-ANOVA). Furthermore, on each of the testing days the effect persisted for the duration of the four hour testing period. By contrast, URB597 did not significantly increase withdrawal thresholds at any time post-treatment ($p>0.05$ vs. vehicle treatment). Likewise, vehicle treatment did not significantly alter withdrawal thresholds.

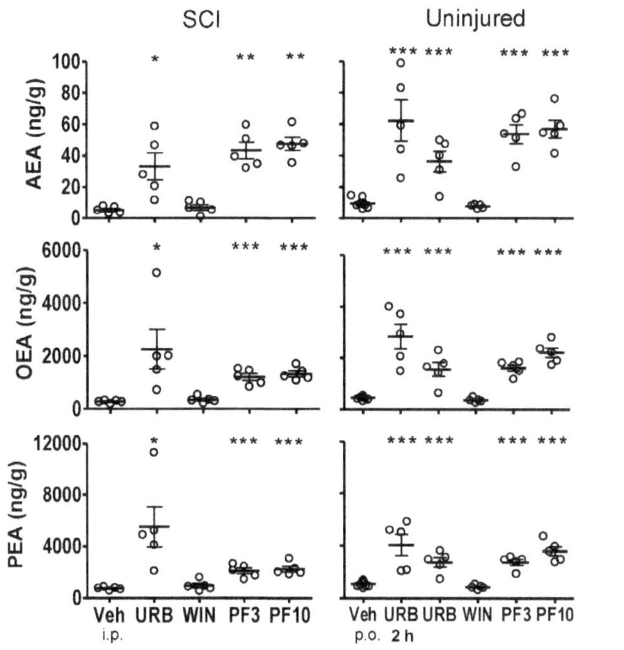

Figure 4. Fatty acid amide concentrations in thoracic spinal cord segments caudal to the spinal injury from SCI rats or comparable spinal cord segments from uninjured rats following treatment with FAAH inhibitors, WIN 55,212-2 and vehicle. Rats were treated with either URB597 (URB; 3 mg/kg, i.p.), WIN 55,212-2 (WIN; 3 mg/kg, s.c.) or vehicle (Veh; 1 ml/kg, i.p.) for seven days and euthanized four hours following the last treatment. One group of uninjured rats was treated once with URB597 and euthanized two hours (2 h) following treatment. Rats that received PF-3845 (PF3, PF10) were treated once (3, 10 mg/kg, p.o.) and euthanized four hours following dosing. Levels of AEA, OEA and PEA from each rat are shown, the dark horizontal line is the mean and the light horizontal lines are the S.E.M. n = 4–10/group. * $p<0.05$, ** $p<0.01$, *** $p<0.001$ vs. vehicle (Student's t-test).

A separate group of SCI rats was dosed once with PF-3845 (Fig. 7). Four weeks following SCI, the mean withdrawal threshold of all rats was 2.3±0.2 g. Increases in withdrawal thresholds were observed with PF-3845 (10 mg/kg) at one and three hours post-treatment ($p<0.05$ vs. vehicle treatment). The increase in withdrawal threshold at one and three hours post-treatment is about a 40% maximum possible effect (100% effect = 15 g). No significant effects on withdrawal threshold were observed with either 3 mg/kg or vehicle ($p>0.05$).

Effect of URB597 and WIN 55,212-2 on below-level motor function in SCI rats

Prior to treatment, the mean BBB Locomotor Scores of all SCI rats was significantly decreased from 21 to 9.8±0.4 ($p<0.05$; Fig. 8). This score means frequent stepping with the dorsal rather than the plantar hind paw and no fore limb-hind limb coordination. After six days of treatment with either URB597, WIN 55,212-2 or vehicle, BBB Locomotor Scores were 9.9±0.6, 10.2±1.3, 10.6±0.5, respectively ($p>0.05$ vs. vehicle treatment). Compared with BBB Scores before treatment, BBB Scores were not significantly changed after six days of treatment in SCI rats ($p>0.05$; Fig. 8). The effect of a single dose of PF-3845 on BBB Locomotor Scores was not assessed.

Discussion

Despite significantly increasing brain and spinal cord tissue levels of FAA in SCI rats, seven day systemic administration of the FAAH inhibitor URB597 did not demonstrate antinociception. Acute treatment with the FAAH inhibitor PF-3845, which also significantly increased CNS levels of FAA, led to a moderate, non-dose dependent antinociception in SCI rats. By contrast, WIN 55,212-2 robustly ameliorated below-level cutaneous hypersensitivity in SCI rats for the duration of the seven-day treatment period. Markedly decreased tissue levels of OEA and PEA were observed at the epicenter and tissue caudal to the epicenter in SCI rats. While both FAAH inhibitors increased tissue FAA in SCI rats, only PF-3845 increased AEA, OEA and PEA at the epicenter, which in part could underlie PF-3845's modest antinociceptive effect. Neither FAAH inhibition nor CB receptor activation over seven days improved hind limb motor function. While direct activation of CB receptors leads to a significant and sustained antinociception, the current data indicate that increasing CNS FAA levels alone may not be sufficient for ameliorating below-level neuropathic SCI pain.

Changes in FAA levels in spinal tissue segments that may be crucial in the initiation and maintenance of neuropathic pain following a SCI were reported in the current study. The current study confirmed a previous finding of no change in levels of AEA and PEA in spinal tissue rostral to the epicenter and at the epicenter four weeks after a SCI [26]. However, the current study observed that PEA was decreased caudal to the epicenter and that OEA was decreased both rostrally and caudally to the epicenter as well as within the epicenter. It is speculated that the loss of tonic FAA-meditated inhibition following SCI could contribute to enhanced excitability of spinal dorsal horn neurons either rostral or caudal to the epicenter [2,27]. In the current study, slight decreases ($p>0.05$; Table 1) in FAA were observed in the lumbar spinal cord, which receives primary afferents that innervate the hind paw. The mechanism that leads to an apparent decrease of FAA in lumbar segment, several segments from the epicenter, has yet to be elucidated, but a consequence could be dorsal horn neuron hyperexcitability. However, lumbar spinal cord FAA were significantly increased following URB597 treatment without being accompanied by significant antinociception. Likewise, FAA levels in lumbar spinal cord were increased following PF-3845, but only a slight antinociceptive effect was obtained. Convincing evidence that the loss of CB_1 receptor-mediated tonic inhibition alone can lead to hyperexcitable lumbar dorsal horn neurons is lacking, but perhaps it is a fusion of diminished functioning of several neurotransmitter systems (e.g. GABA) that leads to the neuropathic pain state following SCI [28,29].

Changes in supraspinal function could also be crucial in the maintenance of neuropathic SCI pain [16,19]. The current study found no significant change in whole brain FAA levels following SCI, but perhaps there are changes in specific pain-related brain nuclei following SCI. It is further speculated that processes involved in cellular function and intercellular signaling could be altered in the brain as well as in the spinal cord following injury [30,31]. Changes in the brain opioid system have been suggested to underlie reduced efficacy of supraspinal injection of morphine in SCI rats [32,33]. By contrast, supraspinal injection of WIN 55,212-2 is fully efficacious in SCI rats [19]. Changes in either brain CB receptors or FAA level have yet to be identified following SCI. Nonetheless, despite a robust increase in whole brain FAA following FAAH inhibition, there was a lack of robust antinociception; a role for brain FAA in SCI pain will need further elucidation.

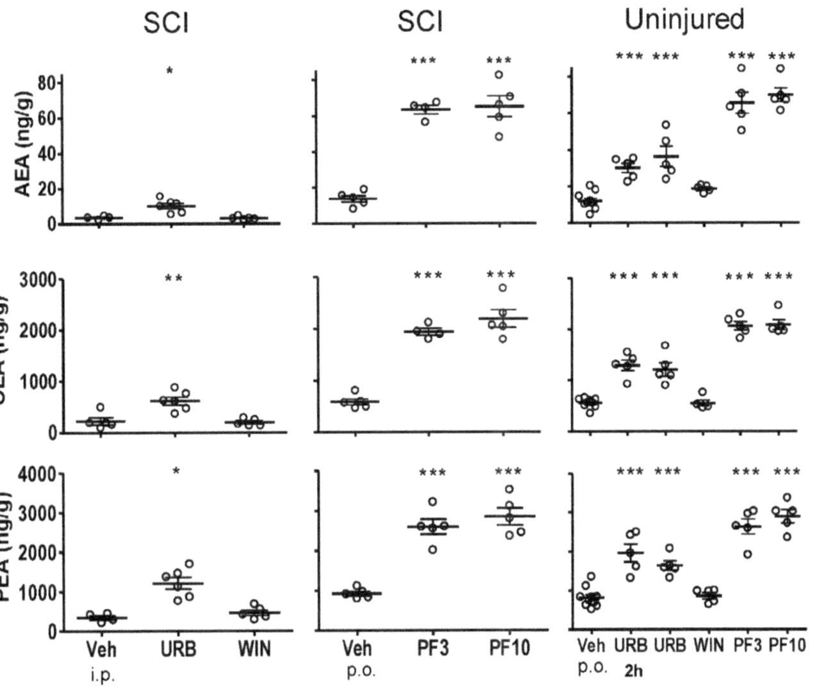

Figure 5. Fatty acid amide concentrations in lumbar spinal cord from SCI rats or uninjured rats following treatment with FAAH inhibitors, WIN 55,212-2 and vehicle. Rats were treated with either URB597 (URB; 3 mg/kg, i.p.), WIN 55,212-2 (WIN; 3 mg/kg, s.c.) or vehicle (Veh; 1.5 ml/kg, i.p.) for seven days and euthanized four hours following the last treatment. One group of uninjured rats was treated once with URB597 and euthanized two hours (2 h) following treatment. Rats that received PF-3845 (PF3, PF10) were treated once (3, 10 mg/kg, p.o.) and euthanized four hours following dosing. Levels of AEA, OEA and PEA from each rat are shown, the thick horizontal line is the mean and the thin horizontal lines are the S.E.M. n = 4–10/group. * $p<0.05$, ** $p<0.01$, *** $p<0.001$ vs. vehicle (Student's t-test).

A number of preclinical neuropathic pain studies have demonstrated marked antinociception following both acute and repeated activation of CB receptors, which appears to be in part mediated through the CB_1 receptor [3,20,34–38]. It is possible that attenuation of specific symptoms, such as hypersensitivity to noxious stimulation (hyperalgesia), could be ameliorated through other CB receptors or non-CB receptors [11,39].

The current study confirms previous findings in neuropathic pain models of a lack tolerance to the antinociceptive effect following repeated treatment with a CB receptor agonist [20,35,36]. By contrast, a loss of efficacy following repeated treatment with morphine in SCI rats has been observed [20]. Thus, a potential advantage of CB1 receptor agonists over, for example, opioid receptor agonists is sustained efficacy over the course of the treatment period. Tolerance to CB receptor agonists does appear however, under specific circumstances. In the case of an acute pain state, as modeled by the hot plate test in uninjured animals, tolerance to the antinociceptive effect appears within five days of daily treatment [20,40]. The mechanism by which CB receptor agonists retain efficacy in some pain states and not in others is currently unknown. While it is possible that the injury state could underlie the development of antinociceptive tolerance, the test stimulus could also influence whether or not tolerance is obtained.

One issue raised by CB receptor agonists is the presence of motoric effects at or near antinociceptive doses. In the case of

Table 1. Summary of Changes in Fatty Acid Amides Four Weeks Following a Spinal Cord Injury in Rats.

	AEA	OEA	PEA
Brain	**n.c.**	**n.c.**	**n.c.**
Spinal cord			
Rostral to epicenter	↓ n.s.	↓*	↓*
Epicenter	↓ n.s.	↓*	↓*
Caudal to epicenter	↓ n.s.	↓*	↓*
Lumbar spinal cord	↓ n.s.	↓ n.s.	↓ n.s.

Changes in fatty acid amides (AEA, *N*-arachidonoylethanolamide; OEA, *N*-oleoyl ethanolamide; PEA, *N*-palmitoyl ethanolamide) four weeks following spinal cord injury compared to that of uninjured rats.
↓, decrease; n.c., no change; n.s., not statistically significant; * $p<0.05$ (Student's t-test).

Table 2. Fold-change of tissue fatty acid amide levels following treatment with URB597 or WIN 55,212-2 relative to vehicle treatment.

Seven days		AEA					OEA					PEA				
Rats	Treatment	Brain	Rostral	Epicenter	Caudal	Lumbar	Brain	Rostral	Epicenter	Caudal	Lumbar	Brain	Rostral	Epicenter	Caudal	Lumbar
SCI	Vehicle	1	1	1	1	1	1	1	1	1	1	1	1	1	1	1
SCI	URB	1.6 (*)	4.3 (**)	0.9 (n.s.)	6.1 (*)	2.9 (*)	5.3 (*)	4.2 (***)	1.2 (n.s.)	8.2 (*)	2.8 (**)	6.5 (***)	3.6 (***)	1.2 (n.s.)	7.5 (*)	3.5 (*)
SCI	WIN	0.5 (n.s.)	1.6 (n.s.)	0.2 (n.s)	1.3 (n.s.)	0.9 (n.s.)	0.4 (n.s.)	1.3 (n.s.)	0.3 (n.s.)	1.2 (n.s.)	0.9 (n.s.)	0.6 (n.s.)	1.3 (n.s.)	0.3 (n.s.)	1.3 (n.s.)	1.3 (n.s.)
One day																
N.I.	Vehicle	1	—	1	—	1	1	—	1	—	1	1	—	1	—	1
N.I.	URB (2 h)	2.7 (*)	—	6.5 (***)	—	2.5 (***)	5.1 (***)	—	6.3 (***)	—	2.3 (***)	5.7 (***)	—	3.8 (***)	—	2.3 (***)
N.I.	URB	1.1 (n.s.)	—	3.8 (***)	—	3.0 (***)	2.5 (***)	—	3.5 (***)	—	2.2 (***)	3.6 (***)	—	2.6 (***)	—	2.0 (***)
N.I.	WIN	0.6 (n.s.)	—	0.8 (n.s.)	—	1.6 (n.s)	0.6 (n.s.)	—	0.8 (n.s.)	—	1 (n.s.)	1 (n.s.)	—	0.8 (n.s.)	—	1 (n.s.)

Values are fold-changes compared to vehicle treatment levels in spinal cord injured (SCI) and non-injured (N.I.) rats. On the seventh day of treatment, tissues were collected 4 hours post-administration with either vehicle, URB597 (URB, 3 mg/kg, i.p.) or WIN 55,212-2 (WIN, 3 mg/kg, s.c.) from SCI rats. Non-injured rats were treated once and tissues collected four hours post-treatment. In one set of non-injured rats (n = 5), tissues were collected two hours (2 h) post-treatment with URB597.
"Epicenter" refers to thoracic spinal cord tissue either from the site of injury from SCI rats or comparable spinal cord tissue from non-injured rats.
n.s., not significant.
*$p<0.05$, **$p<0.01$, ***$p<0.001$ vs. vehicle-treated (Student's t-test).

Table 3. Fold-change of tissue fatty acid amide levels following a single oral treatment with PF-3845 compared to oral vehicle treatment.

		AEA					**OEA**					**PEA**				
Rats	**Treatment**	**Brain**	**Rostral**	**Epicenter**	**Caudal**	**Lumbar**	**Brain**	**Rostral**	**Epicenter**	**Caudal**	**Lumbar**	**Brain**	**Rostral**	**Epicenter**	**Caudal**	**Lumbar**
SCI	Vehicle	1	1	1	1	1	1	1	1	1	1	1	1	1	1	1
SCI	PF, 3	2.9 (**)	9.8 (***)	4.3 (***)	5.7 (***)	4.6 (***)	5.2 (***)	4.1 (***)	2.7 (**)	3.4 (***)	3.3 (***)	4.5 (***)	3.3 (***)	2.0 (**)	2.6 (***)	2.8 (***)
SCI	PF, 10	3.2 (**)	7.7 (***)	5.9 (***)	6.2 (***)	4.7 (***)	4.9 (***)	3.3 (***)	3.9 (***)	3.8 (***)	3.8 (***)	4.2 (***)	2.6 (***)	2.8 (***)	2.8 (***)	3.1 (***)
N.I.	Vehicle	1	—	1	—	1	1	—	1	—	1	1	—	1	—	1
N.I.	PF, 3	6.4 (***)	—	5.6 (***)	—	5.5 (***)	10.2 (***)	—	3.6 (***)	—	3.7 (***)	10.4 (***)	—	2.6 (***)	—	3.1 (***)
N.I.	PF, 10	5.8 (***)	—	6.0 (***)	—	5.8 (***)	8.9 (***)	—	4.9 (***)	—	3.8 (***)	10.1 (***)	—	3.4 (***)	—	3.5 (***)

Values are fold-changes compared to vehicle treatment levels in spinal cord injured (SCI) and non-injured (N.I) rats. Tissues were collected 4 hours post-oral administration of either PF-3845 (3, 10 mg/kg) or vehicle.
"Epicenter" refers to thoracic spinal cord tissue either from the site of injury from SCI rats or comparable spinal cord tissue from non-injured rats.
*$p<0.05$, **$p<0.01$, ***$p<0.001$ vs. vehicle-treated (Student's t-test).

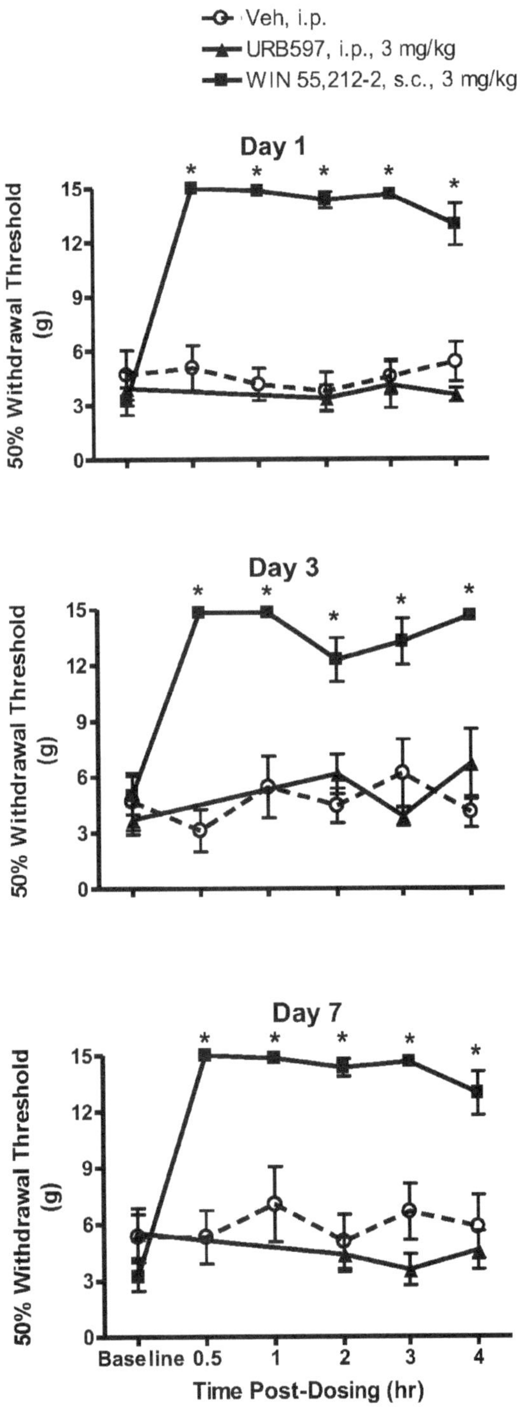

Figure 6. Effects of URB597 and WIN 55,212-2 treatment over seven days on below-level cutaneous hypersensitivity in rats with neuropathic SCI pain. Baseline hind paw withdrawal thresholds were measured prior to treatment with either URB597 (3 mg/kg, i.p.), WIN 55,212-2 (3 mg/kg, s.c.) or vehicle (Veh, 1.5 ml/kg, i.p.). Rats were treated twice daily and tested following the first daily injection. On the first day of testing, a robust antinociception was observed beginning 30 min post-injection of WIN 55,212-2, which was observed also observed on days 3 and 7. By contrast, no antinociceptive effects were observed following treatment with either URB597 or vehicle. Data presented as mean ± S.E.M. n = 8–10/group. * $p<0.05$ vs. vehicle (Two-way repeated measures ANOVA, Student-Newman-Keuls test).

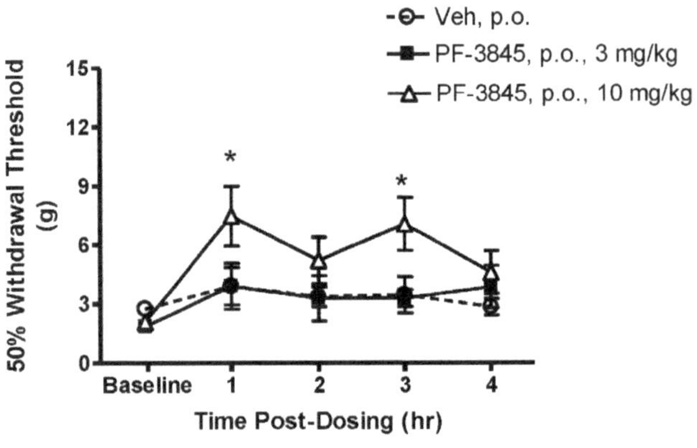

Figure 7. Effect of PF-3845 treatment on below-level cutaneous hypersensitivity in rats with neuropathic SCI pain. Following baseline hind paw withdrawal threshold measurement, SCI rats were treated with either PF-3845 (3, 10 mg/kg, p.o.) or vehicle (Veh; 5 ml/kg, p.o.). An antinociceptive effect was observed 1 and 3 hours following administration of 10 mg/kg, but not 3 mg/kg. Data presented as mean ± S.E.M. n = 8–9/group. * $p<0.05$ vs. vehicle (Two-way repeated measures ANOVA, Student-Newman-Keuls test).

WIN 55,212-2, the 50% antinociceptive dose is 0.9 mg/kg (s.c., 30 min post-dosing) whereas the dose needed to produce 50% disruption on the rotarod test (s.c., 3 hrs. post-dosing) is about the same [14,20]. In a previous study, a sedating dose of the anxiolytic drug diazepam, did not increase hind paw withdrawal thresholds in SCI rats, indicating that the behavioral endpoint is sensitive to antinociceptive treatment rather than to a treatment that merely disrupt motor function [18]. Thus, the increase in withdrawal thresholds observed with WIN 55,212-2 in the current study cannot be entirely attributed to catalepsy or motor dysfunction.

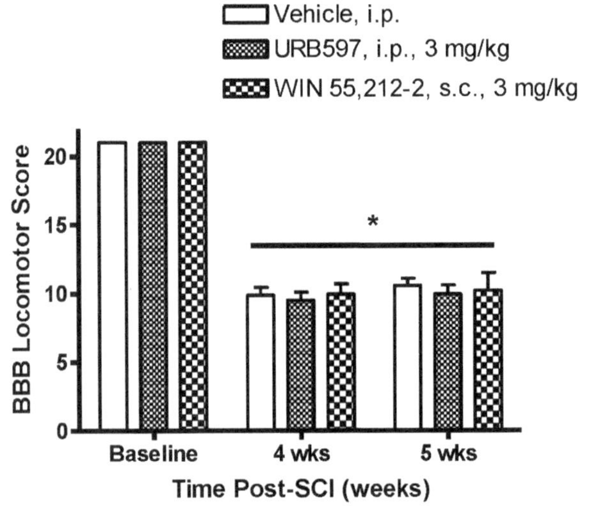

Figure 8. Effects of URB597 and WIN 55,212-2 on BBB Locomotor Scores in SCI rats. Prior to spinal compression surgery ("Baseline"), BBB Locomotor Scores were 21, indicating normal hind limb function. (A Score of "0" indicates no hind limb function.) The mean BBB Locomotor Score obtained the day before initiation of the seven-day treatment procedure ("4 wks" post-SCI) was 9.8±0.4. Spinal cord-injured rats were evaluated again on the sixth day of treatment ("5 wks" post-SCI) and there were no significant changes in BBB Scores. Data presented as mean ± S.E.M. n = 8–10/group. *$p<0.05$ vs. pre-SCI (Two-way repeated measures ANOVA, Student-Newman-Keuls test).

While targeting CB_1 receptors is a promising therapeutic strategy for ameliorating neuropathic SCI pain, prominent psychomotor side effects are associated with CB_1 receptor activation [14,20]. Alternatively, elevating synaptic levels of FAA is antinociceptive and does not appear to induce adverse side effects as the antinociception appears to be mediated through the CB_2 receptor, and possibly through other non-CB mediated mechanisms, such as through activation of the TRPV1 channel, as well as through the CB_1 receptor [9–11,41]. URB597 is a potent FAAH inhibitor—50% of brain FAAH activity is inhibited at a dose of 0.15 mg/kg (i.p.) [10]. At doses higher than 0.3 mg/kg, 1 and 3 mg/kg (i.p.), levels of FAA do not appear to be greatly increased, thus a FAAH inhibition plateau is reached at about 1 mg/kg [42]. In vivo, URB597 inhibits the degradation of AEA within 15 min of injection and significant inhibition of FAAH activity is observed up to 12 hours post-injection [10]. Importantly, no deleterious effect on motor function, as assessed in the rotarod test, was observed at doses of up to 5 mg/kg of URB597 and robust behavioral effects (e.g. antinociception, anxiolytic-like effects) were observed at very low doses (0.1–0.5 mg/kg, i.p.) [13,43]. In the current study, significant spinal tissue levels of FAA were obtained with 3 mg/kg URB597 in both SCI and uninjured rats. Similarly, both doses of PF-3845 significantly raised FAA levels in spinal tissues, including the epicenter of spinal cord from SCI rats as well as spinal tissue from uninjured rats. Thus, the current study demonstrates that it is possible to increase FAA in injured spinal tissue.

Despite significantly increasing CNS FAA levels, no antinociceptive effect was observed with URB597 in SCI rats, following either a single dose (day 1) or multiple doses (at either day 3 or day 7). A single dose of URB597 in peripheral nerve-injured mice resulted in a small antinociceptive effect, but four days of treatment, however, led to an even greater antinociceptive effect [22]. One significant difference between the previous studies showing efficacy with URB597 and the current study is that previous studies utilized models of peripheral neuropathy whereas the current study utilized a model of central pain following a SCI. There are a number of drugs that are efficacious in peripheral neuropathic pain models but are not efficacious in neuropathic SCI models [17,18]. Why this is so is not entirely clear, but the differential pharmacology between peripheral and central neuropathic pain states highly suggests that there are meaningful differences in the substrates that mediate the symptoms presented by these pain states. The differential substrates hypothesized to exist in preclinical models is indirectly supported by clinical findings, as a similar pharmacological divergence also exists between clinical neuropathic SCI and peripheral neuropathic pains [2].

Whereas URB597 lacked efficacy, PF-3845 led to a partial, non-dose dependent amelioration of neuropathic SCI pain. In addition to inhibitory effects on neurons, FAA concurrently suppress the release of pro-inflammatory mediators from immune cells and facilitate the release of anti-inflammatory substances [26]. It is possible that PF-3845 is more potent than URB597 on FAAH expressed in microglia and macrophage or that PF-3845 better penetrates damaged tissue as found at the epicenter to reach these cell types. In fact, 3 mg/kg (p.o.) PF-3845 led to a greater increase of AEA in CNS tissues, including the epicenter, compared to 3 mg/kg (i.p.) URB597. It has been reported elsewhere that FAA levels in mice treated with PF-3845 were higher compared to mice treated with URB597, despite the same dose and route [12]. Following PF-3845 treatment, FAA and anti-inflammatory substances from the epicenter could diffuse to nearby spinal dorsal horn neurons that are hyperexcited following SCI [44]. Perhaps it is the increase in anti-inflammatory substances within and adjacent to the epicenter that is crucial in suppressing hyperexcited central neurons. The antinociceptive effect observed with PF-3845 in neuropathic SCI rats could be partially mediated through a combination of CB receptor-dependent and CB receptor-independent mechanisms [45,46].

While no robust effect was observed on below-level pain in the current study, it is possible that above-level and at-level SCI pain could be attenuated by FAAH inhibition. In addition to significant hyperexcitation of central neurons, there appears to be significant primary afferent hyperexcitation following SCI, which could underlie cutaneous hypersensitivity and spontaneous pain at and above the SCI [44,47,48]. These afferents could be sensitive to FAA through CB receptor or non-CB receptor mediated mechanisms or both. Increased sodium channel expression has been observed in injured peripheral nerves following injury—perhaps a similar increase in sodium channel expression in peripheral nerves following a SCI, as reported in the CNS, underlies at-level pain [49,50]. Indeed, SCI patients have reported relief from at-level pain following application of either capsaicin, a TRPV1 agonist, or lidocaine, a sodium channel blocking local anesthetic [51,52]. Perhaps the slight increase in FAA obtained with PF-3845 would have been sufficient to reduce at-level neuropathic pain. Further studies, however, are needed to characterize the extent of the involvement of primary afferent neurons in SCI pain.

A closer examination of studies that tested FAAH inhibitors on peripheral neuropathic cutaneous hypersensitivity indicates weak to no efficacy. As mentioned earlier, a single treatment of URB597 (10 mg/kg, p.o.) in mice with a chronic constriction injury of the sciatic nerve led to a small antinociceptive effect [22]. In rats with a spinal nerve ligation, URB597 (0.3 mg/kg, i.p.) treatment led to a 42% reversal of hind paw tactile hypersensitivity [42]. It is possible that higher doses of URB597 could yield greater antinociception, even though Karbarz et al. (2009) reported no further increases in FAA with higher doses. In rats with a partial sciatic nerve ligation, no effect was obtained with URB597 (0.3 mg/kg, i.p.), but the same dose was significantly efficacious in rats with a peripheral inflammation [13]. Likewise, significant antinociception and brain FAA levels were obtained in rats with a hind paw inflammation at 3 mg/kg PF-3845 (p.o.) [12]. In FAAH deficient mice, brain AEA levels were about 10-fold higher than that of wild-type mice [53]. Following a sciatic nerve injury, FAAH knockout mice demonstrated marked ipsilateral hind paw hypersensitivity, indicating that increased CNS AEA did not prevent the onset of nerve injury-induced nociception. However, the degree of hind paw carrageenan-induced hypersensitivity in FAAH deficient mice was not as severe as that seen in wild-type mice. While the findings indicate some antinociception following increased CNS FAA in the neuropathic state, the antinociception is not as robust as compared to that obtained in the painful inflammatory state. It is speculated that a SCI that is accompanied by significant inflammation could be sensitive to the effect of FAAH inhibition. Perhaps early treatment, around the time of injury or soon thereafter, will be efficacious.

A potential limitation of the current study is the dose of URB597 used. Perhaps a much greater dose of URB597 would have shown efficacy, even though it appears that there is no further gain in FAA levels in the CNS [42]. In mice with a peripheral nerve injury antinociceptive effects of URB597 were observed at 10 mg/kg (i.p.) and at 50 mg/kg (p.o.) [22,54]. The antinociceptive effects were attenuated with CB_1 receptor antagonist, indicating mediation through CB_1 receptors. Interestingly, Russo et al. (2007) saw only partial attenuation of the effect of

URB597 with CB_2 receptor antagonist treatment whereas Kinsey et al. (2009) observed full attenuation. The different behavioral endpoints and potential off-target activity of a high dose could in part explain the differences between the two findings. Nonetheless, perhaps much higher doses of URB597 in the SCI rats could lead to robust antinociception.

A recent clinical study of the FAAH inhibitor PF-04457845 in osteoarthritis pain [55] showed a lack of analgesic efficacy despite demonstration of significant elevation of FAA in patients' plasma and significant efficacy in preclinical studies in rodent models of non-neuropathic pain [56]. The disconnection between the preclinical findings and clinical outcomes raises issues of translatability, of whether clinical experimental methods in fact parallel preclinical experimental methods and whether preclinical models accurately model the clinical state. On one hand, it is not entirely clear if peripherally measured levels of the biomarker of interest are adequate in order to make predictions on behaviors that are CNS mediated. On the other hand, there may be a tenuous relationship of some preclinical animal models (e.g. the rat hind paw formalin test) to long-standing pathologies such as osteoarthritis. The current study utilized a rat model of neuropathic SCI pain, in which analgesics used for clinical neuropathic SCI pain appear antinociceptive [18]. The current findings suggest that increasing FAA alone may not be an efficacious treatment specifically for below-level SCI neuropathic pain.

While the current study suggests at most a weak antinociceptive effect of FAAH inhibition alone, greater antinociceptive effects could be obtained by combining an FAAH inhibitor with a known analgesic drug, thereby enhancing the efficacy of the analgesic drug [57]. The combination of opioids with AEA leads to a synergistic antinociception [58,59]. A metabolite of acetaminophen has been shown to enhance synaptic AEA by blocking its transporter [60]. Although acetaminophen alone is not antinociceptive in SCI rats, adding it to analgesic drugs led to synergistic antinociception which was CB_1 receptor-mediated [61]. Combination drug therapy, with FAAH inhibitors at the core, could be of great value for neuropathic SCI pain, for which few effective analgesic treatments exist [9,62].

Acknowledgments

We are highly grateful for the technical assistance of Ironwood scientists Rob Busby, Ada Silos-Santiago, Alex Bryant, Gerhard Hannig, Galen Carey and Mark Currie and of University of Miami scientists Maria Collado, Shyam Gajavelli, Stanislava Jergova, and Lyudmila Rusakova. We also thank Kay Ahn and Doug Johnson (Pfizer, Inc.) for the precursor to PF-3845.

Author Contributions

Conceived and designed the experiments: ATH PG GTM JPP JS. Performed the experiments: ATH PG MV. Analyzed the data: MV ATH JPP GTM JS. Contributed reagents/materials/analysis tools: BFC. Wrote the paper: JS ATH GTM JPP.

References

1. Siddall PJ (2009) Management of neuropathic pain following spinal cord injury: now and in the future. Spinal Cord 47: 352–359.
2. Finnerup NB and Jensen TS (2004) Spinal cord injury pain—mechanisms and treatment. Eur J Neurol 11: 73–82.
3. Rahn EJ and Hohmann AG (2009) Cannabinoids as pharmacotherapies for neuropathic pain: from the bench to the bedside. Neurotherapeutics 6: 713–737.
4. Cardenas DD and Jensen MP (2006) Treatments for chronic pain in persons with spinal cord injury: A survey study. J Spinal Cord Med 29: 109–117.
5. Russo EB (2008) Cannabinoids in the management of difficult to treat pain. Ther Clin Risk Mang 4: 245–259.
6. Huestis MA, Gorelick DA, Heishman SJ, Preston KL, Nelson RA, et al. (2001) Blockade of effects of smoked marijuana by the CB1-selective cannabinoid receptor antagonist SR141716. Arch Gen Psychiatry 58: 322–328.
7. Richardson JD, Aanonsen L and Hargreaves KM (1998) Antihyperalgesic effects of spinal cannabinoids. Eur J Pharmacol 345: 145–153.
8. Helyes Z, Nemeth J, Than M, Bolcskei K, Pinter E, et al. (2003) Inhibitory effect of anandamide on resiniferatoxin-induced sensory neuropeptide release in vivo and neuropathic hyperalgesia in the rat. Life Sci 73: 2345–2353.
9. Ahn K, Johnson DS and Cravatt BF (2009) Fatty acid amide hydrolase as a potential therapeutic target for the treatment of pain and CNS disorders. Expert Opin Drug Discov 4: 763–784.
10. Piomelli D, Tarzia G, Duranti A, Tontini A, Mor M, et al. (2006) Pharmacological profile of the selective FAAH inhibitor KDS-4103 (URB597). CNS Drug Reviews 12: 21–38.
11. Starowicz K, Makuch W, Korostynski M, Malek N, Slezak M, et al. (2013) Full inhibition of spinal FAAH leads to TRPV1-mediated analgesic effects in neuropathic rats and possible lipoxygenase-mediated remodeling of anandamide metabolism. PLoS One 8: e60040.
12. Ahn K, Johnson DS, Mileni M, Beidler D, Long JZ, et al. (2009) Discovery and characterization of a highly selective FAAH inhibitor that reduces inflammatory pain. Chem Biol 16: 411–420.
13. Jayamanne A, Greenwood R, Mitchell VA, Aslan S, Piomelli D, et al. (2006) Actions of the FAAH inhibitor URB597 in neuropathic and inflammatory chronic pain models. Br J Pharmacol 147: 281–288.
14. Fox A, Kesingland A, Gentry C, McNair K, Patel S, et al. (2001) The role of central and peripheral Cannabinoid1 receptors in the antihyperalgesic activity of cannabinoids in a model of neuropathic pain. Pain 92: 91–100.
15. Christensen MD and Hulsebosch CE (1997) Chronic central pain after spinal cord injury. J Neurotrauma 14: 517–537.
16. Enomoto M and Hama AT (2012) Pain management following spinal cord injury: clinical and basic science perspectives. In: A. A Martin and J. E Jones, editors. Spinal Cord Injuries: Causes, Risk Factors and Management. Hauppauge, NY: Nova Science Publishers. pp. 49–88.
17. Xu XJ, Hao JX, Aldskogius H, Seiger A and Wiesenfeld-Hallin Z (1992) Chronic pain-related syndrome in rats after ischemic spinal cord lesion: a possible animal model for pain in patients with spinal cord injury. Pain 48: 279–290.
18. Hama A and Sagen J (2007) Behavioral characterization and effect of clinical drugs in a rat model of pain following spinal cord compression. Brain Res 1185: 117–128.
19. Hama A and Sagen J (2011) Activation of spinal and supraspinal cannabinoid-1 receptors leads to antinociception in a rat model of neuropathic spinal cord injury pain. Brain Res 1412: 44–54.
20. Hama A and Sagen J (2009) Sustained antinociceptive effect of cannabinoid receptor agonist WIN 55,212-2 over time in rat model of neuropathic spinal cord injury pain. J Rehabil Res Dev 46: 135–143.
21. Cohen PJ (2009) Medical marijuana: The conflict between scientific evidence and political ideology. Utah Law Review 2009: 35–104.
22. Russo R, Loverme J, La Rana G, Compton TR, Parrott J, et al. (2007) The fatty acid amide hydrolase inhibitor URB597 (cyclohexylcarbamic acid 3′-carbamoylbiphenyl-3-yl ester) reduces neuropathic pain after oral administration in mice. J Pharmacol Exp Ther 322: 236–242.
23. Chaplan SR, Bach FW, Pogrel JW, Chung JM and Yaksh TL (1994) Quantitative assessment of tactile allodynia in the rat paw. J Neurosci Methods 53: 55–63.
24. Basso DM, Beattie MS and Bresnahan JC (1995) A sensitive and reliable locomotor rating scale for open field testing in rats. J Neurotrauma 12: 1–21.
25. Richardson D, Ortori CA, Chapman V, Kendall DA and Barrett DA (2007) Quantitative profiling of endocannabinoids and related compounds in rat brain using liquid chromatography-tandem electrospray ionization mass spectrometry. Anal Biochem 360: 216–226.
26. Garcia-Ovejero D, Arevalo-Martin A, Petrosino S, Docagne F, Hagen C, et al. (2009) The endocannabinoid system is modulated in response to spinal cord injury in rats. Neurobiol Dis 33: 57–71.
27. Drew GM, Siddall PJ and Duggan AW (2004) Mechanical allodynia following contusion injury of the rat spinal cord is associated with loss of GABAergic inhibition in the dorsal horn. Pain 109: 379–388.
28. Gwak YS and Hulsebosch CE (2011) GABA and central neuropathic pain following spinal cord injury. Neuropharmacol 60: 799–808.
29. Liu C and Walker JM (2006) Effects of a cannabinoid agonist on spinal nociceptive neurons in a rodent model of neuropathic pain. J Neurophysiol 96: 2984–2994.
30. Aguilar J, Humanes-Valera D, Alonso-Calvino E, Yague JG, Moxon KA, et al. (2010) Spinal cord injury immediately changes the state of the brain. J Neurosci 30: 7528–7537.
31. Hains BC, Klein JP, Saab CY, Craner MJ, Black JA, et al. (2003) Upregulation of sodium channel Nav1.3 and functional involvement in neuronal hyperexcitability associated with central neuropathic pain after spinal cord injury. J Neurosci 23: 8881–8892.

32. Yu W, Hao JX, Xu XJ and Wiesenfeld-Hallin Z (1997) Comparison of the anti-allodynic and antinociceptive effects of systemic; intrathecal and intracerebroventricular morphine in a rat model of central neuropathic pain. Eur J Pain 1: 17–29.
33. Abraham KE, McGinty JF and Brewer KL (2001) Spinal and supraspinal changes in opioid mRNA expression are related to the onset of pain behaviors following excitotoxic spinal cord injury. Pain 90: 181–190.
34. Sain NM, Liang A, Kane SA and Urban MO (2009) Antinociceptive effects of the non-selective cannabinoid receptor agonist CP 55,940 are absent in CB1(−/−) and not CB2(−/−) mice in models of acute and persistent pain. Neuropharmacol 57: 235–241.
35. Costa B, Colleoni M, Conti S, Trovato AE, Bianchi M, et al. (2004) Repeated treatment with the synthetic cannabinoid WIN 55,212-2 reduces both hyperalgesia and production of pronociceptive mediators in a rat model of neuropathic pain. Br J Pharmacol 141: 4–8.
36. De Vry J, Denzer D, Reissmueller E, Eijckenboom M, Heil M, et al. (2004) 3-[2-cyano-3-(trifluoromethyl)phenoxy]phenyl-4,4,4-trifluoro-1-butanesulfo nate (BAY 59-3074): a novel cannabinoid Cb1/Cb2 receptor partial agonist with antihyperalgesic and antiallodynic effects. J Pharmacol Exp Ther 310: 620–632.
37. Bridges D, Ahmad K and Rice AS (2001) The synthetic cannabinoid WIN55,212-2 attenuates hyperalgesia and allodynia in a rat model of neuropathic pain. Br J Pharmacol 133: 586–594.
38. Chin CL, Tovcimak AE, Hradil VP, Seifert TR, Hollingsworth PR, et al. (2008) Differential effects of cannabinoid receptor agonists on regional brain activity using pharmacological MRI. Br J Pharmacol 153: 367–379.
39. Ahmed MM, Rajpal S, Sweeney C, Gerovac TA, Allcock B, et al. (2010) Cannabinoid subtype-2 receptors modulate the antihyperalgesic effect of WIN 55,212-2 in rats with neuropathic spinal cord injury pain. The Spine Journal: Official Journal of the North American Spine Society 10: 1049–1054.
40. De Vry J, Jentzsch KR, Kuhl E and Eckel G (2004) Behavioral effects of cannabinoids show differential sensitivity to cannabinoid receptor blockade and tolerance development. Behav Pharmacol 15: 1–12.
41. Niforatos W, Zhang XF, Lake MR, Walter KA, Neelands T, et al. (2007) Activation of TRPA1 channels by the fatty acid amide hydrolase inhibitor 3′-carbamoylbiphenyl-3-yl cyclohexylcarbamate (URB597). Mol Pharmacol 71: 1209–1216.
42. Karbarz MJ, Luo L, Chang L, Tham CS, Palmer JA, et al. (2009) Biochemical and biological properties of 4-(3-phenyl-[1,2,4] thiadiazol-5-yl)-piperazine-1-carboxylic acid phenylamide, a mechanism-based inhibitor of fatty acid amide hydrolase. Anesth Analg 108: 316–329.
43. Kathuria S, Gaetani S, Fegley D, Valino F, Duranti A, et al. (2003) Modulation of anxiety through blockade of anandamide hydrolysis. Nat Med 9: 76–81.
44. Drew GM, Siddall PJ and Duggan AW (2001) Responses of spinal neurones to cutaneous and dorsal root stimuli in rats with mechanical allodynia after contusive spinal cord injury. Brain Res 893: 59–69.
45. Brown AJ (2007) Novel cannabinoid receptors. Br J Pharmacol 152: 567–575.
46. Costa B, Comelli F, Bettoni I, Colleoni M and Giagnoni G (2008) The endogenous fatty acid amide, palmitoylethanolamide, has anti-allodynic and anti-hyperalgesic effects in a murine model of neuropathic pain: involvement of CB(1), TRPV1 and PPARgamma receptors and neurotrophic factors. Pain 139: 541–550.
47. Bedi SS, Yang Q, Crook RJ, Du J, Wu Z, et al. (2010) Chronic spontaneous activity generated in the somata of primary nociceptors is associated with pain-related behavior after spinal cord injury. Journal of Neuroscience 30: 14870–14882.
48. Lenz FA, Tasker RR, Dostrovsky JO, Kwan HC, Gorecki J, et al. (1987) Abnormal single-unit activity recorded in the somatosensory thalamus of a quadriplegic patient with central pain. Pain 31: 225–236.
49. Thakor DK, Lin A, Matsuka Y, Meyer EM, Ruangsri S, et al. (2009) Increased peripheral nerve excitability and local NaV1.8 mRNA up-regulation in painful neuropathy. Mol Pain 5: 14.
50. Hains BC, Saab CY and Waxman SG (2005) Changes in electrophysiological properties and sodium channel Nav1.3 expression in thalamic neurons after spinal cord injury. Brain 128: 2359–2371.
51. Wasner G, Naleschinski D and Baron R (2007) A role for peripheral afferents in the pathophysiology and treatment of at-level neuropathic pain in spinal cord injury? A case report. Pain 131: 219–225.
52. Sandford PR and Benes PS (2000) Use of capsaicin in the treatment of radicular pain in spinal cord injury. J Spinal Cord Med 23: 238–243.
53. Lichtman AH, Shelton CC, Advani T and Cravatt BF (2004) Mice lacking fatty acid amide hydrolase exhibit a cannabinoid receptor-mediated phenotypic hypoalgesia. Pain 109: 319–327.
54. Kinsey SG, Long JZ, O'Neal ST, Abdullah RA, Poklis JL, et al. (2009) Blockade of endocannabinoid-degrading enzymes attenuates neuropathic pain. Journal of Pharmacology and Experimental Therapeutics 330: 902–910.
55. Huggins JP, Smart TS, Langman S, Taylor L and Young T (2012) An efficient randomised, placebo-controlled clinical trial with the irreversible fatty acid amide hydrolase-1 inhibitor PF-04457845, which modulates endocannabinoids but fails to induce effective analgesia in patients with pain due to osteoarthritis of the knee. Pain 153: 1837–1846.
56. Ahn K, Smith SE, Liimatta MB, Beidler D, Sadagopan N, et al. (2011) Mechanistic and pharmacological characterization of PF-04457845: a highly potent and selective fatty acid amide hydrolase inhibitor that reduces inflammatory and noninflammatory pain. J Pharmacol Exp Ther 338: 114–124.
57. Tallarida RJ (2007) Interactions between drugs and occupied receptors. Pharmacol Ther 113: 197–209.
58. Tuboly G, Mecs L, Benedek G and Horvath G (2009) Antinociceptive interactions between anandamide and endomorphin-1 at the spinal level. Clin Exp Pharmacol Physiol 36: 400–405.
59. Haller VL, Stevens DL and Welch SP (2008) Modulation of opioids via protection of anandamide degradation by fatty acid amide hydrolase. Eur J Pharmacol 600: 50–58.
60. Hogestatt ED, Jonsson BA, Ermund A, Andersson DA, Bjork H, et al. (2005) Conversion of acetaminophen to the bioactive N-acylphenolamine AM404 via fatty acid amide hydrolase-dependent arachidonic acid conjugation in the nervous system. J Biol Chem 280: 31405–31412.
61. Hama AT and Sagen J (2010) Cannabinoid receptor-mediated antinociception with acetaminophen drug combinations in rats with neuropathic spinal cord injury pain. Neuropharmacol 58: 758–766.
62. Fowler CJ, Naidu PS, Lichtman A and Onnis V (2009) The case for the development of novel analgesic agents targeting both fatty acid amide hydrolase and either cyclooxygenase or TRPV1. Br J Pharmacol 156: 412–419.

8

Imaging Neuroinflammation *In Vivo* in a Neuropathic Pain Rat Model with Near-Infrared Fluorescence and ^{19}F Magnetic Resonance

Kiran Vasudeva[1], Karl Andersen[1], Bree Zeyzus-Johns[1], T. Kevin Hitchens[2], Sravan Kumar Patel[3], Anthony Balducci[4], Jelena M. Janjic[3], John A. Pollock[1]*

1 Biological Sciences, Bayer School of Natural and Environmental Sciences, and Chronic Pain Research Consortium, Duquesne University, Pittsburgh, Pennsylvania, United States of America, **2** NMR Center for Biomedical Research, Carnegie Mellon University, Pittsburgh, Pennsylvania, United States of America, **3** Graduate School of Pharmaceutical Sciences, Mylan School of Pharmacy, and Chronic Pain Research Consortium, Duquesne University, Pittsburgh, Pennsylvania, United States of America, **4** Department of Research and Development, Celsense, Inc., Pittsburgh, Pennsylvania, Unite States of America

Abstract

Chronic neuropathic pain following surgery represents a serious worldwide health problem leading to life-long treatment and the possibility of significant disability. In this study, neuropathic pain was modeled using the chronic constriction injury (CCI). The CCI rats exhibit mechanical hypersensitivity (typical neuropathic pain symptom) to mechanical stimulation of the affected paw 11 days post surgery, at a time when sham surgery animals do not exhibit hypersensitivity. Following a similar time course, TRPV1 gene expression appears to rise with the hypersensitivity to mechanical stimulation. Recent studies have shown that immune cells play a role in the development of neuropathic pain. To further explore the relationship between neuropathic pain and immune cells, we hypothesize that the infiltration of immune cells into the affected sciatic nerve can be monitored *in vivo* by molecular imaging. To test this hypothesis, an intravenous injection of a novel perfluorocarbon (PFC) nanoemulsion, which is phagocytosed by inflammatory cells (e.g. monocytes and macrophages), was used in a rat CCI model. The nanoemulsion carries two distinct imaging agents, a near-infrared (NIR) lipophilic fluorescence reporter (DiR) and a ^{19}F MRI (magnetic resonance imaging) tracer, PFC. We demonstrate that in live rats, NIR fluorescence is concentrated in the area of the affected sciatic nerve. Furthermore, the ^{19}F MRI signal was observed on the sciatic nerve. Histological examination of the CCI sciatic nerve reveals significant infiltration of CD68 positive macrophages. These results demonstrate that the infiltration of immune cells into the sciatic nerve can be visualized in live animals using these methods.

Editor: Jian-Xin Gao, Shanghai Jiao Tong University School of Medicine, China

Funding: Funding for this work was provided by a Hunkele Dreaded Disease Award to JAP, a Samuel and Emma Winters Foundation Award to JAP, a Pennsylvania's Commonwealth Universal Research Enhancement (CURE) Award to JMJ and a Pittsburgh Tissue Engineering Initiative Interface Seed Grant to JMJ & JAP. The funders had no role in study design, data collection and analysis, decision to publish, or preparation of the manuscript.

Competing Interests: Anthony Balducci is employed by Celsense Inc, Pittsburgh, PA. V-Sense DM NIR is produced and marketed by Celsense Inc, Pittsburgh, PA. This relationship with Celsense Inc.

* E-mail: pollock@duq.edu

Introduction

Pain is a public health problem that has deleterious effects on social, mental, physical and economic health of its sufferers [1]. Pain caused by injury or disease associated with the somatosensory nervous system is called neuropathic pain [2]. Recent studies have estimated that at least 6 million Americans suffer from neuropathic pain [3]. Other studies indicate that neuropathic pain is usually associated with nerve inflammation [4], which occurs when leukocytes such as macrophages infiltrate the nerve. Understanding the role of key inflammatory cytokines and immune cells involved in neuropathic pain could lead to a deeper understanding of the signaling mechanisms involved in hypersensitivity as well as better diagnostic and treatment strategies.

The chronic constriction injury (CCI) rat model [5] is a well-characterized example of chronic peripheral neuropathic pain [6]. This model is widely used to simulate Complex Regional Pain Syndrome type II observed in humans (CRPS II, earlier called causalgia) [5]. CRPS II develops when a major peripheral nerve is injured [7] and includes persistent pain and mechanical allodynia [8].

Significant advances have been made in understanding the molecular basis of the diseases and conditions of chronic pain and the hypersensitivity associated with CCI. In many cases, hypersensitivity correlates with changes in the expression of specific ion channels [9]. Among these are cation channel proteins including the Transient Receptor Potential (TRP), a superfamily of receptors [10] that are known for being involved in a variety of sensory processes including nociception and pain [11,12]. In CCI, there is evidence that seven days after the CCI surgery, TRPV1 protein, but not mRNA expression increases in the Dorsal Root Ganglia (DRG) [13,14]. Furthermore, neuroinflammation has been associated with CCI-induced mechanical hypersentivity. Clatworthy and coworkers [15] showed that inflammation plays a key role in pathophysiology of neuropathic pain. Furthermore, macrophages have been shown to play a central role in causing the inflammation that contributes to peripheral neuropathies [16]. It has also been demonstrated that Wallerian degeneration occurs

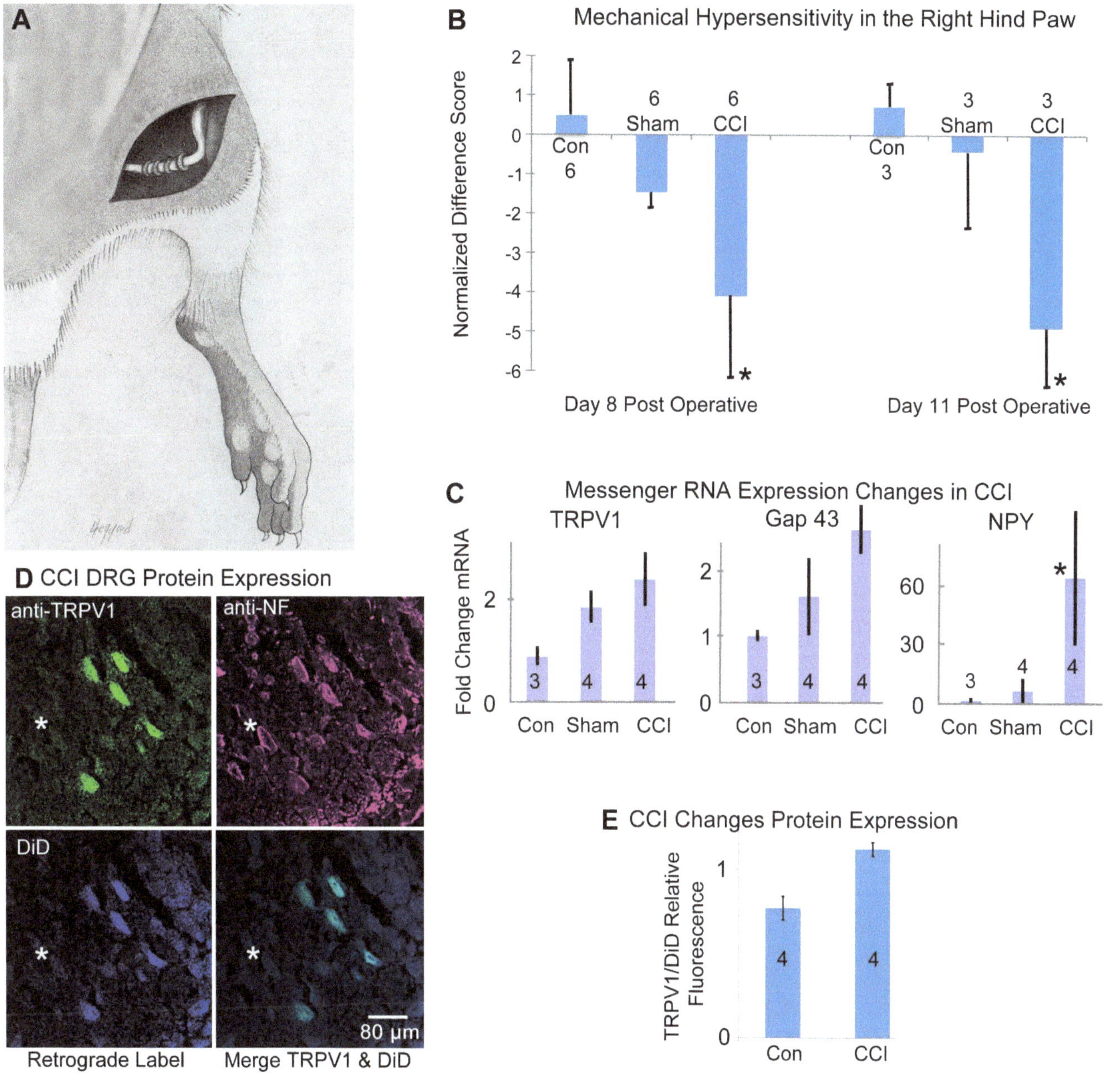

Figure 1. Chronic Constriction Injury (CCI) affects behavior, as well as mRNA and protein expression. A. Sketch of the sciatic nerve with the chronic constriction injury sutures in place. **B.** Mechanical hyperentivity in the right hind paw. Bars represent the mean ± SEM normalized 50% withdrawal threshold from calibrated Semmes-Weinstein monofilaments (g) for each of the treatment groups; un-operated control (Con), sham-operated control (Sham), and chronic constriction injury (CCI). The more negative a mean difference score, the lower the pain threshold in the right hind paw. *Significant difference from un-operated control rats (Kruskal- Wallis 1-way ANOVA by ranks; $P \leq 0.05$). Un-operated and sham-operated control rats did not differ in normalized pain thresholds at day 8 or day 11 post-operative. Sample size representing each mean indicated on the graph. **C.** Relative Expression of mRNA assessed by qPCR (one step direct priming of mRNA). mRNA extracted from dissected L5 ipsilateral dorsal root ganglia for non-surgical control (Con), sham and CCI were used to compare the expression levels of TRPV1, Growth associated protein 43 (Gap43) and Neuropeptide Y (NPY). All three genes exhibit elevated levels of transcript expression in the CCI condition that were significantly different from control, indicating peripheral nerve trauma and neuropathic pain. For TRPV1, these data show that the CCI-treatment group was significantly different from the control groups ($p < 0.05$). The CCI-treatment group was not significantly different from the sham group ($p > 0.05$). For GAP43, these data show that the CCI-treatment group was significantly different from the control groups ($p < 0.05$). The sham-treatment group was not significantly different from the control group ($p > 0.05$). For NPY, these data show that the CCI-treatment group was significantly different from both the sham-treatment group and the control group ($p < 0.001$). Sample size representing each mean indicated on the graph. **D.** DiD retrogradely labeled neurons from the right footpad of a CCI surgical animal. Cell bodies in the L5 doral root ganglia were processed for multi-stain confocal microscopy with anti-TRPV1 and anti-Neurofilament antibodies. The results reveal that some neurons co-label with TRPV1 and DiD, while other neurons identified with anti-Neurofilament antibody (*) lack both DiD and TRPV1. Scale Bar = 80 μm. **E.** Using Leica confocal software, the relative fluorescence of TRPV1 to DiD in co-expressing cells for representative CCI and comparably stained tissue sections from control DRG is shown. Sample size representing each mean indicated on the graph. TRPV1 protein expression is elevated in the CCI condition.

in CCI rat model [17]. During Wallerian degeneration, resident macrophages and the Schwann cells are the first cells to respond to the insult and together they initiate the axonal degeneration phase of the distal portion of the damaged nerve. Within the first three days of nerve injury, acute inflammation is evident with the infiltration of neutrophils reaching the site of injury via diapedesis [18]. The peak in neutrophil infiltration is reached within 24 hours of injury. From day 4 to day 14 post injury, hematogenous macrophages infiltrate the injured nerve area, reaching a peak around 1 week post injury [18]. One of the roles of these macrophages is to remove the degenerating nerve tissue debris and to cause inflammation [18]. The infiltration of these immune cells into damaged nerve tissue is an important component of the inflammatory process. However, the role of inflammatory cell infiltration into the site of neuronal injury and how that initiates chronic pain is not well understood. Understanding this process will ultimately lead to the development of new therapeutic agents and better pain management. To study infiltrating immune cells in a rat chronic pain model, we used a novel NIR (near-infrared) labeled perfluoro-15-crown-5 ether (PCE) nanoemulsion [19], shown to preferentially label macrophages in culture and upon intravenous administration. Perfluoropolyethers (PFPEs), including PCE, have been used for ^{19}F MRI (magnetic resonance imaging) in multiple animal models [20,21,22,23]. Specifically, PFPE nanoemulsions have become a powerful tool for imaging inflammation in varied disease models, from acute organ rejection to rheumatoid arthritis [24]. PFPE nanoemulsion droplets are taken up from the blood stream by phagocytic cells including monocytes and macrophages and carried by these cells to sites of inflammation. PFPEs in the nanoemulsions are biologically and chemically inert, and are not degraded by the phagocytic cells, which gives PFPEs advantage over other imaging modalities [25]. The ^{19}F MR signal remains unchanged during the lifetime of the labeled cell and can be directly correlated to the immune cell number at the site of interest [26]. Further, ^{19}F MR signal is specific for the introduced nanoemulsion and provides an unambiguous signature of monocytes and macrophages *in vivo*. In a recent study [19] we reported *in vivo* inflammation imaging demonstrating that NIR and ^{19}F MRI can be used as complementary imaging modalities for identifying underlying cellular mechanisms in inflammation.

Previously, aspects of the role of inflammation in neuropathic pain have only been established by *ex vivo* techniques [27,28,29,30]. To the best of our knowledge, there are no reports on visualizing neuroinflammation in live animals using the CCI model of neuropathic pain. While ^{19}F MRI has been used previously to image *in vivo* neuroinflammation in the peripheral nervous system [31], we are describing for the first time a novel method to visualize the *in vivo* inflammation associated with nerve injury in the CCI rat. To achieve this, we are using a newly developed nanoemulsion-based dual mode imaging probe [19]. We find that NIR and ^{19}F MRI can be used to monitor inflammation at the site of injury on the sciatic nerve. Using multiple *ex vivo* imaging techniques (NIR, ^{19}F MRI and histology), we demonstrate that macrophages have infiltrated the sciatic nerve following CCI. We discuss the implication of a noninvasive assessment of neuropathic pain for use in studying pain associated with the hypersensitivity caused by CCI.

Materials and Methods

Ethics Statement

This study was carried out in strict accordance with the recommendations in the Guide for the Care and Use of Laboratory Animals of the National Institute of Health, and the Institutional Animal Care and Use Committee (IACUC) at Duquesne University approved the animal protocol (Protocol 1109-10). All surgical procedures were performed under isoflurane anesthesia. Male Sprague-Dawley rats weighing 250–350 g were used in this study (Hilltop Lab Animals, Inc., Scottdale, PA). Rats were maintained on a 12:12 hour light-dark cycle and were given *ad libitum* access to water and purified chow. Purified chow has been demonstrated to reduce non-specific fluorescence caused by plant materials in basic chow in the LI-COR Bioscience Application Note: *In Vivo* Animal Imaging Diet Consideration (http://biosupport.licor.com/docs/InVivoDiet-Considerations.pdf).

Chronic Constriction Injury

The chronic constriction injury (CCI) method developed by Bennett and Xie [5] was used to induce neuropathic pain in the sciatic nerve of rats (Figure 1A). Animals were divided into three groups; CCI, sham and naïve un-operated control. Briefly, under general anesthesia, the common sciatic nerve of the CCI animals was exposed by making an incision through the skin and carefully separating the muscles in the mid thigh region of right hind limb. Four ligatures were tied around the common sciatic nerve using 4-0 chromic gut suture. Care was taken to ensure that the ligatures were secured in place without restricting epineurial blood flow. The muscle layer was closed using 4-0 chromic gut suture followed by skin closure using 9 mm stainless steel wound clips. Sham rats underwent identical surgery except that the ligatures were not tied around the nerve. Naïve control rats did not undergo any surgical procedures and are referred to as un-operated controls.

Behavioral Testing

On the day of surgery, prior to commencement of any surgical procedures, CCI, sham and control rats underwent baseline assessment for mechanical sensitivity. Behavioral testing was repeated on day 8 and day 11 post surgery. Following previously established methods, mechanical pain threshold was assessed by applying calibrated Semmes-Weinstein monofilaments to the plantar surface of both the left and right hind paw, specifically in the cutaneous region that is innervated exclusively by the sciatic nerve [32,33].

A linear regression was used to estimate each rat's 50% withdrawal threshold. As previously described [32], rats were placed on a metal grid and covered with a Plexiglas cover. The lowest-caliber filament (0.41 g) was pushed onto the plantar surface of the right hind paw 5 times until the filament bent; 2 to 3 seconds separated each push. Five minutes later, the left paw of the same rat was similarly assessed. Not less than 5 minutes after the left paw was assessed, the entire procedure was repeated. In this way, the right and left paws were probed with the 0.41 g filament 10 times, and the number of withdrawals was recorded. In ascending order, each filament was so tested until the rat withdrew from all 10 pushes of a single-sized filament or until the largest-caliber filament was tested.

To estimate the force from which the rat withdrew 50% of the time, force (in grams) was regressed on withdrawal frequency for all 5 filaments by using simple linear regression. The force at which the rat withdrew a paw on 5 of 10 pushes (50% withdrawal threshold) was predicted by using the regression equation. If the 50% withdrawal threshold so calculated was greater than 15.13 g, the highest-caliber filament used (15.13 g) was recorded as the gram force. If the rat failed to respond to any of the filaments, 15.13 g was recorded as the 50% withdrawal threshold. The same investigator always performed this test. Threshold levels were then

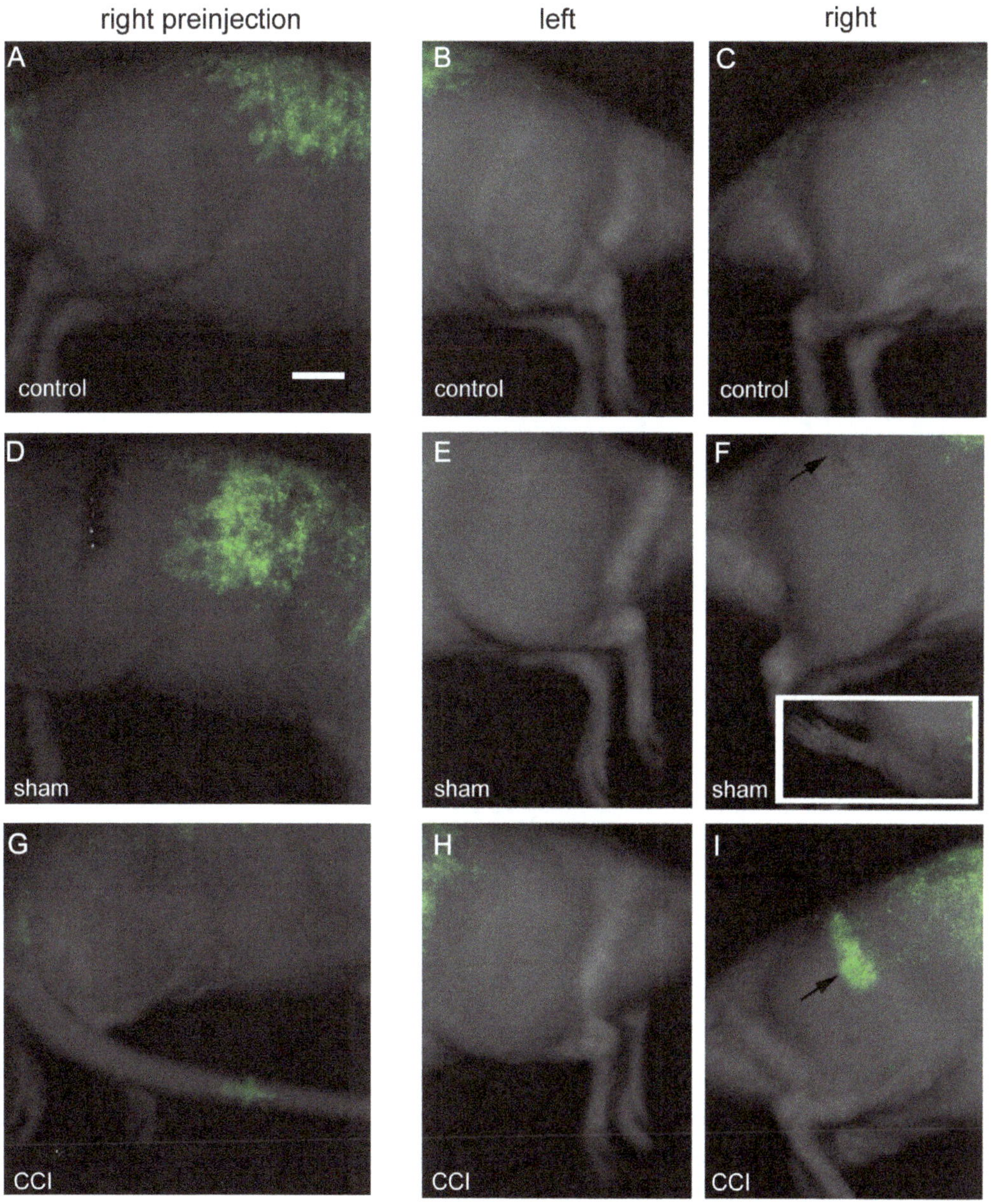

Figure 2. Near Infrared imaging (NIR) of live rats merged with white light images of their body, 2 days post intravenous injection of labeled emulsion on day 11 post surgery. All of these images were acquired on the LiCOR Pearl Live animal imager and processed in the same experiment with linked look-up tables. The control (A, B, C) and sham (D, E, F) exhibit only auto fluorescence over the thoracolumbar region, which is evident prior to injection (A, D, G). The inset in F exhibits a dorsal view of the wound, which lacks any fluorescent signal. The CCI affected right leg (I) exhibits a clear band of fluorescent signal aligned with the position of the sciatic nerve (arrow), which runs parallel to the femur. No signal is evident on the CCI animal's unaffected left leg (H). Note – supplemental data (Figure S3) of a comparable experiment reveals only autofluoresence in sham and naïve controls, while only the CCI exhibits extensive signal along the length of the thigh, parallel to the position of the right sciatic nerve. Bar = 1 cm.

expressed as a difference score between the pain threshold for the right and left hind paws. These values were normalized to differences that existed between the 2 paws at baseline. Statistics were performed using SPSS V12.0 software. We observed significant difference between the CCI condition and the un-operated control rats (Kruskal- Wallis 1-way ANOVA by ranks; $P \leq 0.05$). All behavioral testing was done by experimenter blinded to the surgical treatment. Rats used for the detailed behavioral testing consisted of a separate cohort from those used for the DRG analysis and *in vivo* imaging. All CCI animals were observed to exhibit guarding, paw licking and or paw lifting behaviors by day 8 post-surgery. However, only normal grooming behaviors were seen in the sham and un-operated controls.

Dorsal Root Ganglia Dissection

Nine days post surgery, bilateral L3, L4 and L5 DRG were dissected from CCI rats via laminectomy. These ganglia were chosen because neurons within them provide the sensory component of the sciatic nerve [34,35]. Ganglia were rapidly

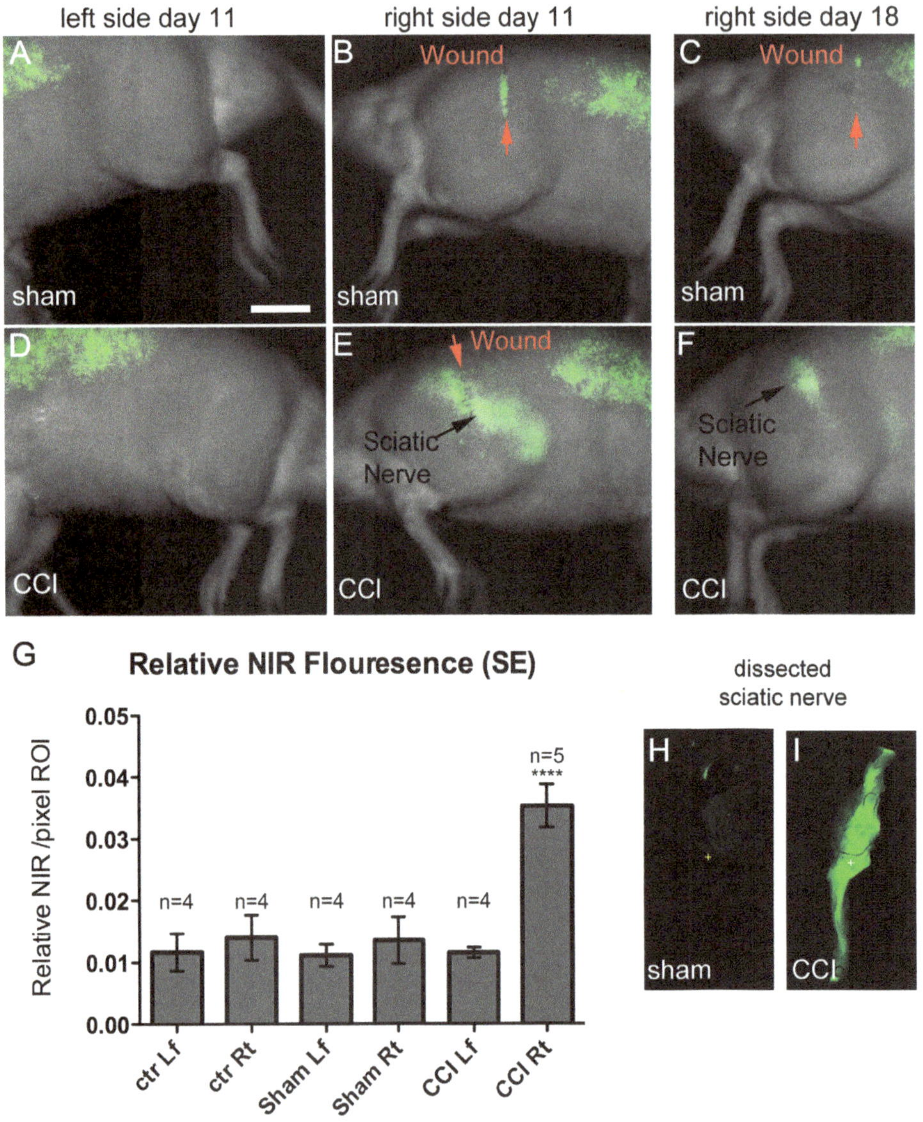

Figure 3. Near Infrared imaging (NIR) of live rats merged with white light images of their body, 2 days post intravenous injection of labeled emulsion on day 11 post surgery compared to day 18 post surgery. All of these images were acquired on the LiCOR Pearl Live animal imager and processed in the same experiment with linked look-up tables. Bar = 1 cm. The sham surgical control (**A**, **B**, **C**) exhibits auto fluorescence over the thoracolumbar region, which is also evident prior to injection. In the sham animal, a superficial fluorescence signal is detected precisely on the surgical wound. That surgical wound signal is dramatically reduced by day 18 (**C**) in the same sham animal. The CCI experimental animal (**D**, **E**, **F**) exhibits auto fluorescence over the thoracolumbar region, which is also evident prior to injection. The CCI affected right leg (**E**) exhibits a clear band of fluorescent signal aligned with the position of the sciatic nerve (black arrow) along the entire length of the thigh. No signal is evident on the CCI animal's unaffected left leg (**D**). On day 18, the signal in the Sham attributed to the wound has nearly completely resolved and no signal is apparent along the sciatic nerve (C). The CCI sciatic nerve associated signal persists in at day 18 (F). Bar = 1 cm. **G.** The relative fluorescence of a region over the sciatic nerve is compared. For each condition ROI measurements were made (Figure S1, Table S2) for the 4 sets of data giving a sample number of 4 to 5. The results of the ANOVA test (Table S3) show that the relative fluorescence in the CCI right is significantly different from the remainder of the samples with a p value <0.0001. Separately, a t-test analysis of the Sham right versus the CCI right revealed a p value of <0.0001. Sciatic nerve dissected from comparable animals imaged simultaneously in the same field of view for NIR fluorescence on the LiCOR Odessey Flatbed Imager (H, I). The CCI sciatic nerve (I) exhibits a strong fluorescent signal in comparison to the sham sciatic nerve (H).

removed and stored in RNA*later* solution (Qiagen) for later use. Rats were sacrificed after completion of DRG extraction.

RNA Isolation and qPCR Analysis

Quantitative PCR (qPCR) and the comparative cycle threshold (CT) method [36] were used to determine if the CCI altered the mRNA expression of TRPV1, Neuropeptide Y (NPY) and Growth-associated Protein 43 (Gap43) relative to Glyceraldehyde 3-phosphate dehydrogenase (GAPDH) in L5 DRG 12 days post surgery (see Table S1 for primers). GAPDH, an important enzyme in glycolysis, serves as a control transcript for comparisons to transcripts from other genes expressed within the same tissue [37]. Tissue samples were removed from the RNA*later* solution, processed over QiaShredder columns and RNA was extracted using the RNeasy kit (Qiagen, Valencia, CA). To prevent any

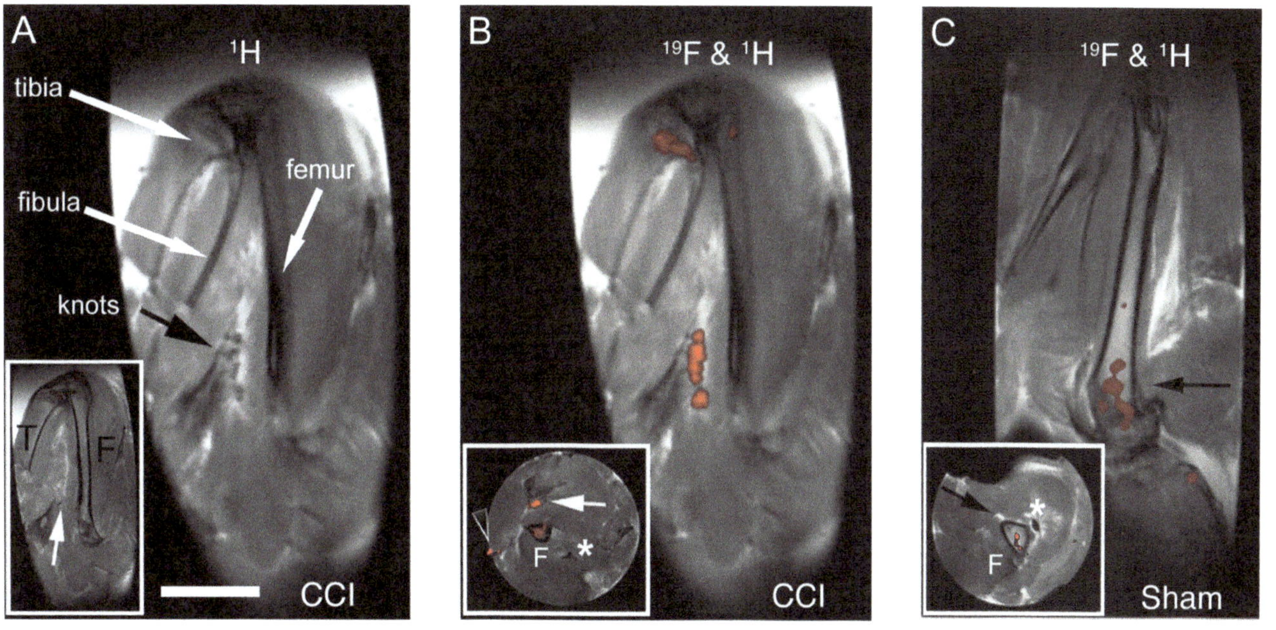

Figure 4. ^{1}H and ^{19}F MRI of the hind limbs for the rats shown in Figure 2F and 2I. Panel **A** shows an anatomical (^{1}H) image of the leg for the animal shown in 2I. The black arrow indicates the sutures used for the chronic constriction injury. The long white arrows indicate the position of the tibia, fibula and femur. The inset image shows the adjacent image slice, giving a clearer view of the tibia (T) and the femur (F). The white arrow in inset panel A points to the sciatic nerve, which appears as a white line. Panel **B** shows a composite ^{1}H/^{19}F image. The ^{19}F image is rendered in pseudo color (red) and is overlaid on the anatomical image shown in **A**. A significant amount of ^{19}F signal is observed at the sutured sciatic nerve. A small amount of fluorine signal is also evident at the head of the tibia and slight in the femur. The inset shows an axial view of the thigh revealing the femur in cross section. A small amount of fluorine signal is observed at the surface aligning with the surgical wound, where minor superficial inflammation is still evident (arrow head). The (F) indicates the femur in cross sections with a low level of ^{19}F signal. The white arrow indicates the sciatic nerve with ^{19}F signal. The asterisk (*) is near the femoral artery. Panel **C** shows a ^{1}H/^{19}F composite image of the sham right leg from the animal shown in Figure 2F. No fluorine signal was observed at the sciatic nerve, however a weak signal was observed in the femur, presumably in the bone marrow (arrow). The inset shows an axial view at the level of the arrow near the head of the femur (F) with ^{19}F signal in the bone marrow. The black arrow points to the femur and the asterisk (*) is near the femoral artery. Bar = 1 cm.

genomic DNA contamination, each RNA sample was treated with DNase I (Invitrogen, Grand Island, NY).

Using RNA as the template, one step qPCR was performed with gene specific primers. Reverse-transcription was performed on the StepOnePlus machine using the *Power* SYBR Green RNA-to-CT *1-Step* Kit (Applied Biosystems). RNA extracted from each rat was analyzed separately in triplicate. Analysis of amplified cDNA products by agarose gel and subsequent DNA sequencing confirmed the identity of the intended PCR product. All statistical tests were performed using SPSS software. Assumptions of ANOVA were met as indicated by Mauchly's Test of Sphericity and Levine's Test for Equality of Variances. Significance of the F statistic was defined as $p \leq 0.05$. TRPV1 mRNA levels in right (ipsilateral to the nerve injury) DRG of CCI rats was compared to right DRG of control (pooled) rats by performing a 1-Way ANOVA with treatment as the between-subjects factor.

Immunohistochemistry and Confocal Microscopy

Dorsal root ganglia from control and CCI rats, were used for immunohistochemistry to explore the protein expression levels of TRPV1. Under general anesthesia, prior to any surgical procedures, the CCI and control rats were injected with DiD Dye (V-22887, Invitrogen, Carlsbad, CA) in the plantar region of the right hindpaw. DiD is a lipophilic retrograde tracer that will stain all neuronal cells innervating the hindpaw. Post-treatment, all DRGs were removed and immediately fixed in 4% paraformaldehyde 1X Phosphate Buffer Saline (PBS) solution. The tissue samples were cryoprotected in 30% sucrose 1X PBS solution for 4 hours. After four hours of incubation, 1/3 of the cryoprotectant solution was replaced with Optimal Cutting Temperature (OCT) compound (Sakura-Finetek, Torrance, CA) and incubated on a rocking shaker overnight. After overnight incubation, samples were embedded in OCT and 20 µm thick sections were made on a cryostat. Sections were postfixed in 4% paraformaldehyde solution 1X PBS, permeabilized with 0.3% Triton X-100 solution and stained with primary and secondary antibodies. The following primary antibodies were used: 1:50 mouse anti-rat Neurofilament-M (Neuromics, Edina, MN), 1:50 rabbit anti-rat TRPV1 (Santa Cruz Biotechnology, Dallas, TX). The sections were then washed and incubated overnight with anti-mouse secondary antibodies conjugated to Alexa-546 (Invitrogen, Carlsbad, CA), and anti-rabbit-FITC (Santa Cruz Biotechnology, Dallas, TX), diluted 1:100 in PBS. Sections were washed in 1X PBS and mounted in Prolong-Gold (Invitrogen, Carlsbad, CA). Relative expression of TRPV1 was determined by comparing the fluorescence intensity for TRPV1 to the fluorescence intensity of DiD, whose fluorescence intensity is not affected by the CCI surgery. This was done for labeled neurons from naïve control DRG and CCI DRG using the Leica TCS SP2 software version 2.3. For a double-labeled cell, the overall TRPV1 mean amplitude was divided by the overall mean DiD amplitude. The results of an unpaired t-test showed $t = -6.45$, sdev = 0.758E-01 degrees of freedom = 6. The probability of this result, assuming the null hypothesis, is 0.0007. An experimenter blind to treatment did staining and quantification of immunohistochemistry.

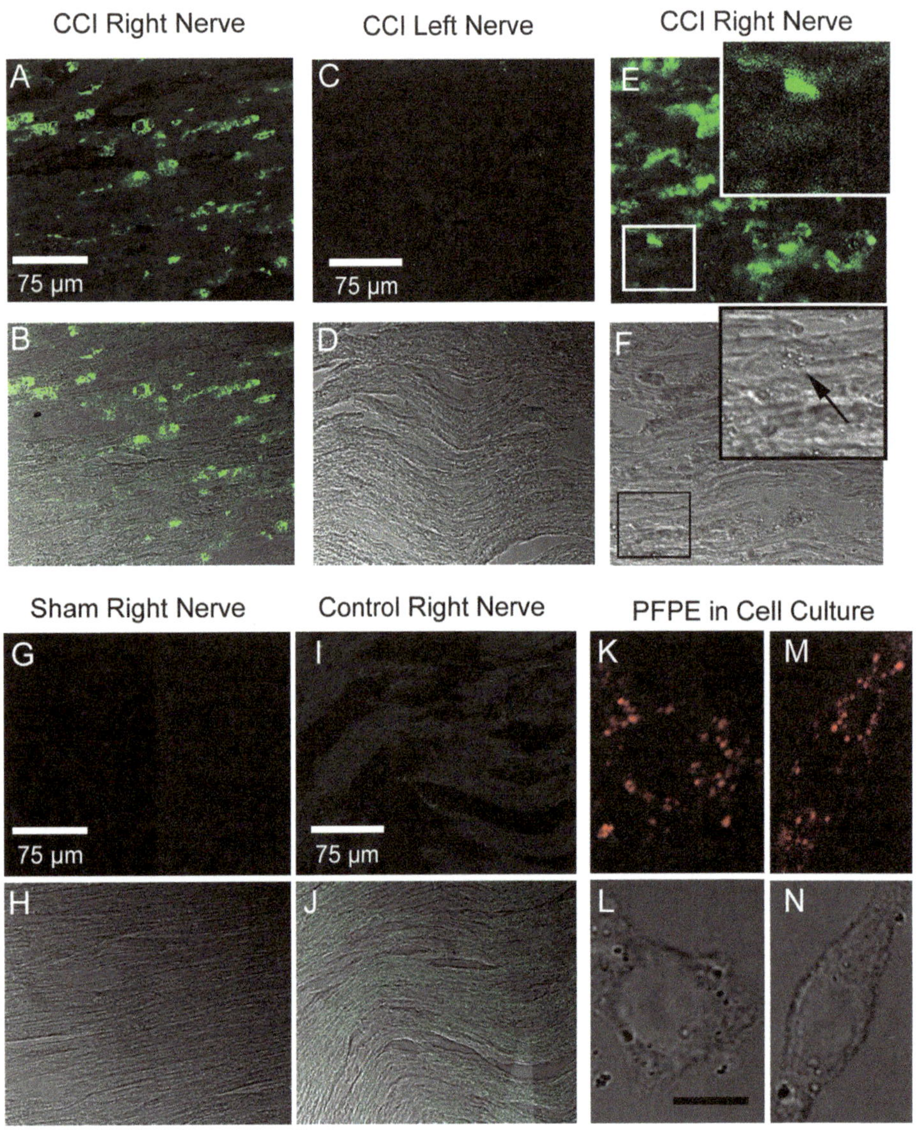

Figure 5. Cryosection of sciatic nerve. A,**B** show the affected right sciatic nerve from the CCI leg shown in Figure 2I stained with anti-CD68 antibody to reveal the presence of macrophages infiltrating the nerve. **C, D** CD68 positive cells are not present in the left leg (contralateral to surgery Figure 2H) of the same CCI animal. **E,F** show a nerve from a separate CCI animal that also exhibits infiltration of CD68 positive cells. The boxed area is enlarged to reveal the granular cytoplasm (black arrow) of the macrophages, indicative of the presence of the nanoemulsion. Sham surgical sciatic nerve and non-surgical control sciatic nerve do not exhibit any CD68 positive cells (**G,H**) and (**I,J**). The fluorescent images A, C, G, and I were all acquired at the same sitting with the exact same image acquisition parameters. Macrophages grown in cell culture take up the nanoemulsion, exhibited as particles evident by both confocal fluorescence emissions 700–850 nm of NIR label (DiR) (**K, M**) as well as transmitted light (**L, N**).

In separate immunohistochemical experiments using comparable protocols, the recovered control, sham and CCI sciatic nerves were prepared for examination using mouse anti rat CD68 antibody (MCA341R, AbD Serotech, Raleigh, NC) and Alexa fluor 488 donkey anti mouse secondary antibody (A-21202, Invitrogen, Carlsbad, CA) to assess the presence of macrophages that infiltrate the nerve.

Cellular uptake of nanoemulsion was performed in the mouse leukemic monocyte macrophage cell line RAW 264.7 (ATCC, Manassas VA) as described by Patel *et al* [38]. Approximately, 0.3 million cells were seeded on cover slips in 6-well plates in 2 mL culture medium per well and grown as adherent macrophages. After 48 h incubation at 37°C and 5% CO_2, medium was aspirated and cells washed with 1X PBS. Cells were exposed to 2 mL of either fresh culture medium alone or dispersed nanoemulsion containing medium (10 μL/mL). Following 5 h incubation, 1 mL medium was aspirated and cells fixed with 1 mL 4% paraformaldehyde in 1X PBS. After 30 minutes at room temperature, the cells were washed with 1X PBS three times. Each coverslip with and without nanoemulsion labeled cells was transferred to glass slides containing a drop of ProLong Gold mounting medium. The nanoemulsion labeled with DiR (Invitrogen, Carlsbad, CA) was detected with 633 nm laser excitation and emission window of 700 nm to 850 nm. Confocal microscopy was performed on a Leica SP2 spectral Laser Scanning Confocal microscope. A transmission DIC image was acquired with each confocal scan.

NIR Labeled PFPE Nanoemulsion

NIR labeled PFPE Nanoemulsion (V-Sense DM NIR) was produced and provided by Celsense Inc (Pittsburgh, PA, USA) and was used without further modifications. Previous studies have demonstrated that the nanoemulsion droplets are on the order of 180–200 nm in size [19].

Live Animal Imaging (NIR)

To follow the localization of emulsion labeled circulating monocytes (monocytes in the blood, macrophages in tissue), NIR imaging of the fluorescent label in live rats was performed on a LiCOR Pearl Impulse (LI-COR Biosciences, Lincoln, NE) small animal imaging system. For the live animal imaging, rats were fed purified chow (D10012G Research Diets, Inc. New Brunswick, NJ), which helps to reduce non-specific fluorescence in the abdominal and thoracic region of the animal caused by certain foods. Tail-vein injection of 300 μL of V-Sense DM nanoemulsion was performed 8 days after surgery under general anesthesia. Within minutes, the injected animals were imaged in the LiCOR imager to establish that the intravenous injection was successful and that the nanoemulsion was not leaking subcutaneously within the tail. On day 11 post surgery, maximum neuroinflammation was predicted based on previous results, and another set of NIR imaging was performed under general anesthesia (xylazine, 7 mg/kg/ketamine, 80 mg/kg) given intraperitoneally. Simultaneous image acquisition of white light (body view) and 785 nm excitation for 820 nm emission were merged and processed in the LiCOR Pearl Impulse Software (version 2.0) with linked look-up-tables (LUT). Relative fluorescence was measured from a region of the same size over the sciatic nerve for both left and right legs for the naïve, sham and CCI conditions. This involved identifying a region of interest (ROI) around the fluorescent signal evident in the CCI. That ROI perimeter was then copied to the other legs for a given experiment. In this way, nearly the same number of pixels of area for the signal is compared within a given paired experiment. The ROI images for each rat (Figure S1) and the tabulation of relative fluorescence from the LiCOR Pearl Impulse software (Table S2) are shown in Supporting Information. Prism software version 5.0 was used to perform analysis of variance (ANOVA) for the entire set of conditions revealing a p value< 0.0001 (Table S3). Furthermore, a t-test specifically comparing the sham right leg to the CCI right leg reveals a p value<0.0001. Dissected sciatic nerves were similarly imaged for NIR fluorescence on a flatbed LiCOR Odyssey Infrared Imaging system. An experimenter blinded to experimental conditions did the analysis of NIR Pearl images.

MRI (^{1}H & ^{19}F) Methods

^{1}H and ^{19}F MRI was performed on rat legs using a Bruker Biospec Avance III 7-T/21-cm system (Bruker Biospin MRI, Billerica MA) and a 35-mm (^{1}H/^{19}F) double resonance birdcage coil (Rapid MR International, Columbus OH). Following perfusion fixation, dissected legs were placed in a 50 mL conical tube and positioned in the magnet. Following pilot scans, the anatomical images were collected using a RARE (Rapid Acquisition with Relaxation Enhancement) sequence with both axial and a double oblique (parallel to the femur/tibia plane) coronal views. The following acquisition parameters were used: TR/TE 4000/7 ms, RARE Factor = 8, NA = 4, 6×6 cm FOV, 256×256 matrix, 2-mm slice thickness, and 22 or 14 contiguous slices for axial or coronal views, respectively. ^{19}F MRI was performed at 282 MHz with the same slice geometry and the following parameters: TR/TE 3000/7 ms, RARE Factor = 4, 6×6 cm FOV, 128×128 matrix, and NA = 256 or 384 for axial or coronal views, respectively. Since the resonance frequencies were centered precisely on the water and the perfluorocarbon resonances, ^{19}F and ^{1}H anatomical images were co-registered without additional image processing.

^{19}F NMR spectra for the PFPE nanoemulsion in the dissected sciatic nerves were acquired following standard protocols with trifluoroacetic acid (TFA) as the internal standard [38]. Nerves were inserted into borosilicate NMR tubes (5 mm diameter) and spectra recorded (Bruker, 470 MHz). ^{19}F NMR peak around −92.5 ppm corresponding to fluorine nuclei was measured with TFA (set at −76.0 ppm) as reference (Figure S2).

Results

In this study, we demonstrate that CCI rats exhibit symptoms of mechanical hypersensitivity, which is a hallmark of chronic pain. We also show that dual mode PFPE nanoemulsion can be used to reveal the focal point of neuroinflammation by both NIR imaging and ^{19}F MRI. Furthermore, we demonstrate that the NIR and ^{19}F signal is arising from CD68 positive macrophage cells carrying the nanoemulsion that infiltrate the CCI injured nerve. Due to anatomical barriers for free nanoemulsion delivery to the site of injury and considering the supporting histological findings, the NIR and ^{19}F MRI signal shown arise from infiltrating cells.

Figure 1B illustrates that in the CCI rat, mechanical hypersensitivity is evident 11 days post surgery. Guarding behavior and other behaviors that are indicators of increased sensitivity were evident in all CCI animals. We also demonstrate that under these conditions, the mRNA expression levels of TRPV1, NPY and Gap43 are elevated on day 12 post surgery (Figure 1C). For TRPV1, the mean fold change values for the CCI-treatment, sham-treatment, and control groups were 2.60±0.352, 2.06±0.30, and 1.11±0.18, respectively. These data show that the CCI-treatment group was significantly different from the control groups ($p<0.05$). The CCI-treatment group was not significantly different from the sham group ($p>0.05$). For GAP43, the mean fold-change values for the CCI-treatment, sham-treatment, and control groups were 2.42±0.32, 1.52±0.51, and 1.00±0.07, respectively. These data show that the CCI-treatment group was significantly different from the sham-treatment and control groups ($p<0.05$). The sham-treatment group was not significantly different from the control group ($p>0.05$). For NPY, the mean fold change values for the CCI-treatment, sham-treatment, and control groups of 64.20±33.79, 6.49±6.21, and 1.44±1.34, respectively. These data show that the CCI-treatment group was significantly different from both the sham-treatment group and the control group ($p<0.001$).

To demonstrate that the expression of the TRPV1 protein is similarly elevated in the L5 dorsal root ganglia of CCI animals as compared to control, we analyzed tissue sections with antibodies against TRPV1 and Neurofilament-M (a neuronal marker). Additionally, the plantar region of the right rear paw of each rat was injected with DiD, a retrograde fluorescent dye that identifies the neurons innervating that specific region of the foot. Not all large diameter neurons in the dorsal root ganglia were positive for the DiD retrograde tracer since only a discrete number of neurons reach that region of the footpad. However, several DiD positive neurons are found and of those, some co-express TRPV1 in both control and CCI tissue. In the control, the immunofluorescent ratio of TRPV1/DiD is 0.787 indicating that under these conditions the DiD signal is brighter than the TRPV1 signal. However, in the CCI the TRPV1/DiD ratio is 1.12 (Figure 1E), indicative of elevated TRPV1 protein expression in these neurons of the dorsal root ganglion.

Figure 2 reveals that after the intravenous injection of the NIR labeled PFPE nanoemulsion, CCI injured rats exhibits NIR fluorescence that is focally localized parallel to the thigh (Figure 2I) at 11 days post CCI. This is in contrast to the autofluorescence evident in sham (Figure 2F) and control (Figure 2C) in the thoracolumbar regions, which is similar to that seen prior to the nanoemulsion injection (Figure 2 A, D, G). In a separate experiment, the surgical wound was occasionally found to exhibit low-level NIR fluorescence (Figure 3 B,C). This indicated that there was some superficial inflammation at the surgical wound as compared to the deeper sciatic nerve signal, which exhibits more scattering along the length of the sciatic nerve (Figure 3 E,F). Using the Li-COR Pearl Impulse software version 2.0 image analysis tools, we identified regions of interest (ROI) over the affected sciatic nerve for the CCI, sham and control animals (Figure S1 and Table S2). By averaging the normalized fluorescence (total relative fluorescence/total area) of the right and left legs, we demonstrate in Figure 3 G, that the CCI fluorescence is significantly brighter than the controls. ANOVA analysis of the entire data set comparing the relative fluorescence detected in the naïve right and left legs, the sham right and left legs and the CCI right and left legs reveals a difference for the CCI affected right leg with a p value<0.0001 (Table S3). A t test specifically comparing the affected CCI right leg to the sham surgical right leg reveals a significant difference with a p value<0.0001 (Table S3). However, given that NIR imaging cannot unequivocally provide spatial localization of the fluorescence, we continued the analysis by assessing the fluorescence of the dissected sciatic nerve from the sham as compared to the CCI animal (Figure 3 H,I). With CCI and sham nerves lying side-by-side and imaged simultaneously on the flatbed Li-COR Odyssey imaging system, only the CCI shows positive signal.

In preparation of the MRI analysis of the tissues, we assessed the NMR spectra of the dissected sciatic nerves to ascertain that the only fluorine signature to be detected was arising from the nanoemulsion and not any contribution that may come from natural sources or from anesthesia. The NMR spectra (Figure S2) show that the only detectable fluorine in the sciatic nerve arises from the PFPE nanoemulsion.

Analysis of the same right legs as those shown in Figure 2F for the Sham and Figure 2I for the CCI condition by proton and ^{19}F MRI show that the PFPE signal is coincident with the ligation of the sciatic nerve (Figure 4). Figure 4A shows that the four suture knots associated with the constriction injury are visible by proton MRI along the sciatic nerve, which is running parallel to the femur. The sciatic nerve (white arrow inset), tibia (T) and femur (F) are clearly visible in the adjacent image slice (Figure 4A – inset). Fluorine signal is evident along the sciatic nerve in the region of the sutures (Figure 4B) as well as in the bone marrow of the proximal head of the tibia. Viewed in cross section (Figure 4B – inset), ^{19}F signal is evident in the sciatic nerve, the femur as well as a slight signal where some minor inflammation persists at the site of the surgical wound. The clips had been removed on day 7 post-surgery. In the sham, a lower level of ^{19}F signal is evident only in the bone marrow near the head of the femur (Figure 4C). A comparable experiment revealed PFPE nanoemulsion labeled inflammation in the region of the CCI sciatic nerve (Figure S3C) as compared to control and sham.

To confirm that the PFPE signal is localized to the site of neuroinflammation byinfiltration of macrophages into the actual nerve, we sectioned the recovered sciatic nerve from the CCI right leg and the left leg of the same animal shown in Figure 2H, I and Figure 4A, B and stained the nerve with anti-CD68 antibody (Figure 5A–D). Similarly, the sciatic nerves from the un-operated control and the sham were also recovered for analysis (Figure 5 G–J). The results clearly demonstrate that macrophages have infiltrated into the CCI nerve, but not any of the controls. In duplicate experiments, examination of the macrophages revealed that they exhibit granular cytoplasm (Figure 5E, F). The nanoemulsion droplets in these cells are consistent with the nature of nanoemulsion droplets detected in macrophages grown in cell culture, which measure at the limit of spatial resolution for the light microscope with a size of 200–300 nm (Figure 5 K, L, M, N), which is consistent with the analytic size measurement of 180–200 nm in diameter [19].

Discussion

Here we report the first live imaging of neuroinflamation in the CCI neuropathic pain model with NIR and ^{19}F labeled nanoemulsion taken up by circulating monocytes that infiltrate into the damaged sciatic nerve and present as macrophages.

Chronic neuropathy in the CCI rat model leads to mechanical hypersensitivity [39]. Figure 1B demonstrates significant induction of mechanical hypersensitivity in ipsilateral hindpaw of CCI rat. We note that the role of TRPV1 as a nociceptor has been widely documented in a variety of acute, chronic, and neuropathic pain models and diseases such as diabetic neuropathy, chronic pancreatitis, cancer pain, osteoarthiritis, and gastrointestinal diseases [40,41,42,43]. NPY is a peptide neurotransmitter released by primary afferent neurons located in the dorsal root ganglia and received by neurons located in the substantia gelatinosa region of the spinal cord [44]. In animal models of neuropathic pain, NPY has been shown to be upregulated [45,46], and can be used as an indicator that trauma to the nerve has occurred. During development, Gap43 is a growth-associated protein that is highly expressed in the growth cones of elongating axons. Its expression decreases after the target has been innervated [47]. In addition to its developmental role, Gap43 is also differently expressed following neuronal tissue damage or inflammation, which has been demonstrated in several animal neuropathy models [47,48,49] and can be used to verify that trauma has occurred in peripheral nerve tissue.

We have demonstrated that in the CCI pain model, changes in mRNA expression levels of TRPV1 as well as NPY and Gap43 are evident in lumbar level five dorsal root ganglia using one-step qPCR analysis (Figure 1C). TRPV1 is known to play a role in inflammatory as well as neuropathic pain models [50]. The increased expression of NPY, a neurotransmitter, is known to play a role in modulating both innate and adaptive immune response [51], including modulating the phagocytic uptake by neutrophils and macrophages [52]. Furthermore, NPY has been shown to modulate neuronal signaling in acute pain, neuropathic pain and inflammatory animal pain models and induces anti-nociceptive effects [44]. The increase in NPY expression provides indirect evidence to support the interpretation that nerve trauma has been induced on the sciatic nerve. We find that mRNA expression of TRPV1 was increased in the ipsilateral dorsal root ganglia level 5 as compared to the control rat (Figure 1C). Furthermore, neurons in the dorsal root ganglia that are retrograde labeled with DiD from the plantar foot pad injection exhibit a relative increase in TRPV1 protein expression in the CCI condition as compared to un-operated control rats (Figure 1D, E). Collectively, these results demonstrate that CCI is inducing a hypersensitivity associated with changes in gene expression for the nerves of the affected DRG and sciatic nerve.

We also reported the *in vivo* imaging of neuroinflammation in the CCI sciatic nerve using dual mode (NIR and ^{19}F MRI) nanoemulsion. Both resident and hematogenous immune cells are involved in causing neuroinflammation at the site of injury in CCI rat model [18]. The infiltration of immune cells into the site of injury results in the release of inflammatory mediators, which then cause changes in the gene expression profile of the affected neurons and leads to peripheral sensitization [53]. *In vivo* imaging of granulomatous inflammation has been previously reported via labeling of macrophages with fluorescent NIR dye [54]. However, optical imaging is compromised due to the absorption and scattering of both the excitation and emitted light [55]. ^{19}F MRI has an advantage in that it is not limited by depth and has no background noise in tissues [56]. ^{19}F MRI has also been successfully used for *in vivo* imaging and quantification of inflammation in various animal disease models [20,31,57]. Previously, we demonstrated *in vitro* phagocytic uptake of a dual labeled nanoemulsion by macrophages in culture [38]. Here, we again demonstrate that a perfluorocarbon nanoemulsion containing both NIR dye and ^{19}F [19] is taken up by macrophages in culture as an assessment of toxicity and uptake as previously measured [19,38], which gave us confidence that we could achieve adequate sensitivity *in vivo* by both imaging modalities (Figure 5 K–N). This nanoemulsion is then used in order that we might achieve maximum sensitivity and specificity *in vivo*, in the analysis of neuroinflammation in CCI.

On day 8 post surgery, an intravenous injection of the nanoemulsion was given to the rats followed immediately by NIR fluorescence assessment to ensure that the injection was not inadvertently released subcutaneously. In the bloodstream, the phagocytic cells evidently engulf these nanoemulsion droplets through a still undetermined mechanism. These labeled immune cells naturally migrate to the site of injury to participate in the inflammatory response. NIR fluorescence emission from the labeling was observed only on the ipsilateral side of the CCI rat overlying the site of sciatic nerve ligation (Figure 2I and Figure 3E, F, I). Fluorescence was absent on hind limbs of sham rat, control rat and the contralateral hind limb of CCI rat (Figure 2 B, C, E, F, Hand Figure 3 A–D). NIR imaging was used to reveal the accumulation of immune cells at the site of sciatic nerve injury in live animals. Macrophages are the primary immune cells that phagocytose perfluorocarbon nanoemulsion droplets and they represent the majority of all the labeled cells [20]. The results from our *in vivo* NIR imaging suggest that the fluorescence signal is associated with neuroinflammation at the site of sciatic nerve injury in CCI rats. To confirm that the observed fluorescence originated in the sciatic nerve, *ex vivo* NIR imaging of the recovered injured sciatic nerves was performed. Fluorescence emission for NIR dye was observed only in the CCI ipsilateral sciatic nerve and not the ipsilateral nerve of the sham animal (Figure 3 H,I). The results complement the findings from the *in vivo* imaging and show that a fluorescence signal is present in the dissected nerve from the CCI rat, which is indicative of the accumulation of labeled macrophages.

To confirm that the fluorescence signal at the site of CCI injury was due to accumulation of nanoemulsion labeled macrophages, highly sensitive ^{19}F NMR spectroscopy and ^{19}F MRI were performed. NMR spectroscopy (Figure S2) demonstrates that in the dissected sciatic nerve, the only fluorine signature arises from the ^{19}F in the PFPE.

The ^{19}F signal localizes at the site of sciatic nerve injury in the CCI rats and no such signal was observed in the sham rat (Figure 4). The presence of ^{19}F signal was also observed in the femur and tibia of CCI and sham rats. Complex regional pain syndrome has previously been associated with osteoporotic changes in human subjects [58]. Furthermore, it has been demonstrated that osteoporotic changes in the ipsilateral tibial bone occur after CCI surgery. These changes are also associated with an increased number of osteoclasts in the bone [59]. Hence, the ^{19}F signal we observed in the bone marrow (Figure 4) could be indicative of the osteoporotic changes in the femur and tibia of CCI rats and is a result of the peripheral nerve injury. It has also been shown that a subset of blood monocytes could serve as osteoclast precursors [60]. Overall, our interpretation is that the ^{19}F signal evident in the bone marrow is due to migration of labeled monocytes to the bone.

Immunohistochemistry performed on the ipsilateral sciatic nerve of CCI rat clearly demonstrates infiltration of macrophages in the sciatic nerve (Figure 5). No such infiltration was observed for the left leg contralateral to the CCI, the ipsilateral sham and the control nerves (Figure 5). Therefore, the ^{19}F signal and the fluorescence observed during *in vivo* and *ex vivo* NIR imaging is due to infiltration of labeled macrophages at the site of injury.

Conclusion

This study demonstrates that the infiltration of immune cells into the CCI affected sciatic nerve can be monitored in live animals. Furthermore, the neuroinflammation caused by the CCI surgery can be imaged using the dual mode nanoemulsion such that both live animal NIR imaging and post-mortem perfluorocarbon ^{19}F MRI generate complementary results demonstrating that this neuroinflammation contributes to the pain associated with CCI surgery. In rats, specifically targeting the immune cells *in vivo* may serve as a treatment for neuroinflammation. The same technique could be used to monitor the effect of therapeutic drugs by assessing the extent of inflammation at the site of injury and to diagnose neuroinflammation without the need for surgical intervention involving a nerve biopsy.

Supporting Information

Figure S1 Near Infrared imaging (NIR) of live rats merged with white light images with the Region of Interest (ROI) indicated. All of these images were acquired on the LiCOR Pearl Live animal imager and processed in the same linked look-up tables. The ROI was set for the right leg CCI condition and then copied to a similar relative position on each of other legs for that experimental set. The LiCOR software tabulates the relative fluorescent signal and area (note Table S2).

Figure S2 ^{19}F NMR spectra for nanoemulsion in dissected CCI sciatic nerve. Exhibits ^{19}F NMR spectrum of dissected right sciatic nerve from CCI animal. TFA (−76.00 ppm) reference standard is shown along with the tissue signal for the nanoemulsion in the sciatic nerve (−92.5 ppm).

Figure S3 Near Infrared imaging (NIR) of live rats merged with white light images of their body, 2 days post intravenous injection of labeled emulsion on day 11 post surgery. All of these images were acquired on the LiCOR Pearl Live animal imager and processed in the same experiment with linked look-up tables. The control, sham and CCI (**A–F**) exhibit auto fluorescence over the thoracolumbar region, which is also evident prior to injection (Note Figure 2). The control animal (**A**) does not exhibit any fluorescence over the right leg. The sham (**B**) similarly does not exhibit any fluorescence in the area of the surgical wound (surgical staples). The CCI animal (**C**) exhibits a wide area of fluorescent signal over much of the thigh. The left side of the control, sham and CCI (**D, E, F**) exhibit only the auto fluorescence in the thoracolumbar region. Bar = 1 cm.

Table S1 Primer Sequences used for this study.

Table S2 LiCOR total relative fluorescence for each ROI. The Mean (Total Relative Fluorescence/Area) for each ROI is used for the analysis of variance (ANOVA) and t-test.

Table S3 1 Way ANOVA of Relative NIR Fluorescence in Live Rats.

Acknowledgments

The authors acknowledge the immunofluorescence contribution of Sophia Williard (BIOL 372 Cell & Systems Physiology course – J.A. Pollock Professor) and members of BIOL 376 Microscopy course (J.A. Pollock Professor). Robert Hoggard provided artwork and Prof. David L. Somers (Rangos School of Health Sciences, Duquesne University) provided assistance with CCI surgery training. ^{19}F NMR analyses performed at Pittsburgh NMR Center for Biomedical Research (Carnegie Mellon University) and at the Center for Molecular Analysis (Carnegie Mellon University).

Author Contributions

Conceived and designed the experiments: KV JMJ JAP. Performed the experiments: KV KA BZ-J SKP TKH JAP. Analyzed the data: KV KA BZ-J SKP TKH JMJ JAP. Contributed reagents/materials/analysis tools: AB TKH JMJ JAP. Wrote the paper: KV JMJ JAP.

References

1. von Hehn CA, Baron R, Woolf CJ (2012) Deconstructing the neuropathic pain phenotype to reveal neural mechanisms. Neuron (73): 638–652.
2. Jensen TS, Baron R, Haanpää M, Kalso E, Loeser JD, et al (2011) A new definition of neuropathic pain. Pain 152: 2204–2205.
3. National Research Council. *Relieving Pain in America: A Blueprint for Transforming Prevention, Care, Education, and Research.* Washington, DC: The National Academies Press, 2011.
4. Tal M (1999) A role for inflammation in chronic pain. Curr Rev Pain 3(6): 440–446.
5. Bennett GJ, Xie YK (1998) A peripheral mononeuropathy in rat that produces disorders of pain sensation like those seen in man. Pain 33: 87–107.
6. Wang LX, Wang ZJ (2003). Animal and cellular models of chronic pain. Adv Drug Deliv Rev 55(8): 949–965.
7. Stanton-Hicks M, Jänig W, Hassenbusch S, Hqddox JD, Boas R, et al. (1995) Reflex sympathetic dystrophy: changing concepts and taxonomy. Pain 63(1): 127–133.
8. Baron R, Wasner G (2001) Complex regional pain syndromes. Curr Pain Headache Rep 5: 114–123.
9. Woolf CJ, Ma Q (2007) Nociceptors–noxious stimulus detectors. Neuron 55: 353–364.
10. Montell C (2005) The TRP superfamily of cation channels. Sci STKE 2005: re3.
11. Voets T, Talavera K, Owsianik G, Nilius B (2005) Sensing with TRP channels. Nat Chem Biol 1: 85–92.
12. Damann N, Voets T, Nilius B (2008) TRPs in our senses. Curr Biol 18: R880–R889.
13. Cortright DN, Szallasi A (2009) TRP channels and pain. Curr Pharm Des 15: 1736–1749.
14. Stucky CL, Dubin AE, Jeske NA, Malin SA, McKemy DD, et al. (2009). Roles of transient receptor potential channels in pain. Brain Res Rev 60: 2–23.
15. Clatworthy AL, Illich PA, Castro GA, Walters ET (1995) Role of peri-axonal inflammation in the development of thermal hyperalgesia and guarding behavior in a rat model of neuropathic pain. Neurosci Lett 184: 5–8.
16. Thacker MA, Clark AK, Marchand F, McMahon SB (2007) Pathophysiology of peripheral neuropathic pain: Immune cells and molecules. Anesthesia and Analgesia 105: 838–847.
17. Myers RR, Heckman HM, Rodriguez M (1996) Reduced hyperalgesia in nerve-injured WLD mice: relationship to nerve fiber phagocytosis, axonal degeneration, and regeneration in normal mice. Exp Neurol 141: 94–101.
18. Gaudet AD, Popovich PG, Ramer MS (2011) Wallerian degeneration: Gaining perspective on inflammatory events after peripheral nerve injury, Journal of Neuroinflammation 8: 110.
19. Balducci A, Wen Y, Zhang Y, Helfer BM, Hitchens TK, et al. (2013) A novel probe for the non-invasive detection of tumor-associated inflammation. OncoImmunology 2: e23034.
20. Ahrens ET, Young WB, Xu H, Pusateri LK (2011) Rapid quantification of inflammation in tissue samples using perfluorocarbon emulsion and fluorine-19 nuclear magnetic resonance. Biotechniques 50(4): 229–234.
21. Srinivas M, Morel PA, Ernst LA, Laidlaw DH, Ahrens ET (2007) Fluorine-19 MRI for visualization and quantification of cell migration in a diabetes model. Magn Reson Med 58(4): 725–734.
22. Srinivas M, Turner MS, Janjic JM, Morel PA, Laidlaw DH, et al. (2009) *In vivo* cytometry of antigen specific T-cells using ^{19}F MRI. Magnetic Resonance in Medicine 62: 747–753.
23. Boehm-Sturm P, Mengler L, Wecker S, Hoehn M, Kallur T (2011) In vivo tracking of human neural stem cells with (19)F magnetic resonance imaging. PLoS ONE 6(12): e29040.
24. Temme S, Bönner F, Schrader J, Flögel U (2012) ^{19}F magnetic resonance imaging of endogenous macrophages in inflammation. WIREs Nanomed Nanobiotechnol, 4: 329–343.
25. Janjic JM, Ahrens ET (2009) Fluorine-containing nanoemulsions for MRI cell tracking. Wiley Interdiscip Rev Nanomed Nanobiotechnol 1(5): 492–501.
26. Chen J, Lanza GM, Wickline SA (2010) Quantitative magnetic resonance fluorine imaging: today and tomorrow. WIREs Nanomed Nanobiotechnol 2: 431–440.
27. Hu P, McLachlan EM (2002) Macrophage and lymphocyte invasion of dorsal root ganglia after peripheral nerve lesions in the rat. Neuroscience 112 (1): 23–38.
28. Ma W, Quirion R (2005) Up-regulation of interleukin 6 induced by prostaglandin E2 from invading macrophages following nerve in- jury: an in vivo and in vitro study. J. Neurochem 93: 664–673.
29. Morin N, Owolabi SA, Hartyetal MW (2007). Neutrophils invade lumbar dorsal root ganglia after chronic constriction injury of the sciatic nerve. Journal of Neuroimmunology 184 (1–2): 164–171.
30. Di Cesare Mannelli L, D'Agostino G, Pacini A, Russo R, Zanardelli M, et al. (2013) Palmitoylethanolamide Is a Disease-Modifying Agent in Peripheral Neuropathy: Pain Relief and Neuroprotection Share a PPAR-Alpha-Mediated Mechanism. Mediators of Inflammation Volume 2013, Article ID 328797. Available: http://dx.doi.org/10.1155/2013/328797.
31. Weise G, Basse-Luesebrink TC, Wessig C, Jakob PM, Stoll G (2011) In vivo imaging of inflammation in the peripheral nervous system by ^{19}F MRI, Experimental Neurology 229: 494–501.
32. Somers DL, Clemente FR (2003) The relationship between dorsal horn neurotransmitter content and allodynia in neuropathic rats treated with high-frequency transcutaneous electric nerve stimulation. Archives of Physical Medicine and Rehabilitation (84): 1575–1583.
33. Swett JE, Woolf CJ (1985) The somatotopic organization of primary afferent terminals in the superficial laminae of the dorsal horn of the rat spinal cord. Journal of Comparative Neurology 231(1): 66–77.
34. Swett JE, Torigoe Y, Elie VR, Bourassa CM, Miller PG (1991) Sensory neurons of the rat sciatic nerve. Experimental Neurololgy 114: 82–103.
35. Ji RR, Samad TA, Jin SX, Schmoll R, Woolf CJ (2002) p38 MAPK activation by NGF in primary sensory neurons after inflammation increases TRPV1 levels and maintains heat hyperalgesia. Neuron 36: 57–68.
36. Livak KJ, Schmittgen TD (2001) Analysis of relative gene expression data using real-time quantitative PCR and the 2(-Delta Delta C(T)) Method. Methods 25 (4): 402–408.
37. Barber RD, Harmer DW, Coleman RA, Clark BJ (2005) GAPDH as a housekeeping gene: analysis of GAPDH mRNA expression in a panel of 72 human tissues, Physiological Genomics 3: 389–395.
38. Patel SK, Zhang Y, Pollock JA and Janjic JM (2013) Cyclooxgenase-2 Inhibiting Perfluoropoly (Ethylene Glycol) Ether Theranostic Nanoemulsions–In Vitro Study. PloS One 8 (2): e55802.
39. Field MJ, Bramwell S, Hughes J, Singh L (1999) Detection of static and dynamic components of mechanical allodynia in rat models of neuropathic pain: are they signaled by distinct primary sensory neurons? Pain 83: 303–311.
40. Hong S, Agresta L, Guo C, Wiley JW (2008) The TRPV1 receptor is associated with preferential stress in large dorsal root ganglion neurons in early diabetic sensory neuropathy. J Neurochem 105: 1212–1222.
41. Xu GY, Winston JH, Shenoy M, Yin H, Pendyala S, Pasricha PJ (2007) Transient receptor potential vanilloid 1 mediates hyperalgesia and is up-regulated in rats with chronic pancreatitis. Gastroenterology 133(4), 1282–1292.
42. Szabó A, Helyes Z, Sándor K, Bite A, Pintér E, et al. (2005) Role of transient receptor potential vanilloid 1 receptors in adjuvant-induced chronic arthritis: in vivo study using gene-deficient mice. J Pharmacol Exp Ther 314, 111–119.
43. Jones RC, Xu L, Gebhart GF (2005) The mechanosensitivity of mouse colon afferent fibers and their sensitization by inflammatory mediators require transient receptor potential vanilloid 1 and acid-sensing ion channel 3. J Neurosci 25: 10981–10989.

44. Smith PA, Moran TD, Abdulla F, Tumber KK, Taylor BK (2007) Spinal mechanisms of NPY analgesia. Peptides 28(2): 464–474.
45. Moran TD, Colmers WF, Smith PA (2004) Opioid-like actions of neuropeptide Y in rat substantia gelatinosa: Y1 suppression of inhibition and Y2 suppression of excitation. J Neurophysiol 92: 3266–3275.
46. Staaf S, Oerther S, Lucas G, Mattsson JP, Ernfors P (2009) Differential regulation of TRP channels in a rat model of neuropathic pain. Pain 144(1–2), 187–199.
47. Leslie TA, Emson PC, Dowd PM, Woolf CJ (1995) Nerve growth factor contributes to the up-regulation of growth-associated protein 43 and preprotachykinin A messenger RNAs in primary sensory neurons following peripheral inflammation. Neuroscience 67: 753–761.
48. Van der Zee CE, Nielander HB, Vos JP, Lopes da Silva S, Verhaagen J, et al. (1989) Expression of growth-associated protein B-50 (GAP43) in dorsal root ganglia and sciatic nerve during regenerative sprouting. J Neurosci 9(10): 3505–3512.
49. Andersen LB, Schreyer DJ (1999) Constitutive expression of GAP-43 correlates with rapid, but not slow regrowth of injured dorsal root axons in the adult rat. Exp Neurol 155: 157–164. doi: S0014-4886(98)96903-5 [pii] 10.1006/exnr.1998.6903.
50. Kanai Y, Nakazato E, Fujiuchi A, Hara T, Imai A (2005) Involvement of an increased spinal TRPV1 sensitization through its up-regulation in mechanical allodynia of CCI rats. Neuropharmacology 49: 977–984.
51. Wheway J, Herzog H, Mackay F (2007) The Y1 receptor for NPY: A key modulator of the adaptive immune system. Peptides 28: 453–458.
52. Bedoui S, von Horsten S, Gebhardt T (2007) A role for neuropeptide Y (NPY) in phagocytosis: Implications for innate and adaptive immunity. Peptides 28: 373–376.
53. Ren K, Dubner R (2010) Interactions between the immune and nervous systems in pain. Nature Medicine 16 (11): 1267–1276.
54. Eisenblatter M, Ehrchen J, Varga G, Sunderkotter C, Heindel W, et al. (2009) In Vivo Optical Imaging of Cellular Inflammatory Response in Granuloma Formation Using Fluorescence-Labeled Macrophages, The Journal of Nuclear Medicine 50 (10): 1676–1682.
55. Mayer-Kuckuk P, Boskey AL (2006) Molecular imaging promotes progress in orthopedic research. Bone 39: 965–977.
56. Srinivas M, Heerschap A, Ahrens ET, Figdor CG, de Vries JM (2010) ^{19}F MRI for quantitative in vivo cell tracking, Trends in Biotechnology 28(7): 363–370.
57. Kadayakkara DK, Ranganathan S, Young W, Ahrens ET (2012) Assaying macrophage activity in a murine model of inflammatory bowel disease using fluorine-19 MRI. Laboratory Investigation 92: 636–645.
58. Moriwaki K, Yuge O, Tanaka H, Sasaki H, Izumi H, Kaneko K (1997) Neuropathic pain and prolonged regional inflammation as two distinct symptomatological components in complex regional pain syndrome with patchy osteoporosis – a pilot study. Pain 72: 277–282.
59. Suyama H, Moriwaki K, Niida S, Maehara Y, Kawamoto M, Yuge O (2002) Osteoporosis following chronic constriction injury of sciatic nerve in rats, Journal of Bone and Mineral Metabolism 20: 91–97.
60. Lari R, Kitchener PD, Hamilton JA (2009) The proliferative human monocyte subpopulation contains osteoclast precursors. Arthritis Research and Therapy 11(1): R23.

Platelet-Derived Growth Factor Receptor-β Antagonism Restores Morphine Analgesic Potency against Neuropathic Pain

Courtney L. Donica[1], Yan Cui[1], Shanping Shi[1], Howard B. Gutstein[1,2]*

1 Department of Anesthesiology, The University of Texas – MD Anderson Cancer Center, Houston, Texas, United States of America, **2** Department of Biochemistry and Molecular Biology, Genes and Development Graduate Program, The University of Texas – MD Anderson Cancer Center, Houston, Texas, United States of America

Abstract

Background: Chronic, intractable pain is a problem of pandemic proportions. Pain caused by nerve injuries (neuropathic pain) is extremely difficult to treat. For centuries, opiates such as morphine have been the first-line treatment for severe chronic pain. However, opiates are often ineffective against neuropathic pain, leaving few options for suffering patients. We previously demonstrated that platelet-derived growth factor- β (PDGFR-β) inhibition completely eliminated morphine tolerance. In these studies, we determined whether PDGFR-β inhibition could improve the effectiveness of morphine for neuropathic pain treatment.

Results and Findings: Spinal nerve ligation was performed in male Sprague-Dawley rats. The clinically used PDGFR antagonist imatinib did not relieve mechanical pain in a nerve injury model as determined by Von Frey assay. Surprisingly, combining imatinib with a previously ineffective dose of morphine led to complete pain relief. Scavenging released PDGF-B also markedly augmented the analgesic effect of morphine.

Conclusions: These findings suggest the novel hypothesis that PDGF-B released by injured nerves renders animals resistant to morphine, implying that PDGFR-β inhibition could potentially eliminate the tremendous suffering caused by neuropathic pain.

Editor: Shilpa J Buch, University of Nebraska Medical Center, United States of America

Funding: This work was funded by grant number RP 120408 from the Cancer Prevention and Research Institute of Texas to H.B.G. The funders had no role in study design, data collection and analysis, decision to publish, or preparation of the manuscript.

Competing Interests: The authors have declared that no competing interests exist.

* E-mail: hgutstein@mdanderson.org

Introduction

In the United States alone, chronic pain afflicts over 100 million people at an estimated yearly cost to society of over 500 billion dollars [1]. Throughout recorded history, opioid drugs such as morphine have been a mainstay of treatment for severe, chronic pain [2]. However, over time tolerance to opioid analgesia develops. Because there are few alternatives to opioids for the treatment of intractable pain, marked increases in opioid dose may be required to compensate for inadequate analgesia as tolerance develops. However, tolerance to the unpleasant or potentially life-threatening side effects of opioids such as respiratory depression, constipation, urinary retention and delirium, does not occur as rapidly as analgesic tolerance [2,3]. Therefore, patients face increased risk as well as suffering when opioids lose effectiveness.

It has been proposed that pain and tolerance utilize common signaling mechanisms [4]. We recently discovered that the platelet derived growth factor beta (PDGFR-β) is a highly selective and specific mediator of morphine tolerance [5]. We established that PDGFR-β signaling is both necessary and sufficient to cause morphine tolerance, and that morphine induced the release of PDGF-B, which caused tolerance to occur. Pain due to nerve injury (neuropathic pain) is particularly resistant to opioids, although high doses of morphine can temporarily relieve neuropathic pain in rodents [6–8]. It is estimated that 40–60% of people suffering from neuropathic pain have inadequate pain relief [9]. It is thought that one of the most difficult features of neuropathic pain to treat is mechanical hypersensitivity caused by nerve injury [10]. We hypothesized that mechanical hypersensitivity could be resistant to the analgesic effects of morphine because the nerve injury itself induced analgesic tolerance. In an animal model of neuropathic pain [11], we found that not only did PDGFR-β inhibition block analgesic tolerance, but also markedly improved the analgesic effectiveness of morphine against mechanical hypersensitivity. Additional experiments suggested the hypothesis that PDGF-B release by injured nerves could render neuropathic pain resistant to the analgesic effects of morphine.

Methods

Animals

Male Sprague Dawley rats (175–200 g, Harlan) were housed in groups of three and were maintained on a 12 hr light/dark cycle with *ad libitum* access to food and water. Rats habituated to the colony room for one week prior to experimental manipulations.

Left L5 spinal nerve ligations were performed as described [11]. All protocols were approved by the MD Anderson Cancer Center Institutional Animal Care and Use Committee.

Drug Administration

Drugs were dissolved in a solution of 10% β-cyclodextrin sulfobutyl ether (Captisol®, CyDex, Lenexa, KS) solution and 0.45% saline. Morphine sulfate was obtained from the MD Anderson Cancer Center Pharmacy, imatinib from LC Laboratories (Woburn, MA) and recombinant human PDGFR-β-Fc from R&D Systems (Minneapolis, MN). PDGFR-β-Fc was re-constituted in phosphate buffered saline (PBS) with 0.1% bovine serum albumin (BSA) at 100 μg/mL and stored at −80°C until use. Drugs were administered daily via subcutaneous injection or lumbar puncture as previously described [12].

Nociceptive Testing

Animals were placed in Plexiglas cages on a mesh surface and habituated for 30 min per day for 3 days prior to testing. Mechanical sensitivity was assessed by Von Frey filaments using the up-down method of Dixon and median 50% threshold determined as described [13,14].

Statistical Analyses

Data were analyzed using GraphPad v 5.0 and was considered statistically significant if $P<0.05$ by two-way analysis of variance (ANOVA).

Results

We initially administered morphine in the presence or absence of the PDGFR inhibitor imatinib [15] daily for 4 days in rats that underwent spinal nerve ligation (SNL). A morphine dose that is analgesic in thermal assays of nociception in non-ligated animals [5] (2 nmol, injected intrathecally (i.t.)) had no effect on mechanical hypersensitivity (Figure 1a). Imatinib alone also had no effect. Surprisingly, administering morphine and imatinib together completely eliminated the mechanical allodynia induced by SNL (Figure 1a; Treatment $F_{(3,31)} = 1009$, Day $F_{(5,155)} = 339.2$, Interaction $F_{(15,155)} = 92.55$; all $p<0.0001$ by two-way ANOVA).

We then determined whether imatinib would block mechanical allodynia from the initiation of nerve injury when given systemically. Animals were treated with a morphine dose that is analgesic in tests of thermal nociception (2.5 mg/kg, injected subcutaneously (s.c.)), imatinib (5 mg/kg, s.c.), the combination, or vehicle starting the day after SNL. Neither morphine nor imatinib alone altered mechanical hypersensitivity. Similar to the results obtained above after a two week surgical recovery (Figure 1a), combining morphine and imatinib produced immediate and complete reversal of mechanical allodynia from the day after nerve injury until the study was concluded 9 days later (Figure 1b; Drug $F_{(4,190)} = 443.9$, Day $F_{(4,190)} = 11.13$, Interaction $F_{(16,190)} = 16.61$; all $p<0.0001$ by two-way ANOVA).

These results suggested the hypothesis that release of PDGF by ligated nerves could render the resulting mechanical hypersensitivity resistant to the analgesic effects of morphine. To test this hypothesis, animals that had undergone SNL were treated with either 2 nmol morphine i.t., 500 ng of a fusion protein constructed of the extracellular domains of the PDGFR-β fused to antibody Fc fragments (PDGFR-β-Fc), which scavenges released PDGF-B (5), the combination, or vehicle. Administering vehicle, morphine, or PDGFR-β-Fc alone had no effect on mechanical hypersensitivity. Remarkably, combining morphine with PDGFR-β-Fc completely eliminated mechanical allodynia (Figure 1c; Treatment $F_{(4,29)} = 186.9$, Day $F_{(9,261)} = 43.29$, Interaction $F_{(36, 261)} = 12.04$; all $p<0.0001$ by two-way ANOVA). Similar to the combination of morphine and imatinib, repeated doses of PDGFR-β-Fc and morphine continued to block mechanical allodynia. These results support the hypotheses that 1) PDGF-B released by injured nerves reduces the effectiveness of morphine against mechanical allodynia and 2) that imatinib augments the effectiveness of morphine against mechanical allodynia by blocking PDGFR-β-mediated signaling.

Discussion

Our findings demonstrate that PDGFR-β inhibition, either spinally or systemically, enhances morphine effectiveness against neuropathic pain. Combining a previously ineffective morphine dose with PDGFR-β antagonists can reverse established allodynia as well as prevent allodynia from developing after nerve injury. In addition, similar to our previously reported results [5], PDGFR-β inhibition prevents tolerance to this effect from developing. Interestingly, imatinib alone does not affect morphine analgesia [5]. Further, repeated administration of morphine with imatinib remains effective through at least 9 days (figure 1B). This suggests that there is no "tolerance" to the PDGFR-β antagonist rescue of morphine effectiveness. These results suggest that lower doses of opioids could be used to treat neuropathic pain if PDGFR-β inhibitors were given concurrently. In addition, the dose escalation that commonly occurs [9] could be avoided. Since tolerance to unpleasant or potentially life-threatening side effects of opioids such as respiratory depression, constipation, urinary retention and delirium, does not occur as rapidly as analgesic tolerance [3], PDGFR-β antagonism could potentially reduce the risks associated with chronic opioid treatment [16] and the suffering that results when opioids lose effectiveness.

We previously demonstrated that administration of PDGF-B to naïve animals rendered them tolerant to subsequent morphine doses [5]. PDGF-B is localized in the dorsal root ganglion and dorsal horn of the spinal cord and PDGFR-β is located in myelinated and unmyelinated nerves, dorsal root ganglion neurons and the spinal dorsal horn [17–20]. Given the distribution of PDGF-B and PDGFR-β, it is possible that PDGFR-β inhibition blocks opioid tolerance by modulating opioid effects on peptidergic primary afferent fibers. It has been suggested that pain and opioid tolerance utilize common signaling pathways [4,21]. Our current observation that PDGF-B scavenging augmented the analgesic effect of morphine against neuropathic pain indicates that nerve ligation also induces PDGF-B release. PDGF-B alone does not appear to induce pain: PDGF-BB administration does not induce thermal sensitivity [5] and scavenging released PDGF-B alone does not alleviate neuropathic pain (Fig 1C). Rather, our data suggests that released PDGF-B affects the ability of morphine to induce analgesia. Taken together, these findings suggest that PDGF-B released by injured nerves causes resistance to the analgesic effect of morphine, possibly through similar translational and post-translational modifications of analgesic effectors induced by prior opioid exposure. In effect, PDGF-B renders animals "pre-tolerant" to morphine analgesia. Previous work has shown that neuropathic pain reduces the efficacy of morphine, supporting this hypothesis [6–8]. Our results also suggest that blockade of PDGFR-β signaling could become an important therapeutic approach for relieving the suffering of untold numbers of patients living with intractable neuropathic pain.

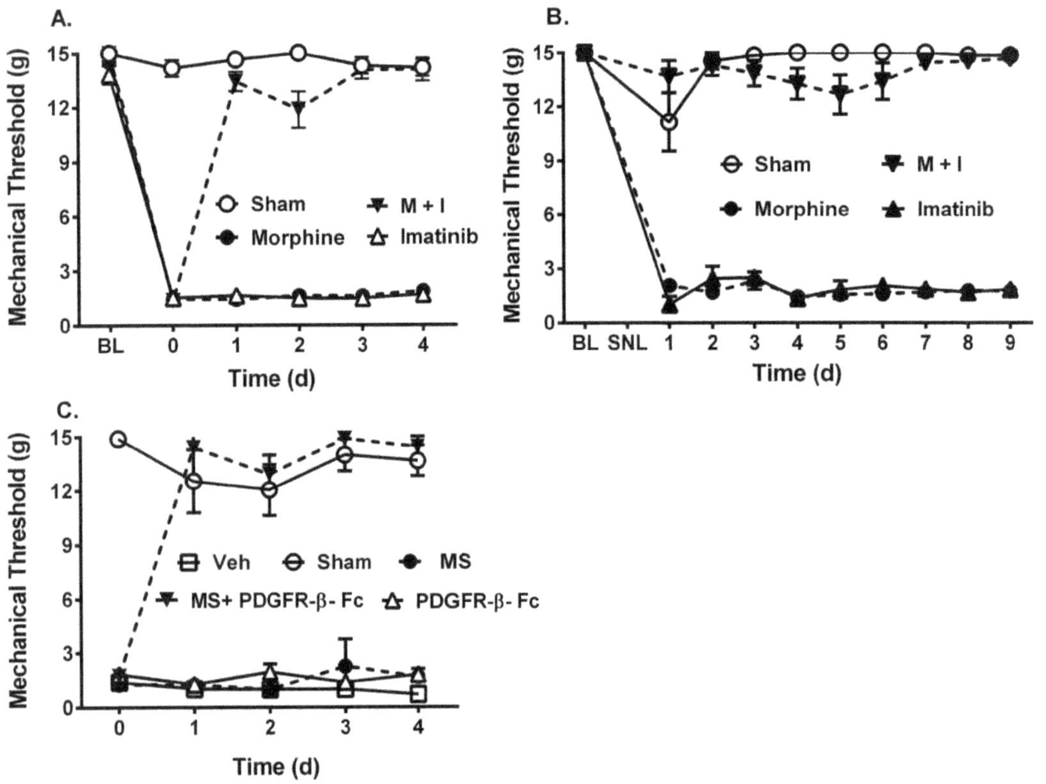

Figure 1. PDGFR inhibition restores morphine efficacy against neuropathic pain. Animals underwent left L5 SNL as described in [11]. Mechanical sensitivity was tested using von Frey filaments and 50% median response threshold determined [13,14]. Sham operated animals underwent the same surgical procedure except a suture was not tied around the L5 nerve root. (**A**) Baseline mechanical sensitivity was determined before surgery (BL). Animals then underwent SNL and were allowed to recover for two weeks. Mechanical sensitivity was tested to confirm that SNL induced mechanical allodynia (day 0). SNL animals received daily intrathecal (i.t.) injections of morphine (2 nmol), imatinib (10 μg), or the combination and mechanical sensitivity was determined. Sham operated animals received injections of vehicle alone. Neither morphine nor imatinib alone were analgesic. Co-administration of morphine and imatinib completely reversed SNL-induced mechanical allodynia. n = 8–9 per group. (**B**) Beginning the day after SNL, animals received daily subcutaneous (s.c.) injections of morphine (2.5 mg/kg), imatinib (5 mg/kg), morphine + imatinib or vehicle and mechanical sensitivity determined. Systemic co-administration of morphine and imatinib completely eliminated allodynia after nerve injury. n = 5–9 per group. (**C**) Following a two week recovery after SNL, animals received daily i.t. injections of morphine (2 nmol), PDGFR-β-Fc scavenger (500 ng), the combination or vehicle. While PDGFR-β-Fc had no effect on mechanical allodynia, co-administration of morphine and PDGFR-β-Fc completely restored the effectiveness of morphine. n = 7–10 per group. All data presented as grams +/− s.e.m; all $p<0.0001$ (2-way ANOVA).

Acknowledgments

We thank Jin Mo Chung and Shao-Rui Chen for instruction in spinal nerve ligation. All animal studies were approved by the M.D. Anderson Cancer Center Institutional Animal Care and Use Committee.

Author Contributions

Conceived and designed the experiments: HBG. Performed the experiments: CLD SS YC. Analyzed the data: CLD SS YC HBG. Wrote the paper: CLD HG.

References

1. Board of Health Sciences Policy (2011) Relieving Pain in America: A Blueprint for Transforming Prevention, Care, Education and Research. Washington, DC: The National Academies Press. 313 p.
2. Gutstein H, Akil H (2006) Opioid Analgesics. In: Brunton L, Lazo J, Parker K, editors. Goodman & Gilman's The Pharmacological Basis of Therapeutics. 11 ed. New York: McGraw-HIll. pp. 547–590.
3. Collett BJ (1998) Opioid tolerance: the clinical perspective. Br J Anaesth 81: 58–68.
4. Mayer D, Mao J, Holt J, Price D (1999) Cellular mechanisms of neuropathic pain, morphine tolerance, and their interactions. Proc Natl Acad Sci 96: 7731–7736.
5. Wang Y, Barker KE, Shi S, Diaz MF, Mo B, et al. (2012) Blockade of PDGFR-β Activation Eliminates Morphine Analgesic Tolerance. Nature Medicine 18: 385–387.
6. Bian D, Nichols ML, Ossipov MH, Lai J, Porreca F (1995) Characterization of the antiallodynic efficacy of morphine in a model of neuropathic pain in rats. Neuroreport 6: 1981–1984.
7. Przewlocka B, Mika J, Labuz D, Toth G, Przewlocki R (1999) Spinal analgesic action of endomorphins in acute, inflammatory and neuropathic pain in rats. Eur J Pharmacol 367: 189–196.
8. Przewlocki R, Przewlocka B (2001) Opioids in chronic pain. Eur J Pharmacol 429: 79–91.
9. Dworkin RH, O'Connor AB, Backonja M, Farrar JT, Finnerup NB, et al. (2007) Pharmacologic management of neuropathic pain: evidence-based recommendations. Pain 132: 237–251.
10. Woolf CJ, Mannion RJ (1999) Neuropathic pain: aetiology, symptoms, mechanisms, and management. Lancet 353: 1959–1964.
11. Chung JM, Kim HK, Chung K (2004) Segmental spinal nerve ligation model of neuropathic pain. Methods Mol Med 99: 35–45.
12. Xu JJ, Walla BC, Diaz MF, Fuller GN, Gutstein HB (2006) Intermittent lumbar puncture in rats: a novel method for the experimental study of opioid tolerance. Anesthesia & Analgesia 103: 714–720.
13. Dixon WJ (1980) Efficient analysis of experimental observations. Annu Rev Pharmacol Toxicol 20: 441–462.
14. Chaplan SR, Bach FW, Pogrel JW, Chung JM, Yaksh TL (1994) Quantitative assessment of tactile allodynia in the rat paw. J Neurosci Methods 53: 55–63.
15. Buchdunger E, Cioffi CL, Law N, Stover D, Ohno-Jones S, et al. (2000) Abl protein-tyrosine kinase inhibitor STI571 inhibits in vitro signal transduction mediated by c-kit and platelet-derived growth factor receptors. J Pharmacol Exp Ther 295: 139–145.

16. Rice ASC, Hill RG (2006) New treatments for neuropathic pain. Annual Review of Medicine 57: 535–551.
17. Eccleston PA, Funa K, Heldin CH (1993) Expression of platelet-derived growth factor (PDGF) and PDGF alpha- and beta-receptors in the peripheral nervous system: an analysis of sciatic nerve and dorsal root ganglia. Dev Biol 155: 459–470.
18. Masuda J, Tsuda M, Tozaki-Saitoh H, Inoue K (2009) Intrathecal delivery of PDGF produces tactile allodynia through its receptors in spinal microglia. Molecular Pain. 2009/05/12 ed. pp. 23.
19. Sasahara A, Kott JN, Sasahara M, Raines EW, Ross R, et al. (1992) Platelet-derived growth factor B-chain-like immunoreactivity in the developing and adult rat brain. Brain Res Dev Brain Res 68: 41–53.
20. Sasahara M, Fries JW, Raines EW, Gown AM, Westrum LE, et al. (1991) PDGF B-chain in neurons of the central nervous system, posterior pituitary, and in a transgenic model. Cell 64: 217–227.
21. Mao J, Price DD, Mayer DJ (1995) Mechanisms of hyperalgesia and morphine tolerance: a current view of their possible interactions. Pain 62: 259–274.

10

Targeting Anti-Inflammatory Treatment Can Ameliorate Injury-Induced Neuropathic Pain

Katsuyuki Iwatsuki*, Tetsuya Arai, Hideyuki Ota, Shuichi Kato, Tadahiro Natsume, Shigeru Kurimoto, Michiro Yamamoto, Hitoshi Hirata

Department of Hand Surgery, Nagoya University Graduate School of Medicine, Showa-ku, Nagoya, Japan

Abstract

Tumor necrosis factor-α plays important roles in immune system development, immune response regulation, and T-cell-mediated tissue injury. The present study assessed the net value of anti-tumor necrosis factor-α treatment in terms of functional recovery and inhibition of hypersensitivity after peripheral nerve crush injury. We created a right sciatic nerve crush injury model using a Sugita aneurysm clip. Animals were separated into 3 groups: the first group received only a skin incision; the second group received nerve crush injury and intraperitoneal vehicle injection; and the third group received nerve crush injury and intraperitoneal etanercept (6 mg/kg). Etanercept treatment improved recovery of motor nerve conduction velocity, muscle weight loss, and sciatic functional index. Plantar thermal and von Frey mechanical withdrawal thresholds recovered faster in the etanercept group than in the control group. On day 7 after crush injury, the numbers of ED-1-positive cells in crushed nerves of the control and etanercept groups were increased compared to that in the sham-treated group. After 21 days, ED-1-positive cells had nearly disappeared from the etanercept group. Etanercept reduced expression of interleukin-6 and monocyte chemotactic and activating factor-1 at the crushed sciatic nerve. These findings demonstrate the utility of etanercept, in terms of both enhancing functional recovery and suppressing hypersensitivity after nerve crush. Etanercept does not impede the onset or progression of Wallerian degeneration, but optimizes the involvement of macrophages and the secretion of inflammatory mediators.

Editor: Allan Siegel, University of Medicine & Dentistry of NJ - New Jersey Medical School, United States of America

Funding: This work was supported by the Health and Labour Sciences Research Grant on Intractable Diseases (Pathogenesis and Diagnostic Accuracy of Neuropathic Pain) from the Ministry of Health, Labour and Welfare of Japan. The funders had no role in study design, data collection and analysis, decision to publish, or preparation of the manuscript.

Competing Interests: The authors have declared that no competing interests exist.

* E-mail: kiwatsuki@med.nagoya-u.ac.jp

Introduction

Tumor necrosis factor (TNF)-α plays important roles in immune system development, immune-response regulation, and T-cell-mediated tissue injury. The immune response to injury coordinates host defense and tissue repair, but also has the inherent capacity to significantly damage host tissues [1]. TNF-α antagonists such as infliximab, etanercept, and adalimumab are indicated for the treatment of refractory rheumatic diseases and inflammatory bowel diseases. In fact, use of these drugs has improved outcomes in the treatment of rheumatoid arthritis, in terms of both symptom severity scores and quality of life measures [2].

After nerve injury, TNF-α is upregulated in activated Schwann cells, macrophages, and other components of the peripheral nervous system. TNF-α has been shown to act as the initiator of Wallerian degeneration (WD) by activating resident Schwann cells and facilitating macrophage recruitment to the injury site [3].

Despite these crucial roles of TNF-α in peripheral nerve repair and regeneration, previous studies have also suggested deleterious effects of TNF-α. For instance, TNF-α released by autoreactive T cells and macrophages may induce immune-mediated demyelinating neuropathies. The proposed pathogenesis of TNF-α-associated neuropathies includes both T-cell and humoral immune attack against peripheral nerve myelin, vasculitis-induced nerve ischemia, and inhibition of signaling support for axons [4]. In fact, experimental results have demonstrated that intraneural injection of TNF-α produces predominantly axonal damage of the sciatic nerve [5]. TNF-α mediates rapid activation of injury-induced binding of nuclear factor (NF)-κB to DNA in Schwann cells, and these events are associated with inhibition of post-injury axonal sprouting [6].

Taken together, TNF-α appears to represent a two-edged sword. In fact, the merits of TNF-α-targeting treatments remain contentious. For example, Chen et al. [7] showed that TNF-α promotes functional motor recovery in crushed peripheral nerves. In contrast, many recent studies have reported that blocking TNF-α prevents nerve degeneration and promotes nerve regeneration, and motor and sensory functional recovery [8,9]. Similarly, evidence has been accumulating indicating that inhibition of TNF-α could reduce inflammatory demyelination in various neuropathies, and TNF-α-knockout mice exhibit nerve preservation after WD induction. These reports strongly imply the central involvement of TNF-α in axonal degradation during WD [10]. In addition, several researchers have successfully demonstrated that selective inhibition of soluble TNF-α is beneficial even in the central nervous system. For example, Branbilla et al. [11] demonstrated enhanced functional recovery after experimental autoimmune encephalomyelitis, while Chio et al. [12] and

Genovese et al. [13] showed neuroprotective effects after brain and spinal cord injuries.

Despite these reports of favorable effects with the use of anti-TNF-α drugs on peripheral nerve disorders, some researchers suspect that such drugs may have negative side effects for patients with peripheral neuropathies. Previous case series have suggested associations between implementation of anti-TNF-α treatment and onset or progression of peripheral nerve disorders such as Guillain-Barré syndrome, Miller Fisher syndrome, chronic inflammatory demyelinating polyneuropathy, multifocal motor neuropathy with conduction block, mononeuropathy multiplex, and axonal sensorimotor polyneuropathies [4]. Furthermore, most of these neuropathies improved over a period of months after withdrawal of the TNF-α antagonist, with or without additional immunomodulatory treatment [4,14]. These reports sounded the alarm that anti-TNF-α therapy should be avoided in patients with pre-existing multiple sclerosis and immediately discontinued when new neurological signs and symptoms arise, pending appropriate evaluation [15].

Another issue regarding the use of TNF-α antagonists for peripheral nerve injuries or disorders is their value as a modulator of pain sensitivity. Neuropathic pain is a recognized pathological pain type where nociceptive responses persist beyond the resolution of damage to the nerve and the surrounding tissue. Satisfactory treatment of chronic pain remains elusive, and novel painkillers rarely reach the modern market [16]. Although consensus is lacking regarding the etiology of neuropathic pain, animal models of this pathology based on various nerve injury types have persistently suggested that TNF-α plays pivotal roles at both the peripheral and central levels of sensitization [17]. Likewise, Kato et al. [8] reported that anti-TNF-α therapy can attenuate neuropathic pain-related behaviors after peripheral nerve injury in a rodent model. Martini et al. [18] proposed the protection of sensory nerve fibers from macrophage attack as a challenging paradigm for the development of putative treatment approaches. In this context, knowledge of the molecular mechanisms underlying Schwann cell-macrophage interactions under pathological conditions is an important prerequisite to developing effective treatment strategies for pain problems associated with peripheral nerve disorders.

WD classically refers to the degeneration of axons distal to a lesion site. WD, the self-destructive set of cellular and molecular processes by which degenerating axons and myelin are cleared after injury, is initiated by macrophages and Schwann cells [1]. Regulating WD is one of the targets in treating central and peripheral nerve disorders and pain [19]. The molecular mechanisms implicated in axonal regeneration and pathfinding after injury are complex, and take into account cross-talk between axons and glial cells, neurotrophic factors, extracellular matrix molecules and their receptors [20]. These varied mechanisms are still not completely understood [21]. Many studies have been made with the help of Wallerian degeneration slow (Wld^S) mice [22,23,24,25,26]. The phenotype in this model is attributed to overexpression of a chimeric protein, Wld^S, which contains the full-length nicotinamide adenine dinucleotide synthetic enzyme, nicotinamide mononucleotide adenylyl-transferase-1 (Nmnat-1) [27,28,29]. Nmnat1 has been reported to protect the axon through NAD-dependent deacetylase sirtuin 1 or local nicotinamide adenine dinucleotide synthesis in neuritis, but Nmnat1 is considerably weaker than Wld^S [30,31,32]. In this mouse mutant, axon stumps distal to the lesion site survive ten times longer than axons in wild-type animals [33,34]. This protein is being studied as a treatment target for central and peripheral nerve disorders, such as trauma [35], Parkinson's disease [36], and Charcot-Marie-Tooth disease [37].

Molecular inflammatory mediators such as interleukin (IL)-1, IL-6, IL-10, TNF-α and NF-κB, the complement system and arachidonic acid metabolites have been shown to modulate these processes. In addition, Schwann cells of the WD following axonal injury can produce TNF-α and IL-1 [38]. NF-κB activation is important for TNF-α secretion from Schwann cells and may play a key role in triggering positive-feedback loops for IL-6 expression [39]. Neurons can synthesize and express molecular inflammatory mediators, and these cytokines may participate in neuronal communication [40,41,42].

The release and activity of TNF-α and other potentially damaging cytokines are controlled at multiple levels to prevent unrestrained collateral tissue damage that can disable, or even kill, the host [43]. As systemic reactions, humoral mechanisms that restrain or inhibit these damaging responses include glucocorticoid hormones, soluble cytokine receptors, IL-10, transforming growth factor-β and other anti-inflammatory cytokines. Activation of cholinergic receptors is also known to regulate immune system activity [38,44].

Direct modulation of voltage-gated sodium channel (Nav) expression by IL-1 and IL-6 is produced by macrophages via activation of purinergic receptor P2X, ligand-gated ion channel (P2RX) 7, and direct activation through a signaling pathway that involves TNF-α acting on TNF receptors. Cytokines produced by inflammatory and glial cells change neuronal excitability and this link contributes directly to the development of intractable pain.

The purpose of the present study was to assess the net value of the anti-TNF-α treatment in terms of functional recovery and inhibition of hypersensitivity after peripheral nerve crush injury using a rat model. In addition, we attempted to elucidate the molecular mechanisms involved, with special emphasis on the effects of TNF-α on macrophage behavior and IL-6 production during WD and axonal regeneration at the injured nerve.

Materials and Methods

Rat Model of Sciatic Nerve Injury

All experimental protocols and animal maintenance procedures were approved by the Animal Ethics Research Committee of Nagoya University (Permit number: 24007), and were in accordance with the Animal Protection and Management Law of Japan (No. 105) and the Ethical Issues of the International Association for the Study of Pain [45].

A total of 138 sciatic nerves of Lewis rats (body weight, approximately 250 g) were used. Animals were anesthetized with an intraperitoneal injection of 5% pentobarbital. Animals were then separated into 3 groups. The first group received only a skin incision (sham group, n = 46). The second group received a nerve crush injury and an intraperitoneal injection of vehicle (solvent saline) (control group, n = 46). The third group received a nerve crush injury and injection of etanercept (Takeda, Osaka, Japan) (etanercept group, n = 46). In both the control and etanercept groups, the right sciatic nerves were dissected from the surrounding tissues and nerve crush injuries [46] were inflicted using a Sugita aneurysm clip (Mizuho Ikakogyo, Tokyo, Japan). The clip was applied for 5 min with approximately 1.5 N of holding force. In the etanercept group, etanercept was administered once intraperitoneally at 6 mg/kg on the day of operation [9].

Electrophysiological Evaluation

According to previous studies, sciatic nerve crush using a Sugita clip for 5 min inevitably leads to complete WD in rats, with spontaneous recovery within 6 weeks. We therefore conducted electrophysiological assessments on days 7, 21 and 35 after crush injury to measure motor nerve conduction velocities (MCVs) of the tibial nerve in the control, etanercept, and sham groups.

Compound muscle action potentials (CMAPs) of the tibialis anterior muscle were measured at room temperature (24°C). Two stainless steel monopolar recording electrodes (H537A; Nihon Kohden, Tokyo, Japan) were placed on the center of the belly of the tibialis anterior muscle after exposing the muscle. The sciatic nerve was exposed and a bipolar stimulating electrode (UM2-5050; Nihon Kohden) was placed around the nerve at the level of the sciatic notch. Electrical pulses (supramaximal; duration, 100 ms; frequency, 1 Hz; square wave) were applied with an isolator (SS-201J; Nihon Kohden) connected to an electronic stimulator. CMAPs were recorded to estimate electrophysiological function and evaluate MCV [47,48].

Wet Muscle Weight Measurement

After euthanasia, tibialis anterior muscle was dissected free from the origin and insertion, and immediately weighed while still wet (n = 5 per group). Tibialis anterior muscle weight was then calculated as a percentage of total body weight [48].

Behavioral Tests

Sensitivity to non-noxious mechanical stimuli was measured using the von Frey test. The rats stood on an elevated platform made of a wide-gauge wire mesh. The von Frey hair was inserted from below, up through the holes in the mesh, and poked through the undersurface of a hind paw. At threshold, the animal quickly responded by flicking its paw away from the hair.

Thermal hyperalgesia was assessed by measuring hind paw withdrawal latency in response to radiant heat using a plantar test apparatus (Ugo Basile, Comerio, Italy). Each rat was placed into a compartment enclosure on a glass surface. A mobile heat source was then positioned under the plantar surface of the hind paw and activated with a light beam [49,50]. Results were calculated as a ratio compared to values in the sham group.

Sciatic Nerve Function

Sciatic functional index (SFI) [51], an index of the functional condition of rat sciatic nerve function based on measurements made from walking tracks, was measured using a CatWalk XT 8.0 automated quantitative gait analysis system (Noldus, Wageningen, the Netherlands) [52,53]. To obtain an overall index of the degree of normal function, the 4 variables measured on each side were entered into the following formula [51]:

$$\boldsymbol{SFI} = [(\boldsymbol{ETOF} - \boldsymbol{NTOF})/\mathrm{NTOF}] + [(\mathrm{NPL} - \mathrm{EPL})/\mathrm{EPL}] + [(\mathrm{ETS} - \mathrm{NTS})/\mathrm{NTS}] + [(\mathrm{EIT} - \mathrm{NIT})/\mathrm{NIT}] \times 220/4,$$

where N is normal, E is experimental, TOF is the distance to the opposite foot, PL is print length, TS is total toe spreading, and IT is the distance between intermediary toes.

Real-time Polymerase Chain Reaction

Total RNA was isolated from crushed sciatic nerves (n = 5 per group) and L5 dorsal root ganglia (DRGs) after crush injury using an RNeasy Lipid Tissue Mini Kit (Qiagen, Valencia, CA), and complementary DNA was made using High-Capacity RNA to cDNA Master Mix (Applied Biosystems, Foster City, CA). Specific primers for TNF-α, IL-6, IL-1β, monocyte chemoattractant protein (MCP)-1, P2RX7 and voltage-gated sodium channels from Nav1.3, 1.8, 1.9 and TaqMan probes (Applied Biosystems) were used. Expression levels of TNF-α, IL-6, IL-1β, MCP-1 and P2RX7 were investigated at the crushed nerves and expression levels of sodium channels were investigated at the DRG.

Samples were subjected to 40 cycles of amplification at 95°C for 15 s and 60°C for 1 min, after holding at 50°C for 2 min and at 95°C for 10 min, and mRNA expression differences among the 3 groups were determined by calculating ΔC_Ts (C_T for each target minus C_T for β-actin for each sample).

Enzyme-linked Immunosorbent Assay for TNF-α and IL-6

A rat TNF-α immunoassay system (RayBio, Norcross, GA) and an IL-6 immunoassay system (Abnova, Taipei, Taiwan) were used. Crushed sciatic nerves (n = 5 per group) at 2, 7, 21, and 35 days after crush injury were homogenized in Tris-buffered saline containing 1% Nonidet P-40, 10% glycerol, and protease inhibitors. Samples were diluted to the same protein concentration. Results were calculated as a ratio compared to values in the sham group.

Immunohistochemistry

Rats were anesthetized as described above and perfused transcardially with fresh 4% paraformaldehyde. Crushed sciatic nerves were removed and postfixed in 4% paraformaldehyde overnight. Tissues were embedded in paraffin, then 10-μm sections were deparaffinized with xylene and rehydrated in graded ethanol. For antigen retrieval, all sections were incubated with protease for 60 min and blocked with 10% goat serum in 0.01-M phosphate-buffered saline with 0.3% Triton X-100 for 2 h at room temperature. Sections were incubated with mouse anti-rat ED-1 (1:100; Abnoba, Taipei, Taiwan) overnight at 4°C, and then goat anti-mouse Alexa 488 fluorescent antibody (1:1,000 A11029; Life Technologies, Gaithersburg, MD) for 1 h.

Statistical Analysis

Statistical analyses were performed using two-way repeated-measures analysis of variance to consider the kinetics-based analyses of the control and etanercept groups. Differences between the three groups were calculated using one-way analysis of variance and the Tukey test for post hoc comparisons when significance was determined by analysis of variance. Values of $p<0.05$ were considered statistically significant.

Results

Electrophysiological Evaluation after Nerve Crush Injury

On day 7, MCVs were not evoked for either the control group or the etanercept group. The results of electrophysiological assessments on days 21 and 35 after crush injury are shown in Figure 1. On day 21, MCVs were significantly slower for the control and etanercept groups than for the sham group, and MCV for the control group was significantly slower than that of the etanercept group. On day 35, MCV of the control group also recovered and significant differences were no longer evident between control and etanercept groups.

Effect of Etanercept on Wet Muscle Weight Measurement after Nerve Crush Injury

The etanercept and control groups exhibited significantly lower percentage wet muscle weights than the sham group on days 21

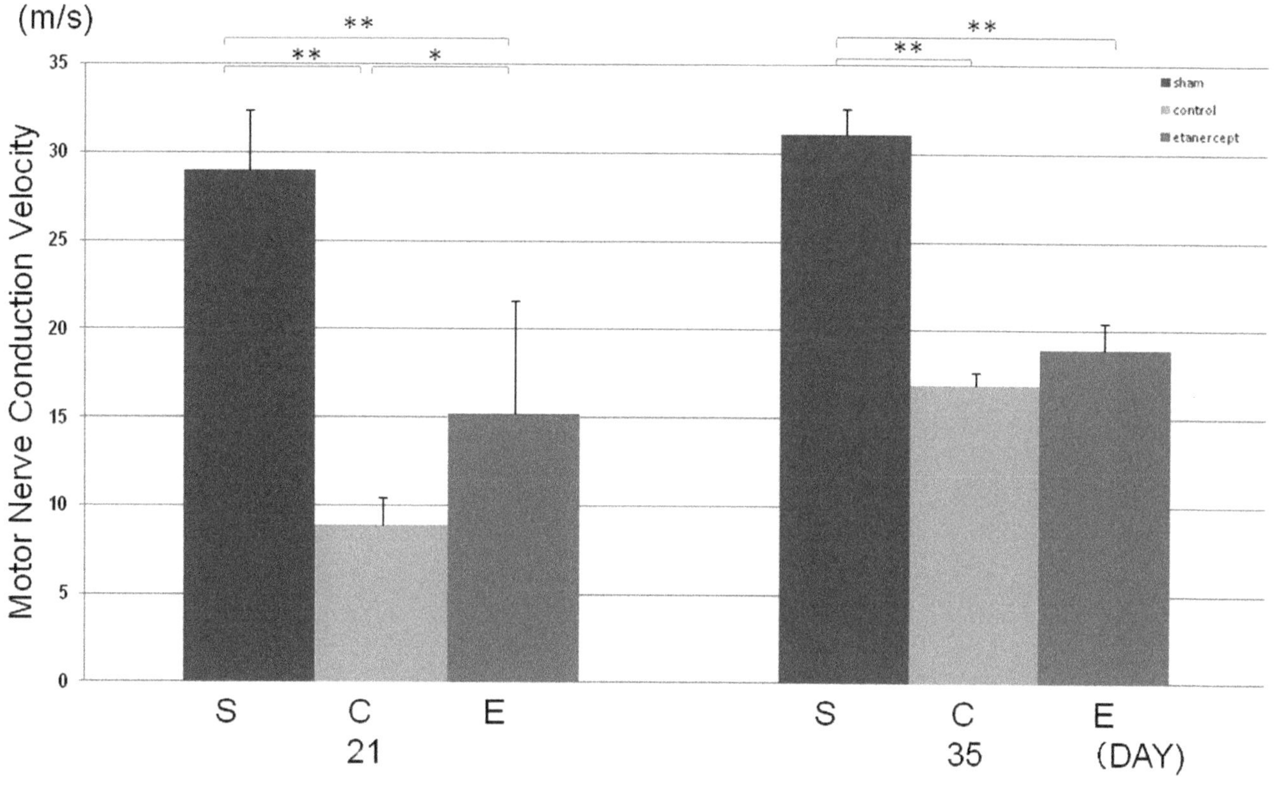

Figure 1. Electrophysiological evaluation after nerve crush injury. Motor nerve conduction velocity of the tibialis anterior muscle was significantly longer in the control group than in the etanercept and sham groups at 21 days post-crush injury (**$p<0.01$; *$p<0.05$).

and 35 (Fig. 2). Furthermore, the control group exhibited a significantly lower percentage wet muscle weight than the etanercept group on day 21. However, on day 35, no significant difference was observed between the etanercept and control groups.

Effects of Etanercept on SFI after Nerve Crush Injury

Although paresis of the right hind paw was observed in the control and the etanercept groups, SFI differed significantly between these 2 groups. Etanercept treatment significantly ameliorated sciatic nerve function on days 21 and 28 after crush injury (Fig. 3).

Effects of Etanercept on Behavioral Tests after Nerve Crush Injury

Mechanical and plantar thermal withdrawal thresholds were measured after nerve crush injury. The von Frey test clearly demonstrated mechanical hyperalgesia in both the control and etanercept groups, but mechanical hyperalgesia resolved faster in the etanercept group than in the control group (Fig. 4A). The plantar test likewise showed thermal hyperalgesia in both control and etanercept groups. Again, thermal hyperalgesia was attenuated by etanercept therapy at 21 days after crush injury, but persisted in the control group (Fig. 4B).

Effects of Etanercept on mRNA Expression after Nerve Crush Injury

The mRNA levels of TNF-α and IL-6 after crush injury were determined by real-time polymerase chain reaction. Expression of TNF-α mRNA in the control and etanercept groups was increased on day 2, but the difference between the 2 groups was not significant, and expression returned to baseline levels by day 7 (Fig. 5A). Expressions of IL-6 mRNA were significantly higher in the control and etanercept groups and remained elevated over 35 days, but etanercept treatment reduced expression of IL-6 mRNA compared to the control group on day 7 (Fig. 5B). Expression of MCP-1 mRNA was significantly higher in the control and etanercept groups on day 2, but etanercept treatment reduced expression of MCP-1 mRNA on days 7 (Fig. 5C). Expression of IL-1β mRNA was upregulated on day 7 after nerve crush, but no significant differences between the control and etanercept groups were identified (Fig. 5D). Expression of P2RX7 mRNA was upregulated after crush injury, and etanercept reduced the P2RX7 expression (Fig. 5E). Crush injury appeared to change the types of sodium channel expressed at the DRG, and etanercept reduced these changes (Fig. 5F–H).

Effects of Etanercept on TNF-α and IL-6 Expression after Nerve Crush Injury

Protein levels were determined in homogenized sciatic nerves by enzyme-linked immunosorbent assay after crush injury. In nerve crush injury groups, TNF-α levels were significantly increased on day 2, but no significant differences were evident between the control and etanercept groups, and both groups returned to baseline levels by day 7. After 7 days, significant differences were apparent between the three groups. However, IL-6 upregulation lasted more than 21 days (Fig. 6A) and returned to baseline by day 35. Etanercept inhibited upregulation of IL-6 on day 7 after crush injury (Fig. 6B).

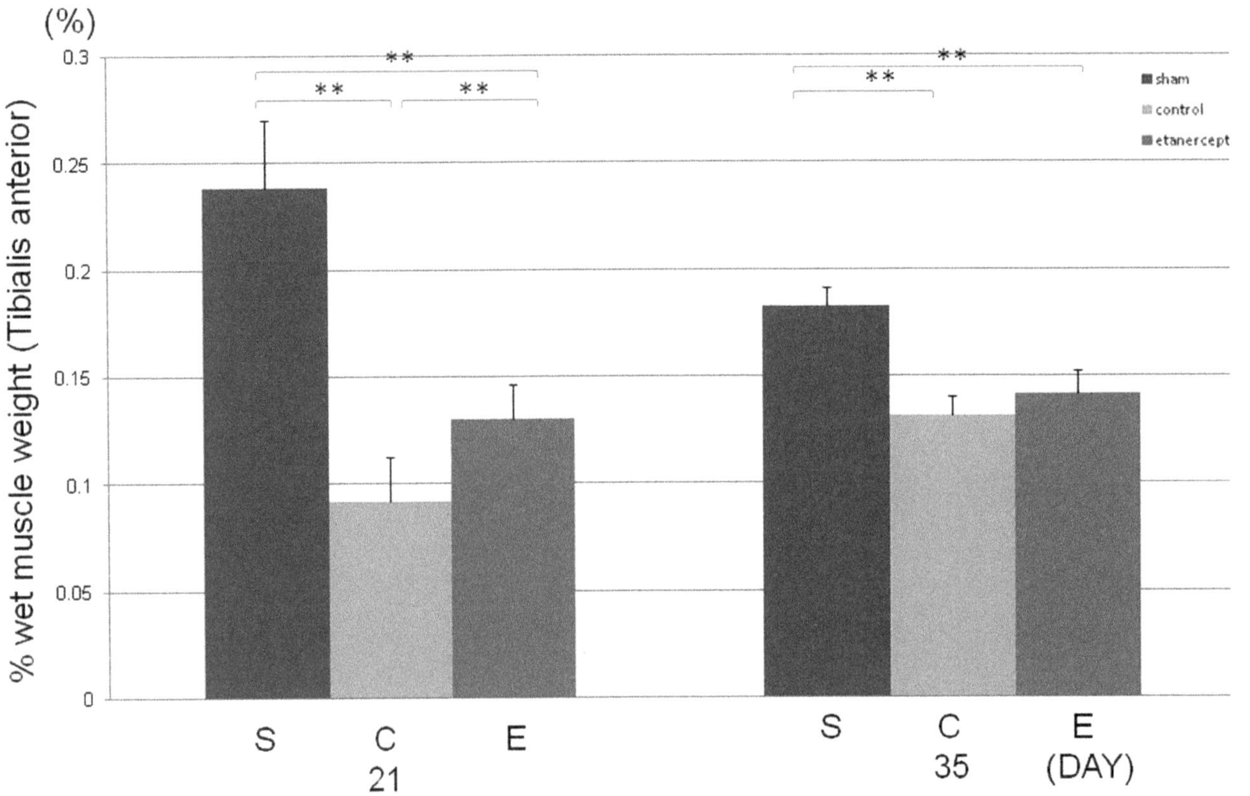

Figure 2. Effect of etanercept on wet muscle weight measurement. Control group showed a significantly lower percentage of wet muscle weight than the etanercept group on day 21 (**$p<0.01$).

Immunostaining for Macrophage Marker ED-1 after Nerve Crush Injury

On day 7 after crush injury, ED-1-positive cells were observed in both control and etanercept groups. This means that macrophages were recruited from the periphery and induced WD by carrying out the removal of myelin debris while Schwann cell proliferation was concomitantly enhanced. After 21 days, ED-1-positive cells had almost disappeared in the etanercept group, whereas the control group still showed abundant ED-1-positive cells within nerve fascicles (Fig. 7).

Discussion

After nerve injury, TNF-α is upregulated in activated cells of the central and peripheral nervous systems. These activated cells are considered to be glia (including Schwann cells), mast cells, endothelial cells, perineurial cells, and both resident and hematogenous macrophages [19].

TNF-α has been shown to act as the initiator of WD by activating resident Schwann cells and facilitating macrophage recruitment to the injury site [3]. TNF-α promotes functional motor recovery in crushed peripheral nerves [7]. Even though TNF-α is needed in peripheral nerve repair and regeneration, anti-TNF-α therapy is also being studied for application in nerve disorders [12]. Anti-TNF-α therapy prevents nerve degeneration and promotes nerve regeneration, and motor and sensory functional recovery [8,9]. These seemingly contradictory reports suggest the complexity and significance of TNF-α involvement in axonal degradation during WD.

Etanercept is a bioengineered dimeric fusion protein consisting of a soluble human 75-kDa TNF-α receptor and the Fc protein of immunoglobulin G1. This protein shows a greatly extended half-life in the bloodstream compared to naturally occurring soluble TNF receptors [54], and can neutralize both human and rat TNF-α [6,8,12]. As mentioned above, TNF-α inhibition can be a two-edged sword. Even pharmaceutical companies distributing anti-TNF-α drugs are proving hesitant to expand the indications to cover neurological problems, instead recommending careful use of these drugs, particularly for patients with demyelinating conditions. The present study therefore aimed to evaluate the net effect of etanercept on axonal regeneration after nerve crush injury.

Scholz and Woolfe [55] recently pointed out many features of neuroimmune disorders in neuropathic pain and suggested the possibility that blockade of reciprocal signaling pathways between neuronal and non-neuronal cells offers new opportunities for more successful pain management. According to Scholz and Woolfe, two different pathways are involved in the sensitization process of nociceptors: direct modulation of Nav expression by IL-1 and IL-6 produced by macrophages via activation of homodimeric P2RX7; and direct activation through a signaling pathway that involves TNF-α acting on TNF receptor 1 [55,56,57]. Isoforms of P2RX2, PR2X3, P2RX4, and P2RX7 are considered to participate in pain perception [58]. These receptor subtypes thus represent promising targets for pain management.

Nociceptive activity is further modulated by activation of the dimeric purinergic receptor comprising P2RX2 and P2RX3, which is mediated in part by voltage-gated sodium channels. P2RX7 dysfunction results in substantially blunted hypersensitivity to mechanical and thermal stimuli in models of neuropathic pain,

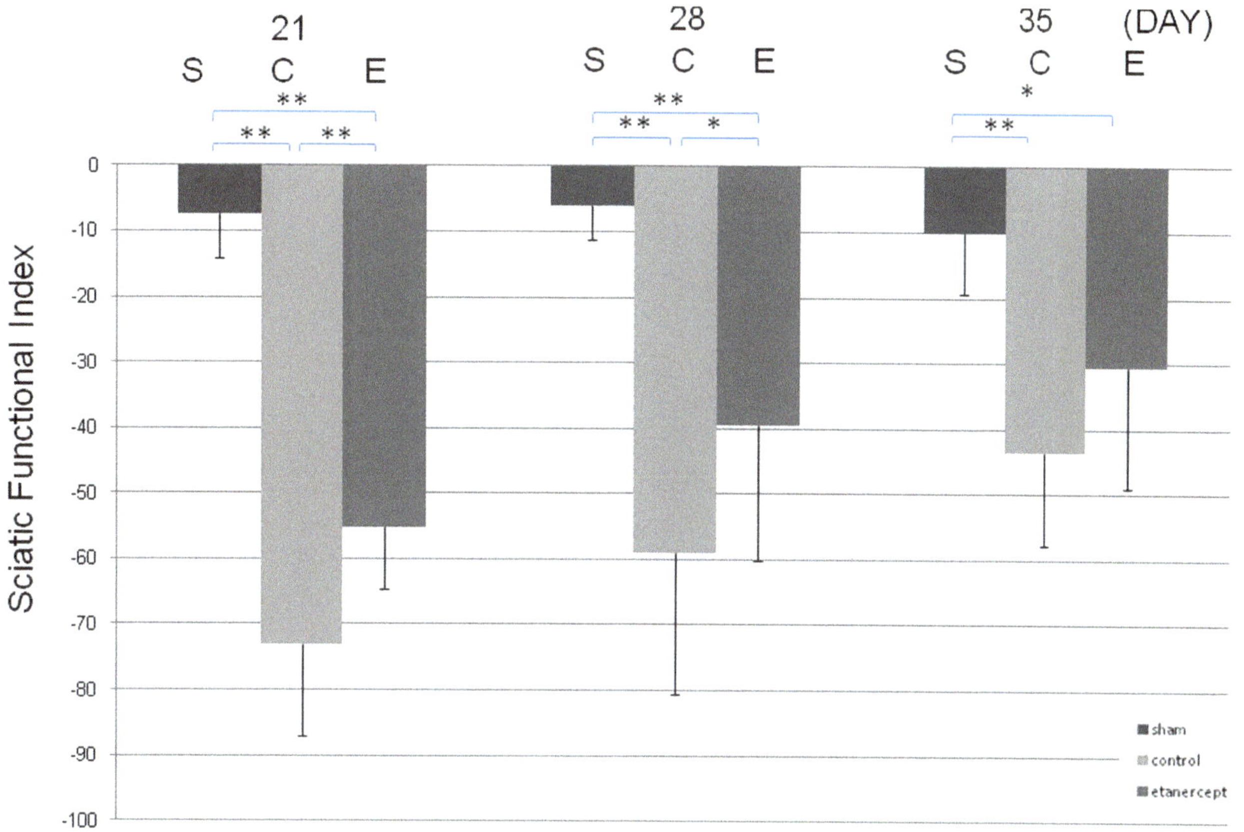

Figure 3. Effects of etanercept on sciatic functional index. Variations in sciatic functional index between groups after nerve crush injury. Sciatic functional index differed significantly between the 3 groups (**$p<0.01$; *$p<0.05$).

presumably because of reduced release of inflammatory cytokines from macrophages and microglia [59]. Crush injury changes the expression levels of cytokines, P2RX, and sodium channels, and after nerve injury the changes of these expressions are similar to those in neuroimmune disorders. The present study aimed to investigate expression changes of these chemical mediators and macrophage activity after anti-TNF-α treatment.

According to George, Sawada, and Kato [9,60,61], who separately studied spatiotemporal expression patterns of TNF-α during WD, TNF-α expression is enhanced promptly after nerve injury in the distal stump, peaking between day 1 and day 3 post-injury, and returning to baseline levels as early as day 7. This temporal expression pattern was reconfirmed in the present study, implying that TNF-α plays roles during the early phase of WD. According to previous studies, TNF-α plays multiple roles in triggering WD. Liefner et al. [62] demonstrated that TNF-α can induce macrophage recruitment from the periphery even without myelin damage or phagocytosis. TNF-α is linked to the development of abnormal blood-nerve barrier permeability [63], monocyte recruitment or residential macrophage activation, and coordination of these inflammatory events with demyelination. Infiltrating macrophages also contribute to the removal of myelin debris, and enhance concomitant Schwann cell proliferation, probably by releasing soluble mitogenic factors [64]. Taking these factors into consideration, we decided to use bolus intraperitoneal injection at the time of nerve crush.

The present study quantified TNF-α expression level in the nerve segment distal to the crush site. As demonstrated above, no significant differences in TNF-α expression were seen at the RNA and protein levels, while significant suppression of IL-6 expression was observed at both RNA and protein levels. This indicates that etanercept did not affect TNF-α production, but instead inhibited its biological function. In fact, immunohistochemical staining for the macrophage marker ED-1 clearly demonstrated that macrophage infiltration inside nerve fascicles took place on day 7 not only in the control group, but also in the etanercept group. This indicates that a single bolus intraperitoneal injection of etanercept does not blockade the onset and progression of WD. However, a marked difference in macrophage distribution between groups was seen on day 21. According to Sommer et al. [65], macrophages are involved in generation of neuropathic pain and the establishment of hyperalgesia following chronic constrictive nerve injury in which Wallerian-like degeneration and macrophage activation take place. Localized WD associated with macrophage influx and proinflammatory cytokine production thus appears to be a critical factor in the development of hyperalgesia in animal models of neuropathic pain. In fact, Sommer and Schafers [66] subsequently emphasized the possibility that macrophage invasion and TNF-α production influence the development of thermal hyperalgesia and that regenerative activity is linked to mechanical allodynia in peripheral mononeuropathy.

TNF-α lies upstream of matrix metalloproteinase-9 in the pathway of macrophage recruitment to injured peripheral nerves [67,68], and stimulates myelin degradation in the distal nerve fragment [69]. In addition, TNF-α also induces other chemotactic factors, such as MCP-1 [70]. MCP-1 plays essential roles in the recruitment of monocytes into lesions of spinal cord contusion and neuroinflammation [71,72,73]. In the present study, etanercept

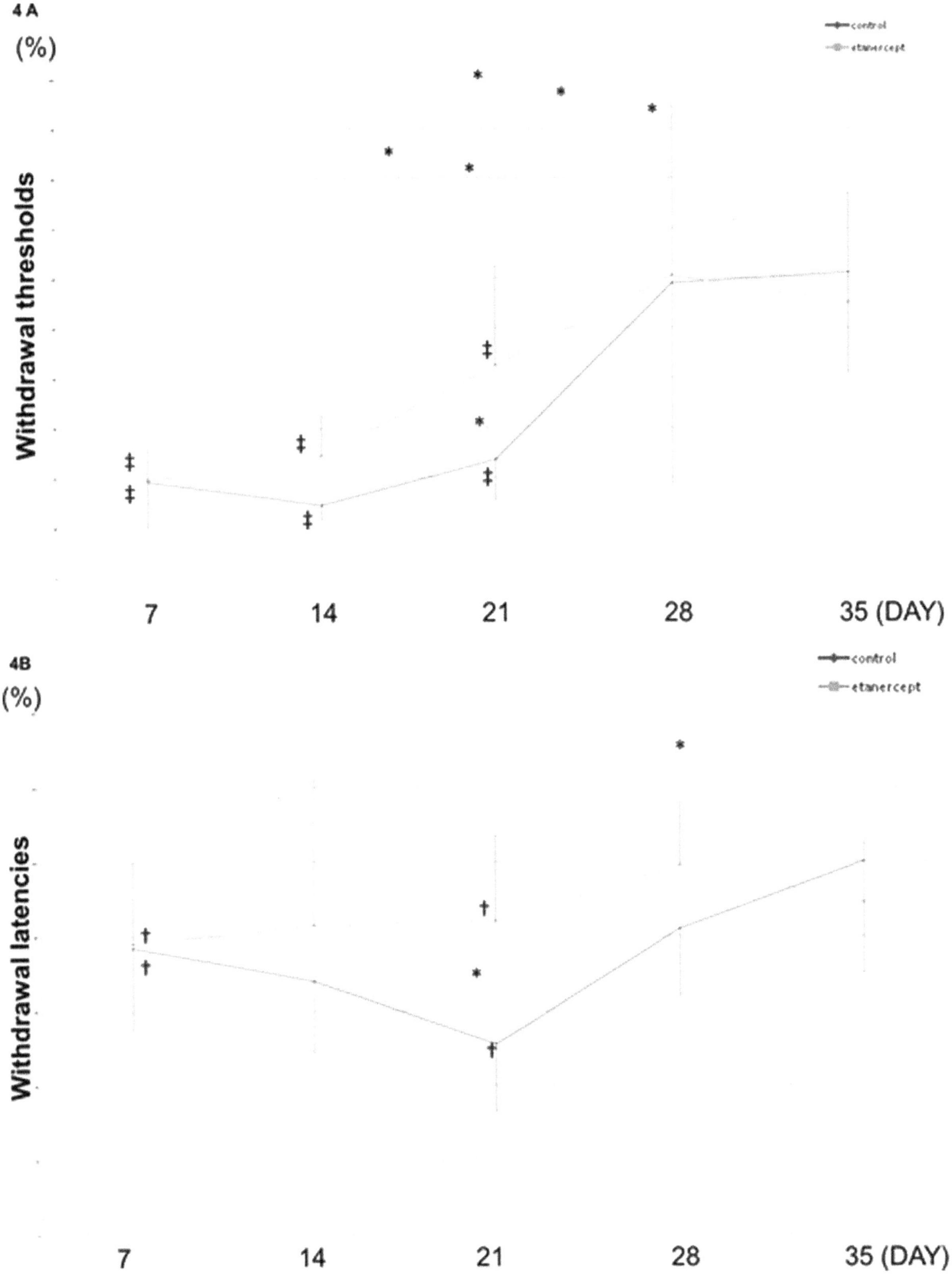

Figure 4. Effects of etanercept on behavioral tests. A) von Frey test **B)** Plantar test The von Frey mechanical withdrawal threshold and plantar thermal withdrawal threshold after crush operation. Control and etanercept groups exhibited mechanical hyperalgesia and thermal hyperalgesia on day 21, with effects attenuated by etanercept therapy (**$p<0.01$; *$p<0.05$; ‡$p<0.01$; †$p<0.05$, compared to sham group).

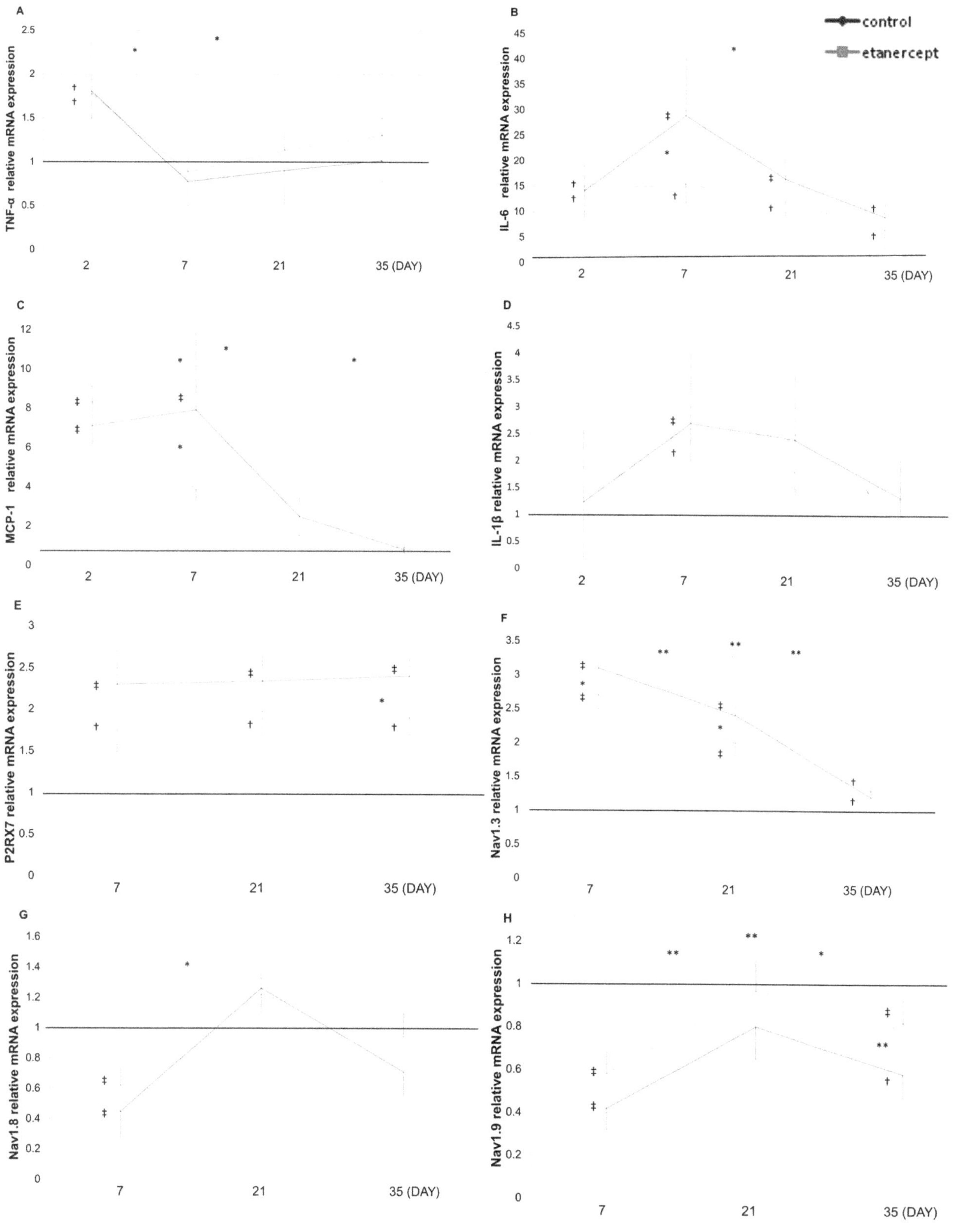

Figure 5. Effect of etanercept on mRNA expressions. The baseline was drawn at a value of 1 (average for the sham group) (**$p<0.01$; *$p<0.05$; ‡$p<0.01$; †$p<0.05$, compared to sham group). **A)** Expressions of TNF-α mRNA at the crushed nerve. **B)** Expression of IL-6 mRNA at the crushed nerve. **C)** Expression of MCP-1 mRNA at the crushed nerve. **D)** Expression of IL-1 mRNA at the crushed nerve. **E)** Expression of P2RX7 mRNA at the crushed nerve. **F)** Expression of Nav1.3 mRNA at the L5 DRG. **G)** Expression of Nav1.8 mRNA at the L5 DRG. **H)** Expression of Nav1.9 mRNA at the L5 DRG.

6A

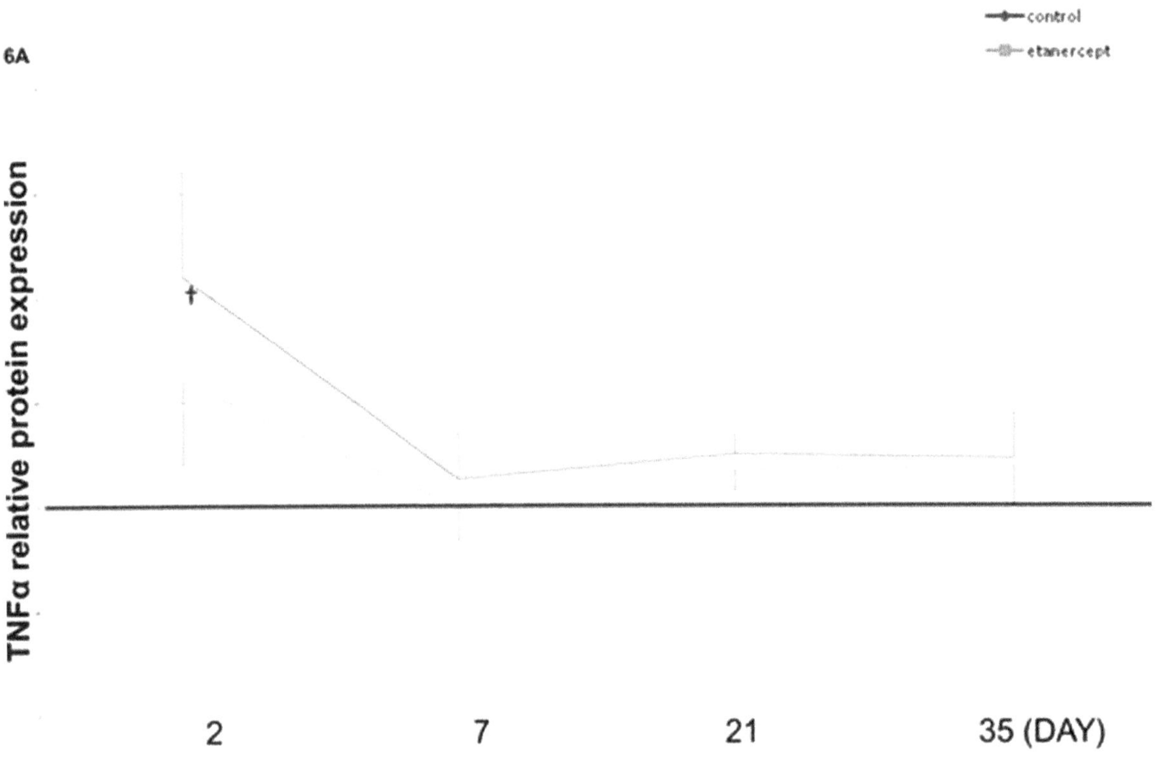

6B

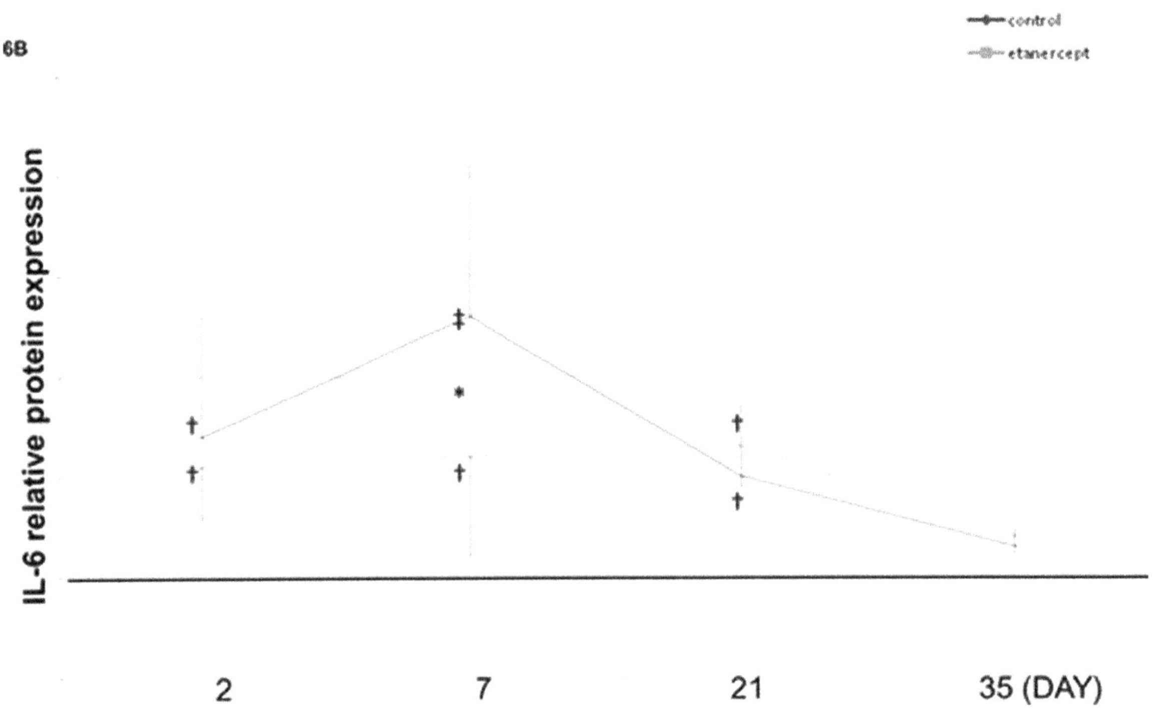

Figure 6. Effects of etanercept on TNF-α and IL-6 expression. Protein levels of TNF-α (**A**) and IL-6 (**B**) were determined in homogenized sciatic nerves. TNF-α levels were significantly increased 2 days after crush injury, but IL-6 upregulation lasted more than 21 days. Etanercept inhibited upregulation of IL-6 levels (***p*<0.01; **p*<0.05; ‡*p*<0.01; †*p*<0.05, compared to the sham group).

reduced MCP-1 expression on days 7 and 21, supporting the results of macrophage recruitment by immunostaining. Endogenous MCP-1, which displays chemotactic activity for monocytes, also plays an important role in the full expression of neuropathic pain. Treatment with anti-MCP-1 neutralizing antibody effectively attenuates neuropathic pain [74,75] following chronic constriction injury of the sciatic nerve [76] and L5 spinal nerve ligation [77].

We consider this a significant observation from a therapeutic perspective. This is because axonal regeneration never takes place without removal of myelin debris (which can strongly repel

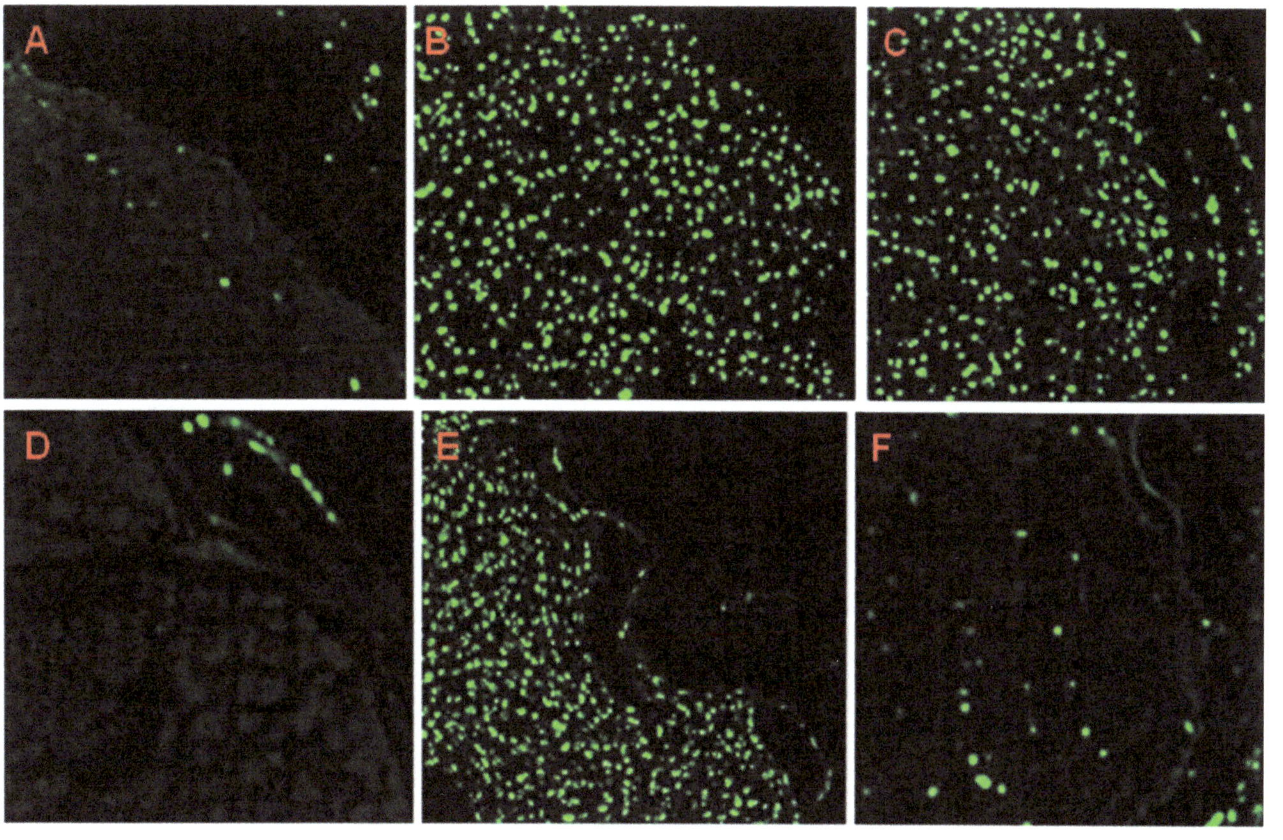

Figure 7. Immunohistochemical staining for macrophage marker ED-1 in crushed sciatic nerve sections. A) Sham-treated 7 days after surgery; **B)** control 7 days after surgery; **C)** etanercept-treated 7 days after surgery; **D)** sham-treated 21 days after surgery; **E)** control 21 days after surgery; and **F)** etanercept-treated 21 days after surgery. By 21 days, ED-1-positive cells had nearly disappeared from the etanercept group.

growing axons) or without formation of a so-called Schwann cell column within the basal lamina, and infiltrating macrophages are responsible for the whole process, as discussed above. Any drug that can completely suppress macrophage infiltration should thus be detrimental to nerve regeneration. We also believe that the prolonged presence of activated macrophages inside the nerve fascicle would also be detrimental to the growth and maturation of regenerating axons, as both electrophysiological and walking track analyses clearly demonstrated significantly quicker functional recovery in the etanercept group.

Macrophage recruitment is an important component of nerve growth factor (NGF) synthesis and of sensory neuron maintenance and axonal regrowth [78]. However, over the past decade, considerable evidence has accumulated indicating that NGF is also a strong mediator of peripheral pain, particularly in chronic pain status [79].

Sensitization to endogenous TNF-α may be essential for the development and maintenance of neuropathic pain [80]. The present study assessed the effects of etanercept on pain status. As demonstrated clearly with both von Frey and plantar thermal tests, both mechanical and thermal hypersensitivity occurred regardless of treatment on Day 7, when macrophage infiltration takes place. However, hypersensitivity improved more rapidly in the etanercept group than in the control group, consistent with the earlier disappearance of infiltrating macrophages.

Etanercept also reduced expression levels of P2RX7. P2RX7 may be an appealing target for pharmacological intervention [56], [81], since this protein may represent a critical communication link between the nervous and immune systems. P2RX7 was originally described in cells of hematopoietic origin, including macrophages, microglia, and certain lymphocytes [82]. P2RX7-knockout animals thus show reductions in IL-1, IL-6, and MCP-1 [59].

Although some reports have examined IL-6 expression after nerve injury [83,84], none have reported serial changes in IL-6 expression in crushed nerves over 5 weeks, and none have reported the role of IL-6 in WD. The present study demonstrated prolonged up-regulation of IL-6 expression even at 35 days after crush injury, but significantly reduced by etanercept. IL-6 belongs to a group of cytokines that control inflammatory responses, in part by regulating the synthesis and release of additional cytokines. IL-6 is a pleiotropic cytokine with robust pro-inflammatory activity. Increased IL-6 expression has been demonstrated during peripheral nerve injury-induced WD following hypoglossal nerve axotomy [83]. In addition, IL-6 was found to be secreted by macrophages and denervated Schwann cells, and is released into the distal nerve stump after nerve injury [85]. IL-6 administration is able to stimulate neurotrophin-dependent neurite outgrowth in cultured dorsal root ganglions [86]. These findings seem to identify IL-6 as an important factor in the onset and progression of axonal regeneration. In addition, IL-6 was recently reported to be involved in neuropathic pain [87]. According to Ohtori et al. [88], epidural administration of an anti-IL-6 receptor monoclonal antibody, tocilizumab, onto the spinal nerve reduced radicular leg pain, numbness, and low back pain without causing any appreciable adverse events. The precise function of IL-6 in WD and axonal regeneration remains to be elucidated [10], but considering the fact that the etanercept group in which IL-6 expression was downregulated showed swifter functional recovery and normalization of pain sensitivity, regulation of IL-6 expression during nerve regeneration may hold promise as a therapeutic strategy [40].

The possibility remains that the whole reaction was affected by more global pain modulating mechanisms [40]. The nervous system can synthesize and express TNF-α, and these cytokines may participate in neuronal communication [41], [42]. This communication is bi-directional, because cytokines can activate hypothalamic-pituitary release of glucocorticoids and, in turn, glucocorticoids suppress further cytokine synthesis [89]. In addition, cells of the immune system can produce neuropeptides, acetylcholine and other neurotransmitters. Acetylcholine interacts with cytokine-producing macrophages in the red pulp and marginal zone to suppress TNF-α release [90]. A prototypical anti-inflammatory neural mechanism is known as the inflammatory reflex [40,91,92]. Action potentials arising in the brainstem are transmitted in the cholinergic vagus nerve to terminate in the celiac ganglion, the site of origin of the adrenergic splenic nerve. Electrical stimulation of either the vagus nerve above the celiac ganglion or the splenic nerve itself significantly inhibits production and release of TNF-α into the circulation by macrophages in the red pulp and marginal zone of the spleen [93]. The spleen is a major organ for the anti-inflammatory effects of efferent vagus nerve signals [1,90].

The mechanism of the inflammatory reflex requires the α7 nicotinic acetylcholine receptor (α7nAChR), a ligand-gated ion channel expressed on macrophages, neurons and other cells [94,95]. Deleting α7nAChR from isolated macrophages impairs the ability of acetylcholine to suppress TNF-α and other cytokines [1]. The importance of the interaction between the nervous system and immune system signaling has been demonstrated in the development of pain. Cytokines produced by inflammatory and glial cells change neuronal excitability and this contributes directly to the development of intractable pain [96]. The inhibition of TNF-α may relate to the inflammatory reflex at the global reflex and regulation of cytokine networks.

While this study specifically focused on local cytokine networks, and the regulation of macrophage activities at the injury site, we are going to look at interactions between the nervous and inflammatory systems in the future.

Conclusion

This study clearly demonstrated that bolus intraperitoneal injection of etanercept, an anti-TNF-α antibody, is useful in terms of both enhancing functional recovery and suppressing hypersensitivity after nerve crush. It should be emphasized that etanercept does not impede the onset or progression of WD, but instead optimizes the involvement of macrophages and the secretion of inflammatory mediators. Treatment protocols in terms of dosage and frequency appear to be important in preventing possible side-effects from jeopardizing the normal process of WD and axonal degeneration.

Author Contributions

Conceived and designed the experiments: KI HH. Performed the experiments: KI TA S. Kato HO TN. Analyzed the data: KI S. Kurimoto. Contributed reagents/materials/analysis tools: KI S. Kurimoto MY. Wrote the paper: KI HH.

References

1. Olofsson PS, Katz DA, Rosas-Ballina M, Levine YA, Ochani M, et al. (2012) alpha7 nicotinic acetylcholine receptor (alpha7nAChR) expression in bone marrow-derived non-T cells is required for the inflammatory reflex. Mol Med 18: 539–543.
2. Choy EH, Panayi GS (2001) Cytokine pathways and joint inflammation in rheumatoid arthritis. N Engl J Med 344: 907–916.
3. Gaudet AD, Popovich PG, Ramer MS (2011) Wallerian degeneration: gaining perspective on inflammatory events after peripheral nerve injury. J Neuroinflammation 8: 110.
4. Stubgen JP (2008) Tumor necrosis factor-alpha antagonists and neuropathy. Muscle Nerve 37: 281–292.
5. Said G, Hontebeyrie-Joskowicz M (1992) Nerve lesions induced by macrophage activation. Res Immunol 143: 589–599.
6. Smith D, Tweed C, Fernyhough P, Glazner GW (2009) Nuclear factor-kappaB activation in axons and Schwann cells in experimental sciatic nerve injury and its role in modulating axon regeneration: studies with etanercept. J Neuropathol Exp Neurol 68: 691–700.
7. Chen LE, Seaber AV, Wong GH, Urbaniak JR (1996) Tumor necrosis factor promotes motor functional recovery in crushed peripheral nerve. Neurochem Int 29: 197–203.
8. Kato K, Kikuchi S, Shubayev VI, Myers RR (2009) Distribution and tumor necrosis factor-alpha isoform binding specificity of locally administered etanercept into injured and uninjured rat sciatic nerve. Neuroscience 160: 492–500.
9. Kato K, Liu H, Kikuchi S, Myers RR, Shubayev VI (2010) Immediate anti-tumor necrosis factor-alpha (etanercept) therapy enhances axonal regeneration after sciatic nerve crush. J Neurosci Res 88: 360–368.
10. Camara-Lemarroy CR, Guzman-de la Garza FJ, Fernandez-Garza NE (2010) Molecular inflammatory mediators in peripheral nerve degeneration and regeneration. Neuroimmunomodulation 17: 314–324.
11. Brambilla R, Ashbaugh JJ, Magliozzi R, Dellarole A, Karmally S, et al. (2011) Inhibition of soluble tumour necrosis factor is therapeutic in experimental autoimmune encephalomyelitis and promotes axon preservation and remyelination. Brain 134: 2736–2754.
12. Chio CC, Lin JW, Chang MW, Wang CC, Kuo JR, et al. (2010) Therapeutic evaluation of etanercept in a model of traumatic brain injury. J Neurochem 115: 921–929.
13. Genovese T, Mazzon E, Crisafulli C, Di Paola R, Muia C, et al. (2006) Immunomodulatory effects of etanercept in an experimental model of spinal cord injury. J Pharmacol Exp Ther 316: 1006–1016.
14. Alshekhlee A, Basiri K, Miles JD, Ahmad SA, Katirji B (2010) Chronic inflammatory demyelinating polyneuropathy associated with tumor necrosis factor-alpha antagonists. Muscle Nerve 41: 723–727.
15. Mohan N, Edwards ET, Cupps TR, Oliverio PJ, Sandberg G, et al. (2001) Demyelination occurring during anti-tumor necrosis factor alpha therapy for inflammatory arthritides. Arthritis Rheum 44: 2862–2869.
16. Roques BP, Fournie-Zaluski MC, Wurm M (2012) Inhibiting the breakdown of endogenous opioids and cannabinoids to alleviate pain. Nat Rev Drug Discov 11: 292–310.
17. Leung L, Cahill CM (2010) TNF-alpha and neuropathic pain–a review. J Neuroinflammation 7: 27.
18. Martini R, Fischer S, Lopez-Vales R, David S (2008) Interactions between Schwann cells and macrophages in injury and inherited demyelinating disease. Glia 56: 1566–1577.
19. Myers RR, Shubayev VI (2011) The ology of neuropathy: an integrative review of the role of neuroinflammation and TNF-alpha axonal transport in neuropathic pain. J Peripher Nerv Syst 16: 277–286.
20. Allodi I, Udina E, Navarro X (2012) Specificity of peripheral nerve regeneration: interactions at the axon level. Prog Neurobiol 98: 16–37.
21. Lingor P, Koch JC, Tonges L, Bahr M (2012) Axonal degeneration as a therapeutic target in the CNS. Cell Tissue Res 349: 289–311.
22. Lunn ER, Perry VH, Brown MC, Rosen H, Gordon S (1989) Absence of Wallerian Degeneration does not Hinder Regeneration in Peripheral Nerve. Eur J Neurosci 1: 27–33.
23. Laser H, Conforti L, Morreale G, Mack TG, Heyer M, et al. (2006) The slow Wallerian degeneration protein, WldS, binds directly to VCP/p97 and partially redistributes it within the nucleus. Mol Biol Cell 17: 1075–1084.
24. Wishart TM, Paterson JM, Short DM, Meredith S, Robertson KA, et al. (2007) Differential proteomics analysis of synaptic proteins identifies potential cellular targets and protein mediators of synaptic neuroprotection conferred by the slow Wallerian degeneration (Wlds) gene. Mol Cell Proteomics 6: 1318–1330.
25. Coleman MP, Freeman MR (2010) Wallerian degeneration, wld(s), and nmnat. Annu Rev Neurosci 33: 245–267.
26. Wang JT, Medress ZA, Barres BA (2012) Axon degeneration: molecular mechanisms of a self-destruction pathway. J Cell Biol 196: 7–18.
27. Wang J, Zhai Q, Chen Y, Lin E, Gu W, et al. (2005) A local mechanism mediates NAD-dependent protection of axon degeneration. J Cell Biol 170: 349–355.
28. Fainzilber M, Twiss JL (2006) Tracking in the Wlds–the hunting of the SIRT and the luring of the Draper. Neuron 50: 819–821.

29. Wishart TM, Brownstein DG, Thomson D, Tabakova AM, Boothe KM, et al. (2009) Expression of the neuroprotective slow Wallerian degeneration (WldS) gene in non-neuronal tissues. BMC Neurosci 10: 148.
30. Araki T, Sasaki Y, Milbrandt J (2004) Increased nuclear NAD biosynthesis and SIRT1 activation prevent axonal degeneration. Science 305: 1010–1013.
31. Conforti L, Fang G, Beirowski B, Wang MS, Sorci L, et al. (2007) NAD(+) and axon degeneration revisited: Nmnat1 cannot substitute for Wld(S) to delay Wallerian degeneration. Cell Death Differ 14: 116–127.
32. Watanabe M, Tsukiyama T, Hatakeyama S (2007) Protection of vincristine-induced neuropathy by WldS expression and the independence of the activity of Nmnat1. Neurosci Lett 411: 228–232.
33. Perry VH, Brown MC, Lunn ER, Tree P, Gordon S (1990) Evidence that Very Slow Wallerian Degeneration in C57BL/Ola Mice is an Intrinsic Property of the Peripheral Nerve. Eur J Neurosci 2: 802–808.
34. Adalbert R, Gillingwater TH, Haley JE, Bridge K, Beirowski B, et al. (2005) A rat model of slow Wallerian degeneration (WldS) with improved preservation of neuromuscular synapses. Eur J Neurosci 21: 271–277.
35. Gillingwater TH, Wishart TM, Chen PE, Haley JE, Robertson K, et al. (2006) The neuroprotective WldS gene regulates expression of PTTG1 and erythroid differentiation regulator 1-like gene in mice and human cells. Hum Mol Genet 15: 625–635.
36. Antenor-Dorsey JA, O'Malley KL (2012) WldS but not Nmnat1 protects dopaminergic neurites from MPP+ neurotoxicity. Mol Neurodegener 7: 5.
37. Meyer zu Horste G, Miesbach TA, Muller JI, Fledrich R, Stassart RM, et al. (2011) The Wlds transgene reduces axon loss in a Charcot-Marie-Tooth disease 1A rat model and nicotinamide delays post-traumatic axonal degeneration. Neurobiol Dis 42: 1–8.
38. Orr-Urtreger A, Kedmi M, Rosner S, Karmeli F, Rachmilewitz D (2005) Increased severity of experimental colitis in alpha 5 nicotinic acetylcholine receptor subunit-deficient mice. Neuroreport 16: 1123–1127.
39. Arima Y, Harada M, Kamimura D, Park JH, Kawano F, et al. (2012) Regional neural activation defines a gateway for autoreactive T cells to cross the blood-brain barrier. Cell 148: 447–457.
40. Tracey KJ (2002) The inflammatory reflex. Nature 420: 853–859.
41. Breder CD, Dinarello CA, Saper CB (1988) Interleukin-1 immunoreactive innervation of the human hypothalamus. Science 240: 321–324.
42. Breder CD, Hazuka C, Ghayur T, Klug C, Huginin M, et al. (1994) Regional induction of tumor necrosis factor alpha expression in the mouse brain after systemic lipopolysaccharide administration. Proc Natl Acad Sci U S A 91: 11393–11397.
43. Tracey KJ (2009) Reflex control of immunity. Nat Rev Immunol 9: 418–428.
44. Matsunaga K, Klein TW, Friedman H, Yamamoto Y (2001) Involvement of nicotinic acetylcholine receptors in suppression of antimicrobial activity and cytokine responses of alveolar macrophages to Legionella pneumophila infection by nicotine. J Immunol 167: 6518–6524.
45. Zimmermann M (1983) Ethical guidelines for investigations of experimental pain in conscious animals. Pain 16: 109–110.
46. Kato N, Nemoto K, Arino H, Fujikawa K (2002) Treatment of the chronic inflammation in peripheral target tissue improves the crushed nerve recovery in the rat: histopathological assessment of the nerve recovery. J Neurol Sci 202: 69–74.
47. Okui N, Yamamoto M, Fukuhira Y, Kaneko H, Hirata H (2010) Artificial perineurium to enhance nerve recovery from damage after neurolysis. Muscle Nerve 42: 570–575.
48. Yamamoto M, Endo N, Ito M, Okui N, Koh S, et al. (2010) Novel polysaccharide-derived hydrogel prevents perineural adhesions in a rat model of sciatic nerve adhesion. J Orthop Res 28: 284–288.
49. Hargreaves K, Dubner R, Brown F, Flores C, Joris J (1988) A new and sensitive method for measuring thermal nociception in cutaneous hyperalgesia. Pain 32: 77–88.
50. Terada T, Hara K, Haranishi Y, Sata T (2011) Antinociceptive effect of intrathecal administration of taurine in rat models of neuropathic pain. Can J Anaesth 58: 630–637.
51. de Medinaceli L, Freed WJ, Wyatt RJ (1982) An index of the functional condition of rat sciatic nerve based on measurements made from walking tracks. Exp Neurol 77: 634–643.
52. Vrinten DH, Hamers FF (2003) 'CatWalk' automated quantitative gait analysis as a novel method to assess mechanical allodynia in the rat; a comparison with von Frey testing. Pain 102: 203–209.
53. Yamamoto M, Okui N, Tatebe M, Shinohara T, Hirata H (2011) Regeneration of the perineurium after microsurgical resection examined with immunolabeling for tenascin-C and alpha smooth muscle actin. J Anat 218: 413–425.
54. Madhusudan S, Muthuramalingam SR, Braybrooke JP, Wilner S, Kaur K, et al. (2005) Study of etanercept, a tumor necrosis factor-alpha inhibitor, in recurrent ovarian cancer. J Clin Oncol 23: 5950–5959.
55. Scholz J, Woolf CJ (2007) The neuropathic pain triad: neurons, immune cells and glia. Nat Neurosci 10: 1361–1368.
56. McGaraughty S, Chu KL, Namovic MT, Donnelly-Roberts DL, Harris RR, et al. (2007) P2X7-related modulation of pathological nociception in rats. Neuroscience 146: 1817–1828.
57. Chessell IP, Hatcher JP, Bountra C, Michel AD, Hughes JP, et al. (2005) Disruption of the P2X7 purinoceptor gene abolishes chronic inflammatory and neuropathic pain. Pain 114: 386–396.
58. Andreev YA, Vassilevski AA, Kozlov SA (2012) Molecules to selectively target receptors for treatment of pain and neurogenic inflammation. Recent Pat Inflamm Allergy Drug Discov 6: 35–45.
59. Skaper SD, Debetto P, Giusti P (2010) The P2X7 purinergic receptor: from physiology to neurological disorders. FASEB J 24: 337–345.
60. George A, Buehl A, Sommer C (2004) Wallerian degeneration after crush injury of rat sciatic nerve increases endo- and epineurial tumor necrosis factor-alpha protein. Neurosci Lett 372: 215–219.
61. Sawada T, Sano M, Omura T, Omura K, Hasegawa T, et al. (2007) Spatiotemporal quantification of tumor necrosis factor-alpha and interleukin-10 after crush injury in rat sciatic nerve utilizing immunohistochemistry. Neurosci Lett 417: 55–60.
62. Liefner M, Siebert H, Sachse T, Michel U, Kollias G, et al. (2000) The role of TNF-alpha during Wallerian degeneration. J Neuroimmunol 108: 147–152.
63. Spies JM, Westland KW, Bonner JG, Pollard JD (1995) Intraneural activated T cells cause focal breakdown of the blood-nerve barrier. Brain 118 (Pt 4): 857–868.
64. Baichwal RR, Bigbee JW, DeVries GH (1988) Macrophage-mediated myelin-related mitogenic factor for cultured Schwann cells. Proc Natl Acad Sci U S A 85: 1701–1705.
65. Sommer C, Lalonde A, Heckman HM, Rodriguez M, Myers RR (1995) Quantitative neuropathology of a focal nerve injury causing hyperalgesia. J Neuropathol Exp Neurol 54: 635–643.
66. Sommer C, Schafers M (1998) Painful mononeuropathy in C57BL/Wld mice with delayed wallerian degeneration: differential effects of cytokine production and nerve regeneration on thermal and mechanical hypersensitivity. Brain Res 784: 154–162.
67. Shubayev VI, Angert M, Dolkas J, Campana WM, Palenscar K, et al. (2006) TNFalpha-induced MMP-9 promotes macrophage recruitment into injured peripheral nerve. Mol Cell Neurosci 31: 407–415.
68. Bosse F (2012) Extrinsic cellular and molecular mediators of peripheral axonal regeneration. Cell Tissue Res 349: 5–14.
69. Chattopadhyay S, Myers RR, Janes J, Shubayev V (2007) Cytokine regulation of MMP-9 in peripheral glia: implications for pathological processes and pain in injured nerve. Brain Behav Immun 21: 561–568.
70. Subang MC, Richardson PM (2001) Influence of injury and cytokines on synthesis of monocyte chemoattractant protein-1 mRNA in peripheral nervous tissue. Eur J Neurosci 13: 521–528.
71. Mahad D, Callahan MK, Williams KA, Ubogu EE, Kivisakk P, et al. (2006) Modulating CCR2 and CCL2 at the blood-brain barrier: relevance for multiple sclerosis pathogenesis. Brain 129: 212–223.
72. Conductier G, Blondeau N, Guyon A, Nahon JL, Rovere C (2010) The role of monocyte chemoattractant protein MCP1/CCL2 in neuroinflammatory diseases. J Neuroimmunol 224: 93–100.
73. Ma M, Wei T, Boring L, Charo IF, Ransohoff RM, et al. (2002) Monocyte recruitment and myelin removal are delayed following spinal cord injury in mice with CCR2 chemokine receptor deletion. J Neurosci Res 68: 691–702.
74. Jeon SM, Lee KM, Cho HJ (2009) Expression of monocyte chemoattractant protein-1 in rat dorsal root ganglia and spinal cord in experimental models of neuropathic pain. Brain Res 1251: 103–111.
75. Jeon SM, Sung JK, Cho HJ (2011) Expression of monocyte chemoattractant protein-1 and its induction by tumor necrosis factor receptor 1 in sensory neurons in the ventral rhizotomy model of neuropathic pain. Neuroscience 190: 354–366.
76. Thacker MA, Clark AK, Bishop T, Grist J, Yip PK, et al. (2009) CCL2 is a key mediator of microglia activation in neuropathic pain states. Eur J Pain 13: 263–272.
77. Gao YJ, Zhang L, Samad OA, Suter MR, Yasuhiko K, et al. (2009) JNK-induced MCP-1 production in spinal cord astrocytes contributes to central sensitization and neuropathic pain. J Neurosci 29: 4096–4108.
78. Brown MC, Perry VH, Lunn ER, Gordon S, Heumann R (1991) Macrophage dependence of peripheral sensory nerve regeneration: possible involvement of nerve growth factor. Neuron 6: 359–370.
79. Pezet S, McMahon SB (2006) Neurotrophins: mediators and modulators of pain. Annu Rev Neurosci 29: 507–538.
80. Schafers M, Lee DH, Brors D, Yaksh TL, Sorkin LS (2003) Increased sensitivity of injured and adjacent uninjured rat primary sensory neurons to exogenous tumor necrosis factor-alpha after spinal nerve ligation. J Neurosci 23: 3028–3038.
81. Romagnoli R, Baraldi PG, Cruz-Lopez O, Lopez-Cara C, Preti D, et al. (2008) The P2X7 receptor as a therapeutic target. Expert Opin Ther Targets 12: 647–661.
82. Skaper SD, Debetto P, Giusti P (2009) P2X(7) Receptors in Neurological and Cardiovascular Disorders. Cardiovasc Psychiatry Neurol 2009: 861324.
83. Hirota H, Kiyama H, Kishimoto T, Taga T (1996) Accelerated Nerve Regeneration in Mice by upregulated expression of interleukin (IL) 6 and IL-6 receptor after trauma. J Exp Med 183: 2627–2634.
84. Murphy PG, Borthwick LS, Johnston RS, Kuchel G, Richardson PM (1999) Nature of the retrograde signal from injured nerves that induces interleukin-6 mRNA in neurons. J Neurosci 19: 3791–3800.
85. Fenrich K, Gordon T (2004) Canadian Association of Neuroscience review: axonal regeneration in the peripheral and central nervous systems–current issues and advances. Can J Neurol Sci 31: 142–156.

86. Golz G, Uhlmann L, Ludecke D, Markgraf N, Nitsch R, et al. (2006) The cytokine/neurotrophin axis in peripheral axon outgrowth. Eur J Neurosci 24: 2721–2730.
87. Noponen-Hietala N, Virtanen I, Karttunen R, Schwenke S, Jakkula E, et al. (2005) Genetic variations in IL6 associate with intervertebral disc disease characterized by sciatica. Pain 114: 186–194.
88. Ohtori S, Miyagi M, Eguchi Y, Inoue G, Orita S, et al. (2012) Efficacy of epidural administration of anti-interleukin-6 receptor antibody onto spinal nerve for treatment of sciatica. Eur Spine J.
89. Besedovsky H, del Rey A, Sorkin E, Dinarello CA (1986) Immunoregulatory feedback between interleukin-1 and glucocorticoid hormones. Science 233: 652–654.
90. Andersson U, Tracey KJ (2012) Reflex principles of immunological homeostasis. Annu Rev Immunol 30: 313–335.
91. Rosas-Ballina M, Tracey KJ (2009) The neurology of the immune system: neural reflexes regulate immunity. Neuron 64: 28–32.
92. Borovikova LV, Ivanova S, Zhang M, Yang H, Botchkina GI, et al. (2000) Vagus nerve stimulation attenuates the systemic inflammatory response to endotoxin. Nature 405: 458–462.
93. Rosas-Ballina M, Olofsson PS, Ochani M, Valdes-Ferrer SI, Levine YA, et al. (2011) Acetylcholine-synthesizing T cells relay neural signals in a vagus nerve circuit. Science 334: 98–101.
94. Pavlov VA, Wang H, Czura CJ, Friedman SG, Tracey KJ (2003) The cholinergic anti-inflammatory pathway: a missing link in neuroimmunomodulation. Mol Med 9: 125–134.
95. Bencherif M, Lippiello PM, Lucas R, Marrero MB (2011) Alpha7 nicotinic receptors as novel therapeutic targets for inflammation-based diseases. Cell Mol Life Sci 68: 931–949.
96. Watkins LR, Maier SF (2002) Beyond neurons: evidence that immune and glial cells contribute to pathological pain states. Physiol Rev 82: 981–1011.

11

Preference for Different Anchor Descriptors on Visual Analogue Scales among Japanese Patients with Chronic Pain

Junya Yokobe[1]*, Masaki Kitahara[1], Masato Matsushima[2], Shoichi Uezono[1]

1 Department of Anesthesiology, The Jikei University School of Medicine, Minato, Tokyo, Japan, **2** Division of Clinical Epidemiology, The Jikei University School of Medicine, Minato, Tokyo, Japan

Abstract

Context: Although many previous studies have examined the preference of patients for different pain measurement scales, preference for anchor descriptors has not been thoroughly discussed.

Objectives: To examine (1) the preferred end-phrases used in the VAS as anchor labels for Japanese patients with chronic pain, and (2) whether the preference differs according to factors such as age, sex, educational level, duration of pain, and pain intensity.

Methods: We performed an observational study in patients suffering from non-cancer chronic pain for more than 3 months at a pain center in Japan. The patients were asked to rate their pain intensity using four types of VAS that used the following different anchor descriptors: "worst pain" ("Worst"), "worst pain bearable" ("Bearable"), "worst pain imaginable" ("Imaginable"), and "worst pain you have ever experienced" ("Experienced"). They were also asked to rank the four scales according to ease of responding, and asked which descriptor best reflected their perceived pain.

Results: In total, 183 patients participated in the study. They consisted of 119 (65.0%) women and 64 (35.0%) men aged 18–84 years with the mean age of 56.9 years. "Experienced" was most preferred (69.8%), followed by "Bearable" (66.3%), "Worst" (48.8%), and "Imaginable" (16.9%). Factors such as age, sex, educational background, duration of pain, and pain intensity did not significantly affect the results. In 83.1% of patients, the preferred descriptor corresponded to the descriptor that best reflected patients' perceived pain.

Conclusion: The frequently used expression "worst pain imaginable" is considered to be difficult to understand for most patients. Widely preferred descriptors, such as "worst pain you have ever experienced" and "worst pain bearable", should be used when evaluating perceived pain. The preference of anchor descriptors was not significantly affected by the factors such as age, sex, educational level, duration of pain, and pain intensity.

Editor: Masahiko Sumitani, The University of Tokyo Hospital, Japan

Funding: The authors have no support or funding to report.

Competing Interests: The authors have declared that no competing interests exist.

* E-mail: yokobejunya@gmail.com

Introduction

The International Association for the Study of Pain (IASP) states that "Pain is always subjective. Each individual learns the application of the word through experiences related to injury in early life" [1]. Pain is thus an individual experience with multi-dimensional aspects [2–4], and, theoretically speaking, pain intensity is impossible to measure objectively and quantitatively [5]. However, accurate quantitative evaluation of perceived pain intensity is a prerequisite for both clinical practice and research purposes [5–8].

Over the past few decades, several self-reporting unidimensional pain scales have been developed, such as the Visual Analogue Scale (VAS), Numerical Rating Scale (NRS), Verbal Rating Scale (VRS), and the Faces Pain Scale. Of these scales, the VAS and NRS have been used most frequently worldwide because of their outstanding simplicity, and their reliability and validity have been proved [6–10]. These scales are designed to measure pain intensity using extremely painful conditions or situations as a point of reference. However, many descriptors have been used as anchor labels with the VAS and NRS in Japanese as well as other languages, and these descriptors have not yet been standardized [11]. Pain intensity cannot be precisely compared without using standardized anchor descriptors, even if the same pain measurement scale is used.

Several studies have investigated the preferred pain assessment tool among the VAS, NRS, VRS, and so on [8,12–16]. However, very few researchers have paid attention to the descriptors used as anchor labels. Many studies have recommended the use of the NRS [6,12,17–25] and VAS [14,26–28] to evaluate pain intensity; nevertheless, patients are sometimes unable to use these scales to correctly rate their perceived pain intensity in clinical and research settings. Some studies have shown that categorical scales such as the VRS are preferred over the VAS or NRS by elderly patients [2,8,14,29], less educated patients [13], cognitively impaired patients [30], and children [31]. These results might be due not only to difficulties with abstract thinking [2,30–32] but also to the ambiguity of anchor descriptors used in the VAS or NRS. Because appropriate quantitative evaluation of patients' pain intensity requires the patients to be able to obtain a clear image of the situations described in the anchor label, investigation of preferred anchor descriptors is expected to contribute to the improvement of pain intensity evaluations.

The two major purposes of this study are to examine (1) the preferred end-phrases used in the VAS as anchor labels for Japanese patients with chronic pain, and (2) whether the preference differs according to factors such as age, sex, educational level, duration of pain, and pain intensity.

Methods

Participants

The subjects for this study were recruited from chronic pain patients who attended the multi-disciplinary outpatient pain clinic of the Jikei University Hospital between June 2012 and May 2013. Most of the patients who attend the clinic were suffering from multiple types of chronic pain. The clinic consists of doctors, nurses, physiotherapists, clinical psychologists, and acupuncturists. The patients were basically treated with medication, therapeutic exercise, psychophysiological approach, and acupuncture. Inclusion criteria were a diagnosis of chronic non-cancer pain with a duration of more than 3 months and age 18 years or older. Patients who had visual disturbance, were unable to speak Japanese, or were suspected to have impaired cognition (Mini-Mental State Examination (MMSE) score $<$ 23 points) were excluded.

Anchor descriptors

The following four commonly used descriptors of the anchor labels used in the VAS in Japan were selected.

"worst pain" (hereafter "Worst")
"worst pain bearable" (hereafter "Bearable")
"worst pain imaginable" (hereafter "Imaginable")
"worst pain you have ever experienced" (hereafter "Experienced")

An American psychologist who was proficient in Japanese validated the translations of anchor descriptors used in Japanese to make sure that they were consistent with the expressions used in English [11].

Questionnaire

A traditional VAS with a straight, horizontal 10-cm line was used, with the anchor label "no pain" at the left side and one of the translated Japanese descriptors at the right side. The four different VASs were placed on a sheet of paper in fixed order. The participants were asked to mark a vertical line on each VAS corresponding to their perceived average pain during the previous 24 hours. The participants were also asked to rank the scales in order of preference, from first to fourth place, on the basis of ease of responding, and they were also asked which descriptor best expressed their own pain.

Ethics Statement

The protocol of this study was approved by the ethics committees of the Jikei University Hospital, and the study was carried out in accordance with the Declaration of Helsinki. Written informed consent was obtained before study entry from all patients who participated in the study.

Data collection

The questionnaire written in Japanese was distributed to the participants when they gave consent after attending the pain clinic, and was collected on the same day. Age, sex, educational background, duration of pain, VAS, VRS, Hospital Anxiety and Depression Scale (HADS) [33–34], and Pain Catastrophizing Scale (PCS) score [35] data, which were administered on the same day, were obtained from medical records. Because the participants of this study are from the multi-disciplinary pain clinic, it is expected that their psychological factors have severely influenced on their pain condition. Therefore, we used HADS and PCS to verify that we could regard the participants to be the representatives of chronic pain patients in Japan. HADS includes two subscales which are anxiety and depression. The total score of each subscale is 21. The cut-off point of the each subscale of HADS is usually set as 8 and 11. The point between 8 and 10 indicates that the patient probably has anxiety or depression; the point of 11 and over definitely has anxiety or depression. The cut-off point of PCS is usually set as 30. The point of 30 and over indicates that the patient is in pain catastrophizing state.

Statistical analysis

All data were analyzed statistically using the SPSS program (version 21.0, SPSS Inc., Chicago, IL, USA). Data treated as a continuous scale are presented as median and range, and categorical and ordinal data are presented as counts and percentages. Wilcoxon signed-rank test and chi-square test was used to compare the values and proportions between elderly and young group (Table 1). Chi-square test was applied to compare the proportions of preference between two groups (Table 2).

Friedman test was used for analyzing the differences in preference among the different descriptors (Figure 1). Bonferroni correction was employed for *post-hoc* comparison of each pair. Wilcoxon signed-rank test was used for analyzing the relationship between the most-preferred descriptor and best-expressing descriptor (Figure 2). Spearman's rank correlation coefficient was calculated to examine whether the reported VAS pain levels using the different anchor descriptors correlate with each other (Table 3). Wilcoxon signed-rank test of the VAS values between the most-preferred descriptor and the least-preferred descriptor, was also performed to examine if the reported pain level significantly differed depending on the anchor descriptor. P-values less than 0.05 were considered statistically significant.

Results

One hundred and eighty-three patients gave consent to participate in the study. Table 1 shows the demographic characteristics of study participants. Almost all of the participants were able to answer the VASs with four different descriptors; only four participants failed to mark at least one of the four VASs. The HADS score suggested that 27.9% of the respondents were in a depressive state, and 26.8% had anxiety. The PCS score indicated that 60.1% of the respondents were catastrophized.

Table 4 shows the characteristics of the participants' pain (some patients have multiple nature of pain). The majority of the participants are suffering from some of musculoskeletal pain.

Table 1. General characteristics of study participants (n = 183).

	Total (n = 183)	Elderly (n = 87)	Young (n = 96)	p-value
Age, years	59 (18–84)	69 (61–84)	46 (18–60)	< 0.0001**
10–19	1 (0.6)			
20–29	9 (4.9)			
30–39	17 (9.3)			
40–49	33 (18.0)			
50–59	32 (17.5)			
60–69	49 (26.8)			
70–79	34 (18.6)			
80-	8 (4.4)			
Sex				0.42
Female	119 (65.0)	54 (62.1)	65 (67.7)	
Male	64 (35.0)	33 (37.9)	31 (32.3)	
Educational level				0.03*
Junior high school	12 (6.8)	7 (8.5)	5 (5.3)	
High school	79 (44.6)	44 (53.7)	35 (36.8)	
College/University	86 (48.6)	31 (37.8)	55 (57.9)	
Duration of pain, months	36 (3–480)	40 (3–240)	33 (3–480)	0.82
HADS (Anxiety)	7 (0–16)	7 (0–15)	7 (0–16)	0.31
HADS (Depression)	7 (0–20)	7 (0–17)	8 (0–20)	0.35
PCS	32.5 (7–51)	32 (9–51)	33 (7–50)	0.58
VRS				0.27
None	3 (1.7)	2 (2.3)	1 (1.1)	
Mild	62 (34.3)	25 (29.1)	37 (38.9)	
Moderate	96 (53.0)	45 (52.3)	51 (53.7)	
Severe	20 (11.0)	14 (16.3)	6 (6.3)	
VAS ("Worst")	59 (0–100)	65 (0–100)	55 (2–100)	0.27
VAS ("Bearable")	61 (0–100)	59 (0–100)	61.5 (2–100)	0.70
VAS ("Imaginable")	58 (0–100)	68 (0–100)	51 (0–100)	0.03**
VAS ("Experienced")	66 (0–100)	73 (0–100)	55.5 (0–100)	< 0.01**

Values are expressed as the median (range) or as number (percentage).
HADS = Hospital Anxiety and Depression Scale; PCS = Pain Catastrophizing Scale;
VRS = Verbal Rating Scale; VAS = Visual Analogue Scale
*chi-square test statistically significant ($p<0.05$).
**Wilcoxon rank sum test statistically significant ($p<0.05$).

Figure 1 shows the rankings given to the four different descriptors used with the VASs in this study. "Experienced" was most preferred by the largest number of participants (38.5%), followed by "Worst" (33.9%), "Bearable" (24.1%), and "Imaginable" (3.4%). The descriptor ranked as least preferred by most participants was "Imaginable" (38.2%), followed by "Worst" (31.2%), "Experienced" (17.6%), and "Bearable" (12.9%). Friedman test demonstrated the differences among the four different descriptors to be statistically significant ($p<0.001$); Bonferroni *post-hoc* tests demonstrated significant differences between "Imaginable" and "Worst", "Bearable", and "Experienced" ($p<0.05$).

Figure 2 compares percentages between the most-preferred and the best-expressing descriptor. Overall, 83.1% of the descriptors were consistent with each other.

Table 2 shows the percentage of participants that ranked each of the descriptors first or second in terms of preference. "Experienced" and "Bearable" were regarded as preferable by 69.8% and 66.3% of the participants, respectively. Almost half of the participants regarded "Worst" as preferable; "Imaginable" was regarded as preferable by only 16.9% of the participants. As Table 2 shows, approximately the same percentage of preference was observed even when the participants were stratified by age, sex, educational level, duration of pain, and pain intensity, with p-values, analyzed by chi-square test, of 0.41, 0.34, 0.74, 0.87, and 0.87, respectively. Table 3 shows pairwise Spearman's rank correlation coefficient between the pain intensity measured by VASs using the four anchor descriptors. The Spearman's rank correlation coefficient indicated that there were strong correlations between each pair of the anchor descriptors. There was a significant difference between the VAS values with the most-preferred descriptor and the least-preferred descriptor, analyzed by Wilcoxon signed-rank test, with the p-value of 0.038.

Table 2. Percentage of participants who considered each descriptor as preferable (sum of 1st and 2nd place).

	A ("Worst")	B ("Bearable")	C ("Imaginable")	D ("Experienced")	p-value
All (n = 183)	48.8%	66.3%	16.9%	69.8%	
Young (n = 96)	46.2%	66.3%	13.2%	75.0%	
					0.41
Elderly (n = 87)	51.9%	66.3%	21.0%	63.8%	
Low education (n = 91)	47.8%	60.4%	20.9%	72.8%	
					0.34
High education (n = 86)	50.0%	72.8%	12.3%	66.3%	
Female (n = 119)	52.2%	62.8%	17.5%	69.3%	
					0.74
Male (n = 64)	42.4%	72.9%	15.5%	70.7%	
Short duration (n = 94)	48.9%	66.7%	14.6%	71.9%	
					0.87
Long duration(n = 89)	48.8%	65.9%	19.3%	67.5%	
Low pain intensity (n = 65)	55.0%	63.9%	18.3%	67.2%	
					0.87
High pain intensity (n = 116)	45.3%	67.6%	17.0%	70.5%	

Elderly, older than 60 years; Young, 60 years or younger;
Low education, junior high school or high school only; high education, college/university or graduate school;
Short duration, thirty six months or less; Long duration, more than thirty six months;
Low pain intensity, sum of "none" and "mild"; High pain intensity, sum of "moderate" and "severe" of Verbal Rating Scale (VRS)

Discussion

The key findings of this study are that (1) Japanese patients with chronic pain show a certain preference concerning the anchor descriptors of extremes; (2) most participants found that one descriptor was both easy to answer and best described their own pain; and (3) preference is not significantly influenced by factors such as age, sex, educational background, duration of pain, and pain intensity of the patient.

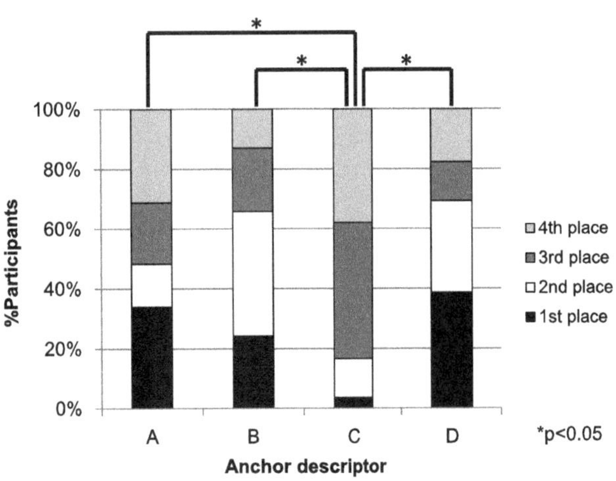

Figure 1. Preference of VAS with the four different descriptors. Friedman test demonstrated a significant difference between the four different descriptors ($p<0.001$); Bonferroni's post-hoc tests demonstrated significant differences between "Imaginable" and "Worst", "Bearable", and "Experienced" ($p<0.05$). A: worst pain ("Worst"). B: worst pain bearable ("Bearable"). C: worst pain imaginable ("Imaginable"). D: worst pain you have ever experienced ("Experienced").

Comparison of preference among different anchor descriptors

We found in this study that Japanese patients with chronic pain show a certain preference concerning the descriptors of extremes (Figure 1). The participants preferred "Experienced" and "Bearable" over the other two descriptors, while "Imaginable" was preferred significantly less often than the other descriptors. "Experienced" represents the "real" pain that an individual has actually experienced; almost all individuals, except for some who

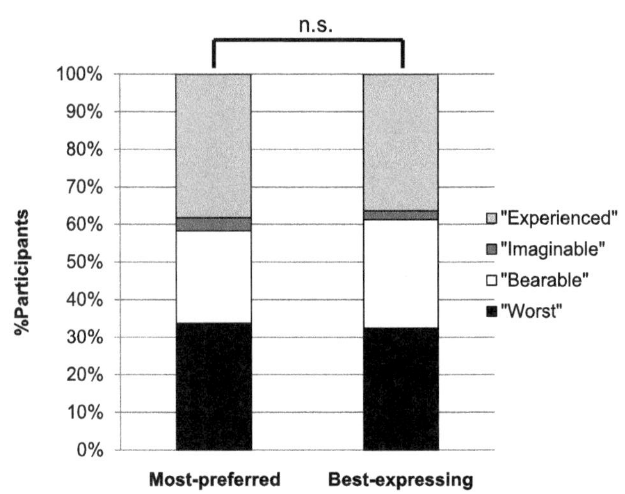

Figure 2. Comparison of percentages between the most-preferred and best-expressing descriptor. n.s., not significant; Wilcoxon's signed rank test, "Worst": worst pain, "Bearable": worst pain bearable, "Imaginable": worst pain imaginable, "Experienced": worst pain you have ever experienced.

Table 3. Pairwise Spearman's rank correlation coefficient between the pain intensity measured by VASs using four anchor descriptors.

	A	B	C	D
A ("Worst")	-			
B ("Bearable")	0.79*	-		
C ("Imaginable")	0.82*	0.78*	-	
D ("Experienced")	0.81*	0.77*	0.87*	-

* Spearman's rank correlation coefficient statistically significant (p<0.05).

may have forgotten episodes of severe pain, should be able to remember and imagine such pain. One plausible explanation for the high preference of the descriptors "Experienced" and "Bearable" is that they are relatively easy to relate to.

On the other hand, "Imaginable" required the participants to imagine unexperienced pain, making it difficult to create a concrete image. Some participants mentioned that rather than imagining unexperienced pain, they remembered pain episodes that they had actually experienced.

Interestingly, approximately half of the participants regarded "Worst" as preferable and half as not preferable. Some participants interpreted "the worst pain imaginable" to mean pain they had experienced, while others interpreted this to mean unexperienced pain. The IASP defines pain as "an unpleasant sensory and emotional experience associated with actual or potential tissue damage, or described in terms of such damage" [1]. "Worst" seems to involve affective and emotional aspects more than the other three descriptors, which may have influenced participants' preference.

We also found in this study that participants tended to regard one descriptor as both easy to answer and best to describe their own pain. We defined "preference" as easiest to answer in this study. Peters et al. found that there was little difference between the scales that patients regarded as best describing, "most easy", and "preferred" [8]. Similarly, our results suggest that the anchor label that best described participants' own pain tended to be the one they answered most easily.

As Table 3 showed, the anchor descriptor did not have a great influence on VAS values of the whole group. However, the result of the Wilcoxon signed-rank test indicated that preference of the anchor descriptor could affect the intra-personal pain intensity. Therefore, the easiest descriptor for each patient to understand should be used to evaluate that patient's pain accurately. Moreover, we had probably better not to use the less preferred anchor descriptor, such as "worst pain imaginable" to obtain precise data.

Table 4. Characteristics of pain (n = 183).

	n
Diagnosis	
Myofascial pain	132
Peripheral neuropathy	19
Spinal degenerative disease	19
Sacroiliac joint dysfunction	18
Failed back syndrome	12
Post-operative pain	9
Postherpetic neuralgia	8
Arthritis	7
Other spinal diseases	6
Complex regional pain syndrome	4
Fibromyalgia	3
Non-specific low back pain	3
Trigeminal neuralgia	3
Headache	2
Type of pain	
Nociceptive	185
Neuropathic	50
Mixed	31
Site of pain	
Face, head, and neck	44
Shoulder and upper extremities	40
Chest and abdomen	16
Back	25
Lumber and buttock	65
Inguinal region and lower extremities	60
Others	5

Comparison of preference by subgroups

Although Table 2 shows that participants who were female, younger, and had a low level of education tended to prefer "Experienced" to "Bearable" and, conversely, that male, older, and highly educated participants tended to prefer "Bearable" to "Experienced", the effect of these factors did not reach statistical significance. Previous studies have found that sex influenced the preference of pain scales to a certain extent [8,14–15]. In any case, the percentage of participants that considered "Experienced" to be preferable was similar to the percentage that preferred "Bearable". On the other hand, few participants preferred "Imaginable", and the rank of preference of "Worst" and "Imaginable" did not differ according to subcategories. One plausible explanation is that some patients may have difficulty with the abstract concepts of inexperienced pain such as "Worst" and "Imaginable".

Although "Imaginable" is a frequently used descriptor in Japan, its use as an anchor label in pain measurement may not provide an appropriate evaluation, because "preference" was defined as ease in understanding or answering in this study. Therefore, we consider it more suitable to use descriptors such as "Experienced" or "Bearable" for the evaluation of pain intensity in Japanese patients with chronic pain.

Many previous studies have investigated the preferences of patients for pain assessment tools. However, to the best of our knowledge, very few studies have dealt with the preference for anchor labels. Hjermstad et al.'s review article concerning pain intensity assessment tools written in English reports the use of 24 different descriptors in 239 papers with the VAS and NRS [11]. Thus, a range of non-standardized descriptors are used to evaluate pain intensity both domestically and internationally. Our study indicates that the preference of patients for descriptors can determine how precisely patients are able to communicate their perceived pain intensity.

These results suggest that anchor descriptors should be standardized as soon as possible for more appropriate evaluation of pain intensity. The findings from this study can contribute to more accurate assessment of the intensity of chronic pain. It should be noted that the participants in this study were from a limited population and that factors such as race, ethnicity, and culture are also known to influence pain perception [36]. To what extent our results extend to patients from other racial and cultural backgrounds is unclear and requires further study.

Study limitations

This study has several limitations. First, patients with other types of pain, such as acute pain and cancer pain, were not included. It remains to be clarified whether the findings from this study can be generalized to all Japanese patients.

Second, participants in this study attended a multi-disciplinary pain clinic, introducing a probable selection bias. However, the range of pain intensity measured by the VAS and VRS, as well as psychometric factors such as the HADS and PCS, were distributed widely, so the participants can be considered to represent common Japanese chronic pain patients.

Third, the meaning of the descriptors in Japanese might not necessarily correspond exactly to their English counterparts. However, as the translated descriptors were checked by an American psychologist who is proficient in Japanese, we do not consider this to be a serious problem.

Conclusions

The result of this study indicate that "worst pain you have ever experienced" and "worst pain bearable" are appropriate descriptors for Japanese chronic pain patients. "Worst pain imaginable", though it is frequently used worldwide, may be inappropriate for evaluating pain intensity, at least among Japanese chronic pain patients. Widely preferred descriptors, i.e., most patients can respond without difficulty, should be used when evaluating perceived pain.

The preference of anchor descriptors was not significantly affected by the factors such as such as age, sex, educational level, duration of pain, and pain intensity.

Acknowledgments

We would like to thank Keiko Kojima, Shumpei Kitamura, Makihiko Hirabayashi, Fumitaka Matsuno, and Jin Shinohara for data collection.

We very much appreciate all the patients who participated in this study.

Author Contributions

Conceived and designed the experiments: JY. Analyzed the data: JY MM. Wrote the paper: JY MK SU.

References

1. Taxonomy ITFo (1994) Part III: Pain Terms: A Current List with Definitions and Notes on Usage. In: Merskey H, Bogduk N, editors. Classification of Chronic Pain. 2nd ed. Seattle: IASP Press. pp. 209–214.
2. Kremer E, Atkinson JH, Ignelzi RJ (1981) Measurement of pain: patient preference does not confound pain measurement. Pain 10: 241–248.
3. Melzack R, Katz J (2006) Pain assessment in adult patients. In: McMahon SB, Klotzenburg M, editors. Wall and Melzack's Textbook of Pain. 5th ed. Philadelphia: Elsevier. pp. 291–304.
4. McQuay HJ, Moore A (2006) Methods of therapeutic trials. In: McMahon SB, Klotzenburg M, editors. Wall and Melzack's Textbook of Pain. 5th ed. Philadelphia: Elsevier. pp. 415–425.
5. Loder E, Burch R (2012) Measuring pain intensity in headache trials: which scale to use? Cephalalgia 32: 179–182.
6. Jensen MP, Karoly P, Braver S (1986) The measurement of clinical pain intensity: a comparison of six methods. Pain 27: 117–126.
7. Flaherty SA (1996) Pain measurement tools for clinical practice and research. AANA J 64: 133–140.
8. Peters ML, Patijn J, Lamé I (2007) Pain assessment in younger and older pain patients: psychometric properties and patient preference of five commonly used measures of pain intensity. Pain Med 8: 601–610.
9. Carlsson AM (1983) Assessment of chronic pain. I. Aspects of the reliability and validity of the visual analogue scale. Pain 16: 87–101.
10. Langley GB, Sheppeard H (1985) The visual analogue scale: its use in pain measurement. Rheumatol Int 5: 145–148.
11. Hjermstad MJ, Fayers PM, Haugen DF, Caraceni A, European Palliative Care Research Collaborative (EPCRC), et al. (2011) Studies comparing Numerical Rating Scales, Verbal Rating Scales, and Visual Analogue Scales for assessment of pain intensity in adults: a systematic literature review. J Pain Symptom Manage 41: 1073–1093.
12. Rodriguez CS, McMillan S, Yarandi H (2004) Pain measurement in older adults with head and neck cancer and communication impairments. Cancer Nurs 27: 425–433.
13. Clark P, Lavielle P, Martínez H (2003) Learning from pain scales: patient perspective. J Rheumatol 30: 1584–1588.
14. Herr KA, Mobily PR (1993) Comparison of selected pain assessment tools for use with the elderly. Appl Nurs Res 6: 39–46.
15. Herr KA, Spratt K, Mobily PR, Richardson G (2004) Pain intensity assessment in older adults: use of experimental pain to compare psychometric properties and usability of selected pain scales with younger adults. Clin J Pain 20: 207–219.
16. de C Williams AC, Davies HT, Chadury Y (2000) Simple pain rating scales hide complex idiosyncratic meanings. Pain 85: 457–463.
17. Paice JA, Cohen FL (1997) Validity of a verbally administered numeric rating scale to measure cancer pain intensity. Cancer Nurs 20: 88–93.
18. Gagliese L, Weizblit N, Ellis W, Chan VW (2005) The measurement of postoperative pain: a comparison of intensity scales in younger and older surgical patients. Pain 117: 412–420.
19. Berthier F, Potel G, Leconte P, Touze MD, Baron D (1998) Comparative study of methods of measuring acute pain intensity in an ED. Am J Emerg Med 16: 132–136.
20. Marquie L, Duarte LR, Marine C, Lauque D, Sorum PC (2008) How patients and physicians rate patients' pain in a French emergency department using a verbally administered numerical rating scale and a visual analog scale. Acute Pain 10: 31–37.
21. Brunelli C, Zecca E, Martini C, Campa T, Fagnoni E, et al. (2010) Comparison of numerical and verbal rating scales to measure pain exacerbations in patients with chronic cancer pain. Health Qual Life Outcomes 8: 42.
22. Downie WW, Leatham PA, Rhind VM, Wright V, Branco JA, et al. (1978) Studies with pain rating scales. Ann Rheum Dis 37: 378–381.
23. Bolton JE, Wilkinson RC (1998) Responsiveness of pain scales: a comparison of three pain intensity measures in chiropractic patients. J Manipulative Physiol Ther 21: 1–7.
24. Grotle M, Brox JI, Vollestad NK (2004) Concurrent comparison of responsiveness in pain and functional status measurements used for patients with low back pain. Spine (Phila Pa 1976) 29: E492–501.
25. Larroy C (2002) Comparing visual-analog and numeric scales for assessing menstrual pain. Behav Med 27: 179–181.
26. Seymour RA (1982) The use of pain scales in assessing the efficacy of analgesics in post-operative dental pain. Eur J Clin Pharmacol 23: 441–444.
27. Price DD, Bush FM, Long S, Harkins SW (1994) A comparison of pain measurement characteristics of mechanical visual analogue and simple numerical rating scales. Pain 56: 217–226.
28. Skovlund E, Bretthauer M, Grotmol T, Larsen IK, Hoff G (2005) Sensitivity of pain rating scales in an endoscopy trial. Clin J Pain 21: 292–296.
29. Closs SJ, Barr B, Briggs M, Cash K, Seers K (2004) A comparison of five pain assessment scales for nursing home residents with varying degrees of cognitive impairment. J Pain Symptom Manage 27: 196–205.
30. Radbruch L, Sabatowski R, Loick G, Jonen-Thielemann I, Kasper M, et al. (2000) Cognitive impairment and its influence on pain and symptom assessment in a palliative care unit: development of a Minimal Documentation System. Palliat Med 14: 266–276.

31. Fanurik D, Koh JL, Harrison RD, Conrad TM, Tomerlin C (1998) Pain assessment in children with cognitive impairment. An exploration of self-report skills. Clin Nurs Res 7: 103-119; discussion 120–124.
32. Gabre P, Sjöquist K (2002) Experience and assessment of pain in individuals with cognitive impairments. Spec Care Dentist 22: 174–180.
33. Zigmond AS, Snaith RP (1983) The hospital anxiety and depression scale. Acta Psychiatr Scand 67: 361–370.
34. Bjelland I, Dahl AA, Haug TT, Neckelmann D (2002) The validity of the Hospital Anxiety and Depression Scale. An updated literature review. J Psychosom Res 52: 69–77.
35. Sullivan MJ, Bishop SR, Pivik J (1995) The Pain Catastrophizing Scale: Development and Validation. Psychological Assessment 7: 524–532.
36. Rahim-Williams B, Riley JL 3rd, Williams AK, Fillingim RB (2012) A quantitative review of ethnic group differences in experimental pain response: do biology, psychology, and culture matter? Pain Med 13: 522–540.

12

Central Administration of C-X-C Chemokine Receptor Type 4 Antagonist Alleviates the Development and Maintenance of Peripheral Neuropathic Pain in Mice

Xin Luo[1,4], Wai Lydia Tai[1,4], Liting Sun[1,4], Qiu Qiu[1,4], Zhengyuan Xia[1,3], Sookja Kim Chung[2,3,4], Chi Wai Cheung[1,3,4]*

1 Department of Anaesthesiology, The University of Hong Kong, HKSAR, China, **2** Department of Anatomy, The University of Hong Kong, HKSAR, China, **3** Research Center of Heart, Brain, Hormone and Healthy Aging, The University of Hong Kong, HKSAR, China, **4** Laboratory and Clinical Research Institute for Pain, The University of Hong Kong, HKSAR, China

Abstract

Aim: To explore the roles of C-X-C chemokine receptor type 4 (CXCR4) in spinal processing of neuropathic pain at the central nervous system (CNS).

Methods: Peripheral neuropathic pain (PNP) induced by partial sciatic nerve ligation (pSNL) model was assessed in mice. Effects of a single intrathecal (central) administration of AMD3100 (intrathecal AMD3100), a CXCR4 antagonist, on pain behavior and pain-related spinal pathways and molecules in the L3-L5 spinal cord segment was studied compare to saline treatment.

Results: Rotarod test showed that intrathecal AMD3100 did not impair mice motor function. In pSNL-induced mice, intrathecal AMD3100 delayed the development of mechanical allodynia and reversed the established mechanical allodynia in a dose-dependent way. Moreover, intrathecal AMD3100 downregulated the activation of JNK1 and p38 pathways and the protein expression of p65 as assessed by western blotting. Real-time PCR test also demonstrated that substance P mRNA was decreased, while adrenomedullin and intercellular adhesion molecule mRNA was increased following AMD3100 treatment.

Conclusion: Our results suggest that central (spinal) CXCR4 is involved in the development and maintenance of PNP and the regulation of multiple spinal molecular events under pain condition, implicating that CXCR4 would potentially be a therapeutic target for chronic neuropathic pain.

Editor: Sam Eldabe, The James Cook University Hospital, United Kingdom

Funding: Funding for this study was provided by the departmental fund, Department of Anaesthesiology, The University of Hong Kong; the department fund, Department of Anaesthesiology, The University of Hong Kong had no further role in study design; in the collection, analysis and interpretation of data; in the writing of the report; and in the decision to submit the paper for publication.

* Email: cheucw@hku.hk

Introduction

Chemokine receptors have been intensively studied for their roles in nociception and considered novel targets for neuropathic pain therapy [1]. C-X-C chemokine receptor type 4 (CXCR4) is the receptor of chemokine (C-X-C motif) ligand 12 (CXCL12), which belongs to the G protein-coupled receptor (GPCR) family. CXCR4 is widely expressed in the peripheral and central nervous system (PNS and CNS) and exerts numerous important functions, such as modulation of neurotransmission, synaptic plasticity, and neuroglial interactions [2]. Increasing number of studies reported roles of CXCR4 in pain processing in the PNS, as CXCR4 is expressed on primary sensory neurons, satellite cells, Schwann cells, and endothelial cells in the peripheral nociceptive structure [3–9]. Recent immunohistochemistry studies also showed that CXCR4 would be involved in the modulation of pain signaling in the CNS. CXCL12 and CXCR4 were positive in neurons, astrocytes, microglia/macrophages, and leukocytes in the lumbar spinal cord and their spinal immunoreactivity was found to be increased in a central neuropathic pain model [10]. The activation of spinal CXCR4 by the intrathecal administration of CXCL12 has been found to induce mechanical allodynia for 3 days, which could be reversed by a CXCR4-neutralizing antibody given intrathecally [9].

Currently, systematic (intraperitoneal) administration of CXCR4 antagonist, AMD3100, was demonstrated to have analgesic effects on opioid-induced hyperalgesia [8] and neuropathic pain induced by peripheral neuropathy [3] and by anti-AIDS therapy [6,7]. These studies implicated the potential application of AMD3100 for analgesia. However, central roles of CXCR4 in pain transduction remain unclear and there has been no study evaluating the effects of pharmacological inhibition of

CXCR4 on central pain signal processing. Therefore, in this study, we aimed to explore the roles and mechanisms of central CXCR4 in pain modulation using specific CXCR4 antagonist AMD3100 and a peripheral neuropathic pain (PNP) model using partial sciatic nerve ligation (pSNL) in mice.

Materials and Methods

Animals

This research was approved by the Committee on the Use of Live Animals in Teaching and Research (CULATR) (Permit Number: 2610-11), the University of Hong Kong, and performed according to the guidelines for the care and use of laboratory animals as established by the Laboratory Animal Unit (LAU) at the University of Hong Kong. The mice were housed at 23±3°C, with humidity ranges between 25% and 45% under a 12-hour light/12-hour dark cycle (lights on at 07:00). The mice were offered free access to water and food. They were fed with Lab Diet 5012 (1.0% calcium, 0.5% phosphorus, and 3.3 IU/g of vitamin D3).

The experiments were conducted using adult male C57BL/6 wild-type mice (25–30 grams). Total number of mice used in this project was 86. In Rotarod test, 20 mice that had not received any operation or behavior test were randomly divided into four groups ($n = 5$ in each group). The mice of four groups were treated intrathecally with AMD3100 1 μg (AMD3100 1 μg group), 5 μg (AMD3100 5 μg group), 25 μg (AMD3100 25 μg group) or saline (saline group). To study the roles of CXCR4 in the development of PNP, the mice were randomly divided into four groups. Two groups received either pSNL (pSNL group, $n = 6$) or sham surgery (sham group, $n = 6$) without intrathecal drug administration. The other two groups were treated 1 hour before pSNL surgery with a single intrathecal injection of either AMD3100 (5 μg, AMD3100 + pSNL group, $n = 12$) or saline (saline + pSNL group, $n = 12$). To study the roles of CXCR4 in the maintenance of PNP, mice were randomly divided into four groups, and all received pSNL surgery. On post-operative day (POD) 7, four groups were treated with a single intrathecal injection of AMD3100 or of saline. The dosages given to the four groups were 1 μg (pSNL + AMD3100 1 μg group, $n = 5$), 5 μg (pSNL + AMD3100 5 μg group, $n = 6$), 25 μg (pSNL + AMD3100 25 μg group, $n = 6$), or saline (pSNL + saline group, $n = 5$). To study the effects of a single intrathecal injection of AMD3100 (intrathecal AMD3100) on pain pathways in the lumbar spinal cords of pSNL-injured mice, the mice were treated with a single injection of either AMD3100 25 μg (AMD3100 group) or saline (saline group) on POD 7 ($n = 8$ per group). To study the effects of intrathecal AMD3100 on pain molecules in the lumbar spinal cords of pSNL-injured mice, the mice were treated with a single injection of either AMD3100 25 μg (AMD3100 group) or saline (saline group) on POD 7 ($n = 6$ per group).

Partial sciatic nerve ligation surgery

A pSNL surgery was used as the PNP model in this study [11]. The mice were anesthetized with halothane in a 1:1 mixture of O_2 and N_2O. Under aseptic conditions, the right sciatic nerve (SN) was exposed by an incision from the right sciatic notch to the distal thigh. The location of the SN ligation was identified using the femoral head as a landmark. Approximately 1/2 of the SN was tightly ligated with a 7-0 silk suture. In the sham-operated mice that were used as controls, the right sciatic nerve was exposed, but not ligated. The incision was closed with 5–0 cotton suture and disinfected with ethanol.

Drug administration

AMD3100 (Sigma), a CXCR4 antagonist, was prepared in saline on the day of the experiment. As the dosage of AMD3100 for intrathecal administration in mice has not been determined, dosages of 1 μg, 5 μg, and 25 μg were used in this study. AMD3100 was administrated as a single dose intrathecally, according to a previous study [12]. Before the injection, the animals were anesthetized using halothane with mixture of oxygen and N_2O as described above. Using a syringe (Hamilton) with a 30-gauge needle, a spinal cord puncture was made between the L3 and L5 levels in order to deliver a total volume of 5 μl to the subarachnoid space. Successful administration was identified by tail swinging or a tail configuration of the "S" type immediately after injection.

von Frey test

Mechanical allodynia is the symptom of PNP, which is indicated by a reduction in the paw withdrawal threshold (PWT). This condition was assessed by von Frey test which was performed in our previous research [13]. For habituation before the experiment, the mice were placed in a transparent plastic dome with a metal mesh floor for 20 to 30 minutes. Their PWT was measured with a series of von Frey filaments (IITC). The filaments were applied perpendicularly to the plantar surface of both hind paws, with sufficient force to bend the filaments into an "S" shape. Quick withdrawal or licking of the paw was considered a positive response.

Rotarod test

To assess whether there would be any the potential side-effect of a single intrathecal injection of AMD3100 (intrathecal AMD3100) on motor function, a rotarod test was conducted to measure the motor coordination and balance of the mice._ENREF_18 Twenty mice that had not received any operation or behavior test were randomly divided into four groups. These animals were habituated to the rotarod apparatus (IITC) for 2 consecutive days at low-speed rotation (5 rpm) for 600 seconds each day before basal measurement. During the experiment, the animals were tested in three accelerating trials of 300 seconds, with the rotarod speed increasing from 5 to 40 rpm over 300 seconds, and with an inter-trial interval of at least 20 minutes. The animals' latency in falling from the rod was recorded for each trial, with a cutoff time at 300 seconds.

Western blotting

The sciatic nerve of C57BL/6 mice is composed from elements of L3 and L4 segments of spinal cord with a smaller contribution from L5 segment [14]. Therefore, after euthanizing each mouse with pentobarbital, the L3-L5 section of its spinal cord was quickly removed and homogenized in ice-cold RIPA lysis buffer. After concentration determination, protein samples were separated in 10% SDS-PAGE and electrotransferred onto PVDF membranes. Protein samples were then probed with antibodies for extracellular signal-regulated kinase (ERK, 4695, Cell Signaling), phosphorylated ERK (pERK, 4511, Cell Signaling), c-Jun N-terminal kinase (JNK, 9258, Cell Signaling), phosphorylated JNK (pJNK, 4668, Cell Signaling), p38 (9212, Cell Signaling), phosphorylated p38 (p-p38, 4511, Cell Signaling), AKT (9272, Cell Signaling), phosphorylated AKT (pAKT, 4060, Cell Signaling), Signal transducer and activator of transcription 3 (STAT3, 9132, Cell Signaling), phosphorylated STAT3 (pSTAT3, 9131, Cell Signaling), or p65 (4764, Cell Signaling) with alpha-tubulin (T5168, Sigma) used as a loading control. The membranes were visualized with horseradish

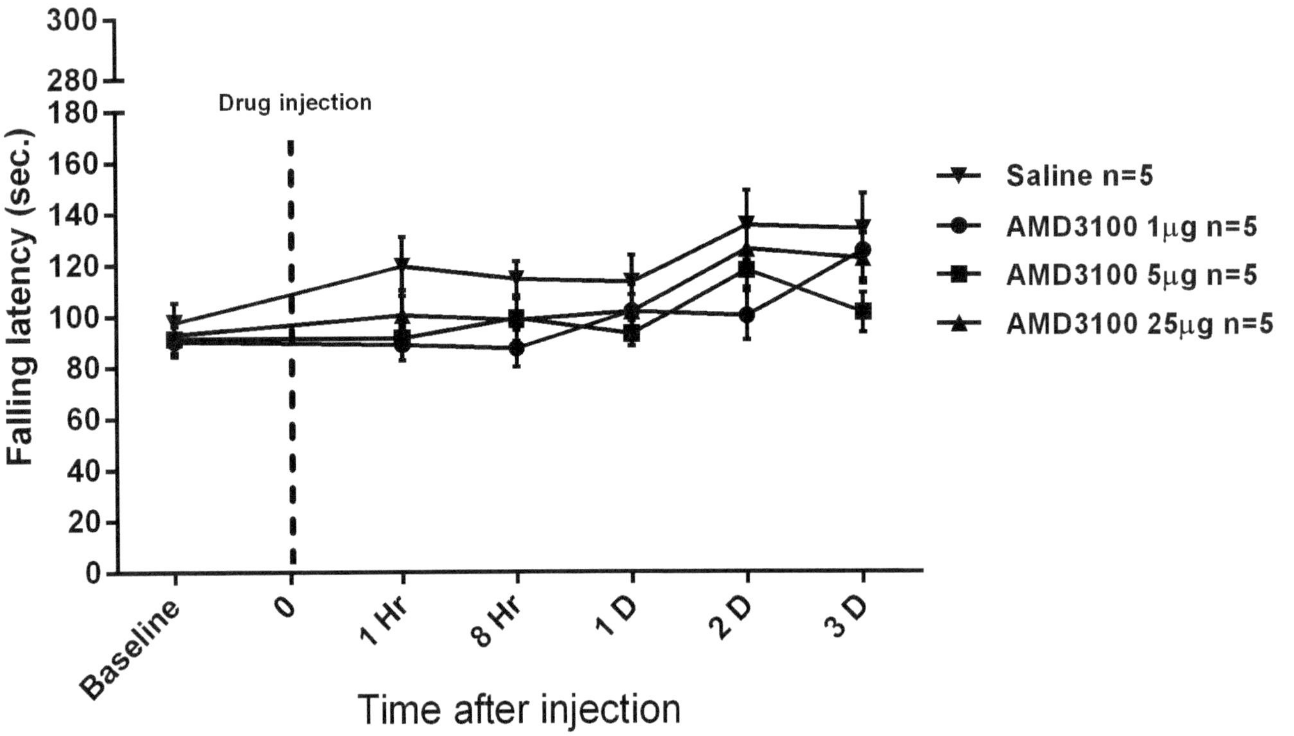

Figure 1. The effects of intrathecal AMD3100 on the motor function of normal mice. There was no significant change in falling latency among the three groups with intrathecal AMD3100, compared to the saline group from hour 1 to day 3 after the injection. Results are mean ± SEM ($n=5$). Sec. = second, D = day, Hr = hour, 0 = time of intrathecal injection.

peroxidase (HRP)-conjugated secondary antibodies (anti-rabbit IgG and anti-mouse IgG, Sigma).

Real time PCR

After euthanizing each mouse with pentobarbital, the L3-L5 section of its spinal cord was quickly removed and stored at −80°C until RNA extraction. mRNA was extracted from homogenized spinal cord segements following the manufacturer's protocol (Takara). After the quality and quantity determination, mRNA samples were made to cDNA library with reverse transcriptase (Life Technologies). Prepared cDNA samples were diluted and stored at −20°C until further tests. Real time PCR reactions were performed with the SYBR green chemistry method or the Taqman chemistry method (Applied biosystems). The specific primers for substance P (SP), adrenomedullin (AM), calcitonin gene-related peptide (CGRP) and 18S rRNA were reported in our previous study [13], and used with Fast SYBR green master mix (Applied Biosystems). The Taqman Probes for mouse Tumor necrosis factor-α (TNF-α, Mm00443258), interleukin-1β (IL-1β, Mm00434228), interleukin-6 (IL-6, Mm00446190), intercellular adhesion molecule (ICAM, Mm00516023), vascular cell adhesion molecule (VCAM, Mm00449197), excitatory amino-acid transporter-2 (EAAT-2, Mm00441457) and actin-β (Mm01205647) were purchased from Applied Biosystems.

Statistical analysis

The data were expressed as means ± SEM. Student's *t* tests was used to analyze Western blot and real time PCR data. Results from von Frey test was analyzed using a student's *t* test or a two-way analysis of variance (ANOVA), followed by a Tukey's multiple comparison post test. Results from the rotarod test were analyzed using a two-way analysis of variance (ANOVA), followed by a Tukey's multiple comparison post test. In all cases, $p<0.05$ was considered as statistically significant.

Results

Effects of intrathecal AMD3100 on the motor function of mice

The effects of intrathecal AMD3100 on motor function had not been studied before. Any impairment in motor function might affect the assessment of pain and intrathecal AMD3100 would not be suitable for potential analgesic treatment if that was the case. Therefore, motor function after intrathecal AMD3100 was assessed by a rotarod test in this study. The falling latency of the three groups with intrathecal AMD3100 showed no significant change compared to the saline group after the injection ($p>0.05$; ANOVA; n = 5; Figure 1). These results indicated that intrathecal AMD3100 did not influence the motor function of mice.

Effects of intrathecal AMD3100 on the development and maintenance of mechanical allodynia in pSNL-injured mice

AMD3100 or saline was given intrathecally at one hour before pSNL surgery, and the involvement of central CXCR4 in the development of PNP was evaluated by von Frey tests. Sham surgery (n = 6) did not affect ipsilateral PWT, but pSNL surgery (n = 6) decreased ipsilateral PWT significantly on POD 1 ($p<0.001$; ANOVA). These results demonstrated that mechanical allodynia was induced immediately by pSNL, but not by sham operation. Pretreatment of a single intrathecal injection of saline (intrathecal saline) did not have any effect on ipsilateral PWT in

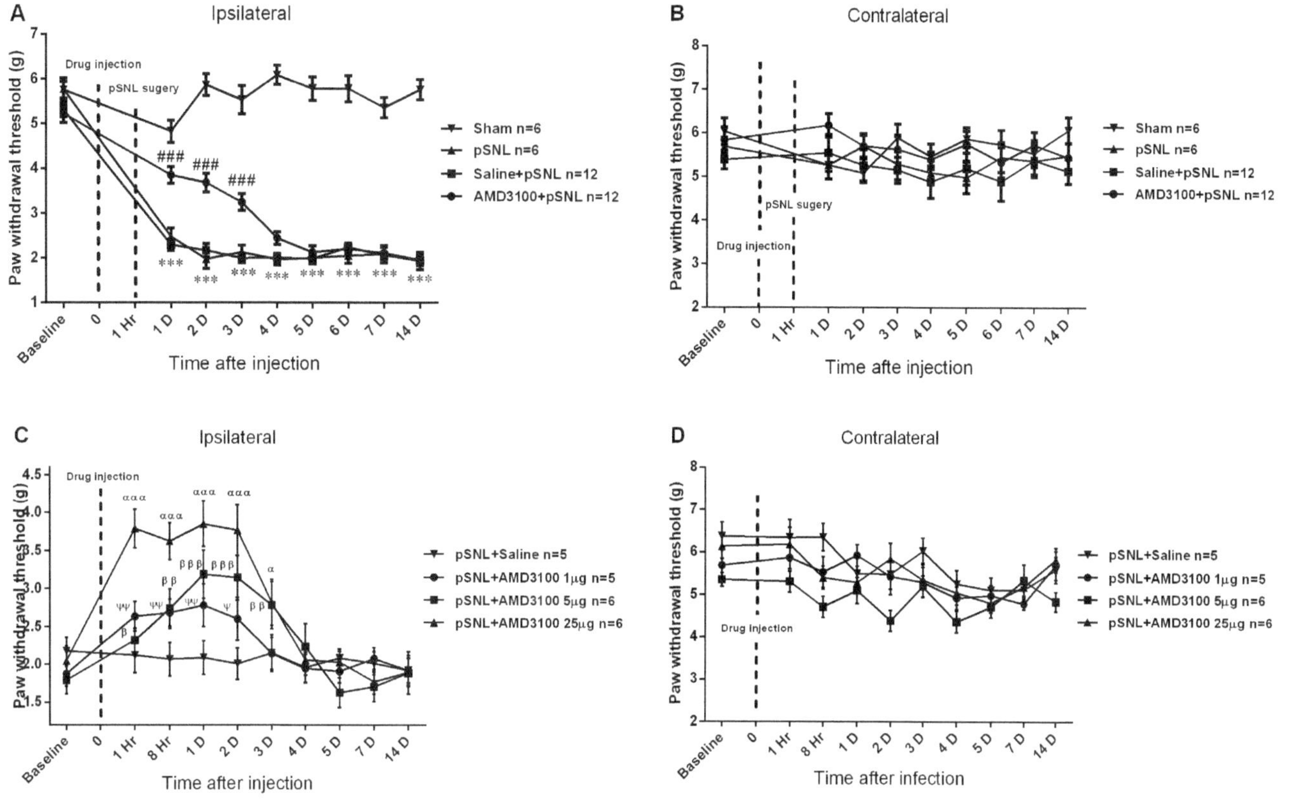

Figure 2. The effects of intrathecal AMD3100 on the development and maintenance of PNP in pSNL-injured mice. The preemptive intrathecal AMD3100, but not intrathecal saline, increased ipsilateral PWT of pSNL mice for 3 days after the surgery (A), but did not affect contralateral PWT (B). On POD 7, intrathecal AMD3100 at dosages of 1 μg, 5 μg and 25 μg increased the ipsilateral PWT of pSNL mice for 2, 3 and 3 days, respectively (C), but did not affect contralateral PWT (D). Results are mean ± SEM ($n = 5$–12). $^{***}p<0.001$ versus the pSNL group at the corresponding timepoints. $^{\#\#\#}p<0.001$ versus the Saline + pSNL group at the corresponding timepoints. $^{\alpha\alpha\alpha}p<0.001$, $^{\alpha}p<0.05$, $^{\beta\beta\beta}p<0.001$, $^{\beta\beta}p<0.01$, $^{\beta}p<0.05$, $^{\Psi\Psi}p<0.01$ and $^{\Psi}p<0.05$ versus the baseline. g = gram, D = day, Hr = hour, 0 = time of intrathecal injection.

the pSNL + saline group (n = 12), as compared with that in the pSNL group without any intrathecal medication ($p>0.05$; ANOVA). However, intrathecal AMD3100 before pSNL surgery increased ipsilateral PWT significantly from day 1 to day 3 ($p<0.001$; ANOVA; n = 12) after drug injection, as compared with the pSNL + saline group (Figure 2A). No difference in contralateral PWT was found among the four study groups ($p>0.05$; ANOVA; Figure 2B). These results suggested that intrathecal AMD3100 could delay the development of mechanical allodynia by pSNL.

To study the role of central CXCR4 in the maintenance of PNP, pSNL-injured mice received either intrathecal AMD3100 or intrathecal saline on POD 7. Mechanical allodynia from hour 1 to day 14 after the injection was assessed by von Frey test. Intrathecal AMD3100 1 μg increased ipsilateral PWT from hour 1 to day 2 ($p<0.01$ or 0.05; student's t test; n = 5; Figure 2C) after the injection. Intrathecal AMD3100 5 μg increased ipsilateral PWT from hour 1 to day 3 ($p<0.001$ or 0.01 or 0.05; student's t test; n = 6; Figure 2C) after the injection. Intrathecal AMD3100 25 μg increased ipsilateral PWT from hour 1 to day 3 ($p<0.001$ or 0.05; student's t test; n = 6; Figure 2C) after the injection. Intrathecal saline did not have any effect on ipsilateral PWT ($p>0.05$; student's t test; n = 5; Figure 2C). No significant difference was shown in contralateral PWT among any of the four groups ($p>0.05$; student's t test; Figure 2D). These results suggested that intrathecal AMD3100 could transiently reverse established mechanical allodynia by pSNL in a dose-dependent way.

Effects of intrathecal AMD3100 on the production of pain molecules in the lumbar spinal cord of pSNL-injured mice

Following the peripheral nerve injury, the central release of neuropeptides (e.g. SP, CGRP and AM), pro-inflammatory cytokines (e.g. TNF-α, IL-1β and IL-6), cellular adhesion molecules (e.g. ICAM and VCAM) and glutamate transporter (e.g. EAAT-2) contribute to neuronal central sensitization and persistent pain [15,16]. Therefore, we also investigated whether intrathecal AMD3100 could affect the spinal production of these neuropeptides and pro-inflammatory cytokines. The mRNA level of SP was decreased but the mRNA level of AM and ICAM were increased significantly on the ipsilateral side of the L3-L5 spinal cord segment in pSNL-injured mice with intrathecal AMD3100 25 μg (n = 6) compared to the saline group (n = 6) at 8 hour after the injection ($p<0.05$; student's t test; Figures 3B, C and G). However, the mRNA levels of CGRP, TNF-α, IL-1β, IL-6, VCAM and EAAT-2 in the L3-L5 spinal cords of pSNL-injured mice were not affected by intrathecal AMD3100 (all $p>0.05$; student's t test; Figures 3A, D, E, F, H and I).

Effects of intrathecal AMD3100 on pain signaling pathways in the lumbar spinal cord of pSNL-injured mice

Spinal mitogen-activated protein kinases (MAPKs), phosphoinositide 3-kinase (PI3K), STAT3 and nuclear factor kappa-light-chain-enhancer of activated B (NF-κB) pathways were shown to be significantly activated on POD 7 using PNP models [17–20]. Our

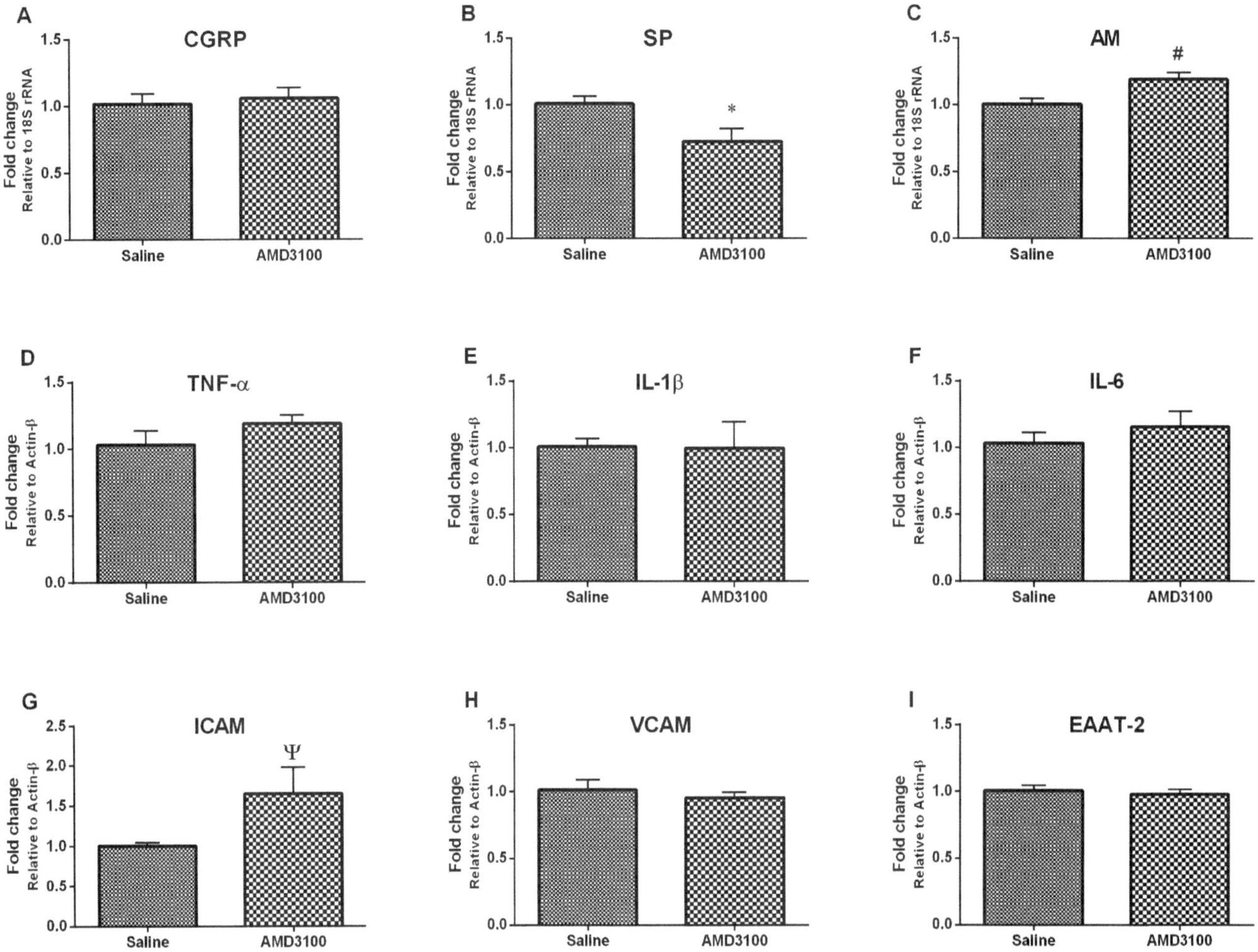

Figure 3. The effects of intrathecal AMD3100 on the production of neuropeptides and pro-inflammatory cytokines, and cellular adhesion molecules in the ipsilateral L3-L5 spinal cord segment of pSNL-injured mice. Real time PCR revealed that intrathecal AMD3100 decreased mRNA level of SP (B) and increased mRNA level of AM (C) and ICAM (G), but did not affect mRNA levels of CGRP (A), TNF-α (D) and IL-1β (E), IL-6 (F), VCAM (H) or EAAT-2 (I) at hour 8 after the injection. Results are means ± SEM (n = 6). *$p<0.01$, $^{\#}p$ and $^{\Psi}p<0.05$ versus the saline group.

result found that intrathecal AMD3100 in all used dosage produced analgesic effects on pSNL-injured mice at hour 8 after the drug injection. Therefore, we harvested lumbar spinal cord sample from this time-point and detected whether intrathecal AMD3100 could affect the activation of members of these pathways. The phosphorylation level of JNK1 ($p<0.01$; student's t test; Figure 4C) and p38 ($p<0.05$; student's t test; Figure 4E) and the expression level of p65 ($p<0.05$; student's t test; Figure 4H) was decreased significantly on the ipsilateral side of the L3-L5 spinal cord segment in pSNL-injured mice with intrathecal AMD3100 25 μg (n = 8), compared to the saline group (n = 8). However, the activation (phosphorylation) levels of ERK1, ERK2, and JNK2 in the L3-L5 spinal cords of pSNL-injured mice were not affected by intrathecal AMD3100 (all $p>0.05$; student's t test; Figures 4A, B, D, F and G).

Discussion

Although recent immunohistochemistry study has suggested the involvement of CXCR4 in pain processing in the CNS [10], central roles of CXCR4 in nociception remain unclear. Therefore, in order to explore the function of CXCR4 in pain modulation in CNS, we studied the pharmacological effects of intrathecal administration of CXCR4 antagonist (AMD3100) on PNP using a pSNL model. The pSNL model is a widely used PNP model, and long-lasted mechanical allodynia is induced following partial sciatic ligation [11]. Our present work employed a single intrathecal injection of AMD3100 before pSNL surgery or on POD 7 with similar methods used in antagonism studies of other chemokine receptors [21,22]. Evidence for the involvement of central CXCR4 in the initiation of PNP came from the observation that the pretreatment of AMD3100 led to an attenuation of pSNL-induced allodynia. Essentially, this CXCR4 antagonist was also effective in alleviating mechanical allodynia when pSNL-induce neuropathy had been established. The results indicated that CXCR4 also contribute to the early maintenance of PNP state. Moreover, the reliability of these behavioral anti-nociceptive effects was enhanced by the facts the intrathecal AMD3100 did not impair any motor function.

Previous studies reported analgesic effects of systematic administration of AMD3100 only lasted for hours [8,10], but the effects of central administration of AMD3100 as used in our current study could last for several days. As CXCR4 is widely distributed on nearly all cell types and plays important roles in the tissue development [23], systematic (intraperitoneal) administration of

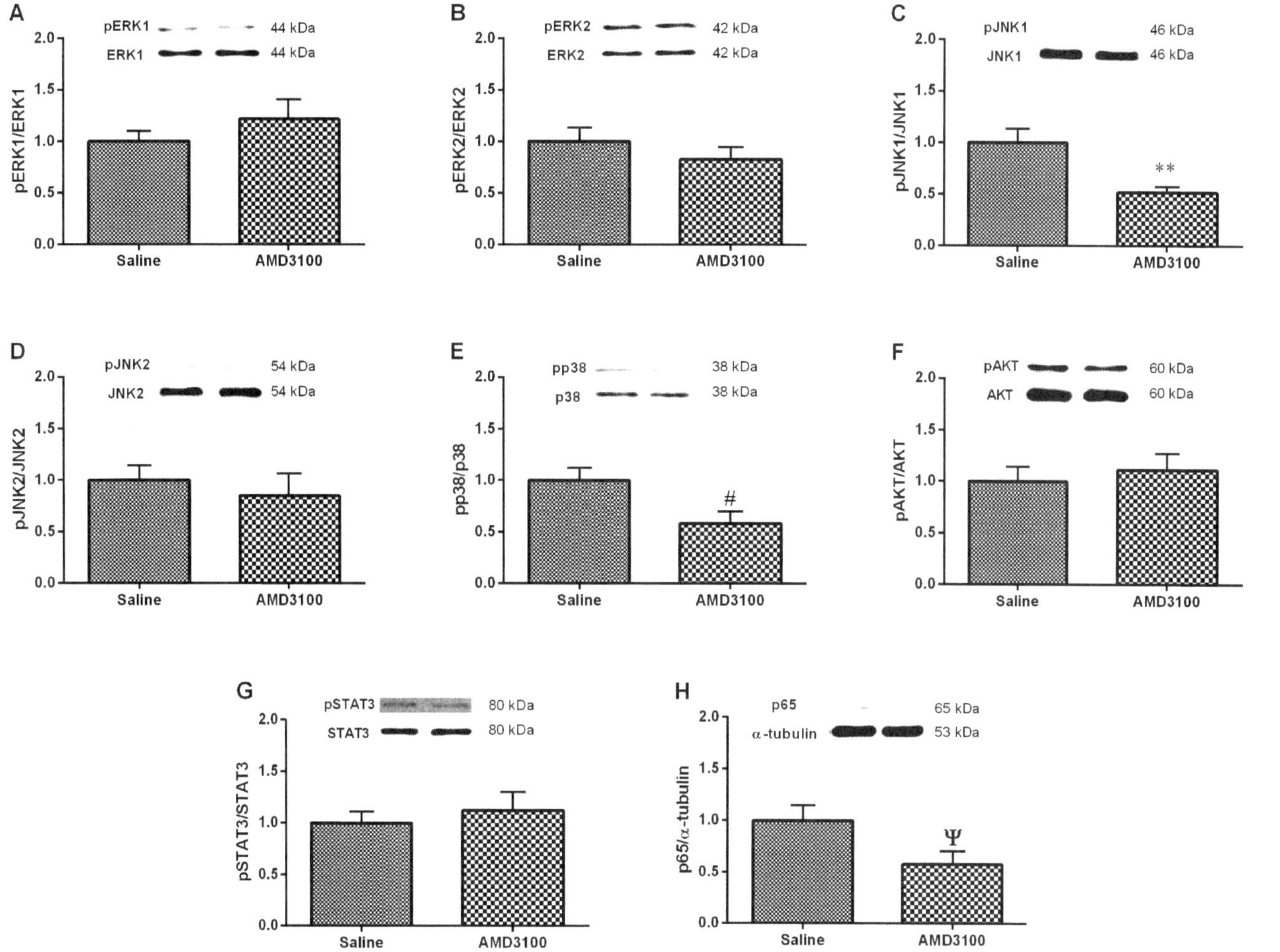

Figure 4. The effects of intrathecal AMD3100 on pain pathways in the ipsilateral L3-L5 spinal cord segment of pSNL-injured mice. Western blotting revealed that intrathecal AMD3100 decreased the phosphorylation level of the JNK1 (C), p38 (E) and p65 (H) pathway, but did not affect the phosphorylation levels of the ERK1 (A), ERK2 (B), JNK2 (D), AKT (F) or STAT3 (G) at hour 8 after the injection. Results are means ± SEM (n = 8). $^{**}p<0.01$, $^{\#}p$ and $^{\Psi}p<0.05$ versus the saline group.

CXCR4 antagonist would be of lower nociceptive structure-specificity and anti-nociceptive efficiency relative to central (intrathecal) administration of AMD3100 theoretically. Moreover, intrathecal delivery of AMD3100 is highly specific to spinal cord, implicating that central (spinal) administration of CXCR4 antagonist for analgesia would be more effective than peripheral injection. While the effects of AMD3100 on DRG have been previously reported [3,4,6–8], its spinal effects have not been studied. Multiple mechanisms would accounts for the anti-nociceptive effects of intrathecal AMD3100, as CXCR4 is expressed on neuron, glia and other cell types in the lumbar spinal cord [9,10]. Therefore, in the current study, we explored its effects on well-known pain pathways and molecules at the lumbar spinal cord.

GPCR coupled signaling, including MAPKs, PI3K, STAT3 and NF-κB pathways, are proposed to function in CXCR4 signaling, and these pathways are also activated in the lumbar spinal cord following peripheral neuropathy [17–20]. As these pathways are activated by different cell type-specific mechanisms, antagonism study of intrathecal AMD3100 on these pathways can explain how CXCR4 signaling works on PNP in the CNS. The present study found that, among MAPK pathways, intrathecal AMD3100 downregulated spinal phosphorylation level of JNK1 and p38, but did not affect ERK1, ERK2 or JNK2. Peripheral neuropathy activates ERK1/2 in neuron, astrocyte and microglia. pSNL-induced activation of JNK1/2 is restricted to spinal astrocyte, while, the activation of p38 is restricted to spinal microglia [17]. This study also uncovered that intrathecal AMD3100 reduced the spinal expression of p65. The family of NF-κB transcription factors is associated with neuropathic pain, and the activation (increase in expression) of these factors is selectively restricted in spinal glial cells (astrocyte and microglia) [18,24]. Peripheral neuropathy also activates STAT3 (restricted to spinal microglia [20]) and AKT (restricted to spinal neuron [19]); however our present study did not found any effect of intrathecal AMD3100 on STAT3 or AKT pathways. Therefore, this research found that, among pain-related CGRP pathways, some pathways activated in spinal glial cells would account for anti-nociceptive effects of intrathecal AMD3100.

This research also studied the effects of intrathecal AMD3100 on pain-related molecules. Our study showed that AMD3100 given intrathecally reduced the spinal production of SP and increased that of AM, but its effects on CGRP were not detectable. SP is locally expressed by secondary sensory neuron at the lumbar spinal cord [25], and spinal SP expression is inducible following neuropathy, implicating that SP may account for the pain signaling to higher level of nociceptive structure [26]. AM is a pain-related neuropeptide with partial homology to CGRP, and recent research with transgenic technology unveiled its central role in pain processing was more complicated than previously surmised [27]. Because the presence of pre-synaptic and post-synaptic CXCR4 receptor implicates the potential interaction of CXCR4 signaling and the release of neurotransmitters [9], our results verified this hypothesis that neuronal CXCR4 may modulate SP and AM-mediated synaptic activity in central nociception. TNF-α, IL-1β and IL-6 are mainly released by spinal glial cells and contribute to the alteration of pain processing centrally [28]. Spinal production of these cytokines was transiently increased at early stage following peripheral neuropathy, implicating that these pro-inflammatory cytokines would be important to the development, but not the maintenance, of neuropathic pain [29]. Therefore, our results indicated that effects of intrathecal AMD3100 on maintenance of PNP did not involve the regulation of these pro-inflammatory cytokines. Moreover, our study found that AMD3100 given intrathecally increased the spinal mRNA level of ICAM. The blood-spinal cord barrier (BSCB) offers a specialized microenvironment for the cellular constituents of the spinal cord, and increasing evidence shows that BSCB is involved in nociception following neuropathic injury [30]. The expression level of ICAM correlates with the permeability of BSCB and the infiltration of immune cells to the CNS [31]. Therefore, this result indicated that central CXCR4 would be involved in the regulation of the permeability of BSCB and the immune response to PNP at the spinal cord. Spinal expression of EAAT-2 is decreased with peripheral neuropahty, and the prevention of downregulated EAAT-2 expression can potentially be an analgesic target [32]. Nevertheless, this studied did not show the involvement of central CXCR4 in the regulation of EAAT-2 expression.

In conclusion, this study firstly reports that central administration of CXCR4 antagonist AMD3100 can attenuate the development and the maintenance of PNP after pSNL without any impairment in motor function. Among well-known pain related pathways and molecules, the analgesic effects of intrathecal AMD3100 involve the downregulation of JNK1, p38 and p65 pathways, with the decrease in SP and the increase in AM and ICAM in the lumbar spinal cord of pSNL-injured mice. This study is an essential step toward understanding the contribution of CXCR4-mediated pain processing in CNS, which can lead to chemokine-targeted analgesia in the future.

Acknowledgments

We would like to thank Dr. Amy Cheuk Yin Lo, who assisted with animal experiments.

Author Contributions

Conceived and designed the experiments: LX CSK CCW. Performed the experiments: LX TWL QQ. Analyzed the data: LX TWL SLT QQ XZY CSK CCW. Contributed reagents/materials/analysis tools: LX TWL SLT XZY CSK CCW. Wrote the paper: LX TLW QQ.

References

1. Rostene W, Dansereau MA, Godefroy D, Van Steenwinckel J, Goazigo ARL, et al. (2011) Neurochemokines: a menage a trois providing new insights on the functions of chemokines in the central nervous system. Journal of Neurochemistry 118: 680–694.
2. Li MZ, Ransohoff RA (2008) Multiple roles of chemokine CXCL12 in the central nervous system: A migration from immunology to neurobiology. Progress in Neurobiology 84: 116–131.
3. Dubovy P, Klusakova I, Svizenska I, Brazda V (2010) Spatio-temporal changes of SDF1 and its CXCR4 receptor in the dorsal root ganglia following unilateral sciatic nerve injury as a model of neuropathic pain. Histochemistry and Cell Biology 133: 323–337.
4. Oh SB, Tran PB, Gillard SE, Hurley RW, Hammond DL, et al. (2001) Chemokines and glycoprotein 120 produce pain hypersensitivity by directly exciting primary nociceptive neurons. Journal of Neuroscience 21: 5027–5035.
5. Bhangoo S, Ren D, Miller RJ, Henry KJ, Lineswala J, et al. (2007) Delayed functional expression of neuronal chemokine receptors following focal nerve demyelination in the rat: a mechanism for the development of chronic sensitization of peripheral nociceptors. Molecular Pain 3: 38.
6. Bhangoo SK, Ren DJ, Miller RJ, Chan DM, Ripsch MS, et al. (2007) CXCR4 chemokine receptor signaling mediates pain hypersensitivity in association with antiretroviral toxic neuropathy. Brain Behavior and Immunity 21: 581–591.
7. Bhangoo SK, Ripsch MS, Buchanan DJ, Miller RJ, White FA (2009) Increased chemokine signaling in a model of HIV1-associated peripheral neuropathy. Molecular Pain 5: 48.
8. Wilson NM, Jung HS, Ripsch MS, Miller RJ, White FA (2011) CXCR4 signaling mediates morphine-induced tactile hyperalgesia. Brain Behavior and Immunity 25: 565–573.
9. Reaux-Le Goazigo A, Rivat C, Kitabgi P, Pohl M, Parsadaniantz SM (2012) Cellular and subcellular localization of CXCL12 and CXCR4 in rat nociceptive structures: physiological relevance. European Journal of Neuroscience 36: 2619–2631.
10. Knerlich-Lukoschus F, von der Ropp-Brenner B, Lucius R, Mehdorn HM, Held-Feindt J (2011) Spatiotemporal CCR1, CCL3(MIP-1 alpha), CXCR4, CXCL12(SDF-1 alpha) expression patterns in a rat spinal cord injury model of posttraumatic neuropathic pain. Journal of Neurosurgery-Spine 14: 583–597.
11. Bennett GJ, Xie YK (1988) A peripheral mononeuropathy in rat that produces disorders of pain sensation like those seen in man. Pain 33: 87–107.
12. Fairbanks CA (2003) Spinal delivery of analgesics in experimental models of pain and analgesia. Advanced Drug Delivery Reviews 55: 1007–1041.
13. Hung VKL, Chen SMY, Tai LW, Chen AYS, Chung SK, et al. (2012) Over-expression of endothelin-1 in astrocytes, but not endothelial cells, ameliorates inflammatory pain response after formalin injection. Life Sciences 91: 618–622.
14. Rigaud M, Gemes G, Barabas ME, Chernoff DI, Abram SE, et al. (2008) Species and strain differences in rodent sciatic nerve anatomy: Implications for studies of neuropathic pain. Pain 136: 188–201.
15. Basbaum AI, Bautista DM, Scherrer G, Julius D (2009) Cellular and Molecular Mechanisms of Pain. Cell 139: 267–284.
16. Chaudhary P, Marracci GH, Bourdette DN (2006) Lipoic acid inhibits expression of ICAM-1 and VCAM-1 by CNS endothelial cells and T cell migration into the spinal cord in experimental autoimmune encephalomyelitis. Journal of Neuroimmunology 175: 87–96.
17. Ji RR, Gereau RW, Malcangio M, Strichartz GR (2009) MAP kinase and pain. Brain Research Reviews 60: 135–148.
18. Chou CW, Wong GTC, Lim G, Wang SX, Irwin MG, et al. (2011) Spatiotemporal Pattern of Concurrent Spinal and Supraspinal NF-kappa B Expression After Peripheral Nerve Injury. Journal of Pain 12: 13–21.
19. Xu JT, Tu HY, Xin WJ, Liu XG, Zhang GH, et al. (2007) Activation of phosphatidylinositol 3-kinase and protein kinase B/Akt in dorsal root ganglia and spinal cord contributes to the neuropathic pain induced by spinal nerve ligation in rats. Experimental Neurology 206: 269–279.
20. Dominguez E, Rivat C, Pommier B, Mauborgne A, Pohl M (2008) JAK/STAT3 pathway is activated in spinal cord microglia after peripheral nerve injury and contributes to neuropathic pain development in rat. Journal of Neurochemistry 107: 50–60.
21. Serrano A, Pare M, McIntosh F, Elmes SJR, Martino G, et al. (2010) Blocking spinal CCR2 with AZ889 reversed hyperalgesia in a model of neuropathic pain. Molecular Pain 6: 90.
22. Milligan ED, Zapata V, Chacur M, Schoeniger D, Biedenkapp J, et al. (2004) Evidence that exogenous and endogenous fractalkine can induce spinal nociceptive facilitation in rats. European Journal of Neuroscience 20: 2294–2302.
23. McGrath KE, Koniski AD, Maltby KM, McGann JK, Palis J (1999) Embryonic expression and function of the chemokine SDF-1 and its receptor, CXCR4. Developmental Biology 213: 442–456.
24. Meunier A, Latremoliere A, Dominguez E, Mauborgne A, Philippe S, et al. (2007) Lentiviral-mediated targeted NF-kappa B blockade in dorsal spinal cord glia attenuates sciatic nerve injury-induced neuropathic pain in the rat. Molecular Therapy 15: 687–697.
25. D'Mello R, Dickenson AH (2008) Spinal cord mechanisms of pain. British Journal of Anaesthesia 101: 8–16.
26. Malmberg AB, Basbaum AI (1998) Partial sciatic nerve injury in the mouse as a model of neuropathic pain: behavioral and neuroanatomical correlates. Pain 76: 215–222.
27. Fernandez AP, Serrano J, Martinez-Murillo R, Martinez A (2010) Lack of Adrenomedullin in the Central Nervous System Results in Apparently Paradoxical Alterations on Pain Sensitivity. Endocrinology 151: 4908–4915.

28. Watkins LR, Milligan ED, Maier SF (2001) Glial activation: a driving force for pathological pain. Trends in Neurosciences 24: 450–455.
29. Lee HL, Lee KM, Son SJ, Hwang SH, Cho HJ (2004) Temporal expression of cytokines and their receptors mRNAs in a neuropathic pain model. Neuroreport 15: 2807–2811.
30. Bartanusz V, Jezova D, Alajajian B, Digicaylioglu M (2011) The Blood-Spinal Cord Barrier: Morphology and Clinical Implications. Annals of Neurology 70: 194–206.
31. Lee SJ, Benveniste EN (1999) Adhesion molecule expression and regulation on cells of the central nervous system. Journal of Neuroimmunology 98: 77–88.
32. Nakagawa T, Kaneko S (2010) Spinal Astrocytes as Therapeutic Targets for Pathological Pain. Journal of Pharmacological Sciences 114: 347–353.

13

Human Mas-Related G Protein-Coupled Receptors-X1 Induce Chemokine Receptor 2 Expression in Rat Dorsal Root Ganglia Neurons and Release of Chemokine Ligand 2 from the Human LAD-2 Mast Cell Line

Hans Jürgen Solinski[1], Franziska Petermann[2], Kathrin Rothe[1], Ingrid Boekhoff[1], Thomas Gudermann[1], Andreas Breit[1]*

1 Walther-Straub-Institut für Pharmakologie und Toxikologie, Ludwig-Maximilians-Universität München, Munich, Germany, **2** Department of Neurology, Klinikum rechts der Isar, Technical University Munich, Munich, Germany

Abstract

Primate-specific Mas-related G protein-coupled receptors-X1 (MRGPR-X1) are highly enriched in dorsal root ganglia (DRG) neurons and induce acute pain. Herein, we analyzed effects of MRGPR-X1 on serum response factors (SRF) or nuclear factors of activated T cells (NFAT), which control expression of various markers of chronic pain. Using HEK293, DRG neuron-derived F11 cells and cultured rat DRG neurons recombinantly expressing human MRGPR-X1, we found activation of a SRF reporter gene construct and induction of the early growth response protein-1 via extracellular signal-regulated kinases-1/2 known to play a significant role in the development of inflammatory pain. Furthermore, we observed MRGPR-X1-induced up-regulation of the chemokine receptor 2 (CCR2) via NFAT, which is considered as a key event in the onset of neuropathic pain and, so far, has not yet been described for any endogenous neuropeptide. Up-regulation of CCR2 is often associated with increased release of its endogenous agonist chemokine ligand 2 (CCL2). We also found MRGPR-X1-promoted release of CCL2 in a human connective tissue mast cell line endogenously expressing MRGPR-X1. Thus, we provide first evidence to suggest that MRGPR-X1 induce expression of chronic pain markers in DRG neurons and propose a so far unidentified signaling circuit that enhances chemokine signaling by acting on two distinct yet functionally co-operating cell types. Given the important role of chemokine signaling in pain chronification, we propose that interruption of this signaling circuit might be a promising new strategy to alleviate chemokine-promoted pain.

Editor: Roland Seifert, Medical School of Hannover, United States of America

Funding: This work was supported by a grant from the "Deutsche Forschungsgemeinschaft" [grant BR 3346/3-1]. The funders had no role in study design, data collection and analysis, decision to publish, or preparation of the manuscript.

Competing Interests: The authors have declared that no competing interests exist.

* E-mail: andreas.breit@lrz.uni-muenchen.de

Introduction

Primate-specific Mas-related G protein-coupled receptors-X1 (MRGPR-X1) have originally been described to be selectively expressed in small-diameter dorsal root ganglia (DRG) neurons [1,2]. However, recently significant MRGPR-X1 mRNA levels were also detected in connective tissue mast cells (CTMC) and the leukaemia-derived human mast cell line (LAD)-2 [3,4]. The endogenous agonist of MRGPR-X1, bovine adrenal medulla (BAM) peptide 8–22, is cleaved from pro-enkephalin, and several studies reported activation of the G_q pathway by MRGPR-X1 in over-expression systems [1,5,6,7]. Studies from our laboratory revealed that MRGPR-X1 engage phospholipase-Cβ to release calcium form the endoplasmatic reticulum and activate the proalgetic transient receptor potential cation channel V1. In sharp contrast to most if not all G_q-coupled receptors MRGPR-X1 do not undergo agonist-promoted endocytosis [6,8]. In line with direct TRPV1 activation by MRGPR-X1 observed at the cellular level, application of BAM8-22 to healthy human volunteers provoked pain-like sensations pointing to acute nociceptive functions of MRGPR-X1 [9]. In contrast, over-expression of MRGPR-X1 in rat dorsal root ganglia (DRG) neurons resulted in BAM8-22-mediated inhibition of voltage-gated calcium currents via $G_{i/o}$ proteins believed to blunt pain perception [10]. Thus, MRGPR-X1 play a significant role in acute human pain perception, but the underlying signaling pathways are still poorly defined. Furthermore, the impact of MRGPR-X1 on gene expression still remains largely elusive. This is of particular interest, because alterations in gene expression are often associated with chronic pain syndromes. In general, G protein-activating neuropeptides have been reported to affect gene expression via cAMP response elements (CRE) or serum response elements (SRE). CRE is activated by means of its interaction with the CRE binding protein (CREB) [11], whereas SRE activity is enhanced after binding to serum response factors (SRF) and to ternary complex factors (TCF) such as the E twenty-six-like transcription factor-1 (ELK-1) [12]. Interactions between CRE and CREB are enhanced after phosphorylation of the latter protein by numerous

Table 1. Primer sequences used for RTQ-PCR experiments.

gene number	name	forward primer	reverse primer
NM_031144.2	β-actin	Ggctcctagcaccatgaaga	atctgctggaaggtggacag
NM_022197.2	c-Fos	Gggacagcctttcctactacc	gatctgcgcaaaagtcctgt
NM_001013146.1	FosB	Acgccgagtcctactccag	tctcctcctcttcgggagac
NM_001109302.1	SRF	Gcacagacctcacgcaga	atgtggccacccacagtt
NM_021836.2	JunB	Gggactgggagctcatacc	aaagggtggtgcatgtgg
NM_012551.2	EGR-1	Cgaacaaccctacgagcac	gcgccttctcgttattcaga
NM_053633.1	EGR-2	Ctacccggtggaagacctc	aatgttgatcatgccatctcc
NM_017086.1	EGR-3	Caatctgtaccccgaggaga	ccgatgtccatcacattctct
NM_019137.1	EGR-4	Gccctcttcaacctcatgtct	ggggaaagggacatccag
NM_024388.1	Nur77	Tgttgatgttcctgcctttg	ggaggccatgtcgatcag
NM_001106009.1	Ldb2	Cagtgctgggaacacaacc	ttggctctcctaccaccatc
NM_017334.1	Crem2	Ctgctttgccacaaggtgt	cgacattctttagcagcttcc
NM_001110860.1	Crem3	Actagcacggggcaatacat	accatcagatcctgggttagaa
NM_153626.1	Npas4	Agggtttgctgatgagttgc	tcccctccacttccatctt
NM_031327.2	Cyr61	Ggatctgtgaagtgcgtcct	ctgcatttcttgccctttt
NM_022266.2	Ctgf	gctgacctagaggaaaacattaaga	ccggtaggtcttcacactgg
NM_021866.1	CCR2	aagaagtatccaagagcttgatgag	tcaccatcatcatagtcatacgg
NM_001007235.1	IP3R-1	Catccagtatggcaacgtga	tcatggcgttcttctccagt
NM_031530.1	CCL2	Agcatccacgtgctgtctc	gatcatcttgccagtgaatgag
NM_017232.3	COX-2	tccaacctctcctactacaccag	tccagaacttcttttgaatcagg
NM_012513.3	BDNF	Agcgcgaatgtgttagtggt	gcaattgtttgcctcttttct

down-stream kinases of GPCR signaling such as protein kinase A or extracellular signal-regulated kinases-1/2 (ERK-1/2) [13]. Likewise, the affinity of the ELK-1/SRF/SRE complex is increased after phosphorylation of ELK-1 by ERK-1/2 [14]. Recent data also suggested a role for calcium/calcineurin-induced activation of nuclear factors of activated T cells (NFAT) in G protein-coupled receptor (GPCR)-promoted gene expression [15,16]. Of note, CREB-, TCF/SRF- or NFAT-dependent gene expression is thought to induce maladaptive processes leading to neuronal dysfunction or pain chronification [16,17,18,19,20,21].

Given the strong link between alterations in gene expression and pain chronification we herein analyzed effects of BAM8-22 on gene expression-regulating signaling pathways in previously reported human HEK293 or F11 (rat DRG neurons × murine NG18TG-2) cells stably expressing MRGPR-X1 and in cultured rat DRG neurons transiently expressing MRGPR-X1 [6,8]. We observed that MRGPR-X1 induce gene expression in all three cell models tested and of particular interest that BAM8-22-induced expression of chemokine receptors 2 (CCR2), which has been linked to neuropathic pain syndromes [22,23]. In LAD-2 mast cells endogenously expressing MRGPR-X1, we detected significant release of the endogenous CCR2 agonist chemokine ligand 2 (CCL2) after BAM8-22 stimulation. Thus, we propose a MRGPR-X1-induced chemokine signaling circuit that involves induction of CCR2 expression in DRG neurons and CCL2 release in mast cells.

Materials and Methods

Materials and Plasmid

All cell culture reagents were purchased from Invitrogen (Darmstadt, Germany). PromoFectin® was from PromoCell (Heidelberg, Germany). Anti-pERK-1/2 (E-4), anti-EGR-1 (C-19) and anti-ERK-2 antiserum (C-14) were obtained from Santa Cruz Biotechnology (Heidelberg, Germany). Monoclonal anti-mouse/rat-CCR2 antibody, conjugated to allophycocyanin (APC) and the CCL2 ELISA kit were obtained from R&D systems (Wiesbaden, Germany) and peroxidase-conjugated anti-mouse or anti-rabbit antibody, both raised in goat, were obtained from Sigma-Aldrich (Deisenhofen, Germany). BSA, forskolin (FSK), poly-L-ornithine and poly-L-lysine were from Sigma-Aldrich and fura2-acetoxymethyl ester was obtained from Fluka (Deisenhofen, Germany). Coelenterazine H was purchased from Biaffin (Kassel, Germany) and firefly luciferase substrate was from Promega (Mannheim, Germany). [^{3}H]-adenine was obtained from PerkinElmer (Rodgau, Germany). BAM8-22 and bradykinin (BK) were purchased from Biotrend (Cologne, Germany) and rat CCL2 from Peprotech (Hamburg, Germany). Cyclosporine A (CsA) was purchased from Sigma-Aldrich and PD-184352 was from Enzo life science (Lörrach, Germany). The generation of expression vectors encoding the human MRGPR-X1 (accession number: AF474990), the rat MRGPR-C (accession number: AF518245) or the murine MRGPR-C (accession number: AY152435) fused at the N-terminus to the Xpress epitope (pcDNA4-MRGPR-X1, pcDNA4-rMRGPR-C and pcDNA4-mMRGPR-C) was previously described [6]. The plasmid pG5α [24] encoding aequorin was kindly provided by Dr. Vladimir Chubanov (Walther-Straub-Institute, Munich, Germany). The reporter gene vector p5xSRE, carrying five repeats of the TCF/SRF-activated SRE-site (5′-GGATGTCCATATTAGGAC-ATC-3′) was kindly provided by Dr. Susanne Muehlich (Walther-Straub-Institute, Munich, Germany). The reporter gene vector p6xCRE carrying six repeats of the CREB-activated CRE site and the reporter gene vector pGL4.30 carrying four repeats of the NFAT-activated transcription site were obtained from Promega.

Cell culture and transfections

HEK293 cells were cultured in DMEM (10% FBS, 2 mM L-glutamine, penicillin/streptomycin) and F11 (rat DRG neurons × murine NG18TG-2) cells in HAM's F-12 (15% FBS, 2 mM L-glutamine, hypoxanthine-aminopterin-thymidine, G-418 and penicillin/streptomycin). F11 cells were generated by Francel et al., [25] and kindly provided by Dr. Mederos y Schnitzler (Philipps University, Marburg, Germany). The CTMC line LAD-2 [26] was kindly provided from Dr. Arnold S. Kirshenbaum (National Institute of Allergy and Infectious Diseases, Bethesda, USA) and cultured in StemPro 34 (2 mM L-glutamine, nutrient supplement, 100 ng/ml recombinant human stem cell factor, penicillin/streptomycin). HEK293-MRGPR-X1, HEK293-rMRGPR-C, HEK293-mMRGPR-C and F11-MRGPR-X1 cells were described previously [6]. HEK293 cells stably expressing either receptor were subjected to a second selection (250 µg/ml G418 and 50 µg/ml zeocin) after transfection with the calcium sensing aequorin-eGFP construct pG5α to give HEK293-MRGPR-X1-Ae, HEK293-rMRGPR-C-Ae and HEK293-mMRGPR-C-Ae cells, respectively. The expression of the fusion proteins was controlled by measuring agonist-induced calcium releases and by fluorescence microscopy. Primary DRG neurons from day 18 embryonic Sprague/Dawley rats were purchased from Innoprot (Derio – Bizkaia, Spain) and cultured in NeuroBasal medium (B-27 supplement, 10% FBS, 2 mM L-glutamine, penicillin/streptomycin/neomycin) on poly-L-ornithine-coated well plates. For transient protein expression in HEK293 cells or DRG neurons PromoFectin® reagent was used according to the manufacturer's protocol. F11 cells were transfected using the Neon® transfection system from Invitrogen accordingly to settings provided by the manufacturer.

Fura2-based single cell calcium imaging

24 h prior to the experiment F11-MRGPR-X1 cells were seeded at a density of 4–6×10^4 cells on glass cover slips in 6-well plates coated with 0.1% poly-L-lysine. Cells were loaded with 5 µM fura2-AM in HEPES-buffered saline (HBS, 10 mM HEPES, 5 mM KCl, 1 mM $MgCl_2$, 140 mM NaCl, 0.1% glucose and 2 mM $CaCl_2$ adjusted to pH 7.4 with 1 M NaOH) supplemented with 0.02% pluronic F-127. Cover slips were washed twice with HBS without BSA and placed in a recording chamber. Cells were analyzed using a Polychrome 5000 monochromator (Till-Photonics, Gräfelfing, Germany) and an Andor charge-coupled device camera coupled to an inverted microscope (IX71, Olympus, Hamburg, Germany) by alternately exciting with 340 nm or 380 nm, respectively, every 0.5 s. Normalized fura2-ratios (340/380) were then plotted against the time in seconds.

Fura2-based calcium measurements with a plate reader

Calcium transients in MRGPR-X1 or rodent MRGPR-C expressing HEK293, F11-MRGPR-X1 or LAD-2 cells were measured with a FLUOstar® Omega plate reader (BMG Labtech, Ortenberg, Germany) as described previously [6] using the fluorescent calcium indicator fura2. To determine concentration-response curves, integrated calcium signals were calculated, normalized to responses to maximal ligand concentrations (100%) and then subjected to curve fitting.

Aequorin-based calcium measurements

Total luminescence in HEK293-MRGPR-Ae cells or DRG neurons transfected with the aequorin encoding plasmid G5α was measured using a FLUOstar® Omega plate reader at 37°C after labelling of the cells with coelenterazine H (5 µM) for 30 min at room temperature. HBS as a control or HBS including BAM8-22 was automatically injected 5 s after starting the measurement. In intervals of 1 s total emission was measured and is given as arbitrary units against the time in seconds.

Western-Blotting

Cells were serum-starved for 24 h, stimulated for the indicated period of time with BAM8-22 or BK and then lysed in laemmli buffer. After SDS-PAGE and protein transfer to nitrocellulose, ERK-1/2 phosphorylation or EGR-1 expression was analyzed by using either a phospho-specific ERK-1/2 (p-ERK-1/2: 1:3,000) or an EGR-1 specific (EGR1: 1:10,000) antiserum and the corresponding peroxidase-coupled secondary antibody (1:10,000). Membranes were stripped and then re-probed with an anti-ERK-2 antibody (t-ERK-2: 1:10,000) and the corresponding peroxidase-coupled secondary antibody (1:10,000). Immuno-reactivity was quantified by densitometry, ratios between p-ERK-1/2 or EGR-1 and t-ERK-2 signals were calculated, and ligand-induced ERK-1/2 phosphorylation/EGR-1 expression was normalized to not stimulated cells.

Reporter gene assays

After transfection of a firefly luciferase reporter gene construct DRG neurons were serum-starved for 1 h and F11 or HEK293 cells for 24 h. Afterwards cells were stimulated with BAM8-22, BK or FSK for the indicated time in serum-free medium. Small molecule inhibitors (concentration as indicated) and the respective carrier control were pre-incubated for 30 minutes before addition of agonist and present during ligand stimulation. After stimulation cells were lysed (25 mM Tris/HCl pH 7.4, 4 mM EGTA, 8 mM $MgCl_2$, 1 mM DTT and 1% Triton-X-100) and luciferase activity measured in white bottom 96-well plates after automatically injecting luciferase substrate and simultaneous detection of total light emission for 7.5 s post injection in a FLUOstar® Omega plate reader. Maximal light emission during this period was recorded and is indicated relative to not stimulated cells.

RT-PCR

DRG neurons were serum-starved for 1 h and F11 or HEK293 cells for 24 h. Afterwards cells were stimulated with BAM8-22 or BK for the indicated period of time in serum-free medium. Total RNA from these cells or from not stimulated LAD-2 cells was isolated using the Tri reagent® (Sigma-Aldrich) according to the manufacturer's instructions. First strand synthesis was carried out with oligo$(dT)_{18}$ primer using 2 µg of total RNA and the RevertAid™ H Minus First Strand cDNA Synthesis Kit (Fermentas, Sankt-Leon Roth, Germany). Quantitative RT-PCR (RTQ-PCR) was done using the LightCycler® 480 SybrGreen I Master Mix (Roche, Mannheim, Germany), 0.08 µl of the first strand synthesis reaction and 1 µM of the primer pairs shown in table 1. Samples were analyzed in a LightCycler® 480 (Roche) using the following conditions: initial denaturation for 15 min at 94°C, 55 cycles of 94°C for 10 sec, 55°C for 10 sec and 72°C for 10 sec. Crossing points (Cp) were determined by the software supplied with the LightCycler® 480 and ligand-induced modulation of target gene expression was calculated relative to β-actin using the ΔΔCp method. Non-quantitative RT-PCR was conducted in cDNA from LAD-2 cells using specific primers for MRGPR-X1 (forward: 5′-tgagtctctgatctgccctct-3′, reverse: 5′-tcaccagctgtatgatctctgatt-3′) or β-actin (forward: 5′-ccaaccgcgagaagatga-3′, reverse: 5′-ccagaggcgtacagggatag-3′). PCR settings were the same as in RTQ-PCR and the number of amplification cycles is indicated in the figure legend.

Flow cytometry

Cells were serum-starved for 4 h and stimulated for 20 h in serum-free medium with BAM8-22, detached with PBS/2 mM EDTA, washed once with PBS/10% FBS and stained with anti-rat-CCR2-APC antibody or the corresponding isotype for 30 minutes at room temperature. After two washing steps cells were resuspended in PBS/10% FBS and analyzed by flow cytometry (CyAn ADP, Beckman Coulter).

cAMP accumulation assay

To determine CCL2-promoted inhibition of forskolin-induced cAMP accumulation, F11 cells were seeded in 12-plates dishes coated with 0.1% polyl-L-lysine 24 h prior to the experiment. Afterwards cells were serum-starved for 4 h, stimulated for 20 h with BAM8-22 or BK in serum-free HAM's F-12 medium containing 2 μCi/ml of [^{3}H] adenine. Cells were stimulated for 30 min at 37°C in HAM's F-12 containing 100 mM HEPES, pH 7.4, 2.5 μM IBMX, 5 μM forskolin alone or along with 100 ng/ml CCL2. The reaction was terminated by removing the medium and adding ice-cold 5% trichloroacetic acid to the cells. [^{3}H] cAMP was then purified by sequential chromatography over dowex resin and aluminium oxide, and the cAMP accumulation expressed as the total amount of [^{3}H] cAMP in DPM/well.

Data analysis

Data were analyzed using Prism4.0 (GraphPad Software Inc., San Diego, CA). Statistical significance of differences was assessed by the two-tailed Student's t-test (two groups) or by one-way analysis of variance and Tukey's honest significance post-hoc test (more than two groups). Asterisks (***$p<0.001$, **$p<0.01$, *$p<0.05$) or dagger signs ($^{\dagger\dagger\dagger}p<0.001$, $^{\dagger\dagger}p<0.01$, $^{\dagger}p<0.05$) were used to indicate significant differences between different experimental groups.

Results

BAM8-22-induced calcium release and ERK-1/2 activation in HEK293-MRGPR-X1 and F11-MRGPR-X1 cells

Binding of the specific agonist BAM8-22 to MRGPR-X1 has been described to activate G_q proteins and thus, to increase intracellular calcium concentrations [1,6,7]. Therefore, we first analyzed BAM8-22-induced calcium signals in previously reported HEK293-MRGPR-X1 or F11-MRGPR-X1 cells that stably express low levels of MRGPR-X1 [6,8]. Stimulation of MRGPR-X1 with BAM8-22 elicited calcium transients with a potency of ~200 nM (Fig. 1A+B) consistent with previous reports [1,5]. ERK-1/2 play a central role in GPCR-promoted gene induction, because ERK-1/2 enhance CREB- and TCF/SRF-dependent gene expression. Thus, we also analyzed BAM8-22-promoted ERK-1/2 phosphorylation in HEK293-MRGPR-X1 and F11-MRGPR-X1 cells. We observed marked, but transient phosphorylation of ERK-1/2 in both cell pools, with a peak at 5 min and a decline thereafter (Fig. 1C+D). Given that calcium has been reported to enhance NFAT-dependent gene expression via calcineurin, and ERK-1/2 via TCF/SRF or CREB, we postulated that BAM8-22 might induce CREB-, TCF/SRF- or NFAT-dependent gene expression in MRGPR-X1 expressing cells.

BAM8-22-induced activation of TCF/SRF- and NFAT-dependent reporters in HEK293-MRGPR-X1 and F11-MRGPR-X1 cells

To test the ability of BAM8-22 to induce gene expression via MRGPR-X1, we used HEK293-MRGPR-X1 and F11-MRGPR-X1 cells to perform reporter gene assays employing constructs that contained binding sites for TCF/SRF, NFAT or CREB. Stimulation of both cell types with BAM8-22 led to activation of the TCF/SRF reporter (Fig. 2A+D) preventable by a specific ERK-1/2 inhibitor (PD-184352), and of the NFAT reporter sensitive to CsA, an inhibitor of the NFAT activator calcineurin (Fig. 2B+E). In contrast, BAM8-22-induced activation of the CREB reporter was not observed in either MRGPR-X1 expressing cell type (Fig. 2C+F).

BAM8-22-induced expression of c-Fos and EGR-1 via ERK-1/2 in F11-MRGPR-X1 cells

To gain deeper insight into BAM8-22-induced expression of TCF/SRF-dependent genes, we analyzed mRNA levels of 15 genes reported to be up-regulated by TCF/SRF in neurons [18]. As shown in figure 3A, mRNA levels of c-Fos and EGR-1 were significantly elevated in F11-MRGPR-X1 cells after 1 h of BAM8-22 stimulation and total EGR-1 protein levels significantly increased after challenging the cells with BAM8-22 for 1 to 2 h (Fig. 3B). Because c-Fos and EGR-1 mRNA induction was blocked by PD-184352 (Fig. 3C and D), we concluded that ERK-1/2 activity is required for BAM8-22-induced expression of TCF/SRF-dependent genes.

BAM8-22-induced expression of IP3R-1 and CCR2 via calcineurin in F11-MRGPR-X1 cells

Recently, it has been reported that CCR2, IP3R-1, CCL2, cyclooxygenase-2 (COX-2) or the brain-derived neurotrophic factor are up-regulated by NFAT in neurons [16,17,27]. Thus, we analyzed effects of BAM8-22 on the mRNA levels of these genes in F11-MRGPR-X1 cells. As shown in figure 4, IP3R-1 and CCR2 were up-regulated after 6 h of BAM8-22 incubation in a CsA-dependent manner, indicating that BAM8-22 induces expression of both genes via calcium/calcineurin-mediated NFAT activation in F11-MRGPR-X1 cells. BAM8-22-induced expression of CCR2 is of particular interest, because enhanced CCR2 expression in DRG neurons is strongly associated with various neuropathic pain syndromes [28]. To further corroborate our observation of BAM8-22-induced CCR2 mRNA expression, we performed flow cytometry experiments with F11-MRGPR-X1 cells and an APC-conjugated CCR2 specific antibody (Fig. 4D). Stimulation of cells with BAM8-22 increased the amount of CCR2 positive cells by 10.8±1.4%, demonstrating that BAM8-22-promoted induction of CCR2 mRNA is translated into increased expression of the CCR2 protein. To test whether BAM8-22-induced CCR2 expression was sufficient to affect the sensitivity of F11-MRGPR-X1 cells to CCL2, we took advantage of the $G_{i/o}$ coupling of CCR2 and performed cAMP accumulation assays with BAM8-22-treated cells. As shown in figure 4E, untreated F11-MRGPR-X1 cells did not respond to CCL2, whereas BAM8-22-pre-treated F11-MRGPR-X1 cells significantly responded to the peptide, such that the CCR2 specific agonist reduced FSK-induced cAMP accumulation by 23.8±4.3%, comparable to the effects of various opioids acting on endogenous opioid receptors constitutively expressed in F11 cells [29]. Therefore, we concluded that BAM8-22 enhances the expression of functional CCR2 in F11-MRGPR-X1 cells, thus enabling CCL2 to engage cognate signaling pathways in DRG neuron-derived cells.

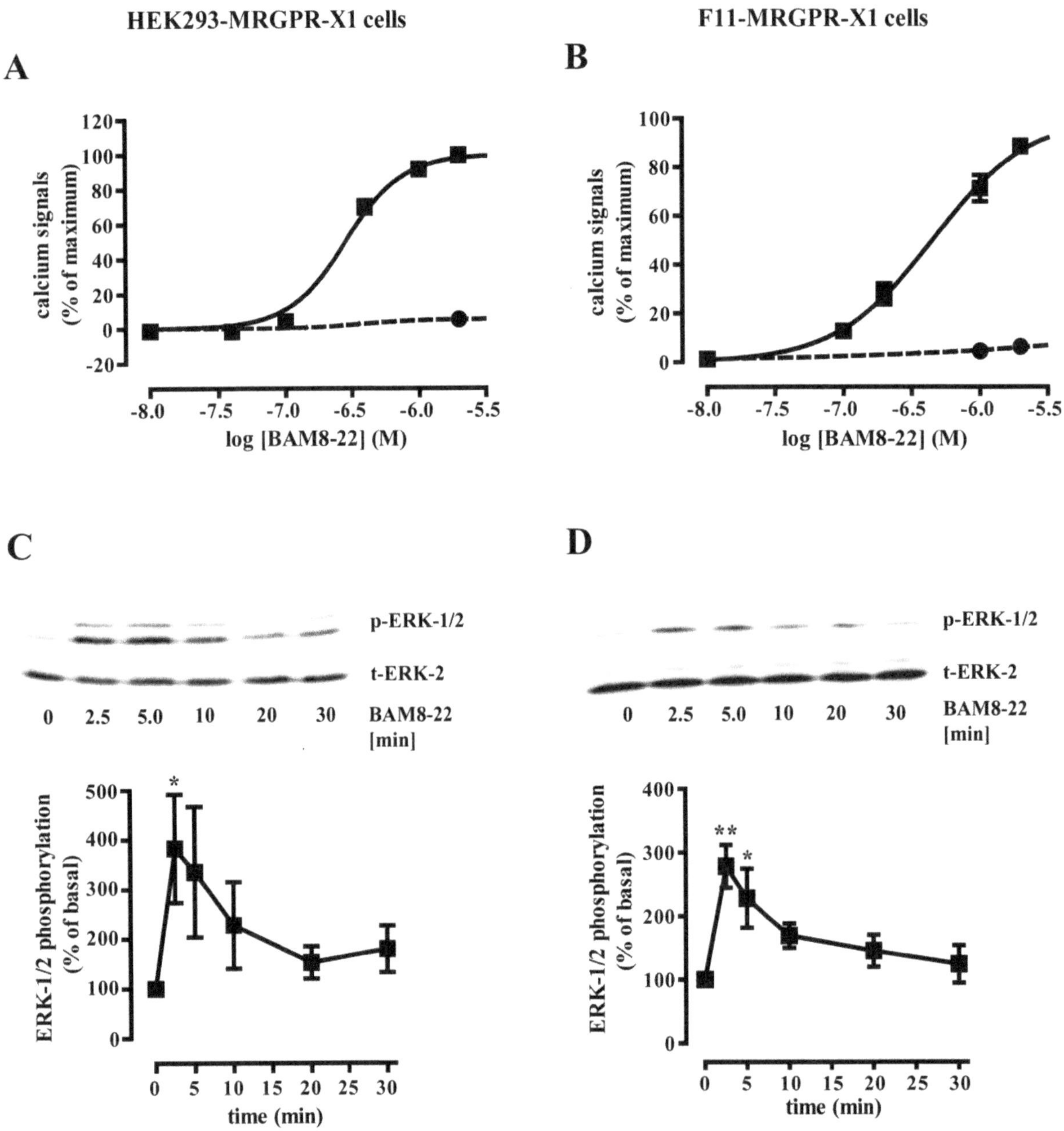

Figure 1. MRGPR-X1 stimulate ERK-1/2 in HEK293- and F11-MRGPR-X1 cells. Concentration response curves of BAM8-22-promoted calcium signals in fura2-loaded HEK293-MRGPR-X1 (A) or in F11-MRGPR-X1 (B) cells (squares) or mock cells (circles) are shown. BAM8-22-induced (1 µM) phosphorylation of ERK-1/2 in HEK293-MRGPR-X1 (C) or in F11-MRGPR-X1 (D) cells was analyzed by western-blotting using a phospho-specific antibody (p-ERK-1/2). Afterwards blots were stripped and re-probed with an antibody against ERK-2 (t-ERK-2). One representative blot is shown. Ligand-induced ERK-1/2 phosphorylation was quantified by densitometry and is given normalized to not stimulated cells. Data from 4 experiments were compiled and expressed as the mean ± S.E.M. Asterisks indicate significant differences to not stimulated cells.

Bradykinin induces EGR-1 expression via ERK-1/2 but not CCR2 expression via NFAT

Next we asked whether other G_q protein activating neuropeptides would also induce EGR-1 and CCR2 expression in a DRG neuron-derived cell model. F11 cells have been reported to endogenously express G_q activating bradykinin-2-receptors (B2R) [25]. Thus, we first compared calcium transients triggered by BAM8-22 or BK. As shown in figure 5A, calcium signals in F11-MRGPR-X1 cells induced by saturated concentrations (EC_{95}) of BK or BAM8-22 were almost identical illustrating that activation of recombinant MRGPR-X1 did not elicit unphysiological high calcium transients. Furthermore, BK induced EGR-1 expression (Fig. 5B+C) in accord with previously observed effects of BK on EGR-1 expression in human fibroblasts or NG108-15 neuroblastoma cells [30,31]. BK also activated the NFAT reporter (Fig. 5D) and also induced IP3R-1 mRNA expression via NFAT (Fig. 5E). However, despite these similarities, BK treatment did neither induce CCR2 mRNA expression (Fig. 5E), nor did it impart CCL2 sensitivity to F11-MRGPR-X1 cells (Fig. 5F), suggesting that CCR2 induction is not a common feature among G_q

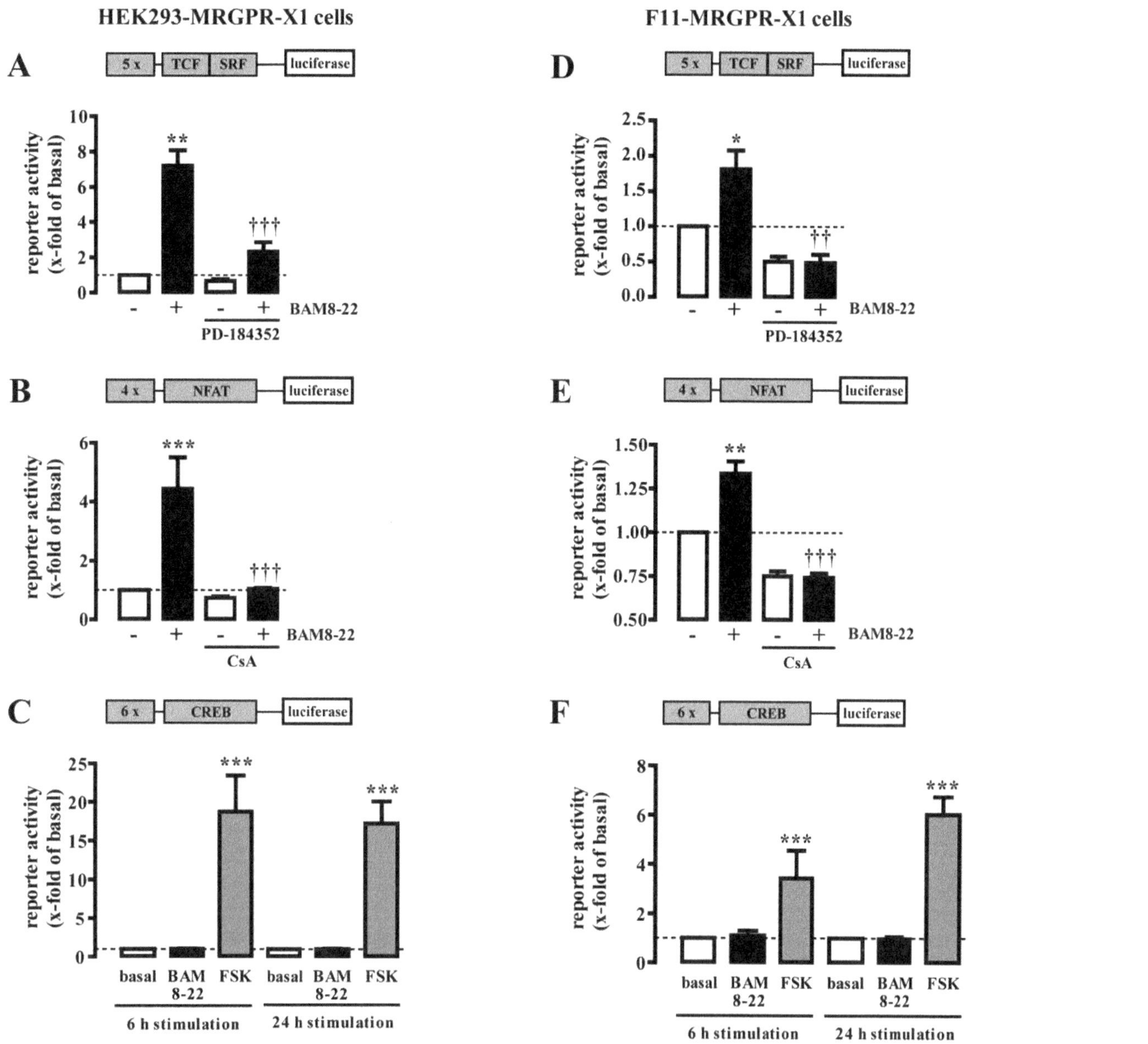

Figure 2. MRGPR-X1 stimulate TCF/SRF- and NFAT-dependent reporter in HEK293- and F11-MRGPR-X1 cells. TCF/SRF-, NFAT- or CREB-dependent reporter gene constructs were transfected into HEK293-MRGPR-X1 (A–C) or in F11-MRGPR-X1 (D–F) cells. Cells were stimulated with 1 μM BAM8-22 for 6 h or as indicated. 5 μM FSK was used as a control for the CREB reporter. CsA (1 μM, 30 min) was used to block the NFAT activator calcineurin and PD-184352 (10 μM, 30 min) to block ERK-1/2 activity. Data from 3–5 independent experiments performed in triplicates were compiled and expressed as the mean ± S.E.M. Asterisks indicate significant differences to not stimulated cells. Dagger signs indicate significant differences between BAM8-22-stimulated inhibitor-treated and untreated cells.

activating neuropeptides, but a characteristic property of MRGPR-X1.

BAM8-22-induced CCR2 and EGR-1 mRNA expression in cultured rat DRG neurons

To substantiate our observations that MRGPR-X1 induce expression of chronic pain markers, we used DRG neurons from day 18 embryonic rats and transfected them with MRGPR-X1 cDNA after 10–14 days in culture. As shown in figure 6A, only MRGPR-X1 expressing DRG neurons reacted to BAM8-22 with robust calcium signals. Furthermore, similar to F11-MRGPR-X1 cells, stimulation of MRGPR-X1 expressing DRG neurons with BAM8-22 increased the activity of the NFAT (Fig. 6B) and the TCF/SRF reporter (Fig. 6C), suggesting that enhancing effects of BAM8-22 on gene expression are not restricted to the F11 cell line, but also occur in cultured DRG neurons. In line with this notion, BAM8-22 also elevated CCR2 mRNA levels in a CsA-sensitive (Fig. 6D) and EGR-1 transcripts in a PD-184352-dependent manner (Fig. 6E), supporting our finding that BAM8-22 induces CCR2 and EGR-1 expression in DRG neurons.

BAM8-22-promoted CCL2 release in LAD-2 cells

So far, MRGPR-X1 are thought to be exclusively expressed in DRG neurons and therefore were originally termed sensory

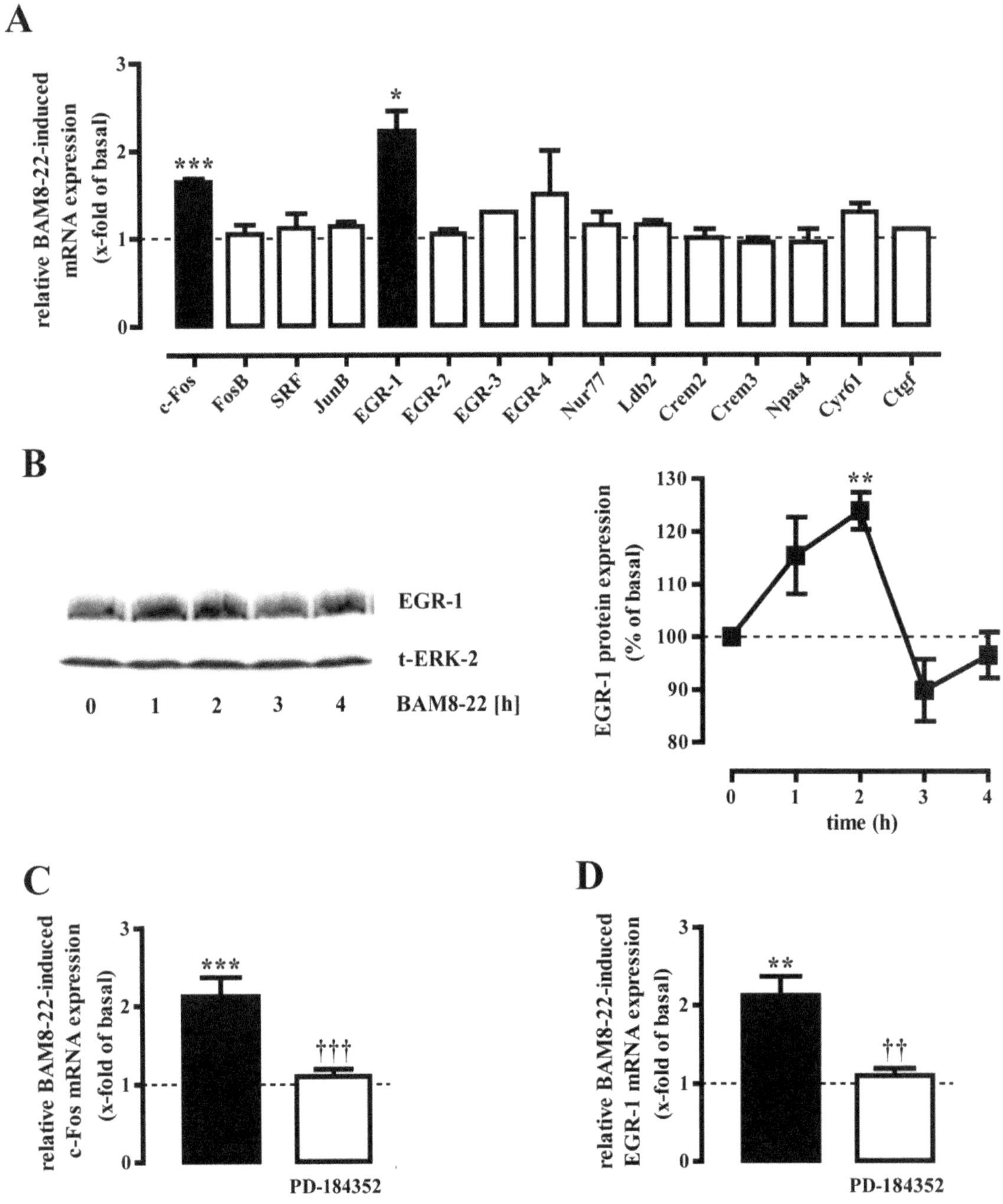

Figure 3. MRGPR-X1 induce EGR-1 via ERK-1/2 in F11-MRGPR-X1 cells. RTQ-PCR experiments were performed with cDNAs derived from serum-starved F11-MRGPR-X1 cells stimulated or not with BAM8-22 (1 μM) for 1 h (A, C and D) using specific primers for 15 distinct genes as indicated in table 1. The name of the analyzed gene is listed beneath the corresponding bar. Genes with a p value <0.05 are show in black bars. In (C and D) cells were treated or not with PD-184352 (30 min, 10 μM). Relative BAM8-22-induced gene expression was normalized to β-actin and calculated using the ΔΔCp method. In (B) serum-starved F11-MRGPR-X1 cells were stimulated or not with BAM8-22 (1 μM) for the indicated period of time and expression of EGR-1 was determined by western-blotting. Afterwards blots were stripped and re-probed with an antibody against ERK-2 (t-ERK-2). One representative blot is shown. Ligand-induced EGR-1 expression was quantified by densitometry and is given normalized to not stimulated cells. Data from 4 independent experiments were compiled and expressed as the mean ± S.E.M. Asterisk indicate a significant difference to not stimulated cells. Dagger signs indicate a significant difference between BAM8-22-stimulated inhibitor-treated and untreated cells.

neuron-specific GPCR [1]. Recently, significant mRNA levels of MRGPR-X1 were detected in native CTMC and in the human LAD-2 mast cell line [4]. In theses lines, we detected significant MRGPR-X1 transcripts in LAD-2-derived cDNA samples (Fig. 7A). However, activation of the MRGPR-X1 protein by its specific agonist BAM8-22 has not been demonstrated yet. Thus, we took advantage of LAD-2 cells and performed fura2-based calcium measurements in order to monitor activation of the MRGPR-X1 protein by its specific agonist BAM8-22. As shown in figure 7B, BAM8-22 induced robust calcium transients in LAD-2 cells, indicating endogenous expression of functional MRGPR-X1. Next, we asked whether BAM8-22-induced signaling would affect

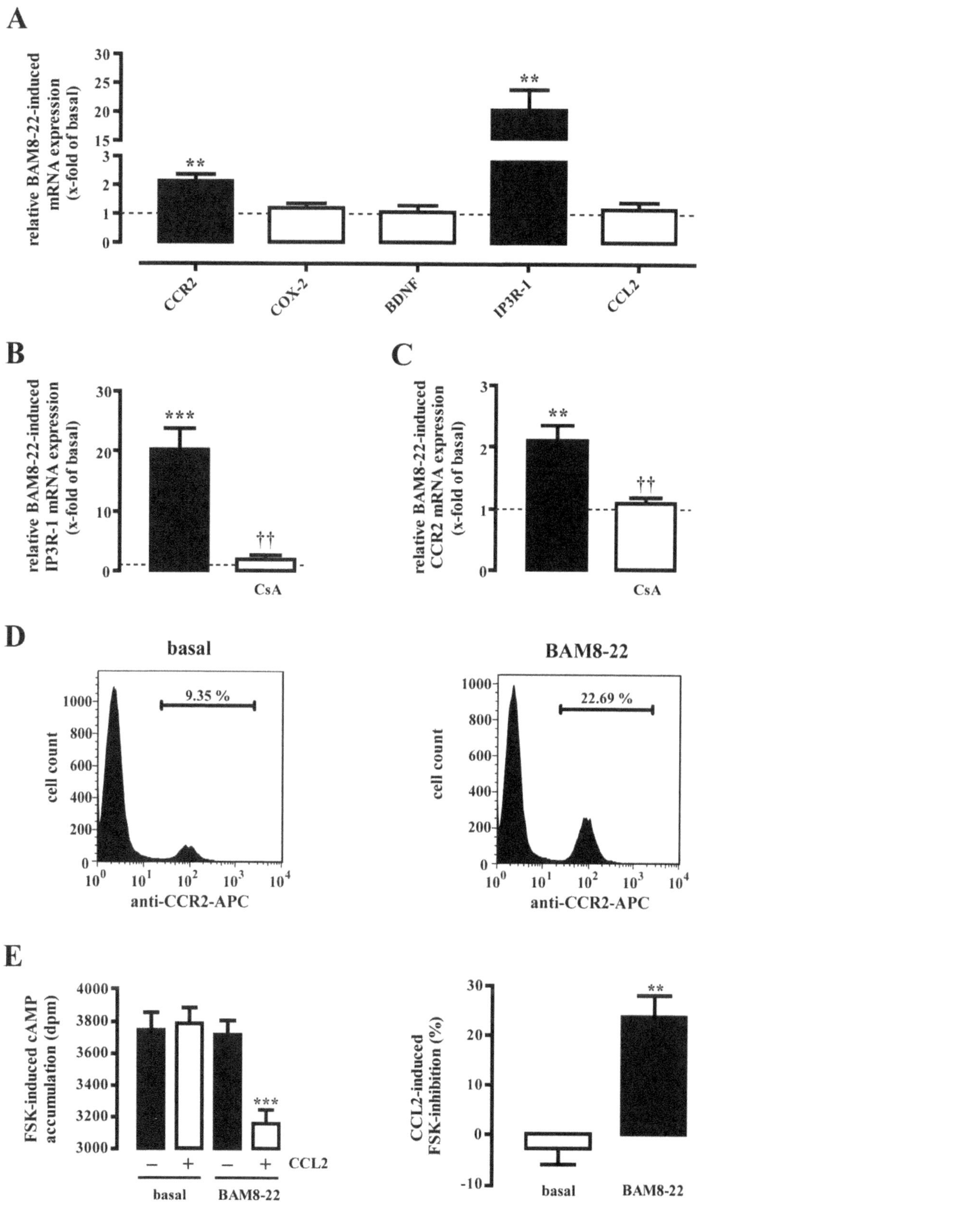

Figure 4. MRGPR-X1 induce CCR2 via NFAT in F11-MRGPR-X1 cells. RTQ-PCR experiments were performed with cDNAs derived from serum-starved F11-MRGPR-X1 cells stimulated or not with BAM8-22 (1 μM) for 6 h (A-C) using specific primers for 5 distinct genes as indicated in table 1. The name of the analyzed gene is listed beneath the corresponding bar. Genes with a p value <0.05 are show in black bars. In (B and C) cells were treated or not with CsA (1 μM, 30 min). Relative BAM8-22-induced gene expression was normalized to β-actin and calculated using the ΔΔCp method. Data from 4 independent experiments were compiled and expressed as the mean ± S.E.M. BAM8-22-induced (1 μM, 20 h) CCR2 protein expression in F11-MRGPR-X1 cells was assessed by flow cytometry (D) or by CCL2-promoted (100 ng/ml) inhibition of FSK-induced (5 μM) cAMP accumulation (E). In (D)

one representative experiment is shown. Accumulation of the data from 5 independent experiments revealed an increase in the number of CCR2 positive cells by 10.8±1.4% after BAM8-22 stimulation. In (E, left panel) one representative experiment is shown and in (E, right panel) data from 5 independent experiments performed in triplicates were compiled and expressed as the mean ± S.E.M. Asterisks indicate a significant difference to not stimulated cells. Dagger signs indicate a significant difference between BAM8-22-stimulated inhibitor-treated and untreated cells.

CCL2 release in LAD-2 cells. Notably, when performing ELISA assays with an antibody specific to human CCL2, we observed that the chemokine was released into the supernatant of LAD-2 cells in response to BAM8-22 (Fig. 7C), indicating that MRGPR-X1 exert their action in cells of the peripheral nervous and the immune system.

Discussion

Primate-specific MRGPR-X1 are selectively expressed in DRG neurons and therefore represent promising targets for innovative pain therapies [1,2]. Interestingly, disease-causing genes are strongly enriched among primate-specific genes [32] and the ligand-binding domain of MRGPR-X1 has been described as a product of strong positive selection [33,34], further underscoring the potential of MRGPR-X1 as therapeutic targets. Despite the high therapeutic potential of MRGPR-X1, hardly any information about the role of this receptor subtype in pain chronification is available. Herein, we analyzed BAM8-22-induced gene expression in HEK293 and F11 cells stably expressing MRGPR-X1. We observed activation of a NFAT- and TCF/SRF-, but not of a CREB-dependent reporter. In-depth analysis of F11-MRGPR-X1 cells confirmed these findings, because BAM8-22-induced ERK-1/2 or calcineurin activation led to significant up-regulation of c-Fos, EGR-1, IP3R-1 and CCR2 mRNA. Thus, our data provide first evidence of BAM8-22-induced gene expression in DRG neuron-derived cells. F11 cells emerged as a valuable biological tool for the analysis of DRG neuron-related signaling pathways, since many studies reported striking similarities to cultured DRG neurons [25,27,35,36,37,38,39,40,41,42,43]. Along these lines, data from our laboratory revealed morphine-induced expression of the early growth response protein-4 via μ opioid receptors in F11 cells and cultured rat DRG neurons [29]. In the same vein, we confirmed BAM8-22-promoted activation of the NFAT or TCF/SRF reporter and enhanced CCR2 or EGR-1 mRNA expression in cultured rat DRG neurons transiently expressing MRGPR-X1.

BAM8-22-induced EGR-1 expression via ERK-1/2

Activated TCF/SRF complexes have been shown to induce immediate early genes such as c-Fos, c-jun or members of the EGR family in neurons of the peripheral or central nervous system and thereby modulate synaptic activity, memory and learning [18]. Herein, we observed BAM8-22-promoted up-regulation of c-Fos and EGR-1 in F11-MRGPR-X1 cells. Induction of c-Fos in the spinal dorsal horn is an established marker of neuronal activity or noxious stimulation [44]. However, less is known about the role of c-Fos induction in DRG neurons. A recent study correlated surgery- or opioid-induced hyperalgesia with ERK-1/2 phosphorylation and c-Fos expression in DRG neurons [45], suggesting that BAM8-22-promoted c-Fos induction is in good agreement with enhanced pain sensations previously reported after BAM8-22 application in humans [9]. So far, induction of the zinc-finger transcription factor EGR-1 (also *zif/268*) in DRG neurons has been described for neurotrophins such as the nerve growth factor or tumor necrosis factor-α [46,47]. Tumor necrosis factor-α-promoted EGR-1 expression plays a significant role in carrageenan-induced inflammatory hyperalgesia [46] and selective knockdown of the EGR-1 protein significantly reduced inflammatory pain induced by complete Freund's adjuvants [48]. Furthermore, elevated EGR-1 protein levels correlate with inflammatory pain in sheep [49], strongly indicating a major contribution of EGR-1 to inflammatory pain in various species.

BAM8-22-induced CCR-2 expression via calcineurin

NFAT-induced gene expression significantly contributes to the differentiation and proliferation of lymphocytes. Recent work suggested that NFAT activation also increases the expression of pro-nociceptive genes such as COX-2 or CCR2 in neurons [17,27], indicating a significant role of NFAT-dependent gene induction for pain chronification [28]. Induction of IP3R-1 via NFAT, as shown herein for G_q-coupled MRGPR-X1, has so far been linked to the activation of receptor tyrosine kinases by neurotrophins in DRG, spinal cord and hippocampal pyramidal neurons [50] or to potassium-induced depolarisation in rat cerebellar neurons [51]. Thus, IP3R-1 is one of the best described targets of NFAT-dependent gene expression in non-immune cells, but cellular or physiological consequences of enhanced IP3R-1 expression levels in neurons have not been sorted out. Chemically induced calcium influx in F11 cells or DRG neurons by ionomycin or high potassium concentrations have been reported to induce CCR2 mRNA expression via NFAT [27]. However, G protein-promoted CCR2 induction via NFAT has not yet been described. Here, we report that stimulation of F11-MRGPR-X1 cells with BAM8-22 not only increased CCR2 mRNA and protein levels, but also imparted sensitivity to the endogenous CCR2 agonist, CCL2, to these cells. MRGPR-X1-induced CCR2 expression is of particular interest, considering that CCL2-induced activation of CCR2 in DRG neurons plays a major role in distinct neuropathic pain syndromes, as demonstrated by significantly diminished neuropathic pain responses found in mice deficient of the CCR2 gene [52] and by abolished neuropathy-induced hyperalgesia and allodynia after application of CCR2 specific antagonists to wild-type mice [22,53]. Therefore, inhibition of CCL2-promoted CCR2 signaling is a promising approach towards a future therapy of neuropathic pain. However, because of versatile physiological roles of chemokines significant side effects are expected when blocking CCR2-induced signaling *in vivo*. Of note, CCR2-deficient mice exhibited normal pain behaviour under physiological conditions and many studies showed that, similar to F11-MRGPR-X1 cells, CCR2 expression levels in DRG neurons are rather low under non-neuropathic conditions [27,28]. Hence, CCR2 up-regulation in DRG neurons emerged as a key event that initiates neuropathic pain syndromes or enhances their progress [22,23,54,55,56,57]. Within this model, controlling CCR2 expression selectively in DRG neurons would be a promising approach to block chemokine-promoted signaling and thus, to alleviate neuropathic pain syndromes without affecting CCL2/CCR2 signaling in other cell types. Herein, we define MRGPR-X1 as endogenous inducers of CCR2 in DRG neurons. Thus, although our conclusions still have to await ultimate proof by *in vivo* studies in primates, we propose a role of MRGPR-X1 in chemokine-promoted pain chronification and consider MRGPR-X1 as promising targets to selectively manipulate CCR2 expression in DRG neurons.

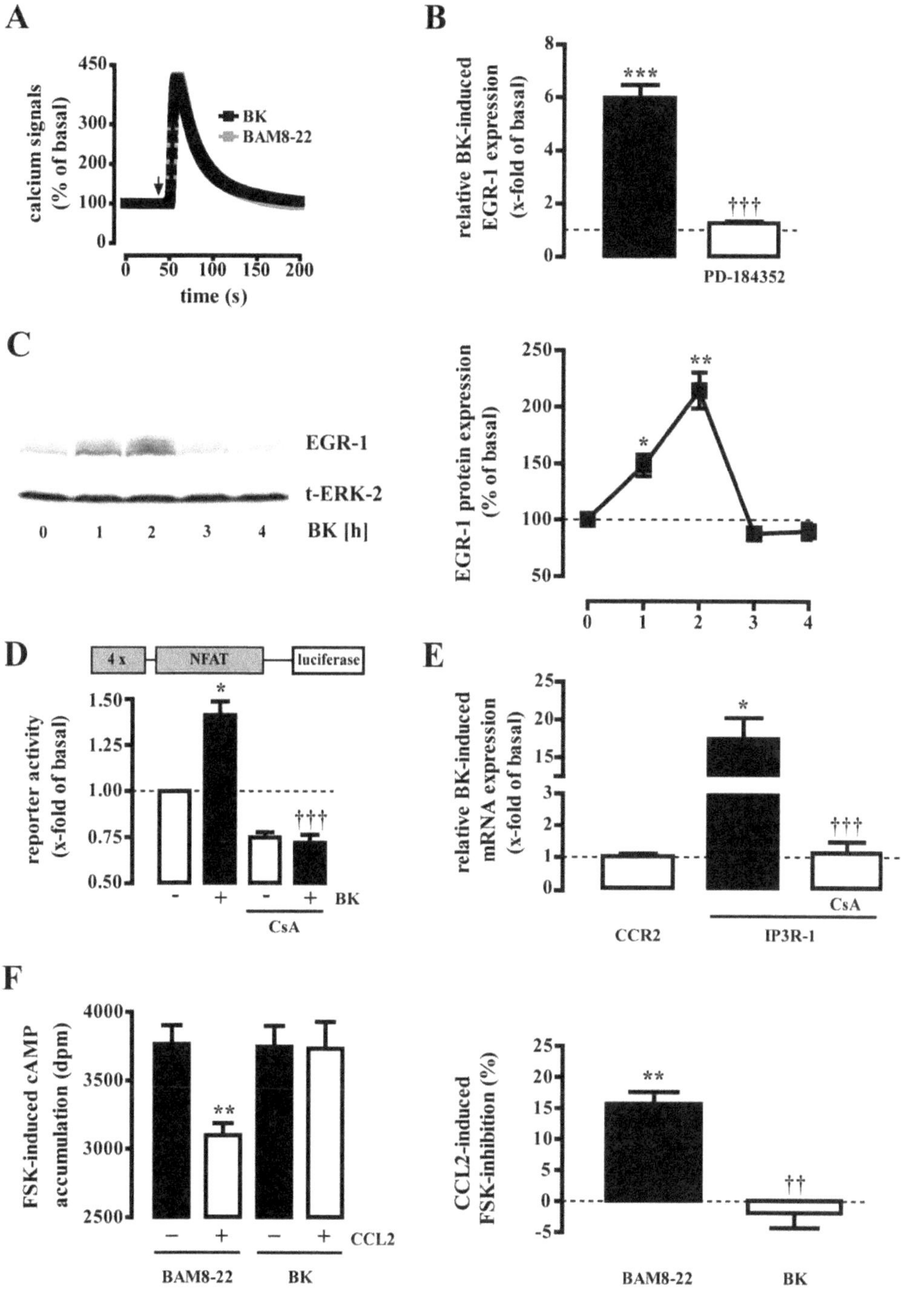

Figure 5. B2R do not induce CCR2 despite NFAT activation. (A) BAM8-22- (2 μM) or BK-induced (1 μM) calcium signals were determined in single fura2-loaded F11-MRGPR-X1 cells by calcium imaging. Data of ~300 cells were compiled and expressed as the mean ± S.E.M. RTQ-PCR experiments were performed with cDNAs derived from serum-starved F11-MRGPR-X1 cells stimulated or not with BK (1 μM) for 1 h in (B) or 6 h in (E). Relative BK-induced gene expression was normalized to β-actin, calculated using the ΔΔCp method, and expressed as the mean ± S.E.M. (C) Serum-starved F11-MRGPR-X1 cells were stimulated or not with BK (1 μM) for the indicated period of time and expression of EGR-1 was determined by western-blotting. Afterwards blots were stripped and re-probed with an antibody against ERK-2 (t-ERK-2). One representative blot is shown. Ligand-induced EGR-1 expression was quantified by densitometry and is given normalized to not stimulated cells as the mean ± S.E.M. (D) BK-induced (1 μM, 6 h) activation of the NFAT reporter is shown in F11-MRGPR-X1 cells. Data are expressed as the mean ± S.E.M. PD-184352 (10 μM, 30 min) was used to inhibit ERK-1/2 activity in (B) or CsA (1 μM, 30 min) to block calcineurin in (D and E). In (B–E) 4 independent experiments were conducted, respectively. In (F) CCR2 protein expression in F11-MRGPR-X1 cells was assessed by CCL2-promoted (100 ng/ml) inhibition of FSK-induced (5 μM) cAMP accumulation after pre-stimulation of the cells with BAM8-22 or BK (1 μM, 20 h). In (F, left panel) one representative experiment is shown and in (F, right panel) data from 5 independent experiments performed in triplicates were compiled and expressed as the mean ± S.E.M. Asterisks indicate a significant difference to not stimulated cells. Dagger signs indicate a significant difference between BK-stimulated inhibitor-treated and untreated cells or between BK- and BAM8-22-stimulated cells.

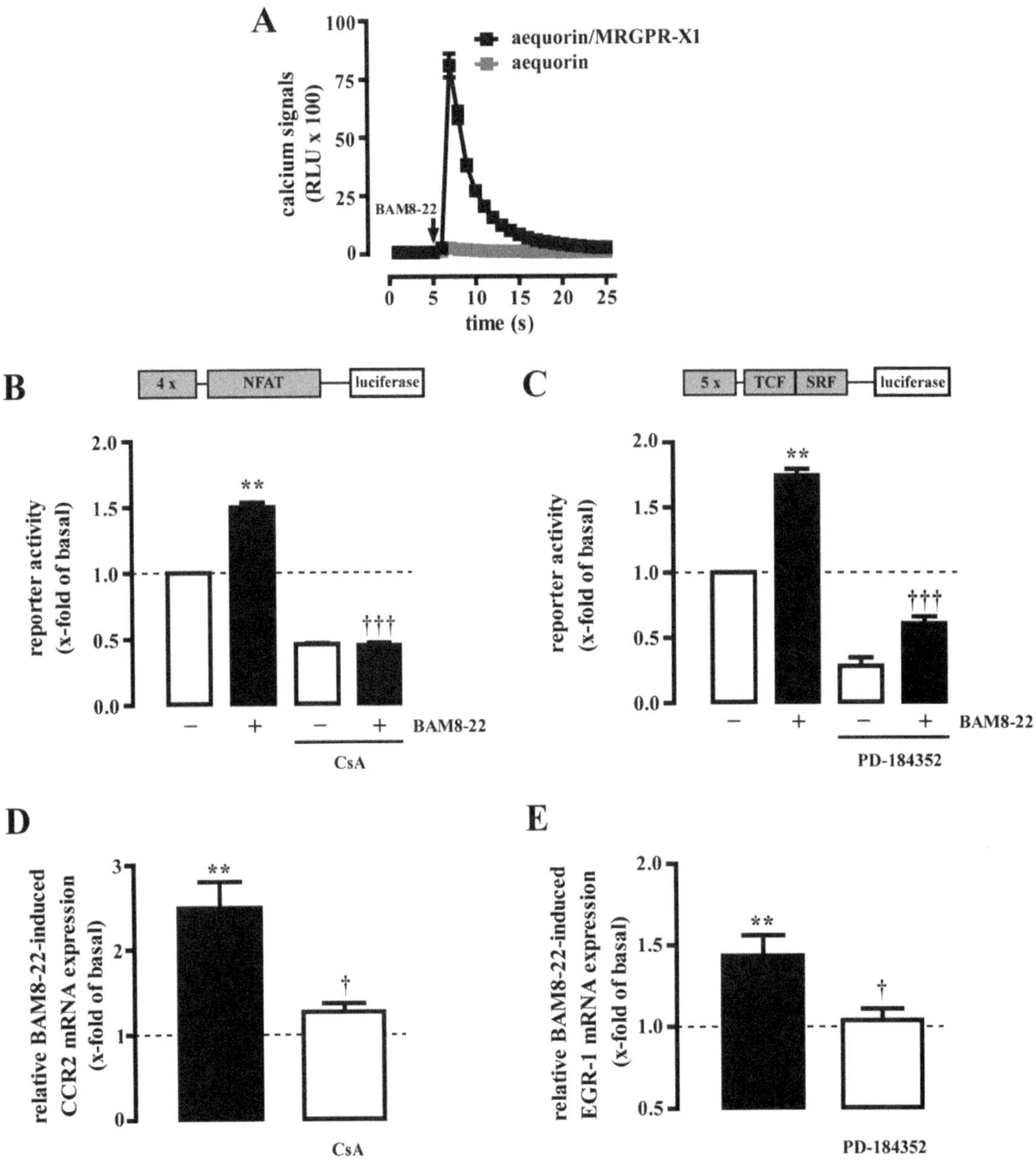

Figure 6. MRGPR-X1 induce EGR-1 via ERK-1/2 and CCR2 via NFAT in primary DRG neurons. BAM8-22-induced (2 μM) calcium signals in rat DRG neurons co-expressing MRGPR-X1 and aequorin or solely aequorin are presented in (A). BAM8-22-induced (2 μM, 8 h) activation of the NFAT (B) or TCF/SRF (C) reporter is shown in rat DRG neurons transiently co-expressing MRGPR-X1. RTQ-PCR experiments were performed with cDNAs derived from serum-starved MRGPR-X1 expressing rat DRG neurons stimulated or not with BAM8-22 (2 μM) for 6 h (D) or 40 min (E). CsA (1 μM, 30 min) was used to block calcineurin in (B and D) or PD-184352 (10 μM, 30 min) to inhibit ERK-1/2 activity in (C and E). Relative BAM8-22-induced gene expression was normalized to β-actin and calculated using the ΔΔCp method. Data from 4 independent experiments were compiled and expressed as the mean ± S.E.M. Asterisks indicate a significant difference to not stimulated cells. Dagger signs indicate a significant difference between BAM8-22-stimulated inhibitor-treated and untreated cells.

CCR-2 expression via calcineurin is not common among G_q activating neuropeptides

Interestingly, BK-promoted NFAT activation did not induce CCR2 expression in F11 cells, although IP3R-1 expression was found to be significantly induced as was COX-2 expression in DRG neurons [16]. *Vice versa*, BAM8-22-induced NFAT activation led to increased CCR2, but not to COX-2 expression (Fig. 4A). Thus, we postulate that NFAT up-regulates pro-nociceptive genes in DRG neurons in concert with other transcription factors and therefore is required, but not sufficient to mediate CCR2 expression via MRGPR-X1 or COX-2 induction via B2R. Further, in contrast to B2R, MRGPR-X1 are resistant against agonist-promoted internalisation and thus, do not interact with arrestins, which have been reported to affect GPCR-promoted gene induction [6,58,59]. Therefore, distinct effects of B2R and MRGPR-X1 on gene expression could either be due to the sustained effects of non-desensitizing MRGPR-X1-promoted signaling or caused by the functional interactions between B2R and arrestins. At last, it has to be mentioned that B2R were endogenously and MRGPR-X1 recombinantly expressed in F11

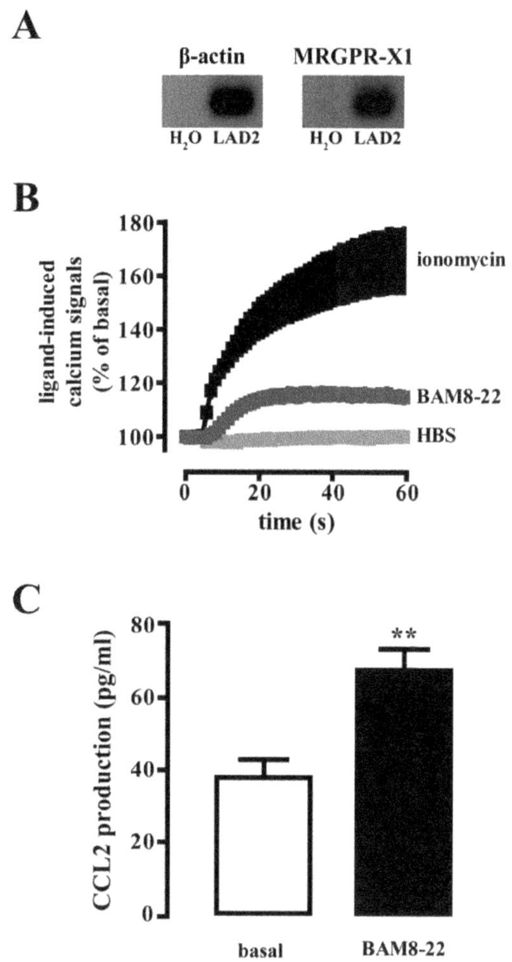

Figure 7. MRGPR-X1-induced CCL2 release in LAD-2 mast cells. (A) MRGPR-X1 (40 cycles) or β-actin (30 cycles) mRNA expression was determined in LAD-2 cells by RT-PCR. As a negative control, RT-PCR was conducted without addition of cDNA (H_2O). (B) Calcium signals in fura2-loaded LAD-2 cells are shown after injection of BAM8-22 (5 μM) or ionomycin (5 μM) or HBS as positive or negative control, respectively. (C) CCL2 release in LAD-2 cells after stimulation with BAM8-22 (5 μM, 18 h) was determined by ELISA. Data from 4 independent experiments performed in triplicates were compiled and expressed as the mean ± S.E.M. Asterisks indicate a significant difference to not stimulated cells.

cells. Recombinant protein expression often leads to significant higher protein levels compared to endogenous expression. Unfortunately, absolute receptor numbers of MRGPR-X1 cannot be determined, because no radiolabeled BAM8-22 is commercially available. Thus, we cannot completely rule out that distinct protein expression levels are responsible for the differences observed. However, it is noteworthy that calcium signaling induced by both receptors and saturated agonist concentrations were almost identical, suggesting comparable numbers of both receptors. Hence, additional work is required to find out how distinct neuropeptides differentially induce NFAT-dependent genes.

BAM8-22-induced CCL2 release in mast cells

Up-regulation of CCR2 in the process of pain chronification is often associated with increased release of its endogenous agonist CCL2 in DRG neurons or immune cells. As shown in figure 4A, BAM8-22 did not induce CCL2 expression in F11-MRGPR-X1 cells, excluding autocrine F11 cell activation via CCL2. Cp have been reported to be associated with DRG neurons and to produce CCL2, leading to paracrine stimulation of CCR2 expressing DRG neurons [60]. Herein, we provide first functional data, indicating that MRGPR-X1 are expressed in the CTMC-derived LAD-2 cell line and thus, exert their action in cells of the peripheral nervous and the immune system. However, so far no data about the physiological role of MRGPR-X1-induced signaling in mast cells are available. Interestingly, we found BAM8-22-promoted CCL2 release in LAD-2 cells and thus, describe the first putatively biological relevant effect of MRGPR-X1 in mast cells. Furthermore our data suggest that MRGPR-X1 may induce a chemokine signaling circuit involving two different mechanisms in distinct, yet functionally co-operating cell types (see figure 8). As mentioned earlier, MRGPR-X1 belong to the small group of GPCR that do not undergo agonist-promoted desensitisation or internalisation [6]. Thus, the predicted effects of BAM8-22 on the chemokine signaling circuit would not be diminished by cellular mechanisms that usually down-regulate GPCR signaling. Hence, one may postulate that prolonged MRGPR-X1-promoted signaling may have sustained effects on CCR2/CCL2 signaling and thus, on chemokine-induced pain chronification in humans.

Pitfalls and Perspectives

Rodents play a central role as *in vivo* models for pain research. Primate-specific expression is therefore the major limitation in the work with human MRGPR-X1, as no ortholog rodent *in vivo* models exist. Of note, there is one receptor subtype in rodents, named mas-related G protein-coupled receptor-C (MRGPR-C) that is also expressed in DRG neurons, activated by BAM8-22 and shares ~50% sequence homology with MRGPR-X1. In addition to BAM8-22, murine MRGPR-C are activated by γ_2-melanocyte stimulating hormone (γ_2-MSH), dynorphin-14 and neuropeptides NPFF or NPAF [61,62]. Overall it is difficult to determine whether rodent MRGPR-C are suitable MRGPR-X1 counterparts. Thus, it has been under debate whether the function of human MRGPR-X1 can be accurately extrapolated from studies with rodent MRGPR-C [7,10]. To obtain more information about the functional characteristics of different MRGPR, we determined the ligand profile of human MRGPR-X1, rat and mouse MRGPR-C in HEK293 cells stably expressing either receptor [6], by monitoring changes in intracellular calcium levels induced by various concentrations of all peptides reported to activate the murine MRGPR-C (Supp. Fig. S1). Thereby we observed that BAM8-22, γ_2-MSH and dynorphin-14 are full agonists and NPFF/NFAF partial agonists of the murine MRGPR-C. Surprisingly, rat MRGPR-C were activated only by γ_2-MSH and BAM8-22, with γ_2-MSH being more potent than BAM8-22, but not by dynorphin-14 or NPFF/NFAF, suggesting differences in the ligand profile between mice and rats. Of all tested peptides, BAM8-22 was the only one that induced significant calcium signals in MRGPR-X1 expressing cells. Thus, these experiments clearly indicate striking differences in the ligand profile between rodent and human MRGPR. Interestingly, differences in the pharmacodynamics of GPCR from distinct species are not restricted to MRGPR but have also been observed for other GPCR such as histamine receptors [63], free fatty acid receptors 2 and 3 [64], G-protein-coupled receptor 35 [65], trace amine-associated receptors 1 [66], kappa opioid receptors [67] and beta-adrenergic receptors [68] and thus, might be an underestimated problem for the development of GPCR-targeting drugs. However, in conjunction with fundamental differences in ligand-promoted desensitization [6] and the lack of MRGPR-C expression in murine mast cells [3],

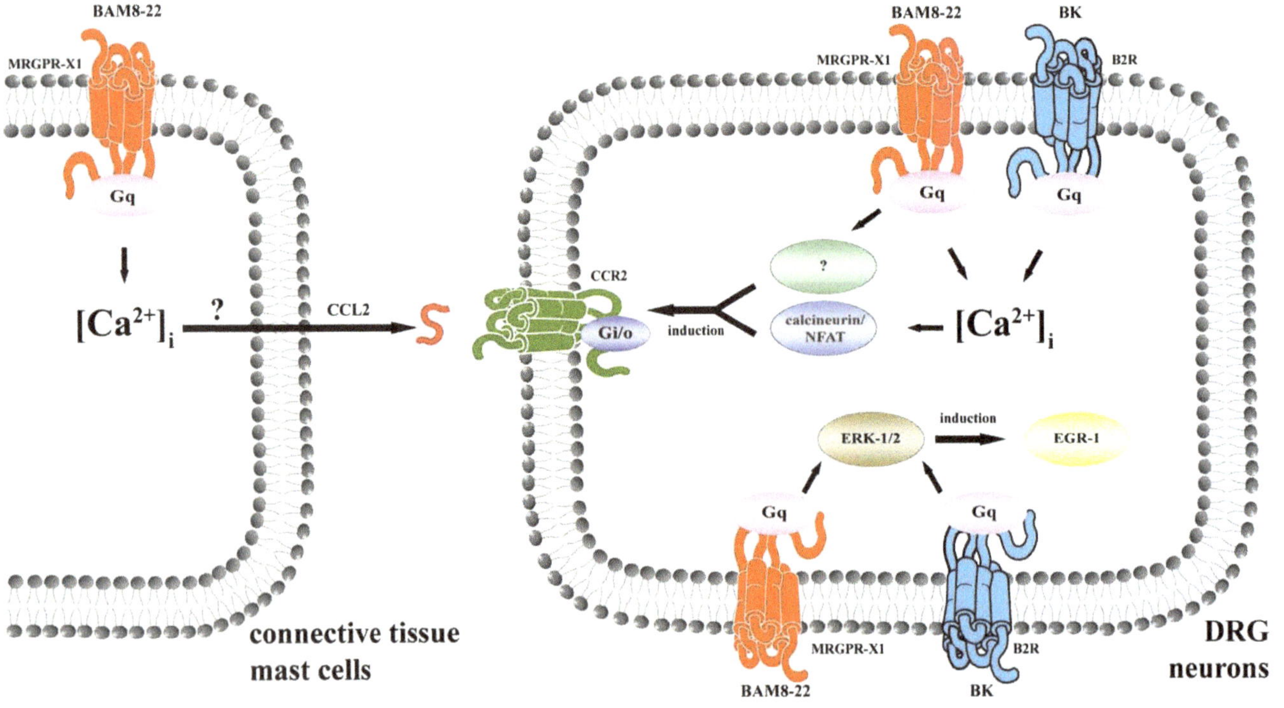

Figure 8. MRGPR-X1-induced signaling in DRG neurons and CTMCs. A cartoon illustrating the signaling circuit by which MRGPR-X1 affect chemokine signaling in DRG neurons and connective tissue mast cells is given.

we reasoned that rodents would not qualify as suitable model systems for our study. Thus, our results obtained at the cellular level still have to await final physiological proof.

Our data define MRGPR-X1 as modulators of gene expression and thereby as inducers of chronic pain markers such CCR2. Furthermore, we identified MRGPR-X1 as positive regulators of CCL2 release in mast cells. Thus, MRGPR-X1 may not only be therapeutic targets for the treatment of acute, but also for chronic pain. Given their exclusive expression in DRG neurons and mast cells, MRGPR-X1-based pain therapy would selectively affect cell types that are pertinent to pain chronification, thereby minimizing the risk of side effects. To validate this hypothesis in the future, it is imperative to establish primate-based, DRG neuron-derived model systems. Furthermore, testing recently described MRGPR-X1 specific antagonists in humans suffering from neuropathic pain may represent an invaluable approach to delineate the pathophysiological role of MRGPR-X1 signaling in human pain chronification [69].

Supporting Information

Figure S1 Distinct ligand profile of human MRGPR-X1 and rodent MRGPR-C. Calcium concentration-response curves in fura2-loaded stably MRGPR-X1 (A), murine MRGPR-C (B) or rat MRGPR-C (C) expressing cells and in coelenterazine H-loaded HEK293-Ae cells stably expressing MRGPR-X1 (D), murine MRGPR-C (E) or rat MRGPR-C (F) were monitored, after injection of various concentrations of BAM8-22 (blue), γ_2-MSH (orange), dynorphin-14 (green), dynorphin-A (black), neuropeptide FF (brown) or neuropeptide AF (red). Background signals induced by injection of HBS were subtracted and responses normalized by defining the calcium transients elicited by the full agonist as 100%. Results are expressed as the mean $\pm$ S.E.M. of at least 4 independent experiments performed in duplicates. Curve fittings were carried out using the sigmoid dose-response (variable slope) algorithm of Prism4.0.
(TIF)

Author Contributions

Conceived and designed the experiments: HJS FP IB TG AB. Performed the experiments: HJS FP KR. Analyzed the data: HJS FP AB. Wrote the paper: HJS IB TG AB.

References

1. Lembo PM, Grazzini E, Groblewski T, O'Donnell D, Roy MO, et al. (2002) Proenkephalin A gene products activate a new family of sensory neuron – specific GPCRs. Nat Neurosci 5: 201–209.
2. Dong X, Han S, Zylka MJ, Simon MI, Anderson DJ (2001) A diverse family of GPCRs expressed in specific subsets of nociceptive sensory neurons. Cell 106: 619–632.
3. Tatemoto K, Nozaki Y, Tsuda R, Konno S, Tomura K, et al. (2006) Immunoglobulin E-independent activation of mast cell is mediated by Mrg receptors. Biochem Biophys Res Commun 349: 1322–1328.
4. Subramanian H, Kashem SW, Collington SJ, Qu H, Lambris JD, et al. (2011) PMX-53 as a dual CD88 antagonist and an agonist for Mas-related gene 2 (MrgX2) in human mast cells. Mol Pharmacol 79: 1005–1013.
5. Breit A, Gagnidze K, Devi LA, Lagace M, Bouvier M (2006) Simultaneous activation of the delta opioid receptor (deltaOR)/sensory neuron-specific receptor-4 (SNSR-4) hetero-oligomer by the mixed bivalent agonist bovine adrenal medulla peptide 22 activates SNSR-4 but inhibits deltaOR signaling. Mol Pharmacol 70: 686–696.
6. Solinski HJ, Boekhoff I, Bouvier M, Gudermann T, Breit A (2010) Sensory neuron-specific MAS-related gene-X1 receptors resist agonist-promoted endocytosis. Mol Pharmacol 78: 249–259.

7. Burstein ES, Ott TR, Feddock M, Ma JN, Fuhs S, et al. (2006) Characterization of the Mas-related gene family: structural and functional conservation of human and rhesus MrgX receptors. Br J Pharmacol 147: 73–82.
8. Solinski HJ, Zierler S, Gudermann T, Breit A (2012) Human sensory neuron-specific Mas-related G protein-coupled receptors-X1 sensitize and directly activate transient receptor potential cation channel V1 via distinct signaling pathways. J Biol Chem.
9. Sikand P, Dong X, Lamotte RH (2011) BAM8-22 Peptide Produces Itch and Nociceptive Sensations in Humans Independent of Histamine Release. J Neurosci 31: 7563–7567.
10. Chen H, Ikeda SR (2004) Modulation of ion channels and synaptic transmission by a human sensory neuron-specific G-protein-coupled receptor, SNSR4/mrgX1, heterologously expressed in cultured rat neurons. J Neurosci 24: 5044–5053.
11. Andrisani OM (1999) CREB-mediated transcriptional control. Crit Rev Eukaryot Gene Expr 9: 19–32.
12. Buchwalter G, Gross C, Wasylyk B (2004) Ets ternary complex transcription factors. Gene 324: 1–14.
13. Shaywitz AJ, Greenberg ME (1999) CREB: a stimulus-induced transcription factor activated by a diverse array of extracellular signals. Annu Rev Biochem 68: 821–861.
14. Davis RJ (1995) Transcriptional regulation by MAP kinases. Mol Reprod Dev 42: 459–467.
15. Seybold VS, Coicou LG, Groth RD, Mermelstein PG (2006) Substance P initiates NFAT-dependent gene expression in spinal neurons. J Neurochem 97: 397–407.
16. Jackson JG, Usachev YM, Thayer SA (2007) Bradykinin-induced nuclear factor of activated T-cells-dependent transcription in rat dorsal root ganglion neurons. Mol Pharmacol 72: 303–310.
17. Groth RD, Coicou LG, Mermelstein PG, Seybold VS (2007) Neurotrophin activation of NFAT-dependent transcription contributes to the regulation of pro-nociceptive genes. J Neurochem 102: 1162–1174.
18. Knoll B, Nordheim A (2009) Functional versatility of transcription factors in the nervous system: the SRF paradigm. Trends Neurosci 32: 432–442.
19. Maldonado R, Blendy JA, Tzavara E, Gass P, Roques BP, et al. (1996) Reduction of morphine abstinence in mice with a mutation in the gene encoding CREB. Science 273: 657–659.
20. Kerr N, Pintzas A, Holmes F, Hobson SA, Pope R, et al. (2010) The expression of ELK transcription factors in adult DRG: Novel isoforms, antisense transcripts and upregulation by nerve damage. Mol Cell Neurosci 44: 165–177.
21. Taylor DA, Fleming WW (2001) Unifying perspectives of the mechanisms underlying the development of tolerance and physical dependence to opioids. J Pharmacol Exp Ther 297: 11–18.
22. Bhangoo S, Ren D, Miller RJ, Henry KJ, Lineswala J, et al. (2007) Delayed functional expression of neuronal chemokine receptors following focal nerve demyelination in the rat: a mechanism for the development of chronic sensitization of peripheral nociceptors. Mol Pain 3: 38.
23. Bhangoo SK, Ripsch MS, Buchanan DJ, Miller RJ, White FA (2009) Increased chemokine signaling in a model of HIV1-associated peripheral neuropathy. Mol Pain 5: 48.
24. Baubet V, Le Mouellic H, Campbell AK, Lucas-Meunier E, Fossier P, et al. (2000) Chimeric green fluorescent protein-aequorin as bioluminescent Ca2+ reporters at the single-cell level. Proc Natl Acad Sci U S A 97: 7260–7265.
25. Francel PC, Harris K, Smith M, Fishman MC, Dawson G, et al. (1987) Neurochemical characteristics of a novel dorsal root ganglion × neuroblastoma hybrid cell line, F-11. J Neurochem 48: 1624–1631.
26. Kirshenbaum AS, Akin C, Wu Y, Rottem M, Goff JP, et al. (2003) Characterization of novel stem cell factor responsive human mast cell lines LAD 1 and 2 established from a patient with mast cell sarcoma/leukemia; activation following aggregation of FcepsilonRI or FcgammaRI. Leuk Res 27: 677–682.
27. Jung H, Miller RJ (2008) Activation of the nuclear factor of activated T-cells (NFAT) mediates upregulation of CCR2 chemokine receptors in dorsal root ganglion (DRG) neurons: a possible mechanism for activity-dependent transcription in DRG neurons in association with neuropathic pain. Mol Cell Neurosci 37: 170–177.
28. White FA, Bhangoo SK, Miller RJ (2005) Chemokines: integrators of pain and inflammation. Nat Rev Drug Discov 4: 834–844.
29. Rothe K, Solinski HJ, Boekhoff I, Gudermann T, Breit A (2012) Morphine activates the ELK-1/SRF pathway via ERK-1/2 in F11 cells derived from dorsal root ganglia neurons. J Pharmacol Exp Ther 342: 41–52.
30. Katayama N, Iwata E, Sakurai H, Tsuchiya T, Tsuda M (1993) Additive induction of Egr-1 (zif/268) mRNA expression in neuroblastoma × glioma hybrid NG108-15 cells via cholinergic muscarinic, alpha 2-adrenergic, and bradykinin receptors. J Neurochem 60: 902–907.
31. Jamieson GA Jr., Mayforth RD, Villereal ML, Sukhatme VP (1989) Multiple intracellular pathways induce expression of a zinc-finger encoding gene (EGR1): relationship to activation of the Na/H exchanger. J Cell Physiol 139: 262–268.
32. Hao L, Ge X, Wan H, Hu S, Lercher MJ, et al. (2012) Human functional genetic studies are biased against the medically most relevant primate-specific genes. BMC Evol Biol 10: 316.
33. Fatakia SN, Costanzi S, Chow CC (2011) Molecular evolution of the transmembrane domains of G protein-coupled receptors. PLoS One 6: e27813.
34. Vallender EJ, Lahn BT (2004) Positive selection on the human genome. Hum Mol Genet 13 Spec No 2: R245–254.
35. Fan SF, Shen KF, Scheideler MA, Crain SM (1992) F11 neuroblastoma × DRG neuron hybrid cells express inhibitory mu- and delta-opioid receptors which increase voltage-dependent K+ currents upon activation. Brain Res 590: 329–333.
36. Jow F, He L, Kramer A, Hinson J, Bowlby MR, et al. (2006) Validation of DRG-like F11 cells for evaluation of KCNQ/M-channel modulators. Assay Drug Dev Technol 4: 49–56.
37. Puttfarcken PS, Manelli AM, Arneric SP, Donnelly-Roberts DL (1997) Evidence for nicotinic receptors potentially modulating nociceptive transmission at the level of the primary sensory neuron: studies with F11 cells. J Neurochem 69: 930–938.
38. McIlvain HB, Baudy A, Sullivan K, Liu D, Pong K, et al. (2006) Pituitary adenylate cyclase-activating peptide (PACAP) induces differentiation in the neuronal F11 cell line through a PKA-dependent pathway. Brain Res 1077: 16–23.
39. Boland LM, Allen AC, Dingledine R (1991) Inhibition by bradykinin of voltage-activated barium current in a rat dorsal root ganglion cell line: role of protein kinase C. J Neurosci 11: 1140–1149.
40. Li Y, Ji A, Weihe E, Schafer MK (2004) Cell-specific expression and lipopolysaccharide-induced regulation of tumor necrosis factor alpha (TNFalpha) and TNF receptors in rat dorsal root ganglion. J Neurosci 24: 9623–9631.
41. Gaudioso C, Hao J, Martin-Eauclaire MF, Gabriac M, Delmas P (2012) Menthol pain relief through cumulative inactivation of voltage-gated sodium channels. Pain 153: 473–484.
42. Eijkelkamp N, Heijnen CJ, Willemen HL, Deumens R, Joosten EA, et al. (2010) GRK2: a novel cell-specific regulator of severity and duration of inflammatory pain. J Neurosci 30: 2138–2149.
43. Fioravanti B, De Felice M, Stucky CL, Medler KA, Luo MC, et al. (2008) Constitutive activity at the cannabinoid CB1 receptor is required for behavioral response to noxious chemical stimulation of TRPV1: antinociceptive actions of CB1 inverse agonists. J Neurosci 28: 11593–11602.
44. Bullitt E (1989) Induction of c-fos-like protein within the lumbar spinal cord and thalamus of the rat following peripheral stimulation. Brain Res 493: 391–397.
45. Romero A, Gonzalez-Cuello A, Laorden ML, Campillo A, Vasconcelos N, et al. (2012) Effects of surgery and/or remifentanil administration on the expression of pERK1/2, c-Fos and dynorphin in the dorsal root ganglia in mice. Naunyn Schmiedebergs Arch Pharmacol 385: 397–409.
46. Utreras E, Futatsugi A, Rudrabhatla P, Keller J, Iadarola MJ, et al. (2009) Tumor necrosis factor-alpha regulates cyclin-dependent kinase 5 activity during pain signaling through transcriptional activation of p35. J Biol Chem 284: 2275–2284.
47. Kendall G, Ensor E, Brar-Rai A, Winter J, Latchman DS (1994) Nerve growth factor induces expression of immediate-early genes NGFI-A (Egr-1) and NGFI-B (nur 77) in adult rat dorsal root ganglion neurons. Brain Res Mol Brain Res 25: 73–79.
48. Ko SW, Vadakkan KI, Ao H, Gallitano-Mendel A, Wei F, et al. (2005) Selective contribution of Egr1 (zif/268) to persistent inflammatory pain. J Pain 6: 12–20.
49. Dolan S, Hastie P, Crossan C, Nolan AM (2011) Co-induction of cyclooxygenase-2 [correction of cyclooxyenase-2] and early growth response gene (Egr-1) in spinal cord in a clinical model of persistent inflammation and hyperalgesia. Mol Pain 7: 91.
50. Groth RD, Mermelstein PG (2003) Brain-derived neurotrophic factor activation of NFAT (nuclear factor of activated T-cells)-dependent transcription: a role for the transcription factor NFATc4 in neurotrophin-mediated gene expression. J Neurosci 23: 8125–8134.
51. Genazzani AA, Carafoli E, Guerini D (1999) Calcineurin controls inositol 1,4,5-trisphosphate type 1 receptor expression in neurons. Proc Natl Acad Sci U S A 96: 5797–5801.
52. Abbadie C, Lindia JA, Cumiskey AM, Peterson LB, Mudgett JS, et al. (2003) Impaired neuropathic pain responses in mice lacking the chemokine receptor CCR2. Proc Natl Acad Sci U S A 100: 7947–7952.
53. Serrano A, Pare M, McIntosh F, Elmes SJ, Martino G, et al. (2012) Blocking spinal CCR2 with AZ889 reversed hyperalgesia in a model of neuropathic pain. Mol Pain 6: 90.
54. Sun JH, Yang B, Donnelly DF, Ma C, LaMotte RH (2006) MCP-1 enhances excitability of nociceptive neurons in chronically compressed dorsal root ganglia. J Neurophysiol 96: 2189–2199.
55. White FA, Sun J, Waters SM, Ma C, Ren D, et al. (2005) Excitatory monocyte chemoattractant protein-1 signaling is up-regulated in sensory neurons after chronic compression of the dorsal root ganglion. Proc Natl Acad Sci U S A 102: 14092–14097.
56. Wang CH, Zou LJ, Zhang YL, Jiao YF, Sun JH (2010) The excitatory effects of the chemokine CCL2 on DRG somata are greater after an injury of the ganglion than after an injury of the spinal or peripheral nerve. Neurosci Lett 475: 48–52.
57. Jung H, Bhangoo S, Banisadr G, Freitag C, Ren D, et al. (2009) Visualization of chemokine receptor activation in transgenic mice reveals peripheral activation of CCR2 receptors in states of neuropathic pain. J Neurosci 29: 8051–8062.
58. Zimmerman B, Simaan M, Akoume MY, Houri N, Chevallier S, et al. (2011) Role of ssarrestins in bradykinin B2 receptor-mediated signalling. Cell Signal 23: 648–659.
59. Pierce KL, Lefkowitz RJ (2001) Classical and new roles of beta-arrestins in the regulation of G-protein-coupled receptors. Nat Rev Neurosci 2: 727–733.

60. Skaper SD, Giusti P, Facci L (2012) Microglia and mast cells: two tracks on the road to neuroinflammation. Faseb J.
61. Grazzini E, Puma C, Roy MO, Yu XH, O'Donnell D, et al. (2004) Sensory neuron-specific receptor activation elicits central and peripheral nociceptive effects in rats. Proc Natl Acad Sci U S A 101: 7175–7180.
62. Brinkmann M, Lutkemeyer D, Gudermann F, Lehmann J (2002) New technologies for automated cell counting based on optical image analysis; The Cellscreen'. Cytotechnology 38: 119–127.
63. Strasser A, Wittmann HJ, Buschauer A, Schneider EH, Seifert R (2013) Species-dependent activities of G-protein-coupled receptor ligands: lessons from histamine receptor orthologs. Trends Pharmacol Sci 34: 13–32.
64. Hudson BD, Tikhonova IG, Pandey SK, Ulven T, Milligan G (2012) Extracellular ionic locks determine variation in constitutive activity and ligand potency between species orthologs of the free fatty acid receptors FFA2 and FFA3. J Biol Chem 287: 41195–41209.
65. Jenkins L, Brea J, Smith NJ, Hudson BD, Reilly G, et al. (2012) Identification of novel species-selective agonists of the G-protein-coupled receptor GPR35 that promote recruitment of beta-arrestin-2 and activate Galpha13. Biochem J 432: 451–459.
66. Wainscott DB, Little SP, Yin T, Tu Y, Rocco VP, et al. (2007) Pharmacologic characterization of the cloned human trace amine-associated receptor1 (TAAR1) and evidence for species differences with the rat TAAR1. J Pharmacol Exp Ther 320: 475–485.
67. Li J, Li JG, Chen C, Zhang F, Liu-Chen LY (2002) Molecular basis of differences in (−) (trans)-3,4-dichloro-N-methyl-N-[2-(1-pyrrolidiny)-cyclohexyl]benzeneacetamide - induced desensitization and phosphorylation between human and rat kappa-opioid receptors expressed in Chinese hamster ovary cells. Mol Pharmacol 61: 73–84.
68. Moore JJ Jr., Whitsett JA (1982) The beta-adrenergic receptor in mammalian placenta: species differences and ontogeny. Placenta 3: 257–268.
69. Kunapuli P, Lee S, Zheng W, Alberts M, Kornienko O, et al. (2006) Identification of small molecule antagonists of the human mas-related gene-X1 receptor. Anal Biochem 351: 50–61.

14

Spinal SIRT1 Activation Attenuates Neuropathic Pain in Mice

Haijun Shao[1], Qingsheng Xue[1], Fujun Zhang[1], Yan Luo[1], Hao Zhu[2], Xiaoqing Zhang[1], Honghai Zhang[3], Wenlong Ding[2], Buwei Yu[1]*

1 Department of Anesthesiology, Ruijin Hospital, School of Medicine, Shanghai Jiao Tong University, Shanghai, PR China, **2** Department of Anatomy, School of Medicine, Shanghai Jiao Tong University, Shanghai, PR China, **3** Department of Anesthesiology, Hangzhou First People's Hospital, Nanjing Medical University, Zhejiang, PR China

Abstract

Abnormal histone acetylation occurs during neuropathic pain through an epigenetic mechanism. Silent information regulator 1 (sir2 or SIRT1), a NAD-dependent deacetylase, plays complex systemic roles in a variety of processes through deacetylating acetylated histone and other specific substrates. But the role of SIRT1 in neuropathic pain is not well established yet. The present study was intended to detect SIRT1 content and activity, nicotinamide (NAM) and nicotinamide adenine dinucleotide (NAD) in the spinal cord using immunoblotting or mass spectroscopy over time in mice following chronic constriction injury (CCI) or sham surgery. In addition, the effect of intrathecal injection of NAD or resveratrol on thermal hyperalgesia and mechanical allodynia was evaluated in CCI mice. Finally, we investigated whether SIRT1 inhibitor EX-527 could reverse the anti-nociceptive effect of NAD or resveratrol. It was found that spinal SIRT1 expression, deacetylase activity and NAD/NAM decreased significantly 1, 3, 7, 14 and 21 days after CCI surgery as compared with sham group. In addition, daily intrathecal injection of 5 µl 800 mM NAD 1 h before and 1 day after CCI surgery or single intrathecal injection of 5 µl 90 mM resveratrol 1 h before CCI surgery produced a transient inhibitory effect on thermal hyperalgesia and mechanical allodynia in CCI mice. Finally, an intrathecal injection of 5 µl 1.2 mM EX-527 1 h before NAD or resveratrol administration reversed the anti-nociceptive effect of NAD or resveratrol. These data indicate that the reduction in SIRT1 deacetylase activity may be a factor contributing to the development of neuropathic pain in CCI mice. Our findings suggest that the enhancement of spinal NAD/NAM and/or SIRT1 activity may be a potentially promising strategy for the prevention or treatment of neuropathic pain.

Editor: Shao-Jun Tang, University of Texas Medical Branch, United States of America

Funding: This work was supported by the National Natural Sciences Foundation of China (grant number 30400421). The funders had no role in study design, data collection and analysis, decision to publish, or preparation of the manuscript.

Competing Interests: The authors have declared that no competing interests exist.

* Email: yubuwei_1958@163.com

Introduction

Neuropathic pain is characterized by both negative symptoms and positive symptoms including hyperalgesia, allodynia, paresthesia and spontaneous pain [1]. Many studies [2,3,4,5] suggest that the symptoms of neuropathic pain can be attributed to a variety of alterations in pain-related gene expression and modification in primary afferent or spinal cord neurons. One of the characteristic alterations in gene modification is abnormal histone acetylation, which is believed to be one of the transcription factor-mediated epigenetic mechanisms underlying neuropathic pain [6,7]. Several classes of histone deacetylases (HDACs) are expressed in the spinal cord that is a critical structure of the nociceptive pathway [8,9]. Silent information regulator (SIRT) can act as a HDAC deacetylating acetylated histone.

Sir2 or SIRT1, a member of SIRT family, is a NAD-dependent deacetylase. It was initially identified as a mediator of longevity in yeast [10]. Its mammalian homologue, SIRT1, is a class III HDAC and plays important roles in many physiopathological conditions such as diabetes, cardiovascular disorders, cancer and neurodegeneration [11,12,13,14]. The specificity of SIRT1 catalytic activity relies on two domains of the substrate binding site: a Rossmann -like domain that binds to NAD [15], and an alpha-helix domain with a zinc ribbon for zinc binding. SIRT1 deacetylation needs NAD as a cofactor, which is consumed by SIRT1 and then into NAM [16]. In addition, NAM inhibits genome silencing and accelerates aging by regulating yeast sir2 at 50–150 µM concentrations, and maintaining the NAD/NAM ratio may be crucial for the normal SIRT1 catalytic activity [17]. In addition, SIRT1 is a major effector of axonal protection mediated by increased NAD biosynthesis [18]. Resveratrol (3,4′,5-trihydroxystilbene), a phytoalexin naturally present in plants, binds to SIRT1 at the N-terminal and then increases SIRT1 activity [19], showing promising potential for the treatment of pain mediated by nucleus pulposus [20] and the attenuation of neuropathic pain [21,22] and inflammatory pain [23]. EX-527 (6-chloro-2, 3, 4, 9-tetrahydro-1-H-carbazole-1-carboxamide), a SIRT1 inhibitor that is more potent and selective than other current SIRT1 inhibitors [24], can induce p53 acetylation and cell death through targeting SIRT1 [25]. Recently, SIRT1 has been implicated in the pathologic process in lumbar segment of the spinal cord in a $SOD1^{G93A}$ transgenic mouse model of amyotrophic lateral sclerosis [26], suggesting that SIRT1 may

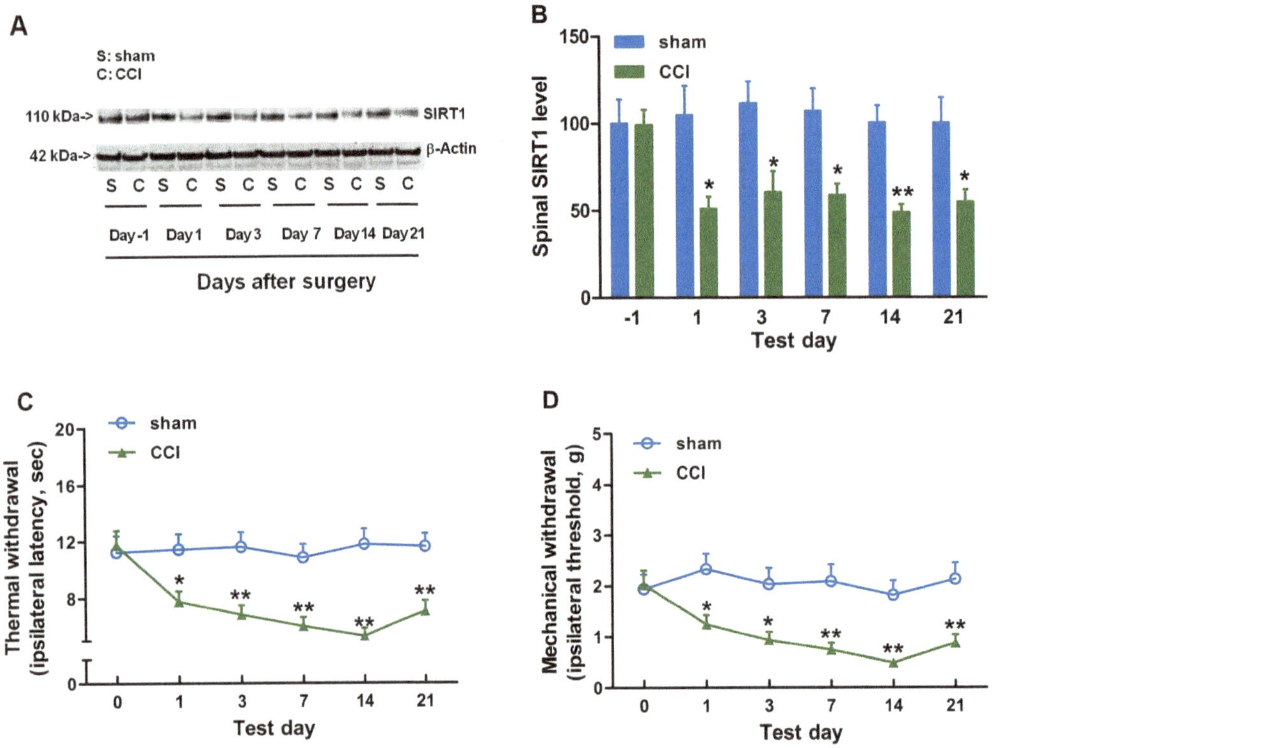

Figure 1. CCI surgery decreases spinal SIRT1 content and this is associated with an increase in pain-related behaviors. (A) Spinal SIRT1 content is decreased 1, 3, 7, 14 and 21 days after CCI surgery as compared with that after sham surgery. (B) Quantification of the immunoblots shows that SIRT1 levels are decreased after CCI surgery. CCI surgery induces (C) thermal hyperalgesia and (D) mechanical allodynia in ipsolateral hind paw. $n = 12$ in each group for behavioral test and $n = 6$ at each time point in each group for SIRT1 analysis; $^{*}P<0.05$, $^{**}P<0.01$ *vs.* sham group at each time point. CCI, chronic constriction injury; SIRT1, silent information regulator 1.

play some role in pain modulation. However, the role of SIRT1 in neuropathic pain is not well established yet.

We therefore hypothesized that the decreased SIRT1 deacetylase activity may be a contributing factor of the development of neuropathic pain. We set out to observe the SIRT1 content and activity, NAM and NAD in the spinal cord using immunoblotting or mass spectroscopy over time in mice following chronic constriction injury (CCI) or sham surgery. The effect of intrathecal injection of NAD or resveratrol on thermal hyperalgesia and mechanical allodynia in CCI mice was then evaluated. Finally, we investigated whether SIRT1 inhibitor EX-527 could reverse the anti-nociceptive effect of NAD or resveratrol. It was found that CCI surgery decreased SIRT1expression/activity and the NAD/NAM ratio in mice. The intrathecal injection of 5 µl 800 mM NAD or 90 mM resveratrol might be effective to modulate the CCI-induced development of neuropathic pain by promoting NAD-dependent SIRT1 deacetylase activity. In addition, an intrathecal injection of 5 µl 1.2 mM EX-527 1 h before the NAD or resveratrol administration reversed the anti-nociceptive effect of increased spinal NAD or exogenous resveratrol, suggesting that the SIRT1 activation may be essential for the effect of NAD or resveratrol. Our data suggest that the enhancement of SIRT1 activity may be a potentially promising pharmacological strategy for the prevention or treatment of neuropathic pain.

Materials and Methods

Subjects

All experimental protocols were approved by the Animal Care and Use Committee of Shanghai JiaoTong University School of Medicine (Shanghai, China). All surgical procedures were performed under general anaesthesia, and every effort was made to minimize stress. Adult male Kunming mice ($n = 384$) weighing 20–25 g (SLAC Laboratory Animal Co., Ltd., Shanghai, China) were housed in a temperature-controlled (22°C) colony room under a 12 h/12 h light/dark cycle regime, with food and water available *ad libitum.* All behavioral testing was performed during the light cycle between 10:00 AM and 3:00 PM. The mice were randomly allocated to drug- or vehicle-treated groups. Each behavioral test group included 10 or 12 mice and each molecular detection group included 6 mice.

Intrathecal injection

Drugs or vehicles were intrathecally injected into mice as the method described by Hylden et al [27]. Briefly, a 30 gauge stainless steel needle attached to a 10-µl Hamilton microsyringe was inserted at an angle about 20° above the vertebral column into L4 or L5 spinous space, and then advanced carefully to the intervertebral space as the angle of the syringe was decreased to about 10° until a sudden slight flick of the tail was observed, indicating the tip of the needle had entered the subarachnoid space. The drug or the vehicle was then injected in a 5 µl volume over a 30 s period into the subarachnoid space and the needle was left in place for further 15 s before withdrawl. NAD

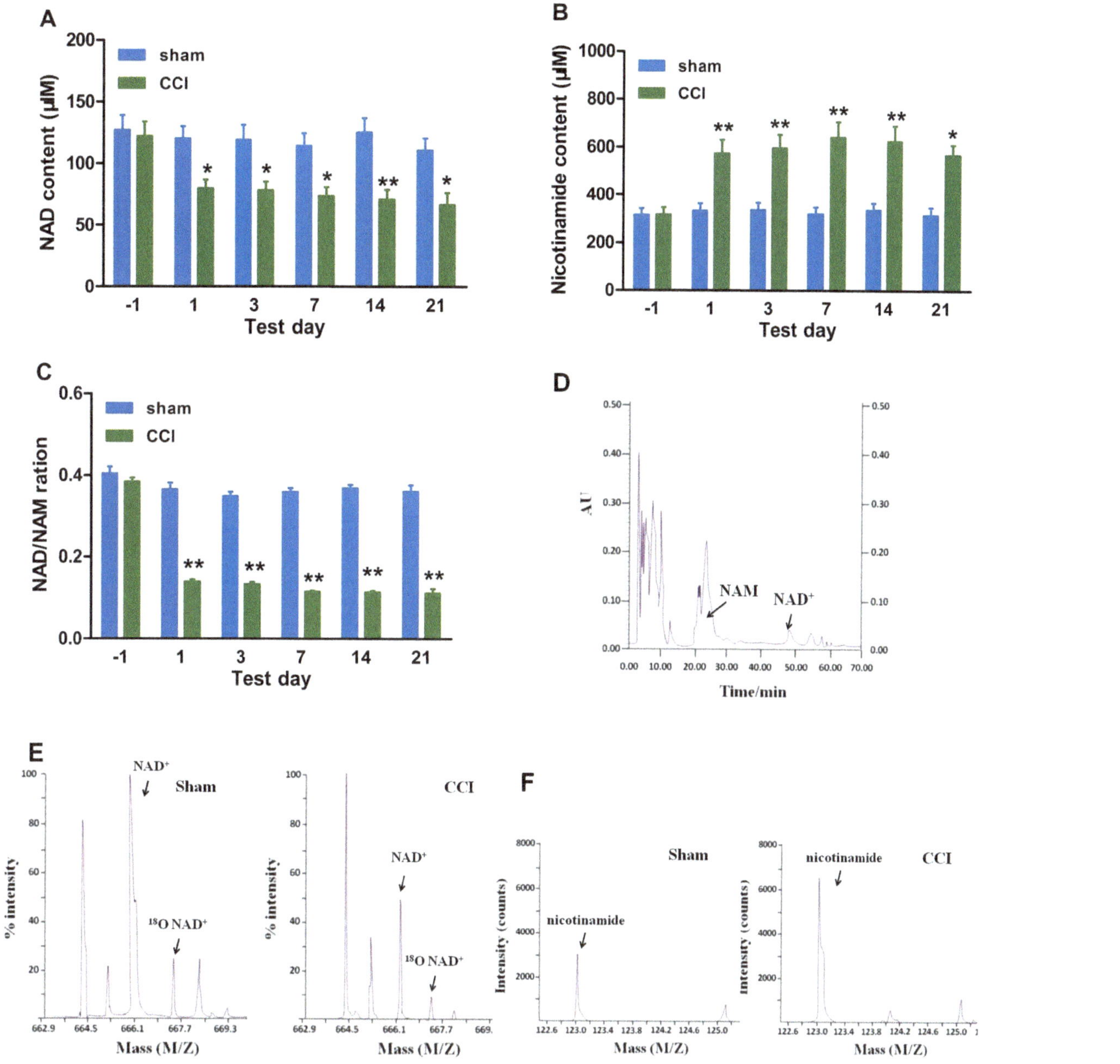

Figure 2. CCI surgery decreases NAD and increases NAM in the spinal cord. CCI surgery decreases (A) NAD and increases (B) NAM as compared with sham surgery. (C) The ratio of NAD/NAM is decreased in CCI mice as compared with that in sham group. (D) NAM and NAD fractions are collected according to HPLC method. The arrows show the retention time of NAM and NAD, which is at around 21 min and 48 min, respectively. The NAM peaks are mixed with those of other impurities. (E) Spectrograms of NAD with MALDI-MS are representative results from a sham-treated (left) and a CCI-treated (right) mouse. The position of NAD and ^{18}O NAD are indicated. (F) Spectrograms of NAM with ESI-MS are representative results from a sham-treated (left) and a CCI-treated (right) mouse. The position of NAM is indicated. $n=6$ at each time point in each group; $^{*}P<0.05$, $^{**}P<0.01$ *vs.* sham group at each time point. NAM, nicotinamide; NAD, nicotinamide adenine dinucleotide; CCI, chronic constriction injury; MALDI-MS, matrix-assisted laser desorption ionization-mass spectroscopy; ESI-MS, electrospray ionization-mass spectrometry.

and resveratrol were purchased from Sigma (St. Louis, MO) and EX-527 was a gift from Lei Zhang (the Ninth People's Hospital, Shanghai, China). The doses of NAD, resveratrol and EX-527 were selected according to previous reports and our preliminary experiments. Specifically, 400 mM and 800 mM NAD was prepared in saline [18,28,29], 45 mM and 90 mM resveratrol was dissolved in 20% DMSO [21,30,31] and 1.2 mM EX-527 was prepared in 20% DMSO [24]. The dosing schedule of drugs or vehicles was present in the Results or Figures. Motor functions were cursorily evaluated by observing the placing/stepping reflexes and righting reflex 5 min before the next nociceptive test or drug administration. Animals with signs of motor impairment were excluded from the experiment.

Neuropathic pain model

After a pre-evaluation of pain, mice received either chronic constriction injury of the sciatic nerve or sham surgery by only

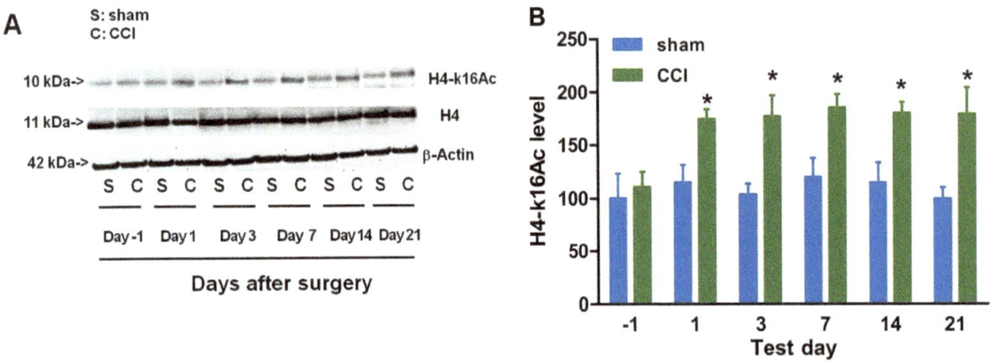

Figure 3. CCI surgery increases acetylation of H4-k16. (A) The levels of H4-k16Ac, but not total H4, are increased 1, 3, 7, 14 and 21 days after CCI surgery as compared with those after sham surgery. (B) Quantification of the immunoblots shows that H4-k16Ac is increased after CCI surgery. $n=6$ at each time point in each group; $^{*}P<0.05$, $^{**}P<0.01$ *vs.* sham group at each time point. CCI, chronic constriction injury; SIRT1, silent information regulator 1; H4-k16Ac, H4-k16 acetylation.

exposing the sciatic nerve without ligation as described previously [32]. Briefly, the left sciatic nerve was exposed at the mid-thigh level under sodium pentobarbital anesthesia (65 mg kg^{-1}, i.p.). Three ligations (4–0 chromic gut, with a distance about 1 mm apart) were loosely constricted around the nerve proximal to the trifurcation by blunt dissection through the biceps femoris. The tension of the constriction was guided by the occurrence of a short flick of the ipsilateral hind limb.

Assessment of thermal hyperalgesia and mechanical allodynia

The investigator was unaware of the drug or vehicle administration that the mouse had received. Thermal hyperalgesia was evaluated by radiant heat paw withdrawal test as described by Hargreaves et al [33]. Briefly, the mouse was individually placed on a 1 mm thick and smooth glass surface surrounded by a plastic chamber (7×9×11 cm) and the heat source was provided by an analgesia meter located below the

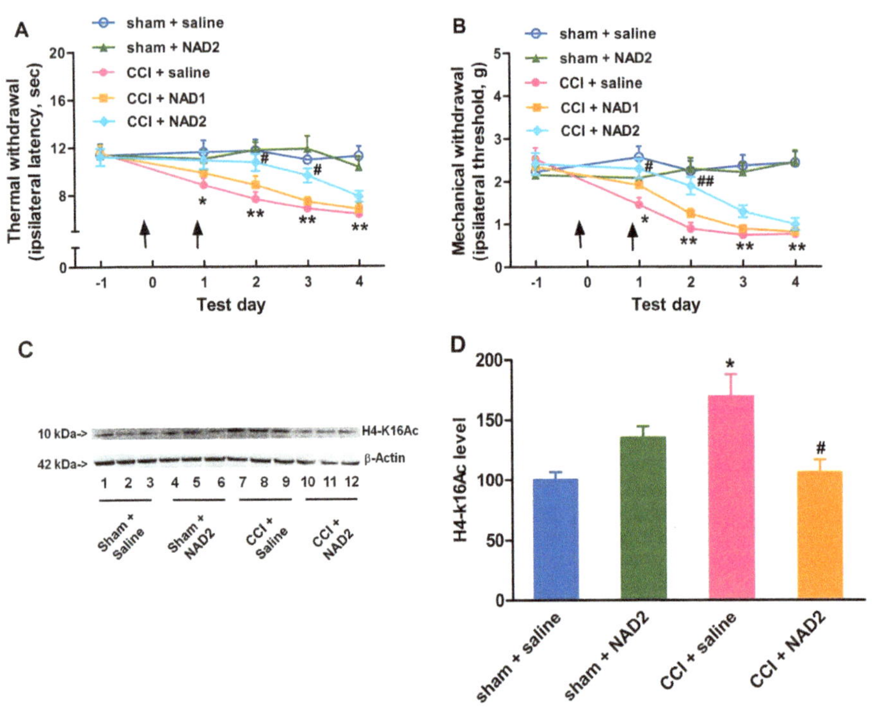

Figure 4. NAD attenuates the development of neuropathic pain by alleviating the reduction of SIRT1 deacetylase activity. Daily intrathecal injections of 5 μl 800 mM NAD into mice 1 h before and 1 day after CCI surgery, but not 400 mM, produce transient inhibition of the development of (A) thermal hyperalgesia and (B) mechanical allodynia induced by CCI surgery. (C) 800 mM NAD attenuates CCI-induced elevation of H4-K16Ac 2 days after CCI surgery. (D) Quantification of the immunoblots shows that 800 mM NAD attenuates CCI-induced increase in H4-K16Ac. An arrow indicates an intrathecal injection. $n=10$ in each group for behavior test and $n=6$ in each group for H4-K16Ac analysis; $^{*}P<0.05$, $^{**}P<0.01$ *vs.* saline-treated sham group; $^{\#}P<0.05$, $^{\#\#}P<0.01$ *vs.* saline-treated CCI group. NAD1, 400 μM nicotinamide adenine dinucleotide; NAD2, 800 μM nicotinamide adenine dinucleotide; CCI, chronic constriction injury; H4-k16Ac, H4-k16 acetylation.

glass surface. The mouse was placed in the chamber to acclimatize to the environment for 45 min before behavior tests. The heat source was focused on a portion of the ipsilateral hind paws of the mouse and an automatic 20-s cutoff was used to prevent tissue damage. Each hind paw was tested three times with a of 5-min interval between two measurements to avoid habituation. Mechanical allodynia was determined by observing the occurrence of foot withdrawal in response to mechanical indentation of the plantar surface of each hind paw with Von Frey filaments (North Coast Medical Inc., CA, USA). Before starting the experiments, we tested the actual forces of the series of 8 von Frey filaments (actual force: 0.31, 0.38, 0.45, 0.6, 1.0, 1.4, 2.0, and 4.0 g). The mouse was placed individually in a 20×25×15 cm plastic box on a wire mesh floor and then allowed to acclimate for 45 min. The filaments were perpendicularly presented to 10 designated loci distributed over the plantar surface of the hind paws with a force to cause slight bending against the hind paw, and held for 4–5 s. The filaments were applied in order of ascending force, starting with 0.31 g and ending with 4.0 g as cutoff value with a 10–15 s interval. Each filament was applied alternately to each foot and locus. The incidence of foot withdrawal was expressed as the number of positive responses multiplied by 10 and the percentage of response of each filament was then plotted as a function of force. For each mouse, ascending forces were tested either until the maximum stimulus (4.0 g) was reached or until a hair force was achieved that caused 10 positive responses. The mechanical allodynia was defined as the force that produced a minimum detectable withdrawal observed on 50% of the tests at the same force level. In cases where none of the specific filaments exactly produced 5 positive withdrawals in 10 tests, the linear interpolation was calculated as the threshold.

Immunoblotting

The animals were sacrificed by overdose urethane after the supposed survival time. The L4–5 spinal cord was dissected and removed, and the dorsal horn of the left half of L4 and L5 was isolated and then frozen immediately in liquid nitrogen. Tissue samples were homogenized in lysis buffer (12.5 μl mg^{-1} tissue) containing (in mM) Tris 20.0, sucrose 250.0, Na_3VO_4 0.03, $MgCl_2$ 2.0, EDTA 2.0, EGTA 2.0, phenylmethylsulfonyl fluoride 2.0, dithiothreitol (DTT) 1.0, and protease inhibitor cocktail 0.02% (v/v), pH 7.4. The homogenate was centrifuged at 13,000 rpm for 15 min at 4°C and the supernatant was collected for protein concentration determination by using Bradford method [34]. Primary antibody SIRT1 (1:2000; Abcam, Cambridge, UK), H4-k16Ac (1:2000) and H4 (1:1000) (Cell Signaling Technology, Danvers, Massachusetts) were used to detect SIRT1, H4-16Ac and H4.

Assessment of NAD and NAM

An aliquot of the frozen spinal cord was lysed in 200 μl $HClO_4$ (1.0 M) containing 3.2 nmol [^{18}O] NAD and 1.4 nmol [^{18}O] NAM. The supernatant was collected after centrifugation at 12,000 rpm for 10 min at RT, neutralized with NaOH and injected on a C-18 semipreparative column. NAD and NAM fractions were collected according to the retention time of authentic standards, lyophilized and redissolved in 50% acetonitrile. Matrix-assisted laser desorption ionization-mass spectroscopy (MS) (positive mode) was used to detect NAD, and ESI-MS (positive mode) was used to measure NAM signal. Peak areas for NAD were determined by integration of total ion at mass 646 amu and at 666 amu, and the peak was calculated with the formula: ^{16}O pmol = (646 ion area/666 ion area –0.035) ×^{18}O pmol. The peak ratio of 123/125 provided quantity of the nmol of NAM. ^{16}O pmol = (123 ion area/125 ion area –0.035) ×^{18}O pmol. The NAD or NAM concentrations in tissue were obtained from NAD and NAM contents divided by the tissue volume (density, 1.0 μl mg^{-1} of tissue). Appropriate blanks and controls were also analyzed together.

Statistical Analysis

Data were presented as means ± SEM. Comparisons in withdrawal latencies over time were performed by using two-way analysis of variance (ANOVA) with repeated measures followed by Bonferroni post hoc tests. Western blot and MS data between the groups were analyzed by student's *t* test or one-way analysis of variance. The results of all analyses were considered significant at $P<0.05$.

Results

Down-regulation of SIRT1 and NAD in the spinal cord of CCI mice

The decreased SIRT1 expression or activity in CCI-induced neuropathic pain is a prerequisite of our hypothesis. Mice were sacrificed for molecular detection before, and at 1, 3, 7, 14 and 21 days after CCI or sham surgery. It was found that CCI surgery induced a decrease in SIRT1 protein content (Fig. 1A and 1B) in the spinal cord, accompanied with an increase in thermal hyperalgesia (Fig. 1C) and mechanical allodynia (Fig. 1D), as compared with sham group. However, sham surgery had no significant effect on SIRT1 content (Fig. 1A and 1B). Knowing that SIRT1 consumes NAD and then releases NAM, we further investigated the effect of CCI surgery on NAD and NAM content. The content of NAD was decreased (Fig. 2A) and the content of NAM was increased (Fig. 2B) in CCI mice as compared with those in sham group. Thus, the NAD/NAM ratio (Fig. 2C) was decreased in CCI mice as compared with that in sham group, which was equal to the aberration of SIRT1 content. NAM and NAD fractions were collected with HPLC method at around 21 min and 48 min, respectively (Fig. 2D). Then, NAD and NAM were detected with MALDI-MS (Fig. 2E) and ESI-MS (Fig. 2F), respectively. The decrease in SIRT1 protein content and NAD/NAM ratio in the spinal cord of CCI mice coincided with a marked reduction in the SIRT1 deacetylase activity as represented by an apparent elevation in acetylation level of SIRT1 substrate H4-k16Ac (acetylation of H4-k16) (Fig. 3A and 3B) in the spinal cord, as determined by immunoblots using an antibody specific for H4-k16Ac residue [35]. Similarly, no significant effect of sham surgery on SIRT1 deacetylase activity was observed (Fig. 3A and 3B), suggesting that CCI surgery, but not exposure of the sciatic nerve, decreased the SIRT1 activity. One of the possible explanations for the observed elevation of immunoreactive H4-k16Ac content was an increase in total H4 content. In contrast, the total H4 content in the spinal cord did not undergo significant change in CCI mice as compared with sham group (Fig. 3A), indicating that the increase in immunoreactive H4-K16Ac content in the spinal cord was attributed to the reduction in deacetylation. Accordingly, we did not further detect total H4 protein content in the subsequent parts of the study. Additionally, H3-k9Ac (acetylation of H3-k9) levels were also increased in CCI mice relative to those before CCI surgery (data not shown). Our data were consistent with other studies demonstrating that SIRT1 deacetylated histone polypeptides with a preference for H4-k16Ac and H3-K9Ac [35]. In this study, H4-k16Ac signaling was used as the specific indicator for

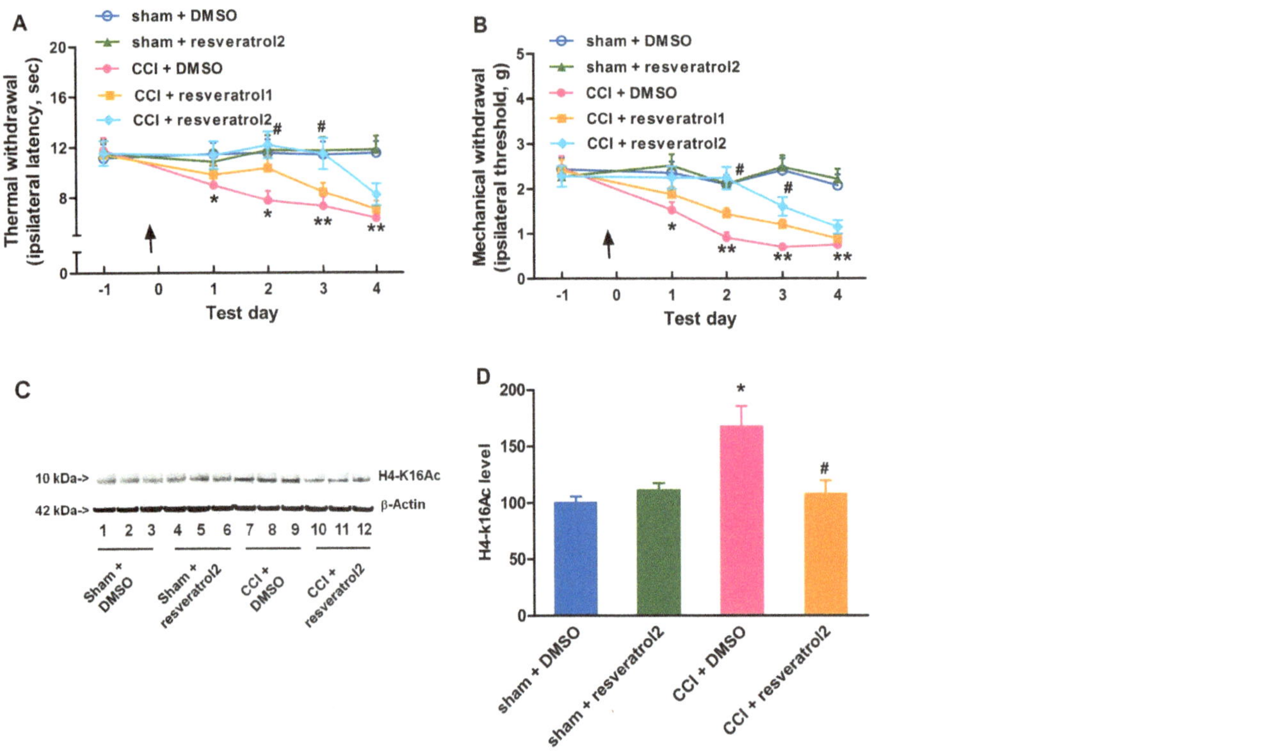

Figure 5. Resveratrol attenuates the development of neuropathic pain by alleviating the reduction of SIRT1 deacetylase activity. An intrathecal administration of 5 μl 90 mM resveratrol 1 h before CCI surgery, but not 45 mM suppresses the development of (A) thermal hyperalgesia and (B) mechanical allodynia induced by CCI surgery. (C) 45 mM resveratrol attenuates CCI-induced elevation of H4-K16Ac 2 days after CCI surgery. (D) Quantification of the immunoblots shows that 45 mM resveratrol attenuates CCI-induced increase in H4-K16Ac 2 days after surgery. An arrow indicates an intrathecal injection. $n = 10$ in each group for behavior test and $n = 6$ in each group for H4-K16Ac analysis; $^{*}P<0.05$, $^{**}P<0.01$ *vs.* DMSO-treated sham group; $^{\#}P<0.05$, $^{\#\#}P<0.01$ *vs.* DMSO-treated CCI group. Resveratrol1, 45 μM resveratrol; resveratrol2, 90 μM resveratrol; CCI, chronic constriction injury; H4-k16Ac, H4-k16 acetylation.

SIRT1-mediated deacetylase activity. Taken together, CCI surgery decreases SIRT1 content/activity and NAD/NAM in the mouse spinal cord.

NAD attenuates the CCI-induced development of neuropathic pain

Neuronal cells express membrane proteins which can bind and transport extracellular NAD into the cell [36]. Therefore, we investigated whether the exogenous NAD could attenuate the CCI-induced neuropathic pain. Daily intrathecal injection of 5 μl 800 mM NAD [28,29] into mice 1 h before and 1 day after CCI surgery, but not 400 mM, produced transient inhibition on the development of thermal hyperalgesia (Fig. 4A) and mechanical allodynia (Fig. 4B), with the degree of pain returning within 48 h after the last injection, as compared with the saline-treated CCI group. Additionally, 800 mM NAD attenuated the CCI-induced elevation of H4-k16Ac (Fig. 4C and 4D) 2 days after CCI surgery in mice as compared with the saline-treated CCI group. Taking into account that the levels of H3 or H4 acetylation can be used to evaluate the deacetylase activity of SIRT1 [35], our data suggested that abundant exogenous NAD injected intrathecally attenuated the development of neuropathic pain through an epigenetic mechanism in the mouse spinal cord.

Resveratrol attenuates the CCI-induced development of neuropathic pain

Knowing that resveratrol has an anti-nociceptive effect in some pain models [20,21,22,23] and works as an activator of SIRT1 as reported in the literature [37,38], we further asked whether resveratrol could delay the development of neuropathic pain. It was found in our study that an intrathecal administration of 5 μl 90 mM resveratrol [21,30,31] 1 h before CCI surgery, but not 45 mM, delayed the onset of thermal hyperalgesia (Fig. 5A) and mechanical allodynia (Fig. 5B), as comparable to the effect of exogenous NAD (Fig. 4A and 4B). Meanwhile, 90 mM resveratrol injected intrathecally reversed the CCI-induced elevation of H4-k16Ac (Fig. 5C and 5D) 2 days after CCI surgery in mice, as compared with the DMSO-treated CCI group. However, resveratrol had no significant effects on sham-operated mice. These results tempted us to conclude that resveratrol may delay the development of neuropathic pain induced by CCI and the reduction of SIRT1 activity may be one of the responsible factors contributing to the CCI-induced neuropathic pain.

Normal SIRT1 activity is essential for the anti-nociceptive effect of NAD and resveratrol

To confirm that SIRT1 was a key factor through which NAD or resveratrol attenuated the development of neuropathic pain, we further observed the effect of SIRT1 inhibitor EX-527 on the anti-nociceptive effect of NAD or resveratrol. It was found that an intrathecal injection of 5 μl EX-527 (1.2 mM) [24] 1 h before

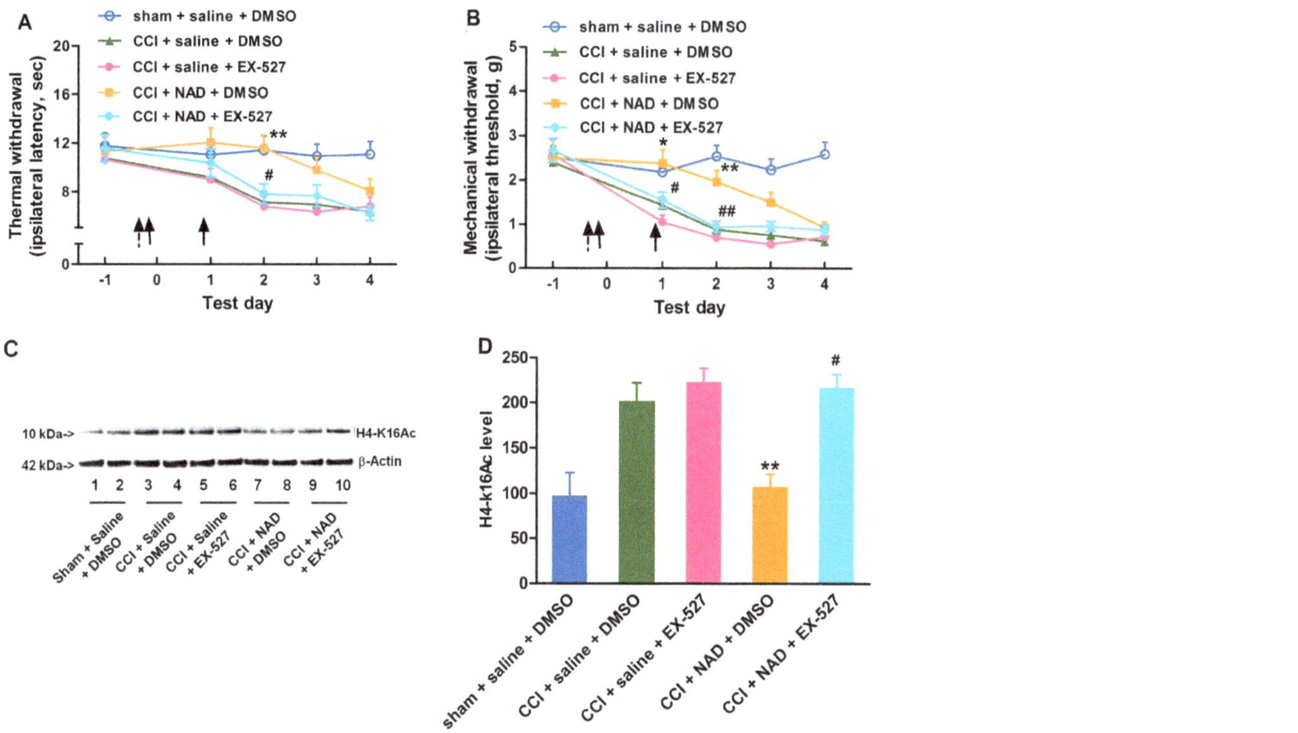

Figure 6. EX-527 inhibits the anti-nociceptive effect of NAD. An intrathecal injection of 5 µl EX-527 (1.2 mM) 1 h before NAD administration effectively reverses the effect of NAD (800 mM) delaying the onset of (A) thermal hyperalgesia and (B) mechanical allodynia produced by CCI surgery. (C) EX-527 inhibits the effect of NAD attenuating CCI-induced elevation of H4-K16Ac 1 day after CCI surgery. (D) Quantification of the immunoblots shows that EX-527 inhibits the effects of NAD on H4-K16Ac. An arrow indicates a NAD injection and a dotted arrow indicates an EX-527 injection. $n = 10$ in each group for behavior test and $n = 6$ in each group for H4-K16Ac analysis; $^{*}P<0.05$, $^{**}P<0.01$ *vs.* saline-DMSO-treated CCI group; $^{\#}P<0.05$, $^{\#\#}P<0.01$ *vs.* NAD-DMSO-treated CCI group. NAD, nicotinamide adenine dinucleotide; CCI, chronic constriction injury; H4-k16Ac, H4-k16 acetylation; DMSO, dimethyl sulfoxide.

NAD administration effectively blocked the anti-nociceptive effect of 800 mM NAD as compared with the DMSO-treated NAD-CCI group (Fig. 6). Additionally, an intrathecal injection of 5 µl EX-527 (1.2 mM) 1 h before resveratrol administration also effectively blocked the anti-nociceptive effect of 90 mM resveratrol as compared with the DMSO-treated resveratrol-CCI group (Fig. 7). These results indicated that SIRT1 may be the major effector of the exogenous NAD or resveratrol that prevented the development of neuropathic pain induced by CCI. Furthermore, the requirement of SIRT1 about 24 h prior to CCI surgery for NAD and resveratrol and SIRT1's predominant nuclear location [39] suggested that SIRT1 regulated a genetic program of the anti-nociceptive effect of NAD or resveratrol in the CCI-induced neuropathic pain.

Discussion

The present study has demonstrated that the SIRT1 content/activity and NAD/NAM ratio in the spinal cord were decreased in CCI mice. Additionally, the elevation of spinal SIRT1 deacetylase activity after the intrathecal administration of NAD or resveratrol transiently inhibited the onset of CCI-induced thermal hyperalgesia and mechanical allodynia in mice. Finally, we found that an intrathecal injection of SIRT1 inhibitor EX-527 before NAD or resveratrol administration reversed the anti-nociceptive effect of NAD or resveratrol in CCI mice. Nevertheless, these findings only represent our pilot investigation and preliminary assumption that SIRT1 and NAD may be involved in neuropathic pain. The long-term goal is to further determine the most effective modulated way of SIRT1 in attenuating neuropathic pain and the underlying mechanism.

SIRT1 may play some role in an epigenetic mechanism underlying CCI-induced neuropathic pain. The anatomical analysis of SIRT1 immunoreactivity highlights the presence of SIRT1 in all four major divisions of both adult rodent and human spinal cord including the cervical, thoracic, lumbar and sacral columns [39]. SIRT1 has been implicated in molecular pathways associated with pain [40] and nerve injury [18]. CCI produced by sciatic nerve ligature [32] enables nerve cells to mobilize a reprogramming process, which involves a variety of alternations in gene modification or gene mRNA expression [4,41]. It was found in this study that the SIRT1 expression and activity were decreased in CCI mice (Fig. 1 and 3) and modulations of SIRT1 activity by NAD (Fig. 4) or resveratrol (Fig. 5) ameliorated the development of neuropathic pain, suggesting that SIRT1 and its substrates [42] may be involved in the reprogramming process of the development of neuropathic pain. However, further studies are needed to observe pain behavioral changes in spinal SIRT1 (−/−) mice so as to clarify the direct contributions of SIRT1 to pain.

The decline in NAD and the resultant loss of genome silencing cause alternations in the related gene expression [43]. We demonstrated that NAD was decreased after CCI surgery (Fig. 2) and the exogenous NAD could ameliorate the development of neuropathic pain induced by CCI surgery (Fig. 4), suggesting that the pain neural circuit in the spinal cord may be susceptible to the NAD aberration. To further clarify the direct effect of reduced

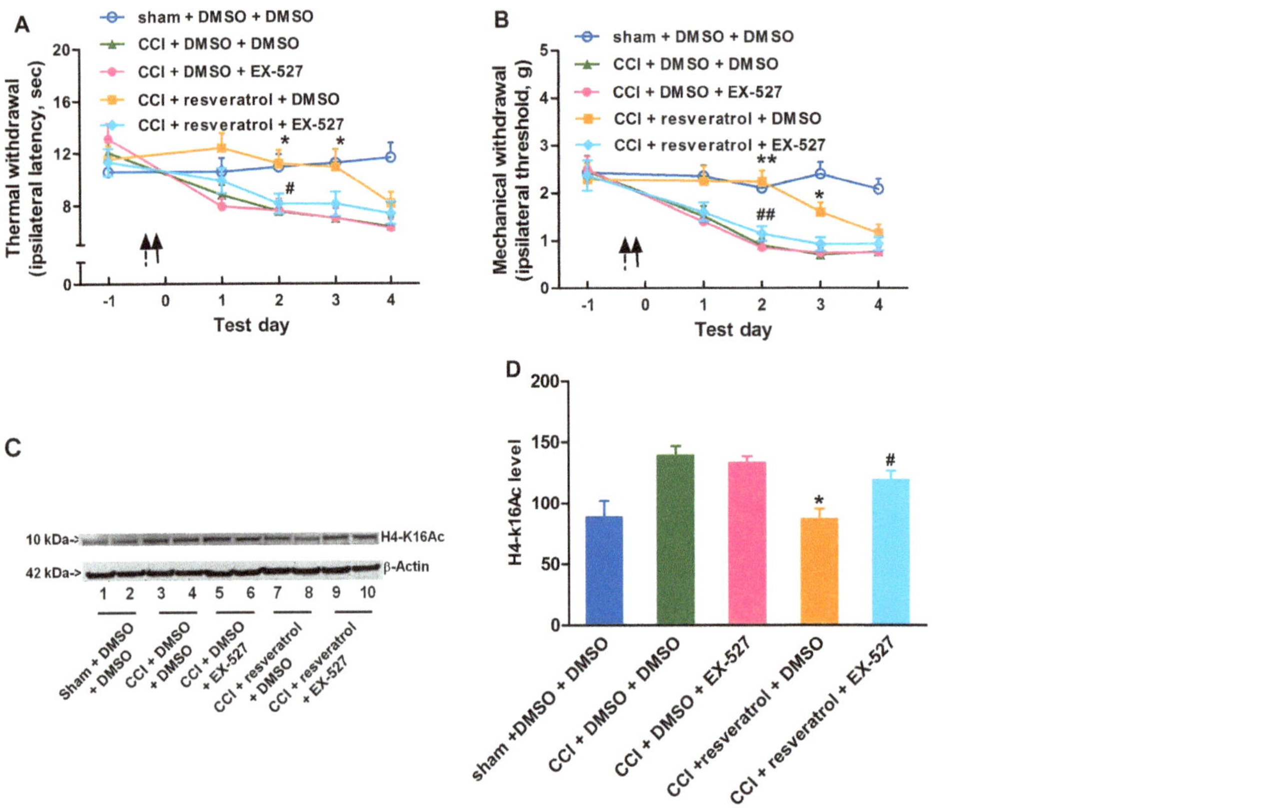

Figure 7. EX-527 inhibits the anti-nociceptive effect of resveratrol. Intrathecal injection of 5 μl EX-527 (1.2 mM) 1 h before resveratrol administration effectively reverses the effect of resveratrol (45 mM) delaying the onset of (A) thermal hyperalgesia and (B) mechanical allodynia produced by CCI surgery. (C) EX-527 inhibits the effect of resveratrol attenuating CCI-induced elevation of H4-K16Ac 1 day after CCI surgery. (D) Quantification of the immunoblots shows that EX-527 inhibits the effects of resveratrol on H4-K16Ac. An arrow indicates a resveratrol injection and a dotted arrow indicates an EX-527 injection. $n = 10$ in each group for behavior test and $n = 6$ in each group for H4-K16Ac analysis; $^{*}P<0.05$, $^{**}P<0.01$ *vs.* DMSO-DMSO-treated CCI group; $^{\#}P<0.05$, $^{\#\#}P<0.01$ *vs.* resveratrol-DMSO-treated CCI group. CCI, chronic constriction injury; H4-k16Ac, H4-k16 acetylation; DMSO, dimethyl sulfoxide.

NAD on hyperalgesia, further study in nicotinamide nucleotide adenylyltransferase 1 (Nmnat1) (−/−) mice may be helpful. It was reported [44] that the calorie restriction (CR) treatment increased the NAD/NAM ratio in the brain and prevented experimental amyloid neuropathology, but it was not clear whether CR could increase NAD in the spinal cord and attenuate neuropathic pain. Our ongoing study will focus on the effect of some different living habits such as CR and environmental enrichment on the NAD content and neuropathic pain in mice.

Knowing that resveratrol has poor bioavailability when given systemically such as via oral administration [45], we administered resveratrol intrathecally and observed its local pharmacology in the spinal cord. Some studies [46,47] reported that resveratrol was not a direct activator of SIRT1 in neuroprotection. Although resveratrol had multiple effects on many mammalian enzymes which complicated the interpretation of its effects, many effects of resveratrol in mice were consistent with the activation of SIRT1. Resveratrol was reported to extend lifespan in invertebrate organisms through activating SIRT1 homologues [37]. Specifically, resveratrol had beneficial effects in mice, which depended on SIRT1 [38]. In addition, these studies were carried out in *vitro*, and therefore it was possible that resveratrol might activate SIRT1 through some intermediate factors. Our *vivo* study showed that EX-527 as a SIRT1 inhibitor could reverse the effect of resveratrol, suggesting that the anti-nociceptive effect of resveratrol may be due to, at least in part, resveratrol-induced SIRT1 activation. However, it could not be excluded that resveratrol might attenuate the elevation of H4-k16Ac induced by CCI surgery through other pathways other than the SIRT1 pathway. To further clarify whether SIRT1 activation could attenuate neuropathic pain, our ongoing study will focus on the effect of other specific SIRT1 activators on CCI mice. The effects of NAD and resveratrol were delayed almost 2 days by paradigm pretreatment (Fig. 4, 5), suggesting that the drug effect and epigenetic modification may be transient and reversible if the drugs are given for only one or two times, indicating that continual intrathecal injections of NAD or resveratrol are needed to achieve a long-lasting anti-hyperalgesic effect. Whether the post-treatment of NAD or resveratrol could inhibit the established CCI-induced pain also needs further study. Knowing that SIRT1 is a NAD-dependent protein deacetylase and NAD is only a co-factor in SIRT1's deacetylation, a single or two administrations of NAD may not be able to produce long-lasting effects. Additionally, our data showed that the intrathecal injections of NAD were done 2 times at 24 h intervals while resveratrol was injected once and showed longer and stronger anti-hyperalgesic effects. There may be two underlying reasons. Firstly, NAD was quickly consumed to NAM by SIRT1, while resveratrol activated SIRT1 for a longer time. Secondly, resveratrol was more hydrophobic than NAD, and was easier to go through the cell membrane and then reach the target site, showing stronger action than NAD.

Both of the above presumptions need to be further studied. A most recent study [21] reported that the SIRT1 content was decreased after CCI surgery in rats, and this decrease was consistent with the behavioral change. However, they did not investigate the effect of the increased SIRT1 activity on attenuating CCI-induced neuropathic pain, and therefore their finding could not strongly support that CCI-induced hyperalgeisa was attributed to the reduction of SIRT1. In addition, their study did not show the effect of sham surgery on SIRT1 content and activity. Our study demonstrated that SIRT1 content and activity were decreased in CCI mice, but not in sham surgery mice (Fig. 1 and 3). We also found that the elevation of SIRT1 activity by exogenous NAD or resveratrol ameliorated the development of neuropathic pain induced by CCI surgery and SIRT1 inhibitor EX-527 reversed the anti-nociceptive effect of NAD or resveratrol, suggesting that SIRT1 may be a key factor contributing to CCI-induced neuropathic pain. Our future study will investigate the down-stream mechanism through which SIRT1 attenuates neuropathic pain.

In conclusion, our in *vivo* results have provided some evidence that SIRT1 plays a role in ameliorating the development of neuropathic pain, which may be a novel mechanism underlying neuropathic pain. It may be possible that the manipulation of SIRT1 activity by NAD and/or resveratrol in epidural anaesthesia combined with local anesthetics could provide new therapeutic opportunities for the treatment of neuropathic pain induced by nerve injuries associated with some surgical procedures such as amputation or thoracic operation.

Acknowledgments

We would like to thank Lei Zhang for his gift of EX-527.

Author Contributions

Conceived and designed the experiments: HS BY. Performed the experiments: HS QX FZ YL H. Zhu XZ H. Zhang. Analyzed the data: H. Zhang HS. Contributed reagents/materials/analysis tools: WD. Wrote the paper: HS BY.

References

1. Baron R (2006) Mechanisms of disease: neuropathic pain – a clinical perspective. Nat Clin Pract Neurol 2: 95–106.
2. Uchida H, Ma L, Ueda H (2010) Epigenetic gene silencing underlies C-fiber dysfunctions in neuropathic pain. J Neurosci 30: 4806–4814.
3. Uchida H, Sasaki K, Ma L, Ueda H (2010) Neuron-restrictive silencer factor causes epigenetic silencing of Kv4.3 gene after peripheral nerve injury. Neuroscience 166: 1–4.
4. Adilakshmi T, Sudol I, Tapinos N (2012) Combinatorial action of miRNAs regulates transcriptional and post-transcriptional gene silencing following in vivo PNS injury. PLoS One 7: e39674.
5. Wang Y, Nowicki MO, Wang X, Arnold WD, Fernandez SA, et al. (2012) Comparative effectiveness of antinociceptive gene therapies in animal models of diabetic neuropathic pain. Gene Ther.
6. Uchida H, Matsushita Y, Ueda H (2013) Epigenetic regulation of BDNF expression in the primary sensory neurons after peripheral nerve injury: implications in the development of neuropathic pain. Neuroscience 240: 147–154.
7. Kiguchi N, Kobayashi Y, Maeda T, Fukazawa Y, Tohya K, et al. (2012) Epigenetic augmentation of the macrophage inflammatory protein 2/C-X-C chemokine receptor type 2 axis through histone H3 acetylation in injured peripheral nerves elicits neuropathic pain. J Pharmacol Exp Ther 340: 577–587.
8. Chiechio S, Zammataro M, Morales ME, Busceti CL, Drago F, et al. (2009) Epigenetic modulation of mGlu2 receptors by histone deacetylase inhibitors in the treatment of inflammatory pain. Mol Pharmacol 75: 1014–1020.
9. Denk F, Huang W, Sidders B, Bithell A, Crow M, et al. (2013) HDAC inhibitors attenuate the development of hypersensitivity in models of neuropathic pain. Pain 154: 1668–1679.
10. Tissenbaum HA, Guarente L (2001) Increased dosage of a sir-2 gene extends lifespan in Caenorhabditis elegans. Nature 410: 227–230.
11. Finkel T, Deng CX, Mostoslavsky R (2009) Recent progress in the biology and physiology of sirtuins. Nature 460: 587–591.
12. Nakahata Y, Kaluzova M, Grimaldi B, Sahar S, Hirayama J, et al. (2008) The NAD+-dependent deacetylase SIRT1 modulates CLOCK-mediated chromatin remodeling and circadian control. Cell 134: 329–340.
13. Nakahata Y, Sahar S, Astarita G, Kaluzova M, Sassone-Corsi P (2009) Circadian control of the NAD+ salvage pathway by CLOCK-SIRT1. Science 324: 654–657.
14. Kim D, Nguyen MD, Dobbin MM, Fischer A, Sananbenesi F, et al. (2007) SIRT1 deacetylase protects against neurodegeneration in models for Alzheimer's disease and amyotrophic lateral sclerosis. EMBO J 26: 3169–3179.
15. Bellamacina CR (1996) The nicotinamide dinucleotide binding motif: a comparison of nucleotide binding proteins. FASEB J 10: 1257–1269.
16. Blander G, Guarente L (2004) The Sir2 family of protein deacetylases. Annu Rev Biochem 73: 417–435.
17. Bitterman KJ, Anderson RM, Cohen HY, Latorre-Esteves M, Sinclair DA (2002) Inhibition of silencing and accelerated aging by nicotinamide, a putative negative regulator of yeast sir2 and human SIRT1. J Biol Chem 277: 45099–45107.
18. Araki T, Sasaki Y, Milbrandt J (2004) Increased nuclear NAD biosynthesis and SIRT1 activation prevent axonal degeneration. Science 305: 1010–1013.
19. Milne JC, Denu JM (2008) The Sirtuin family: therapeutic targets to treat diseases of aging. Curr Opin Chem Biol 12: 11–17.
20. Wuertz K, Quero L, Sekiguchi M, Klawitter M, Nerlich A, et al. (2011) The red wine polyphenol resveratrol shows promising potential for the treatment of nucleus pulposus-mediated pain in vitro and in vivo. Spine (Phila Pa 1976) 36: E1373–1384.
21. Yin Q, Lu FF, Zhao Y, Cheng MY, Fan Q, et al. (2013) Resveratrol Facilitates Pain Attenuation in a Rat Model of Neuropathic Pain Through the Activation of Spinal Sirt1. Reg Anesth Pain Med.
22. Tillu DV, Melemedjian OK, Asiedu MN, Qu N, De Felice M, et al. (2012) Resveratrol engages AMPK to attenuate ERK and mTOR signaling in sensory neurons and inhibits incision-induced acute and chronic pain. Mol Pain 8: 5.
23. Tsai RY, Chou KY, Shen CH, Chien CC, Tsai WY, et al. (2012) Resveratrol regulates N-methyl-D-aspartate receptor expression and suppresses neuroinflammation in morphine-tolerant rats. Anesth Analg 115: 944–952.
24. Napper AD, Hixon J, McDonagh T, Keavey K, Pons JF, et al. (2005) Discovery of indoles as potent and selective inhibitors of the deacetylase SIRT1. J Med Chem 48: 8045–8054.
25. Peck B, Chen CY, Ho KK, Di Fruscia P, Myatt SS, et al. (2010) SIRT inhibitors induce cell death and p53 acetylation through targeting both SIRT1 and SIRT2. Mol Cancer Ther 9: 844–855.
26. Lee JC, Shin JH, Park BW, Kim GS, Kim JC, et al. (2012) Region-specific changes in the immunoreactivity of SIRT1 expression in the central nervous system of SOD1(G93A) transgenic mice as an in vivo model of amyotrophic lateral sclerosis. Brain Res 1433: 20–28.
27. Hylden JL, Wilcox GL (1980) Intrathecal morphine in mice: a new technique. Eur J Pharmacol 67: 313–316.
28. Klaidman LK, Mukherjee SK, Hutchin TP, Adams JD (1996) Nicotinamide as a precursor for NAD+ prevents apoptosis in the mouse brain induced by tertiary-butylhydroperoxide. Neurosci Lett 206: 5–8.
29. Hoane MR, Pierce JL, Holland MA, Anderson GD (2008) Nicotinamide treatment induces behavioral recovery when administered up to 4 hours following cortical contusion injury in the rat. Neuroscience 154: 861–868.
30. Perez-Severiano F, Bermudez-Ocana DY, Lopez-Sanchez P, Rios C, Granados-Soto V (2008) Spinal nerve ligation reduces nitric oxide synthase activity and expression: effect of resveratrol. Pharmacol Biochem Behav 90: 742–747.
31. Bermudez-Ocana DY, Ambriz-Tututi M, Perez-Severiano F, Granados-Soto V (2006) Pharmacological evidence for the participation of NO-cyclic GMP-PKG-K+ channel pathway in the antiallodynic action of resveratrol. Pharmacol Biochem Behav 84: 535–542.
32. Bennett GJ, Xie YK (1988) A peripheral mononeuropathy in rat that produces disorders of pain sensation like those seen in man. Pain 33: 87–107.
33. Hargreaves K, Dubner R, Brown F, Flores C, Joris J (1988) A new and sensitive method for measuring thermal nociception in cutaneous hyperalgesia. Pain 32: 77–88.
34. Bradford MM (1976) A rapid and sensitive method for the quantitation of microgram quantities of protein utilizing the principle of protein-dye binding. Anal Biochem 72: 248–254.
35. Vaquero A, Scher M, Lee D, Erdjument-Bromage H, Tempst P, et al. (2004) Human SirT1 interacts with histone H1 and promotes formation of facultative heterochromatin. Mol Cell 16: 93–105.
36. Bruzzone S, Guida L, Zocchi E, Franco L, De Flora A (2001) Connexin 43 hemi channels mediate Ca2+-regulated transmembrane NAD+ fluxes in intact cells. FASEB J 15: 10–12.
37. Wood JG, Rogina B, Lavu S, Howitz K, Helfand SL, et al. (2004) Sirtuin activators mimic caloric restriction and delay ageing in metazoans. Nature 430: 686–689.
38. Baur JA, Sinclair DA (2006) Therapeutic potential of resveratrol: the in vivo evidence. Nat Rev Drug Discov 5: 493–506.
39. Zakhary SM, Ayubcha D, Dileo JN, Jose R, Leheste JR, et al. (2010) Distribution analysis of deacetylase SIRT1 in rodent and human nervous systems. Anat Rec (Hoboken) 293: 1024–1032.

40. Renthal W, Kumar A, Xiao G, Wilkinson M, Covington HE 3rd, et al. (2009) Genome-wide analysis of chromatin regulation by cocaine reveals a role for sirtuins. Neuron 62: 335–348.
41. Imai S, Saeki M, Yanase M, Horiuchi H, Abe M, et al. (2011) Change in microRNAs associated with neuronal adaptive responses in the nucleus accumbens under neuropathic pain. J Neurosci 31: 15294–15299.
42. Borrelli E, Nestler EJ, Allis CD, Sassone-Corsi P (2008) Decoding the epigenetic language of neuronal plasticity. Neuron 60: 961–974.
43. Imai S (2009) From heterochromatin islands to the NAD World: a hierarchical view of aging through the functions of mammalian Sirt1 and systemic NAD biosynthesis. Biochim Biophys Acta 1790: 997–1004.
44. Qin W, Yang T, Ho L, Zhao Z, Wang J, et al. (2006) Neuronal SIRT1 activation as a novel mechanism underlying the prevention of Alzheimer disease amyloid neuropathology by calorie restriction. J Biol Chem 281: 21745–21754.
45. Larrosa M, Azorin-Ortuno M, Yanez-Gascon MJ, Garcia-Conesa MT, Tomas-Barberan F, et al. (2011) Lack of effect of oral administration of resveratrol in LPS-induced systemic inflammation. Eur J Nutr 50: 673–680.
46. Pacholec M, Bleasdale JE, Chrunyk B, Cunningham D, Flynn D, et al. (2010) SRT1720, SRT2183, SRT1460, and resveratrol are not direct activators of SIRT1. J Biol Chem 285: 8340–8351.
47. Tang BL (2010) Resveratrol is neuroprotective because it is not a direct activator of Sirt1-A hypothesis. Brain Res Bull 81: 359–361.

15

Palliation of Bone Cancer Pain by Antagonists of Platelet-Activating Factor Receptors

Katsuya Morita[1,2,4], Seiji Shiraishi[2], Naoyo Motoyama[2,3], Tomoya Kitayama[4], Takashi Kanematsu[4], Yasuhito Uezono[2], Toshihiro Dohi[5]*

1 Department of Pharmacology, Faculty of Nursing, Hiroshima Bunka Gakuen University, Hiroshima, Japan, **2** Cancer Pathophysiology, Division National Cancer Center Research Institute, Tokyo, Japan, **3** Department of Dental Science for Health Promotion, Division of Integrated Health Sciences, Institute of Biomedical and Health Sciences, Hiroshima University, Hiroshima, Japan, **4** Department of Cell and Molecular Pharmacology, Division of Basic Life Science, Institute of Biomedical and Health Sciences, Hiroshima University, Hiroshima, Japan, **5** Department of Pharmacotherapy, Pharmaceutical Sciences, Nihon Pharmaceutical University, Saitama, Japan

Abstract

Bone cancer pain is the most severe among cancer pain and is often resistant to current analgesics. Thus, the development of novel analgesics effective at treating bone cancer pain are desired. Platelet-activating factor (PAF) receptor antagonists were recently demonstrated to have effective pain relieving effects on neuropathic pain in several animal models. The present study examined the pain relieving effect of PAF receptor antagonists on bone cancer pain using the femur bone cancer (FBC) model in mice. Animals were injected with osteolytic NCTC2472 cells into the tibia, and subsequently the effects of PAF receptor antagonists on pain behaviors were evaluated. Chemical structurally different type of antagonists, TCV-309, BN 50739 and WEB 2086 ameliorated the allodynia and improved pain behaviors such as guarding behavior and limb-use abnormalities in FBC model mice. The pain relieving effects of these antagonists were achieved with low doses and were long lasting. Blockade of spinal PAF receptors by intrathecal injection of TCV-309 and WEB 2086 or knockdown of the expression of spinal PAF receptor protein by intrathecal transfer of PAF receptor siRNA also produced a pain relieving effect. The amount of an inducible PAF synthesis enzyme, lysophosphatidylcholine acyltransferase 2 (LPCAT2) protein significantly increased in the spinal cord after transplantation of NCTC 2472 tumor cells into mouse tibia. The combination of morphine with PAF receptor antagonists develops marked enhancement of the analgesic effect against bone cancer pain without affecting morphine-induced constipation. Repeated administration of TCV-309 suppressed the appearance of pain behaviors and prolonged survival of FBC mice. The present results suggest that PAF receptor antagonists in combination with, or without, opioids may represent a new strategy for the treatment of persistent bone cancer pain and improve the quality of life of patients.

Editor: Theodore John Price, University of Arizona, United States of America

Funding: This work was supported in part by Grants-in Aid for Scientific Research (B) 22390349, (C) 21592421 and (C) 24592798 from the Japanese Society for Promotion of Sciences and by the National Cancer Center Research and Development Fund (23-A-30). The funders had no role in study design, data collection and analysis, decision to publish, or preparation of the manuscript.

Competing Interests: The authors have declared that no competing interests exist.

* E-mail: t-dohi@nichiyaku.ac.jp

These authors contributed equally to this work.

Introduction

Pain in cancer is produced by pressure on, or chemical stimulation of, specialized pain-signalling nerve endings called nociceptors (nociceptive pain) or it may be caused by damage or illness affecting nerve fibers themselves (neuropathic pain) which is responsive to stimuli that are normally non-painful; allodynia. Bone cancer pain is one of the most common and usually serious pain conditions in cancer patients [1].

Opioids remain the mainstay of cancer pain management, but in addition to the acute side effects the long-term consequences of tolerance, dependency, hyperalgesia and the suppression of the hypothalamic/pituitary axis should be acknowledged. Because the current available treatments are relatively ineffective against bone cancer pain, almost half of cancer patients have inadequate pain control [2,3]. Thus, the development of novel analgesics effective at treating bone cancer pain are required.

We have previously suggested that platelet-activating factor (PAF) may be a mediator of neuropathic pain. PAF injection into the mouse spinal cord caused thermal hyperalgesia and tactile allodynia, which were at least in part mediated by spinal dysfunction of glycine receptor α3 (GlyRα3) and were blocked by PAF receptor antagonists [4,5]. Subsequent studies showed PAF receptor blockade reduced pain behaviors elicited in nerve injury models. A PAF receptor antagonist, CV-3988, injected near the dorsal root ganglion (DRG) in rats or mice lacking PAF receptors showed a reduction in tactile allodynia following spinal nerve injury [6]. Intrathecal injection of the PAF receptor antagonist, WEB 2086, a benzodiazepine derivative for 9 days post-surgery in rats suppressed the development of mechanical allodynia in a rat spared nerve injury model [7]. PAF receptor antagonists, TCV-309 (PAF related), BN 50739 (natural product related compound), and WEB 2086, produced profound and long lasting anti-allodynia effects in several different neuropathic pain models in mice, including a partial sciatic nerve ligation injury model, a partial infraorbital nerve ligation model, a chronic constriction of the infraorbital nerve injury model (CCI model) and a streptozotocin (STZ)-induced diabetes model [8]. The evidence suggests that PAF contributes to neural tissue damage and pain behavior after nerve injury.

The animal models above investigated pain due to bone cancer, in which tumor cells are injected locally into the bone. The present study used the femur bone cancer (FBC) model in mice [9]. Animals were injected with osteolytic NCTC2472 cells, and subsequently the effects of PAF receptor antagonists on pain behaviors were evaluated.

Materials and Methods

Experimental Animals

The experiments were performed using male C3H/HeN mice (CLEA Japan, Inc., Tokyo), weighing 20–25 g. All experimental procedures and animal handling were performed according to both the Guiding Principles for the Care and Use of Laboratory Animals approved by the Japanese Pharmacological Society and the guidelines of Hiroshima University, Hiroshima, Japan and the guidelines of National Cancer Center Research Institute, Tokyo, Japan. The protocol was approved by the committee on the Ethics of Animal Experiments of the Hiroshima University (Permit Number: A-09-17 and A-11-16), and of the National Cancer Center (Permit Number: T11-004-M02). All surgery was performed under sodium pentobarbital anesthesia, and all efforts were made to minimize suffering. The animals were used for only one measurement in each experiment.

The Mouse Femur Bone Cancer (FBC) Model

For the FBC model, NCTC 2472 tumor cells (American Type Cuiture Collection, ATCC; Manassas, VA, USA) were injected into the medullary cavity of the distal femur of C3H/HeN mice [9]. The NCTC 2472 cells were maintained in Dulbecco's Modified Eagle's Medium, supplemented with 10% Fetal bovine serum, 100 unit/ml penicillin, and 100 μg/ml streptomycin (all products from Gibco Laboratories); and cultured at 37°C in a humidified atmosphere of 5% CO_2 then passaged weekly according to ATCC guidelines. For administration, cells were detached by scraping and then centrifuged at 900 rpm for 3 min. The pellet was suspended in Hank's balanced salt solution (HBSS) and then used for intratibial injection.

For implantation, tumor cells were injected following the protocol described previously by Honore et al. [9] with slight modification. In brief, C3H/HeN mice were anesthetized with a sodium pentobarbital (60 mg/kg) i.p. injected. For intratibial inoculation of cells, the right knee of each mouse was bent and placed facing the experimenter and a minimal skin incision was made exposing the tibial plateau. A 25 gauge dental reamer was used to perforate the tibial plateau and, once removed, a 30 gauge needle coupled to a Hamilton syringe filled with the cell suspension was carefully introduced into the medullary cavity of the tibia. Then, 10^5 NCTC 2472 cells suspended in 5 μl of HBSS were slowly injected (living cells). Control groups were injected with 5 μl of HBSS or HBSS containing 10^5 NCTC 2472 cells killed by quickly freezing and thawing them twice without cryoprotection and then washing with fresh HBSS (deaden cells). Finally, Caviton EX, a dental-grade hydraulic temporary sealant (GC Dental Products, Co. Ltd., Tokyo, Japan) was applied to the tibial plateau incised area and the surgical procedure was completed with stitching of the knee skin. Body weights were recorded for each mouse every 3 days throughout the study. The animals were euthanized following weight loss greater than 20% of body weight or upon demonstrating related symptoms such as serious ataxic movements or other neurological abnormalities due to ethical concerns.

Drug Administration

Gabapentin (1-(aminomethyl)-cyclohexaneacetic acid) was obtained from Sigma-Aldrich (St. Louis, MO). Morphine was obtained from Takeda Pharmaceutical Co., (Osaka, Japan). WEB 2086 (3-[4-(2-chlorophenyl)-9- methyl-6*H*-thieno[3,2-*f*][1,2,4]triazolo-[4,3-*a*][1,4]-diazepin-2-yl]-1-(4-morpholinyl)-1-propanone) was obtained from Tocris Bioscience (Ellisville, MO). TCV-309 (3-bromo-5-[*N*-phenyl-*N*-[2-[[2-(1,2,3,4-tetrahydro-2-isoquinolyl- carbonyloxy)ethyl]carbamoyl]ethyl]carbamoyl]-1-propylpyridinium nitrate), and BN 50739 (tetrahydro-4,7,8,10methyl-(chloro-2phenyl)6[dimethoxy-3,4- phenylthio]-methylthiocarbonyl-9 pyrido[4′,3′-4,5]thieno[3,2-*f*]triazolo-1,2,4[4,3-*a*]diazepine-1,4) were donated from Takeda Pharmaceutical Co., and Institute Henri Beaufour, respectively.

TCV-309 and WEB 2086 were each dissolved in sterile artificial cerebrospinal fluid (ACSF) or saline solution. BN 50739 was dissolved in a solvent containing 25% 2-hydroxypropyl-β-cyclodextrin (Sigma/RBI, Natick, MA) and distilled water, pH adjusted to ~6 using 1 N NaOH, and diluted appropriately with ACSF or saline. Other reagents were dissolved in ACSF or saline. The drug solutions were freshly prepared on each experimental day. ACSF composition (in mM) was NaCl 142, KCl 5, $CaCl_2$ $2H_2O$ 2, $MgCl_2{\cdot}6H_2O$ 2, NaH_2PO_4 1.25, D-glucose 10, HEPES 10, pH 7.4. TCV-309, BN70329, or WEB 2086 was administered intravenously 30 min-3 hr before pain assessment.

Knockdown of PAF Receptor in the Spinal Cord

Knockdown of PAF receptor was performed according to a previous report [5]. siRNAs were incorporated into the hemagglutinating virus of the Japan (HVJ)-Envelope Vector according to the manufacturer's instructions. Briefly, after mixing 40 μl (1 assay unit, AU) of HVJ-Envelope Vector with 4 μl of the enclosing factor, the mixture was centrifuged (10,000×*g*, 10 min, 4°C), and the pellet suspended in 10 μl of buffer solution. Then, 10 μl of a mixture of 3 siRNAs solution (#1, #2 and #3, 1 μg/μl each) was added, and the mixture was kept on ice for 5 min. Sterile ACSF (10 μl) containing synthetic siRNA duplexes (0.45 pmole/animal) was injected into the subarachnoid space between the L5 and L6 vertebrates of conscious mice. The sequences of the siRNA oligonucleotide (sense) were as follows: PAF receptor (#1, 5′-CACCUCAGUGAGAAGUUUUACAGCA-AG-3′; #2, 5′-AC-CCUUCCAAGAAACUAAAUGAGAU-AG-3′; #3, 5′-CAACU-UCCAUCAGGCUAUUAAUGAU-AG-3′; targeting sequences around position 1005 to 1029, 232 to 256, 893 to 917, respectively, in *pafr*, GenBank accession no. D5087). Moreover, mismatched siRNA with three or four nucleotide mismatches was prepared to examine nonspecific effects of siRNA duplexes (siRNA#4, 5′-AC<u>U</u>CU<u>G</u>CCAAGA<u>G</u>ACUA<u>C</u>AUGAGAU-AG-3). These selected sequences were also submitted to a BLAST search (Bioinformatics Center Institute for Chemical Research, Kyoto University, Japan) against the mouse genome sequence to ensure that only one gene in the mouse genome was targeted. siRNAs were purchased from iGENE Therapeutics Inc. (Tsukuba, Japan).

Behavioral Analysis in the FBC Model

The behavioral analysis was preformed following the protocol described previously [5,10]. The pain-related behaviors in the FBC model were evaluated before and after drug administration on 11 days after tumor implantation. The experimental and sham operated animals were evaluated for on-going pain based on guarding behavior, for ambulatory pain based on limb-use abnormality, and for allodynia-like behavior based on the von Frey filament test and paintbrush test. Guarding behavior, limb-use abnormality and allodynia-like pain were assessed in the same animals. The mice were placed in a clear plastic observation box and allowed to habituate for 15 min. Then, spontaneous guarding behavior was assessed during a 2-min observation period. The lifting time of the hind paw on the ipsilateral side during ambulation was measured as guarding behavior. Limb-use abnormality was scored on a scale of 0 to 4: 0, normal use of limb; 1, slight limp; 2, clear limp; 3, partial non-use of limb; and 4, complete non-use of limb. Allodynia-like behavior was assessed by lightly stroking the injured leg with a paintbrush (allodynia score) or evaluated by measuring the paw withdrawal threshold in response to probing with a series of calibrated fine filaments (allodynia threshold) as reported previously [5]. The allodynia score was ranked as described by Minami et al. [11]: 0, no response; 1, mild squeaking with attempts to move away from the stroking probe; 2, vigorous squeaking, biting the stroking probe and strong efforts to escape from the stroking probe. Values are the average of the total score evaluated 3 times at each time point (possible maximum score at each time point: 2/mouse). The guard times were significantly prolonged at 5 and 6 days after tumor implantation compared with the values at pre-implantation. Similarly, animals also started to exhibit abnormal limb-use at 5 days after tumor implantation, and such abnormal behavior was more prominent in the later days. The allodynia threshold was evaluated by measuring the paw withdrawal threshold in response to probing with von Frey monofilaments, and significant threshold declines were observed after the 3rd day post tumor implantation compared with the values at pre-implantation, and the decrease reached a peak after 5 and 7 days. The allodynia score was evaluated by measuring the ranked response to lightly stroking with a paintbrush, and significant score rises were observed after the 4-day post tumor implantation compared with the values at pre-implantation, and the increase reached a peak after 6 and 8 days. Throughout the experiment, behavioral testing was performed under blind conditions by a single experimenter. Injections were performed blind by another person. Intrathecal injection was performed as described previously [4].

Determination of Lyso-PAF-Acetyltransferase (Lyso-PAF AT)/Lysophospha- tidylcholine Acyltransferase 2 (LPCAT2), a PAF Synthesis Enzyme

The lumbar regions of the spinal cord (L2-L6) were obtained from sham-operated (deaden cells implanted) or tumor-bearing mice. The spinal cord tissues (4.8–5.0 mg) were homogenized in 20 mM Tris-HCl (pH 7.5) containing 1 mM EDTA, 1 mM EGTA, 10 mM NaF, 10 mM β-glycerophosphate and 1 μg/ml of various protease inhibitors (benzamdine, leupeptin and antipain). The homogenate was reacted with 0.6% NP-40 for 5 min at 4°C, followed by centrifugation at 15,000 rpm for 5 min at 4°C and the supernatant was obtained. The supernatant was mixed at a volume ration of 4:1 in 10 mM Tris-HCl (pH 6.8) containing 10% (v/v) glycerol, 2% sodium dodecylsulfate (SDS), 0.01% bromophenol blue and 0.5% β-mercaptoethanol, with subsequent boiling at 70°C for 30 min.

Immunoblotting Assays

The obtained samples were electrophoresed for 2 hr at room temperature on polyacrylamide gels (stacking gel 3% and separating gel 10%) and then blotted to polyvinylidene fluoride membranes previously treated with 100% methanol. The transferred proteins on the membranes were blocked by incubating with blocking solution, a 5% skim milk-containing wash buffer (20 mM Tris-HCl (pH 7.5), 137 mM NaCl and 0.1% Tween 20), at 25°C for 1 hr. The membranes were exposed to the primary antibody as follows: against LPCAT2 (1:1,000; Sigm); against β-actin (1:1,000; IMGENEX Innovations in Functional Genomics, SanDiego, CA) diluted with the wash buffer containing 1% skim milk overnight at 4°C, followed by washing three times with the wash buffer, and then incubation with a secondary antibody as follows: for the LPCAT2 antibody and β-actin antibody, an anti-rabbit IgG antibody conjugated with horseradish peroxidase (1:2,000; DakoCytomation, Glostrup, Denmark) at room temperature for 1 hr. The membranes were again rinsed three times with the wash buffer and developed with an enhanced chemiluminescence (ECL) western detection system (ECL reagents, purchased from Thermo Fisher Scientific, and Nacalai Tesque Inc., Kyoto Japan; ImageQuant^{TM} LAS 4000 mini detection system, GE healthcare Japan, Tokyo, Japan). The density of each band was analyzed using NIH Image software, and the densitometric units were corrected using the value of β-actin. The data are expressed as the mean ± SEM.

Morphine-induced Constipation

Mice were provided food and water ad libitum before the test period, and both (with or without TCV-309) groups consumed comparable amounts of food prior to the test as measured over a 24-hr period in the test environment. No food or water was available during the test. Mice were caged in acrylic boxes with grid floors suspended over filter paper. Fecal boli were collected from each group of mice every hour for 1 hr following the injection of saline or various doses of morphine and the weight of fecal boli was recorded as an index of the constipating effects of morphine.

Generation of Kaplan–Meier Survival Curves

The health of the mice was examined daily. Mice that presented with signs of ill health were killed by cervical dislocation according to the recommendations of our Ethical Committee. In our experience, these signs precede the time of death by a couple of days. The time of death was recorded for each mouse that was found dead or was killed. Kaplan–Meier survival curves were generated using Graphpad Prism software (version 4; Graphpad, Inc, San Diego, CA).

Statistical Analyses

All data are reported as values of the mean ± SEM (standard error of the mean). Graphpad Prism software version 4 was used to perform the statistical analysis. Regarding the statistical analysis of the pain-related behaviors, comparisons of the allodynis score, withdrawal threshold, guarding behavior and limb-use abnormality of the differences between the drug-treated groups and the vehicle-treated group were evaluated using two-way ANOVA followed by Tukey-Kramer test, or an unpaired Student's *t*-test. Comparisons of median survival were performed using log-rank and Gehan–Breslow–Wilcoxon tests. A probability value (P) of <0.05 was considered statistically significant.

Results

Effects of Systemic Administration of Specific PAF Receptor Antagonists on Tactile Allodynia and Pain Behaviors in FBC Model Mice

Effects of TCV-309 on allodynia and pain behaviors (guarding behavior and limb-use abnormality) were examined in FBC model mice. TCV-309 with a range of 10–300 μg/kg by i.v. dose-dependently reduced the allodynia score (Figure 1A) and increased the withdrawal threshold (Figure 1B) at 11 to 15 days after tumor implantation in the mice. The effects of TCV-309 were quite long lasting. For instance, TCV-309 significantly ameliorated mechanical allodynia by a single injection of 100 μg/kg, i.v. with a peak effect at 1 to 2 days after the injection up to 6 days. Guarding behavior was continuously aggravated during the observation period, while limb-use abnormality reached a maximal response and continued during the period (Figure 1C, 1D). Guarding behavior and limb-use abnormality were also improved by TCV-309. TCV-309 up to 1 mg/kg did not affect general behavior or motor function estimated by the RotaRod test (data not shown). Other PAF receptor antagonists, BN 50739 and WEB 2086, also ameliorated the allodynia and pain behaviors in the FBC model mice (Figure1E–1H).

Effects of Blockade of Spinal PAF Receptors on Allodynia and Pain Behaviors in FBC Model Mice

To confirm the site of cancer pain palliation by PAF antagonists, the effects of intrathecal injection of TCV-309 and WEB 2086, and also interference in the expression of spinal PAF receptors using siRNA of PAF receptor mRNA were examined. Spinal administration of 10 pg of these drugs 13 days post-tumor implantation produced rapid and marked suppression of tactile allodynia with the maximal effect at 1 day post-implantation and significantly suppressed the allodynia within 4 days (Figure 2A). Pain release effects evaluated by withdrawal threshold, guarding behavior and limb-use abnormality of intrathecal injection of TCV-309 and WEB 2086 were also achieved (Figure 2B–2D).

Knockdown of the expression of spinal PAF receptor protein was achieved by intrathecal transfer of PAF receptor siRNA in mice. As previously reported, a significant reduction in PAF receptor expression in normal mice and mice 15 days after surgery on the sciatic nerve, reaching 37.5±5.4% and 29.9±4.9% of the control at 3 days after siRNA transfection, respectively, while the expression was not altered by the HVJ-E vector alone or mismatched siRNA [5]. By siRNA transfection 13 days post-tumor implantation, the allodynia score, withdrawal threshold, guarding behavior an limb-use abnormality were improved with the peak effect at 2 to 3 days after siRNA transfection, while the pain-relief action gradually disappeared over 9 days (Figure 3E–3H). Injection of mismatched siRNA had no effect on the development of allodynia and pain behaviors. The amount of LPCAT2 protein significantly increased in the spinal cord at 8, 15 and 30 days after transplantation of NCTC 2472 tumor cells into mice tibia (Figure 3). The results support the concept that PAF increase in the spinal cord of tumor-bearing mice may relate to pain production and that the site of pain-relief action of the PAF receptor antagonists involve the spinal cord in FBC mice.

Potentiation of the Analgesic Effect by Combination of PAF Receptor Antagonists with Morphine

Bone cancer pain is one of the most severe types of cancer pain and is often resistant to treatment even with opioid analgesics. Combinations of opioids and non-opioid analgesics are usual practice to obtain a better analgesic effect in clinical practice. Combined administration of morphine with TCV-309 was examined (Figure 4A). Morphine 0.1 and 0.3 mg/kg injection 1 day after TCV-309 3 and 10 μg/kg administration produced a marked reduction in the allodynia score at 30 min after morphine

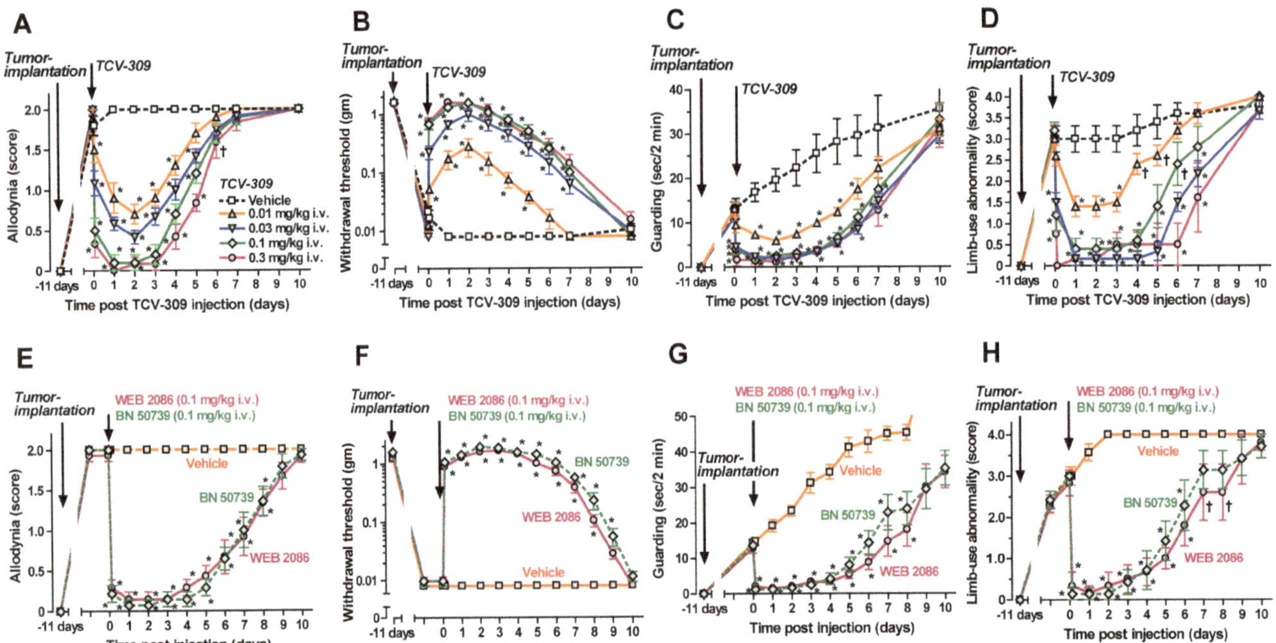

Figure 1. Effects of PAF-receptor antagonists on tactile allodynia (A, B, E, F), guarding behavior (C, G) and limb-use abnormality (D, H) in the femur bone cancer (FBC) mice. TCV-309 0.01-0.3 mg/kg, WEB 2086 0.1 mg/kg, BN 50739 0.1 mg/kg or a vehicle were intravenously injected at 11 days post tumor transplantation. Control mice received injections with a vehicle: saline or 25% 2-hydroxypropyl-β-cyclodextrin. The pain-related behaviors that developed after tumor implantation in mice were not affected by vehicle treatments. Values represent the mean ± SEM. n = 11 mice per group. †P<0.05, *P<0.01 compared with the corresponding control (vehicle treated) values, as determined by analysis of variance followed by Tukey-Kramer test.

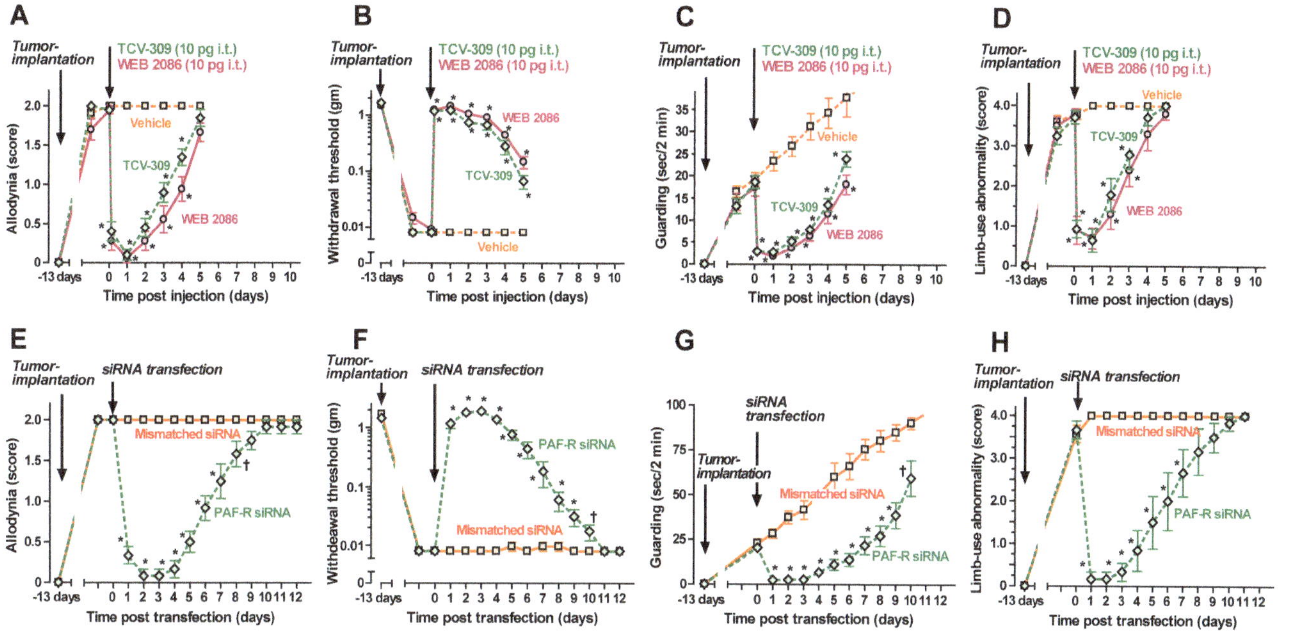

Figure 2. Effects of blockade of PAF receptors by intrathecal injection of PAF receptor antagonists (A–D) or knockdown of spinal PAF receptors by siRNA (E–H) on tactile allodynia (A, B, E, F), guarding behavior (C, G) and limb-use abnormality (D, H) in FBC mice. (A–D); Tumor cells were implanted into the intramedulla of left femur bone 13 days before the intrathecal (i.t.) injection of PAF receptor antagonists. TCV-309 (10 pg/mouse), WEB 2086 (10 pg/mouse) or the vehicle were injected intrathecally at time "0". Data are expressed as the mean ± SEM., n = 8–12 mice per group. *P<0.01 compared with the corresponding control (vehicle treated) values, as determined by analysis of variance followed by Tukey-Kramer test. Control mice received injections with a vehicle: ACSF. The pain-related behaviors that developed after tumor implantation in mice were not affected by the vehicle treatments. (E–H); siRNA or mismatched siRNA of PAF-receptor mRNA were transfected into the spinal cord 13 days after tumor implantation. Data are expressed as the mean ± SEM. n = 8–10 mice per group. †P<0.05, *P<0.01 compared with the corresponding control (mismatched siRNA transfection) values, as determined by analysis of valiance followed by an unpaired Student's *t*-test. Control mice received injections with mismatched siRNA or a vehicle: HVJ-envelope only. The pain-related behaviors that developed after tumor implantation in mice were not affected by mismatched siRNA or vehicle treatments.

injection and the effect returned to each level of TCV-309 alone at 3 to 4 hrs after the administration. The combination of morphine 1 mg/kg with gabapentin 10 mg/kg i.v. had no significant anti-allodynia effect (Figure 4B). A large dose of gabapentin, 30 mg/kg, was required to produce a transient anti-allodynia effect. Morphine alone had little analgesic effect at 0.3 to 3 mg/kg, s.c. and a small effect at 10 mg/kg in the FBC model. A higher dose of 30 mg/kg of morphine was less effective (Figure 4C).

The dose-response relation of TCV-309 and morphine in combination is shown in Figure 4D and Figure 4E. Morphine 0.3 mg/kg and TCV-309 0.1–1.0 µg/kg at each dose alone had no anti-allodynia effect, but in combination, the allodynia score decreased by more than 90% depending on the dose of TCV-309 (Figure 4D). Morphine in combination with TCV-309 10 µg/kg as low as 0.03 mg/kg produced a significant anti-allodynia effect and abolished the allodynia response at 0.3 mg/kg (Figure 4E). Eight days after the injection of TCV-309, WEB 2086 and BN 50739, pain relieving effect of these compounds became not significant (Figure 5). However, the additional administration of morphine 0.3 mg/kg still markedly ameliorated allodynia and pain behaviors (Figure 5). These results showed that PAF receptor antagonists achieves long-lasting potentiation of the analgesic effect when morphine was administered.

Effect of PAF Receptor Antagonists on Morphine-induced Constipation

Constipation is one of the most common side-effects of morphine and it appears in almost all patients treated with morphine. If the obstacle effect of morphine on intestinal activity is not potentiated, this side effect of morphine could be reduced by reducing the dosage of morphine without disturbing the analgesic effect. Morphine reduced the amount of feces from 1 mg/kg s.c. and abolished it more than 10 mg/kg. The dose-dependent constipation effect of morphine was not affected by TCV-309 10 µg/kg (Figure 6).

Repeated Administration of TCV-309 Protected Against the Appearance of Pain-like Behavior

As the anti-allodynia effect of TCV-309 was long-lasting, the effect of the repeated administration was examined. In control mice, tactile allodynia appeared at 3 days after tumor implantation and reached to peak response at 8 days. Guarding behavior appeared at 10 days post tumor implantation and gradually increased over 30 days, while limb-use abnormality appeared at 8 days and reached a maximum at about 16 days post implantation (Figure 7A–7D). Injection of TCV-309 at 0.3 mg/kg, i.v. was started on the day mice were implanted with the tumor and was continued every 4 days for 28 days. Pain behaviors evaluated by allodynia score, withdrawal threshold, guarding behavior and limb-use abnormality did not appear during dosing (Figure 2). Thus, the treatment with TCV-309 before pain arose protected against crisis of pain and tolerance to TCV-309 analgesia did not develop.

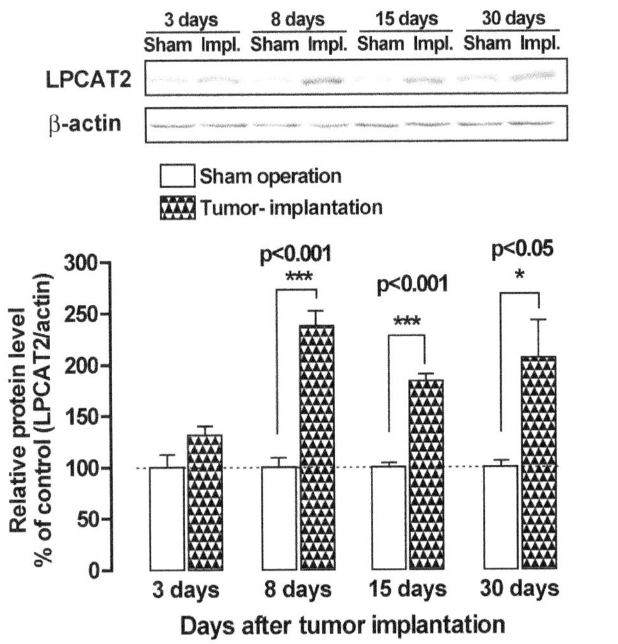

Figure 3. Changes in lysophosphatidylcholinr acyltransferase 2 (LPCAT2), an inducible PAF synthesis enzyume, in the spinal cords of mice after implantation of tumor cells. Alteration of spinal LPCAT2 expression 3, 8, 15, and 30 days after the levels of immunoreactivity were normalized to that of β-actin and represented as % induction compared with the values of sham-operated (deaden cells implanted) mice (mean ± SEM., n = 5–7). *P<0.05, ***P<0.001 versus the corresponding values in sham-operated mice (unpaired Student's *t*-test).

Treatment with TCV-309 Prolonged the Survival of FBC Mice

The effect of treatment with TCV-309 was evaluated in FBC mice (Figure 8). Median survival was significantly prolonged by repeated treatment with TCV-309; about 50% of FBC mice receiving saline died up to 26 days after tumor implantation, while about 50% of FBC mice receiving TCV-309 at 0.3 mg/kg every 4 days died up to 50 days. Gain of body weight by tumor-bearing mice was small during the observation period and the change in body weight was similar between control and TCV-308 treated mice (Figure 8 insert).

Discussion

Bone cancer pain is often very complex; bone is highly innervated with C fibers, which are triggered by an inflammatory infiltrate secondary to cancer cells and others including acids, cytokine, growth factors, etc along with primary afferent destruction following osteoclast activation. Additionally, bone resorption weakens the bone under torsion, thus exciting mechanosensitive fibers within mineralized bone. The most intractable pain is often neuropathic in origin. However, in bone cancer pain, there is a unique neurochemical reorganization of the spinal cord, as well peripheral sensitization of afferent fibers innervating the cancerous bone, while spinal synaptic transmission mediated through Aδ and C fibers is enhanced in the substantia gelationsa across a wide area of lumbar levels following sarcoma implantation in the femur [12]. As the disease progresses, analgesics effective to treat inflammatory or neuropathic pain, even opioids, are frequently insufficient in this pain state [13,14]. It has been reported that toll-like receptor (TLR) 4, which plays an important role in glial activation in neuropathic pain increased in the spinal expression of a rat model of cancer-induced bone pain and intrathecal injection of TLR4 siRNA or TLR4 signaling pathway blockers led to a pain relieving effect at an early stage, but not at day 16 of cancer-induced bone pain [15]. The present study demonstrated that intravenous administration of PAF receptor antagonists, TCV-309, BN 50739 and WEB 2086, effectively ameliorated allodynia and pain behaviors such as guarding and limb-use abnormalities in FBC mice. The pain relieving effects of PAF receptor antagonists are long lasting. We have previously suggested that the anti-allodynia effect of PAF antagonists in sciatic nerve injured mice is at least in part mediated by spinal relief of PAF-induced dysfunction of GlyRα3 [8]. In agreement with this concept, the present results showed that the intrathecal introduction of siRNA of PAF receptor mRNA effectively improved bone cancer pain behaviors in FBC mice. DRG contains a PAF synthesis enzyme, LPCAT2, and PAF receptor mRNA was increased in the ipsilateral DRG after nerve injury [6]. LPCAT2 mRNA and PAF receptor mRNA were increased in the spinal microglia after nerve injury in a rat spared nerve injury model [7]. Several studies have showed the ability of several cancer cell types to produce PAF and express PAF receptors on their membranes [16–20]. In the present study, the amount of LPCAT2 protein increased in the spinal cord of FBC mice, although in which cells the increase occurred remains to be elucidated. Therefore, PAF signaling in the microenvironment of the spinal pain transduction system may be increased by bone cancer due to peripheral nerve injury. We have further revealed a unique mode of action of TCV-309; TCV-309 is a specific competitive inhibitor of PAF receptors [21], but the potency of TCV-309 intensified as a function of time after administration, and the mode of action changed from a competitive manner within several hours after the injection of TCV-309 to a non-competitive manner later [8]. The intensification of the anti-allodynia potency of TCV-309 and change in its mode of action to a non-competitive manner as a function of time led us to speculate about a different mechanism of action; such as down-regulation of PAF receptors by binding TCV-309 to PAF receptors in the later stage of after nerve injury. This idea may explain the long lasting pain relieving effect of TCV-309.

The dose of morphine to block bone cancer pain was ten times that required to block inflammatory pain behaviors [12]. Morphine became less effective than oxycodone in FBC mice [22,23]. Differential attenuation of μ-opioid receptor activation between morphine and oxycodone in FBC mice was reported, the former was significant whereas the latter was limited [24]. According with the evidence, morphine at 10 mg/kg s.c. had a tiny anti-allodynia effect in the present study, and the analgesic effect of a higher dose of 30 mg/kg of morphine was underestimated due to increased locomotion.

The essential finding in the present study is the enhanced pain reliving effect by combined administration of PAF receptor antagonists and morphine. For example, the combination of TCV-309 as low as 1 μg/kg i.v. and morphine 0.3 mg/kg s.c. (each drug had no pain relieving effect by itself) produced a significant anti-allodynia effect in FBC mice. Guarding behavior and limb-use abnormality were also reversed by the combined administration (data not shown). It is interesting that the enhanced pain relieving effect of PAF receptor antagonists, TCV-309, BN 50739 and WEB 2086 on morphine still remained at 8 days after the administration of these PAF receptor antagonists.

Constipation resulting from treatment with opioids is the most common component of a more general condition – opioid-induced

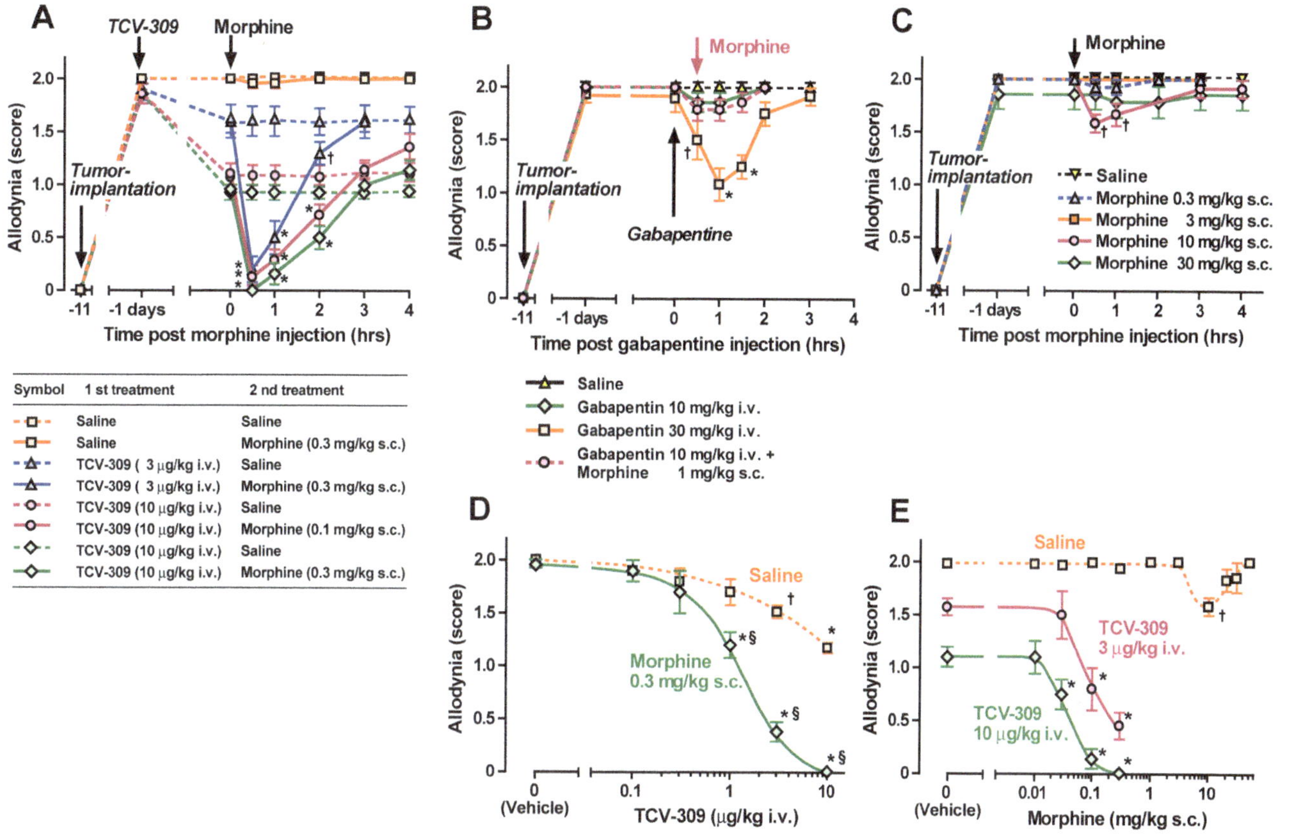

Figure 4. Enhanced pain reliving effect with a combination of TCV-309 and morphine in FBC mice. TCV-309, 3 and 10 µg/kg were injected i.v. at 10 days post tumor implantation and morphine 0.1 mg/kg and 0.3 mg/kg were injected s.c. 1 day after the injection of TCV-309 (A). Gabapentine 10 and 30 mg/kg i.v. were injected 11 days post tumor transplantation and morphine, 1 mg/kg was injected at 30 min after gabapentin injection (B). Morphine 0.3–30 mg/kg was injected at 11days post tumor transplantation (C). Pain-like behaviors were evaluated at 20 min after morphine injection. Various doses of TCV-309 were injected i.v. at 11 days post tumor implantation and morphine 0.3 mg/kg were injected s.c. 1 days after the injection of TCV-309 (D). One day after the injection of TCV-309, various doses of morphine were injected (E). Control mice received injections with a vehicle: saline. The pain-related behaviors that developed after tumor implantation in mice were not affected by vehicle treatments. Each group contained 11 mice. $^{\dagger}P<0.05$, $^{*}P<0.01$ compared with the corresponding control (vehicle treated) values, as determined by analysis of variance followed by Tukey-Kramer test. $^{\S}P<0.01$ compared with the corresponding control (vehicle treated without morphine) values, as determined by analysis of variance followed by an unpaired Student's *t*-test.

bowel dysfunction [25]. Tolerance commonly develops to opioids during long-term use, requiring increased doses to achieve the same analgesia. Although some tolerance develops against the effects of opioids on gastrointestinal motility, constipation often persists unless remedial measures are taken [26]. Using lower doses of opioids will not prevent constipation because the dose that produces constipation is approximately 4-fold less than the analgesic dose [25,27]. Therefore, some patients may discontinue opioids to avoid constipation. The present study showed that while a dose of morphine 10 mg/kg s.c. exhibited only a tiny pain relieving effect, 0.1 and 0.3 mg/kg of morphine in combination with PAF receptor antagonists produced a significant pain relieving effect. This result suggests that the combination use of morphine with PAF receptor antagonists may reduce the effective dose of morphine needed to below constipating dose. Activation of µ-receptors by morphine can have any of several effects depending on receptor location. Mu-opioid receptors in the central nervous system modulate pain perception and can depress respiratory function, while those in the gastrointestinal tract reduce bowel motility [26]. If µ-receptor-mediated signaling in the gastrointestinal tract was enhanced by PAF receptor antagonists, it would make defecation more difficult. The dose-response curve of morphine-induced defecation was not affected at all by 0.3 mg/kg of TCV-309, which is the dose producing the maximal analgesic effect and thus the possibility to avoid the appearance of morphine-induced constipation is suggested. On the other hand, PAF antagonists may cause side effects by interfering with the physiological roles of PAF, such as regulation of blood pressure, immunological or inflammatory responses, Ca^{2+} mobilization in polymorphonuclear leucocyte, or implantation of embryos, as shown by the creation of PAF receptor-transgenic and PAF receptor-deficient mice [28]. The possible side effects of PAF receptor antagonists could be reduced by combination with morphine. Therefore, good quality management of bone cancer pain could be achieved with a combination of morphine and PAF receptor antagonists. The long lasting effects of PAF receptor antagonists make it possible to relieve pain by repeated treatment at 4 day intervals and the results showed that these antagonists were effective from an early stage to a late stage, 30 days after tumor implantation at which point more than 50% of control mice died. The results further showed no formation of tolerance to repeated treatment with PAF receptor antagonists.

A role for PAF in tumor development has been suggested by the spontaneous development of skin tumors in transgenic mice

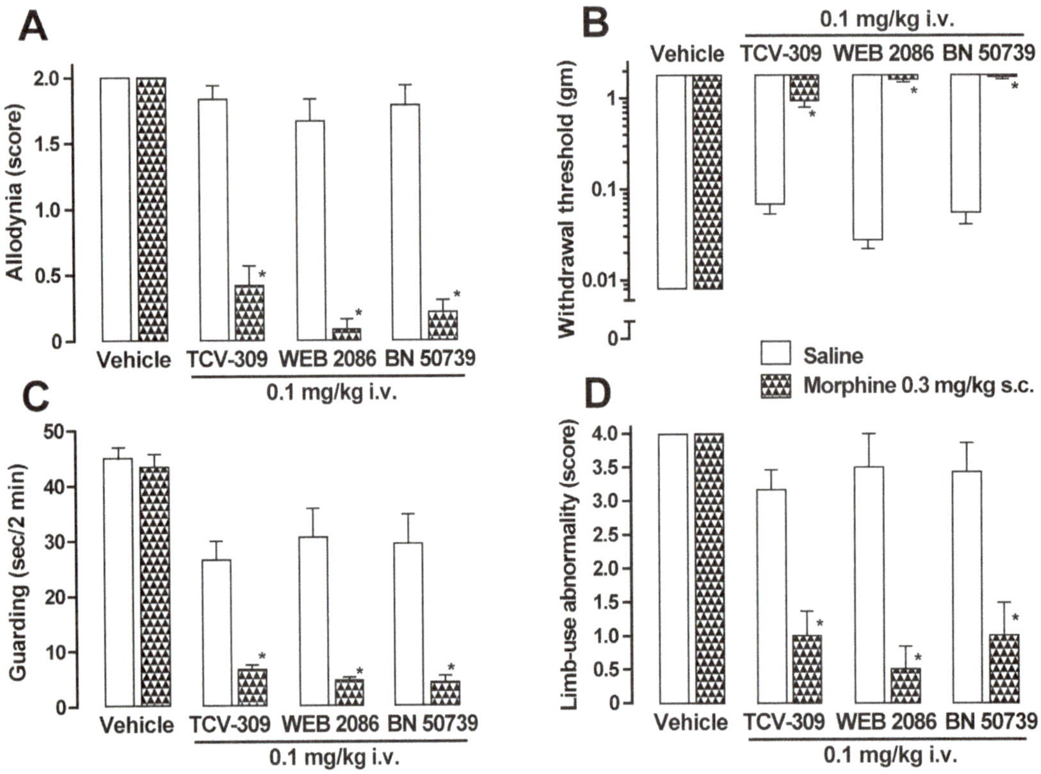

Figure 5. Enhanced pain reliving effect of TCV-309, WEB 2086, BN 50739 and morphine in FBC mice. TCV-309, WEB 2086 and BN 50739 were administered at 11 days post tumor implantation. Morphine 0.3 mg/kg s.c. was injected at 8 days after the injection of PAF receptor antagonists. Allodynia (A, B), guarding behavior (C) and limb-use abnormality (D) were evaluated at 20 min after the injection of morphine. Values represent the mean ± SEM. n = 11 mice per group. *P<0.01 compared with the corresponding control values, as determined by analysis of variance followed by an unpaired Student's *t*-test.

overexpressing PAF receptors [29]. PAF also induced an autocrine proliferative loop in an endometrial cancer cell line HEC-1A [30], induced migration of Kaposi's cells [31], promoted migration and proliferation of tumor cells and neo-angiogenesis [17], acted as a promoter of melanoma metastasis [32], while PAF receptor-dependent pathways control tumor growth [33]. In addition, PAF receptor antagonists suppress cancer growth, proliferation and metastasis [20,32–34]. The improvement in the survival of femoral

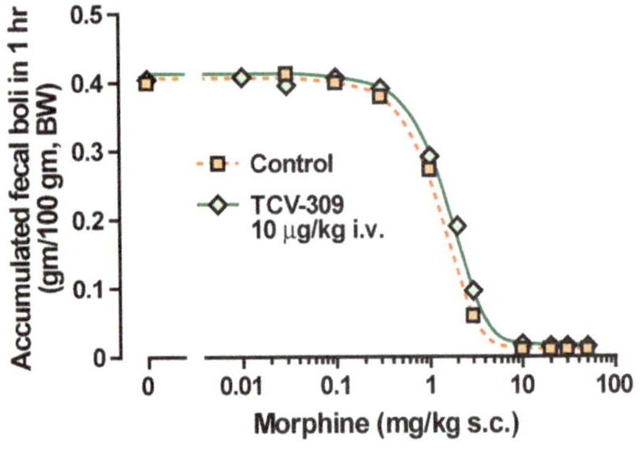

Figure 6. Morphine-induced constipation with or without TCV-309. Normal mice received with various doses of morphine and the accumulated feces on the floor over 60 min were weighed. TCV-309 was injected 1 day before morphine administration. Data are expressed as the mean. n = 10 mice per group.

bone tumor-bearing mice with TCV-309 may be due to its tumor suppressive action. As an another possibility, pain is an exquisite stressor and a cause for potential immune dysfunction, as shown in immunosuppression during the perioperative period, and thus poor pain control is assumed to promote tumor growth. Lilleme et al. [35] reported that patients with preexisting pain who received chemical splanchnicectomy with alcohol showed a significant improvement in survival. The authors reported that the achievement of better pain control with chemical splanchnicectomy may prolong life. Whether the improvement in survival by PAF receptor antagonist may include its indirect effect via suppression of pain is remained to be clarified.

Although the possibility could not be entirely ruled out that the tumor suppressive action of PAF antagonists may partly participate in the pain relieving effect of the repeated treatment of PAF antagonists in the FBC model, the acute pain relieving effect of PAF antagonists may be independent from anti-tumor action because the effect developed shortly after the intravenous injection and even by intrathecal injection.

Opiates in which their mechanisms of analgesia include the enhancement of the descending inhibitory pathway connected to the inhibitory inter-neurons such as glycinergic and GABAergic neurons. Recent findings emphasize that a reduction in the $GABA_A$ receptor– and glycine receptor-mediated synaptic inhibition; ie., disinihibition of inhibitory neurotransmission within the dorsal horn, is implicated in the generation of neuropathic pain and may be a cause for insufficiency of morphine analgesia. Thus, reinforcement of the glycinergic neurotransmission by glycine transporter inhibitors are proposed as a novel drug discovery

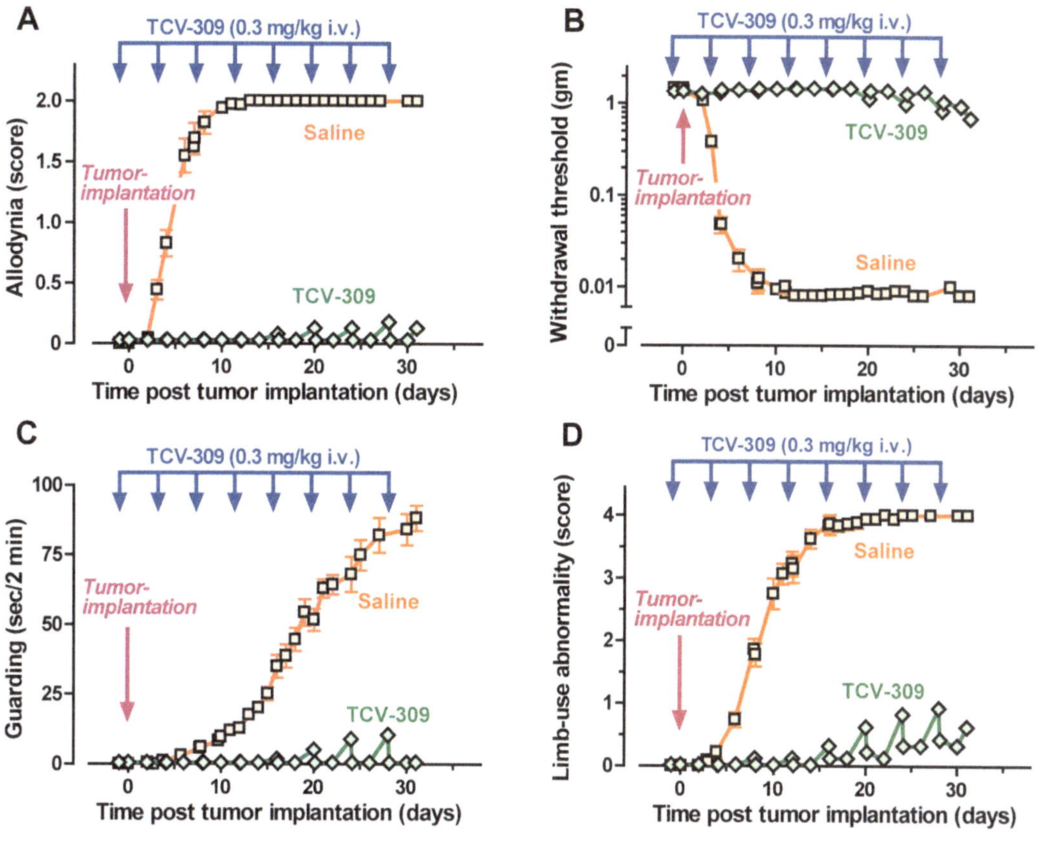

Figure 7. Effect of the repeated administration of TCV-309 on the pain-like behaviors in FBC mice. The administration of TCV-309 0.3 mg/kg i.v. was started 6 hr before the tumor implantation, given once a day and continued every 4 days up to 28 days. Allodynia (A, B), guarding behavior (C) and limb-use abnormality (D) were evaluated at 3 hr and 1, 2, 3 days after TCV-309 injection. Data are expressed as the mean ± SEM. n = 15 mice per group.

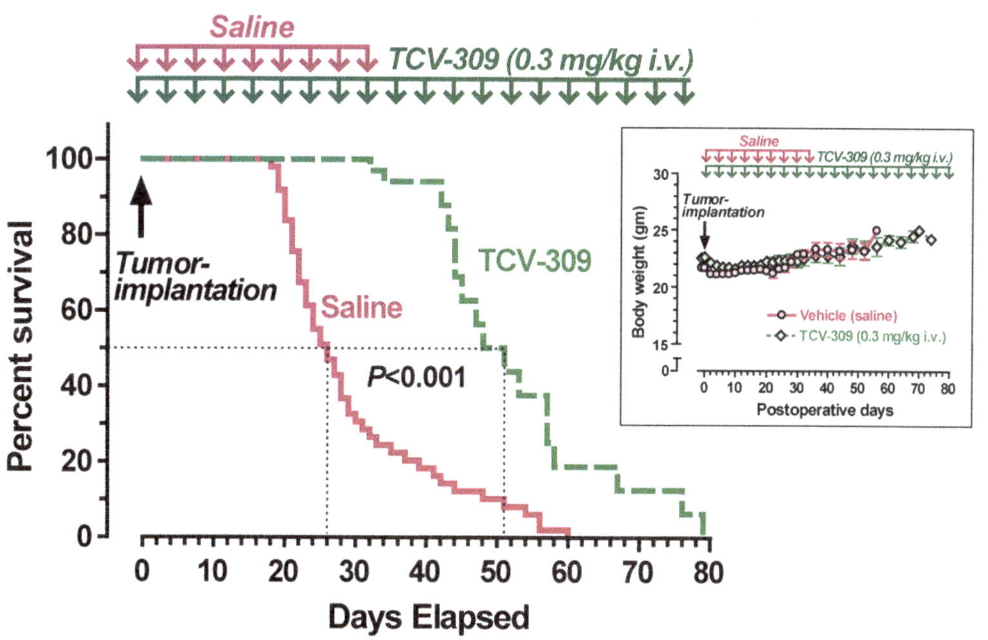

Figure 8. The Kaplan-Mayer survival curve of FBC mice and the change of body weight (insert). For the survival experiments, TCV-309 and saline were given once a day and continued every 4 days until the animals died (n = 17 and 50, respectively). Control mice received saline for 32 days. Days for 50% of mice died after receiving TCV-309 were significantly prolonged compared to the saline-treated control, $P<0.001$. Statistical analysis was performed by log-rank and Gehan–Breslow–Wilcoxon tests.

strategy for neuropathic pain [36]. Taking that PAF via an increase in nitric oxide/cyclic GMP cascade reduces GlyRα3 function in the spinal cord [5], the combination of PAF receptor antagonists and opioids, the former protects from disfunction of PAF-induced inhibitory neurotransmission and the latter enhances descending inhibitory pathway may represent a new strategy for the treatment of persistent cancer pain and the quality/quantity of life of patients.

Acknowledgments

The authors wish to thank Dr. Z. Terashita (Takeda Pharmaceutical Co. Kyoto, Japan) and Dr. P. Braquet (Institute Henri Beaufour, Le Plessis Robinson, France) for generously donating TCV-309 and BN 50739, respectively. This work was carried out with equipment from the Natural Science Center for Basic Research and Development, Hiroshima University, and the National Cancer Center Research Institute.

Author Contributions

Conceived and designed the experiments: KM TD NM SS. Performed the experiments: KM NM T. Kitayama SS. Analyzed the data: KM NM T. Kanamatsu SS YU. Contributed reagents/materials/analysis tools: NM KM T. Kanematsu. Wrote the paper: TD KM NM.

References

1. Mundy GR (2002) Metastasis to bone: causes, consequences and therapeutic opportunities. Nat Rev Cancer 2: 584–593.
2. Portenoy RK, Lesage P (1999) Management of cancer pain. Lancet 353: 1695–1700.
3. de Wit R, van Dam F, Loonstra S, Zandbelt L, van Buuren A, et al. (2001) The amsterdam pain management index compared to eight frequently used outcome measures to evaluate the adequacy of pain treatment in cancer patients with chronic pain. Pain 91:339–349.
4. Morita K, Morioka N, Abdin J, Kitayama S, Nakata Y, et al. (2004) Development of tactile allodynia and thermal hyperalgesia by intrathecally administered platelet-activating factor in mice. Pain 111: 351–359.
5. Morita K, Kitayama T, Morioka N, Dohi T (2008) Glycinergic mediation of tactile allodynia induced by platelet-activating factor (PAF) through glutamate-NO-cyclic GMP signalling in spinal cord in mice. Pain 138: 525–536.
6. Hasegawa S, Kohro Y, Shiratori M, Ishii S, Shimizu T, et al. (2010) Role of PAF receptor in proinflammatory cytokine expression in the dorsal root ganglion and tactile allodynia in a rodent model of neuropathic pain. PLoS One 5, e10467.
7. Okubo M, Yamanaka H, Kobayashi K, Kanda H, Dai Y, et al. (2012) Up-regulation of Platelet-activating factor synthases and its receptor in spinal cord contribute to development of neuropathic pain following peripheral nerve injury. Mol Pain 8: 8.
8. Motoyama N, Morita K, Kitayama T, Shiraishi S, Uezono Y, et al. (2013) Pain-releasing action of Platelet-activating factor (PAF) antagonists in neuropathic pain animal models and the mechanisms of action. Eur J Pain 17: 1156–1167.
9. Honore P, Mantyh PW (2000) Bone cancer pain: from mechanism to model to therapy. Pain Med 1: 303–309.
10. Luger NM, Sabino MA, Schwei ML, Mach DB, Pomonis JD, et al. (2002) Efficacy of systemic morphine suggests a fundamental difference in the mechanisms that generate bone cancer vs inflammatory pain. Pain 99: 397–406.
11. Minami T, Nishihara I, Ito S, Sakamoto K, Hyodo M, et al. (1995) Nitric oxide mediates allodynia induced by intrathecal administration of prostaglandin E_2 or prostaglandin $F_{2\alpha}$ in conscious mice. Pain 61: 285–290.
12. Yanagisawa Y, Furue H, Kawamata T, Uta D, Yamamoto J, et al. (2010) Bone cancer induces a unique central sensitization through synaptic changes in a wide area of the spinal cord. Mol Pain 6: 38.
13. Portenoy RK, Rayne D, Jacobsen P (1999) Breakthrough pain: characteristics and impact in patients with cancer pain. Pain 81: 129–134.
14. Becker R, Jakob D, Uhle EI, Riegel T, Bertalanffy H (2000) The significance of intrathecal opioid therapy for the treatment of neuropathic cancer pain conditions. Stereotact Funct Neurosug 75: 16–26.
15. Li X, Wang X-W, Feng X-M, Zhou W-J, Wang Y-Q, et al. (2013) Stage-dependent anti-allodynia effects of intrathecal Toll-like receptor 4 antagonists in a rat model of cancer induced bone pain. J Physiol Sci DOI 10.1007/s12576-D12-0244-5.
16. Bussolino F, Arese M, Montrucchio G, Barrs L, Primo L, et al. (1995) Platelet-activating factor produced in vitro by Kaposi's Sarcoma cells induces and Sustains in vivo angiogenesis. J Clin Invest 96: 940–952.
17. Bussolati B, Biancone L, Cassoni P, Russo S, Rola-Pleszczynski M, et al. (2000) PAF produced by human brest cancer cells promotes migration and proliferation of tumor cells and neo-angiogenesis. Am J Pathol 157: 1713–1725.
18. Bussolati B, Russo S, Deambrosis I, Cantaluppi V, Volpe A, et al. (2002) Expression of CD154 on renal cell carcinomas and effect on cell proliferation, motility and platelet-activating factor synthesis. Int J Cancer 100: 654–661.
19. Fallani A, Grieco B, Barletta E, Mugnai G, Giorgi G, et al. (2002) Synthesis of platelet-activating factor (PAF) in transformed cell lines of a different origin. Prostaglandins Other Lipid Mediat 70: 209–226.
20. Tsoupras AB, Iatrou C, Frangia C, Demopoulos CA (2009) The implication of platelet-activating factor in cancer growth and metastasis: Potent beneficial role of PAF-inhibitors and antioxidants. Infectious Disorders-Drug Targets 9: 390–399.
21. Terashita Z-I, Kawamura M, Takatani M, Tsushima S, Imura Y, et al. (1992) Beneficial effects of TCV-309, a novel potent and selective platelet-activating factor antagonist in endotoxin and anaphylaxis shock in rodents. J Pharmacol Exp Ther 260: 748–755.
22. Narita M, Nakamura A, Ozaki M, Imai S, Miyoshi K, et al. (2008) Comparative Pharmacological profiles of morphine and oxycodone under a neuropathic pain-like state in mice: evidence for less sensitivity to morphine. Neuropsychopharmacology 33: 1097–1112.
23. Minami K, Hasegawa M, Ito H, Nakamura A, Tomii T, et al. (2009) Morphine, oxycodone, and fentanyl exhibit different analgesic profiles in mouse pain models. J Pharmacol Sci 111:60–72.
24. Nakamura A, Hasegawa M, Minami K, Kanbara T, Tomii T, et al. (2013) Differential activation of the µ-opioid receptor by oxycodone and morphine in pain-related brain regions in a bone cancer pain model. Br J Pharmacol 168: 375–388.
25. Yuan C-S (2005) Handbook of opioid bowel syndrome. New York: Haworth Medical Press: Haworth Reference Press. 256 p.
26. Akil H, Owens C, Gutstein H, Taylor L, Curran E, et al. (1998) Endogenous opioids: overview and current issues. Drug Alcohol Depend 51: 127–140.
27. Yuan C-S, Foss JF (2000) Antagonism of gastrointestinal opioid effects. Reg Anesth Pain Med 25: 639–642.
28. Honda Z, Ishii S, Shimizu T (2002) Platelet–activating factor receptor. J Biochem 131: 773–779.
29. Ishii S, Nagase T, Tashiro F, Ikuta K, Sato S, et al. (1997) Bronchial hyperreactivity, increased endotoxin lethality and melanocytic tumorigenesis in transgenic mice overexpressing platelet-activating factor receptor. EMBO J 16: 133–142.
30. Maggi M, Bonaccorsi L, Finetti G, Carioni V, Muratori M, et al. (1994) Platelet-activating factor mediates an autocrine proliferative loop in the endometrial adenocarcinoma cell line HEC-1A. Cancer Res 54: 4777–4784.
31. Biancone L, Cantaluppi V, Boccellino M, Bussolati B, Del Sorbo L, et al. (1999) Motility induced by human immunodeficiency virus-1 Tat on Kaposi's sarcoma cells requires platelet-activating factor synthesis. Am J Pathol 155: 1731–1739.
32. Melnikova V, Bar-Eli M (2007) Inflammation and melanoma growth and metastasis: The role of platelet-activating factor (PAF) and its receptor. Cancer Metastasis Rev 26: 359–371.
33. de Oliveira SI, Andrade LNS, Onuchic AC, Nonogaki S, Fernandes PD, et al. (2010) Platelet-activating factor receptor (PAF-R)-dependent pathways control tumor growth and tumor response to chemotherapy. BMC Cancer 10:200
34. Im SY, Ko HM, Kim JW, Lee HK, Ha TY, et al. (1996) Augmentation of tumor metastases by platelet-activating factor. Cancer Res 56: 2662–2665.
35. Lillemoe KD, Cameron JL, Kaufman HS, Yeo CJ, Pitt HA, et al. (1993) Chemical splanchnicectomy in patients with unresectable pancreatic cancer. A prospective randomized trial. Annals Surgery 217: 447–457.
36. Dohi T, Morita K, Kitayama T, Motoyama N, Morioka N (2009) Glycine transporter inhibitors as a novel drug discovery strategy for neuropathic pain. Pharmacol Ther 123: 54–79.

16

Spinal Cord Transection-Induced Allodynia in Rats – Behavioral, Physiopathological and Pharmacological Characterization

Saïd M'Dahoma[1,2]*, Sylvie Bourgoin[1,2], Valérie Kayser[1,2], Sandrine Barthélémy[1,2], Caroline Chevarin[1,2], Farah Chali[3], Didier Orsal[3], Michel Hamon[1,2]

1 Centre de Psychiatrie et Neurosciences, Institut National de la Santé et de la Recherche Médicale, INSERM U894, Université Paris Descartes, Paris, France, **2** Neuropsychopharmacologie, Faculté de Médecine Pierre et Marie Curie, site Pitié-Salpêtrière, Paris, France, **3** Laboratoire de Neurobiologie des Signaux Intercellulaires, Centre National de la Recherche Scientifique, CNRS UMR 7101, Université Pierre et Marie Curie, Paris, France

Abstract

In humans, spinal cord lesions induce not only major motor and neurovegetative deficits but also severe neuropathic pain which is mostly resistant to classical analgesics. Better treatments can be expected from precise characterization of underlying physiopathological mechanisms. This led us to thoroughly investigate (i) mechanical and thermal sensory alterations, (ii) responses to acute treatments with drugs having patent or potential anti-allodynic properties and (iii) the spinal/ganglion expression of transcripts encoding markers of neuronal injury, microglia and astrocyte activation in rats that underwent complete spinal cord transection (SCT). SCT was performed at thoracic T8–T9 level under deep isoflurane anaesthesia, and SCT rats were examined for up to two months post surgery. SCT induced a marked hyper-reflexia at hindpaws and strong mechanical and cold allodynia in a limited (6 cm^2) cutaneous territory just rostral to the lesion site. At this level, pressure threshold value to trigger nocifensive reactions to locally applied von Frey filaments was 100-fold lower in SCT- versus sham-operated rats. A marked up-regulation of mRNAs encoding ATF3 (neuronal injury) and glial activation markers (OX-42, GFAP, P2×4, P2×7, TLR4) was observed in spinal cord and/or dorsal root ganglia at T6-T11 levels from day 2 up to day 60 post surgery. Transcripts encoding the proinflammatory cytokines IL-1β, IL-6 and TNF-α were also markedly but differentially up-regulated at T6–T11 levels in SCT rats. Acute treatment with ketamine (50 mg/kg i.p.), morphine (3–10 mg/kg s.c.) and tapentadol (10–20 mg/kg i.p.) significantly increased pressure threshold to trigger nocifensive reaction in the von Frey filaments test, whereas amitriptyline, pregabalin, gabapentin and clonazepam were ineffective. Because *all* SCT rats developed *long lasting, reproducible and stable* allodynia, which could be alleviated by drugs effective in humans, thoracic cord transection might be a reliable model for testing innovative therapies aimed at reducing spinal cord lesion-induced central neuropathic pain.

Editor: Mohammed Shamji, Toronto Western Hospital, Canada

Funding: This research has been supported by grants from Institut National de la Santé et de la Recherche Médicale (INSERM), University Pierre and Marie Curie (UPMC), Agence Nationale de la Recherche (Contract ANR 11BSV4 017 04, TrkBDNFarmod), and Institut pour la Recherche sur la Moelle Epinière et l'Encéphale (IRME, Contract "M.Hamon, 2010–2011"). Saïd M'Dahoma was supported by fellowships from the Ministère de la Recherche et de l'Enseignement Supérieur (France) during performance of this work. The funders had no role in study design, data collection and analysis, decision to publish, or preparation of the manuscript.

Competing Interests: The authors have declared that no competing interests exist.

* Email: said.mdahoma@yahoo.fr

Introduction

Spinal cord injury (SCI) is a debilitating state which causes not only severe motor dysfunctions, loss of bladder control and impairment of sexual function, but also chronic pain, especially neuropathic pain [1,2]. Pain can be so severe that some SCI patients would be ready to privilege pain relief at the expense of further deficits in bladder control or sexual function. SCI-induced central neuropathic pain can be localized above-, at- or below- the level of injury and is mostly characterized by allodynia refractory to conventional treatments [2,3].

Several animal models of SCI-induced neuropathic pain have been developed (through spinal cord contusion, compression, ischemia, section; see [4]), each of them displaying different characteristics in terms of localization, duration, type of pain and even responses to drugs. Although some studies did provide relevant data regarding treatment efficacy and underlying molecular mechanisms [5–7], they focused mostly on pain below the lesion produced by contusion or clip compression of the spinal cord. Yet, despite the fact that these SCI models reproduce adequately some types of spinal cord injuries seen in humans, they suffer from limitations because of unavoidable, large, interindividual variations in the extent and severity of evoked lesions [8,9]. Furthermore, lesion-induced neuroinflammatory processes could be highly variable among SCI rats which underwent the very same lesion procedure [10], so that characterization of actual physiopathological mechanisms underlying neuropathic pain might be a real challenge in, at least, some SCI models.

In contrast to these models, complete transection of the spinal cord would be cleared of such limitations due to unavoidable interindividual variations in the extent and severity of the lesion. Indeed, spinal cord transection (SCT) has already been widely used to study the mechanisms of subsequent locomotor recovery [11–13] and reorganization of the somatosensory system [14–15] in medullary lesioned rats. However, to date, only few studies showed that the SCT model could be used to investigate spinal lesion-induced neuropathic pain [16], and, indeed, some authors even reported that no neuropathic pain develops in rats with complete SCT [17,18].

These discrepant data led us to reinvestigate whether or not the rat model consisting of complete SCT at the thoracic level could be a relevant model of central neuropathic pain, allowing studies of underlying physiopathological mechanisms and responses to drugs with patent or potential alleviating properties. Nocifensive responses to mechanical and thermal stimulations were assessed using the validated von Frey filaments test and the paw immersion and acetone drop tests, respectively. We then investigated whether responses to these tests could be affected by acute treatments with various drugs (opioids, antidepressants, anticonvulsants and others) known to alleviate neuropathic pain in SCI patients. Finally, we analyzed by real time quantitative RT-PCR, at different times after thoracic cord transection, the expression of mRNAs encoding proteins implicated in neuroinflammation and neuroplasticity, with particular focus on markers of microglia and astrocyte activation, pro- and anti-inflammatory cytokines (Interleukins IL-1β, IL-6 and IL-10, Tumor Necrosis Factor alpha,TNF-α), Brain-Derived Neurotrophic Factor (BDNF) and nociceptive signaling pathways in dorsal root ganglia (DRG) and spinal cord tissues, for comparison with previous studies aimed at unveiling physiopathological mechanisms associated with neuropathic pain in other SCI models.

Materials and Methods

Animals and Ethics Statements

Male Sprague–Dawley rats, weighing 225–250 g (7–8 weeks old) on arrival in the laboratory, were purchased from Janvier Breeding Center (53940 Le Genest Saint Isle, France). They were housed under standard controlled environmental conditions (22±1°C, 60% relative humidity, 12:12 h light–dark cycle, lights on at 7:00 am), on ground corn cobs (GM-12, SAFE, 89290, Augy, France), with complete diet for rats/mice/hamster (105, SAFE, 89290, Augy) and tap water available *ad libitum*. Before surgery, rats were housed 5 per cage (40×40 cm, 20 cm high) and allowed to habituate to the housing facilities without any handling for at least 1 week before being used. After surgery, all efforts were made to minimize suffering. In particular, SCT rats were housed under the very same conditions, except that each cage was for only two operated rats, so as to avoid as much as possible allodynic contacts between them. All animals were thoroughly examined each day, and in case of any sign of abnormal physiological alterations or suffering appeared, they were immediately sacrificed by a lethal dose of pentobarbital (150 mg/kg i.p.), strictly following the recommendations of the Ethical Committee of the French Ministry of Research and High Education (articles R.214–124, R.214–125). Both the Ethics and Scientific Committee of the French *Institut pour la Recherche sur la Moelle Epinière et l'Encéphale* (IRME; contract to M.H., 2010–2011) and the national (French) Committee for Animal Care and Use for Scientific Research (registration nb.01296.01; official authorization B75-116 to M.H., 31 December 2012) specifically approved the study.

In addition, the Ethical Guidelines of the Committee for Research and Ethical Issues of the International Association for the Study of Pain [19] and the Institutional Guidelines in compliance with French and international laws and policies (Council directive 87–848, October 19, 1987, *Ministère de l'Agriculture et de la Forêt, Service vétérinaire de la santé et de la protection animale*, permissions nb A752128 to S.M., 006228 to S.B., nb 00482 to V.K.) were strictly followed.

Spinal Cord Transection

Animals underwent surgery under deep isoflurane anaesthesia (3%). Paravertebral muscles were cut bilaterally and the T8 vertebra was opened using a gouge-forceps. Local anaesthesia was made by cooling the spinal cord with cryoflurane (Promedica, France) a few seconds before the lesion. Complete transverse section with ophthalmic scissors at the T8–T9 spinal cord segments level was performed following the procedure described by Antri et al. [11], then sterile absorbable haemostatic gel foam (Surgicel; Ethicon, Somerville, NJ, USA) was inserted into the lesion. Sham-operated animals underwent laminectomy only. At the last step of surgery, muscles were sutured and the skin was closed up by skin clips. Both SCT and sham-operated rats then received antibiotic treatments to prevent staphylococcic infection (oxacillin, Bristol Myers Squibb S.P.A., Italy, 0.3 mg/100 g s.c. once a day during 7 days) and urinary infection (gentamicin, Panpharma, France, 0.2 mg/100 g s.c., immediately after the surgery). No further treatment was administered to operated animals, to avoid potential interference with the development of allodynia and hyperalgesia. For recovery, SCT and sham rats were housed two per cage. The bladder of SCT rats was emptied manually once daily until reappearance of the voiding reflex (usually before the 10th day post surgery) (see Results).

Tests with Von Frey Filaments

Assessment of At-Level Mechanical Allodynia. For assessment of SCT-induced neuropathic-like pain in the cutaneous territory bordering surgery scar, rats were placed individually into a plastic cage (42×24×15 cm) and allowed to adapt to this environment for 1 hour before any stimulation. Tactile allodynia was then looked for with a graded series of von Frey filaments (Bioseb, 92370 Chaville, France) producing a bending force ranging between 0.008 g and 100 g. The threshold pressure to trigger a response (see below) was determined using the "up-down" method [20]. The stimuli were applied 3 times (3 seconds apart) for each filament, within a cutaneous territory of about 6 cm^2 just rostral to the lesion (see Results). When positive nociceptive behaviors, consisting of either a shake, an attack (filament biting), or an escape reaction [5,20], occurred, the next lower pressure-von Frey filaments were tested down to the filament producing no response. Then, the next higher pressure-filaments were applied back to the one triggering a response. The minimal force filament causing at least one of these responses (usually biting) allowed determination of the mechanical pressure threshold value. The 100 g filament, chosen as cut-off to prevent tissue injury, induced no nociceptive behavior in the majority (> 90%) of naïve rats. To avoid nonspecific responses, only these "non-reactive" rats were selected for surgery and included in the study.

Assessment of Mechanical Sensitivity in Body Territories Outside the Allodynic Area. SCT and sham-operated rats were also subjected to mechanical stimulation with von Frey filaments to assess evoked responses at the level of forepaws, hindpaws, vibrissae pad and other body territories outside the allodynic 6 cm^2 area just rostral to the surgery scar. For these tests, each rat was placed on a wire grid platform (5×5 mm mesh) under a small plastic (35×20×15 cm) cage for 2 hours, and mechanical sensitivity was determined with a graded series of 9 von Frey filaments (bending force of 4, 6, 8, 10, 12, 15, 26, 60 and 100 g). The "up-down" method [20] was also used at all of these sites. At paw level, stimuli were applied onto the lateral plantar surface of the right forepaw or hindpaw 3 times (3 seconds apart) for each filament. The minimal force filament for which animals presented either a brisk paw withdrawal and/or an escape attempt allowed determination of the mechanical pressure threshold [21]. Usually, the mechanical pressure threshold value to trigger a (non nocifensive) response in naïve healthy rats was around 60 g. Because SCT rats presented large time-dependent changes in mechanical sensitivity (see Fig. 1), higher pressures were also tested, with cut-off fixed at 100 g to avoid any tissue injury.

Assessment of Thermal Sensitivity

Paw Immersion Test. Because variations in skin temperature can affect the responses in nociceptive tests [22], we systematically performed control experiments that consisted of measuring hindpaw skin temperature just before the paw immersion test. The rat was left in its cage and a thermistor probe (Thermocouple thermometer Digi-Sense, Model N°8528-10; Cole-Parmer Instrument Company, Chicago, IL; 15 mm in diameter) was applied onto the plantar surface of hindpaw. Stable temperature readings were obtained after 10 sec with a precision measure of 0.1°C [23].

Thermal sensitivity at the hindpaw level was determined using the paw immersion test in both SCT and sham-operated rats [24]. Briefly, the right hindpaw was immersed into a water bath maintained at 46°C (Polystat, Bioblock Scientific, Illkirch-Graffenstaden, France) for heat stimulation or at 10°C (Ministat, Bioblock Scientific) for cold stimulation, and the latency to struggle reaction (paw withdrawal) was measured to the nearest 0.1 sec.

At-Level Cold Allodynia. Cold allodynia in SCT rats was assessed at day 15 post-surgery using a procedure slightly adapted from the acetone drop test described by Baastrup et al. [5]. Four drops of 10 μL acetone were gently deposited within two seconds all around the surgery scar in SCT and sham-operated rats. The number of trunk shakes and the time spent in escape or licking behavior were determined for one min after acetone drops application.

Pharmacological Treatments

Gabapentin and pregabalin were purchased from Sequoia (Pangbourne, UK). Amitriptyline, baclofen, ketamine and 8-OH-DPAT [(±)-8 hydroxy-2-dipropylamino-tetralin] were from Sigma-Aldrich (Saint-Quentin Fallavier, France). Other compounds

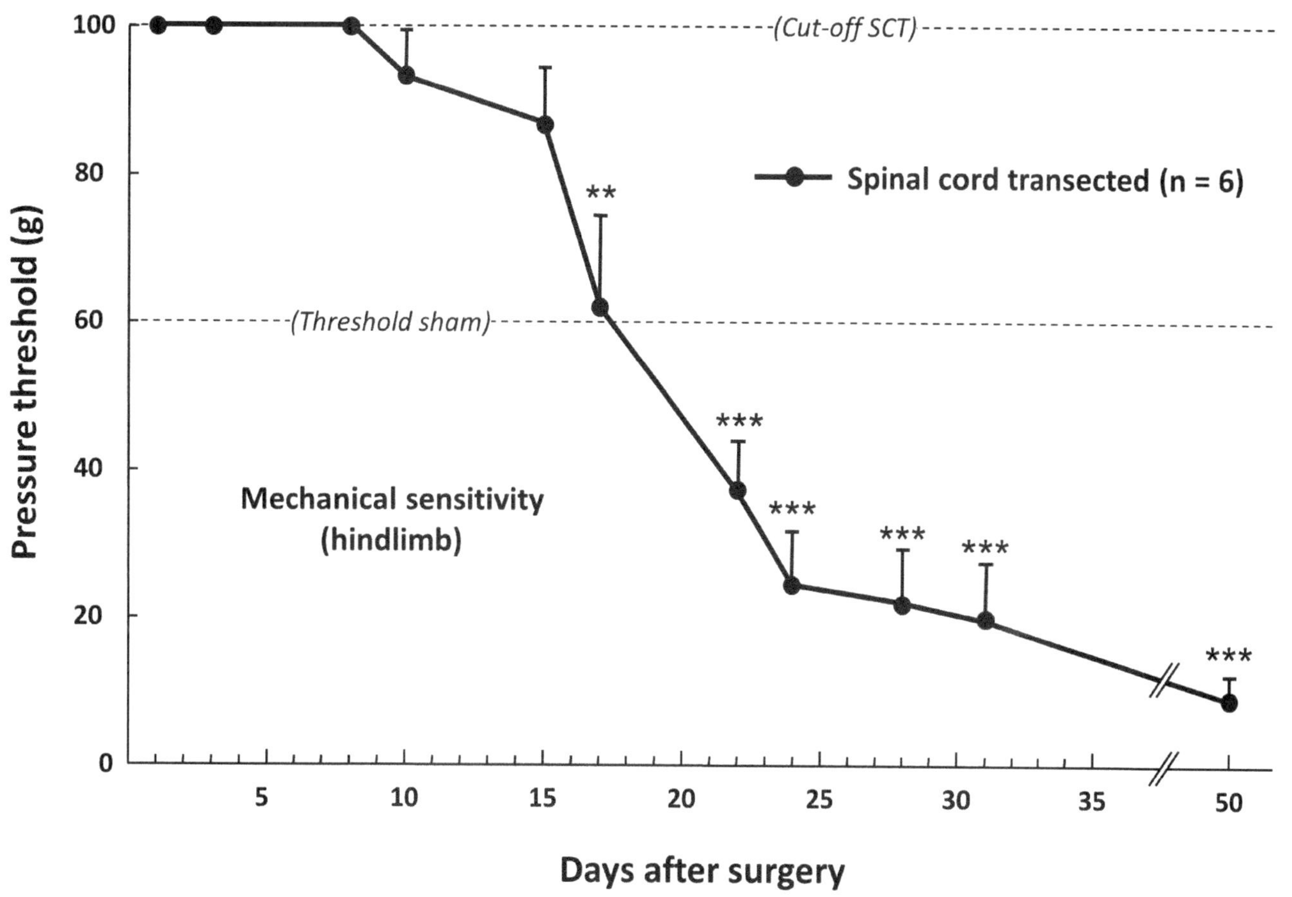

Figure 1. Time-course changes in the pressure threshold value to trigger hindpaw withdrawal in spinal cord-transected rats. Pressure threshold values were determined using a graded series of von Frey filaments applied onto hindpaw. Each point is the mean + S.E.M. of independent determinations in 6 rats. « Cut-off SCT » corresponded to the maximal pressure tested in spinal cord-transected rats; even at this high pressure level (100 g), no response of hindpaws was evoked for the first 9 days post-surgery. The « Threshold sham » corresponded to the minimal pressure (60 g) to which sham-operated animals start to respond by hindpaw withdrawal. ** P<0.01, *** P<0.001, significantly different from 100 g « cut-off SCT » value. One-way ANOVA for repeated measures followed by Dunnett's test.

were clonazepam (Roche, Basel, Switzerland), cyclotraxin B (BIO S&T, Montreal, Canada), morphine (Pharmacie Centrale des Hôpitaux de Paris, France), tapentadol (Grünenthal, Aachen, Germany), naratriptan and ondansetron (Glaxo Wellcome, Harlow, UK).

All treatments were administered between 2 pm and 4 pm. Routes of administration and doses (as free bases; see Table 1) were chosen according to previous data in the literature (see appropriate references in sections of Results and Discussion). All drugs were dissolved in saline (0.9% NaCl) except baclofen which was dissolved in dimethyl-sulfoxide (DMSO):0.9% NaCl (50:50) and clonazepam in ethanol:water (50:50). Drugs or their vehicles were injected acutely 30 days after thoracic cord transection, when mechanical allodynia had fully developed in the 6 cm^2 area just rostral to the lesion (see Results). For intrathecal injections (of ondansetron), rats were briefly anaesthetized with isoflurane (3% in air), and the needle (26 G) was inserted into the lumbar space between the L5 and L6 vertebrae [25] for administration of the appropriate dose in 20 µL of saline. Von Frey filaments test was then applied (by a skilled experimenter blind to treatments) at various times after acute drugs administration to determine the time course of drug-induced changes in pressure threshold value to trigger nocifensive response (biting of the filament, see Results), until the drug effect completely disappeared. In all experiments, only one treatment was administered per rat.

Real Time Quantitative RT-PCR Measurements

SCT- and sham-operated rats were decapitated at various times, from 2 to 60 days, after surgery. DRG, thoracic cord segments below (T9–T11) and above (T6–T8) the lesion, along with cervical and lumbar enlargements, were rapidly dissected out at 0–4°C, and immediately frozen in liquid nitrogen to be stored at −80°C. In some experiments, spinal cord samples were further sectioned by a medio-vertical cut to separate dorsal and ventral halves. Total RNA was extracted using the NucleoSpin RNA II extraction kit (Macherey-Nagel, 67722 Hoerdt, France) and quantified using NanoDrop. First-stranded cDNA synthesis (from 660 ng total RNA per 20 µL reaction mixture) was carried out using High Capacity cDNA reverse transcription kit (Applied Biosystems, Courtaboeuf, France). PCR amplification, in triplicate for each sample, was performed using ABI Prism 7300 (Applied Biosystems), TaqMan Universal PCR Master Mix No AmpErase UNG (Applied Biosystems) and Assays-on-Demand Gene Expression probes (Applied Biosystems) for targets'genes: *ATF3* (assay ID Rn00563784_m1), *GFAP* (Rn01460868_m1), *OX-42* (Rn00709342_m1), *IL-1β* (Rn00580432_m1), *IL-6* (Rn00561420_m1), *TNF-α* (Rn00562055_m1), *IL-10* (Rn00563409_m1), *BDNF* (Rn02531967_s1), *TLR4* (Rn00569848_m1), *P2×4* (Rn00580949_m1), *P2×7* (Rn00570451_m1). mRNA determinations were made with reference to the reporter gene encoding glyceraldehyde 3-phosphate dehydrogenase (*GaPDH*; Rn99999916_s1). The polymerase activation step at 95°C for 15 min was followed by 40 cycles of 15 s at 95°C and 60 s at 60°C. The validity of the results was checked by running appropriate negative controls (replacement of cDNA by water for PCR amplification; omission of reverse transcriptase for cDNA synthesis). Specific mRNA levels were calculated after normalizing from *GaPDH* mRNA in each sample. Data are presented as relative mRNA units compared to control (sham) values (see [21]).

Statistical Analyses

All values are expressed as means ± S.E.M. For von Frey filaments tests, the data were analyzed by one-way ANOVA for repeated measures (effect of a drug over time) followed by Dunnett's test. Statistical evaluations of SCT-induced changes in behavioral responses to thermal stimulations were made using the Student's t test. For qRT-PCR data, the $2^{-\Delta\Delta Ct}$ method [26] was used for analysis of the relative changes in specific mRNA levels and for graphic representations (RQ Study Software 1.2 version; Applied Biosystems). For analysis of the time course expression of the targets'genes, a two-way ANOVA was performed, followed by Bonferroni test for comparison of SCT rats versus respective

Table 1. Pharmacological treatments tested for potential anti-allodynic effects in spinal cord-transected rats.

Drugs	Pharmacological effect	Dose	Efficacy on biting behavior
Morphine	Opioid receptor agonist	1, 3, 10 mg/kg s.c.	+++
Tapentadol	Opioid receptor agonist and noradrenaline reuptake inhibitor	10, 20 mg/kg i.p.	+++
Ketamine	NMDA receptor antagonist	50 mg/kg i.p.	++
Baclofen	GABA B receptor agonist	10 mg/kg i.p.	+
Clonazepam	Benzodiazepine (agonist)	0.25, 2 mg/kg i.p.	-
Gabapentin	Blockade of calcium channel α2δ subunit	30, 100, 300 mg/kg i.p.	-
Pregabalin	Blockade of calcium channel α2δ subunit	30 mg/kg i.p.	-
Amitriptyline	Tricyclic antidepressant	10 mg/kg i.p.	-
Amitriptyline + Gabapentin	Tricyclic antidepressant + Blockade of calcium channel α2δ subunit	10 mg/kg i.p. +100 mg/kg i.p.	-
Cyclotraxin B	TrkB receptor blocker	20 mg/kg i.p.	-
Naratriptan	$5\text{-HT}_{1B/D}$ receptor agonist	0.1 mg/kg i.p.	-
Ondansetron	5-HT_3 receptor antagonist	20 µg i.t.	-
8-OH-DPAT	$5\text{-HT}_{1A/7}$ receptor agonist	0.25 mg/kg i.p.	-

+++: potent anti-allodynic effect (complete recovery of control mechanical sensitivity);
++: potent but short lasting anti-allodynic effect;
+: modest but significant anti-allodynic effect; -: inactive treatment.

(sham) controls at each time. The critical level of statistical significance was set at $P<0.05$.

Results

Physiological State of Spinal Cord Transected Rats

After full recovery from anaesthesia, SCT rats first showed hindlimb paralysis and flabbiness. Although they moved in their cage without major difficulty and could access food and water as readily as before the surgery, SCT rats stopped gaining weight for the first week after surgery (−6.3±3.8 g, mean ± S.E.M., n = 8), in contrast to sham-operated animals (+43±2 g, mean ± S.E.M., n = 8); but, afterwards, weight gain was parallel in both SCT- and sham-operated rats (+175.4±28.3 g and +171.2±12.5 g from day 7 to day 30 post-surgery, respectively, means ± S.E.M., n = 8 in each group).

Most striking symptoms were urinary retention and/or hematuria. Hematuria disappeared after 3 or 4 days without any specific treatment. To deal with urinary retention, we had to trigger off the miction reflex by rubbing the bladder once a day during 8–9 days on average. Then, the reflex recovered completely. It also happened that some SCT rats had an accelerated gut transit with diarrhea for the first 3 days post surgery. Later on, such gut disorders were only exceptionally observed. On the other hand, SCT rats had their fur a little bit more tousled than sham animals, but it stayed very clean in areas located both rostrally and caudally of the lesion site, most probably through grooming (that we regularly noted) by their cage mate. Abnormal suffering (with signs such as skin scratching) and/or autotomy were never observed when SCT rats were housed two per cage, as always used for these studies.

Immediately after the surgery and during usually 9–10 days, SCT rats showed paraplegia, first characterized by a total absence of reaction when hindlimbs were mechanically stimulated with von Frey filaments exerting pressure up to the cut-off value (100 g) (Fig. 1). This was followed by a hypo-reflexia which progressively vanished up to normal-like response (as in control unoperated rats) to mechanical stimulation which was usually recovered two weeks post surgery. Later on, SCT rats developed a hyper-reflexia with a pressure threshold value to trigger brisk hindpaw withdrawal strikingly lower (−80%) than that determined in sham rats up to at least 7 weeks post-surgery (Fig. 1). All along the observation period, SCT rats had paralyzed hindlimbs with spasticity, rigidity and tonicity. They also had frequent spontaneous movements of the tail and hindlimbs (shaking), and developed uncoordinated flexion and extension movements.

Development and Localization of Mechanical Allodynia

Among all the body areas tested, only the lesion site on the back and the hindlimbs (see above) showed altered behavioral responses in the von Frey filaments test in SCT- compared to sham-operated rats.

Within a few days after SCT, supersensitivity to mechanical stimulation appeared at the lesion site. From day 2 to day 9, such supersensitivity was mostly rostro-lateral to the lesion site within small areas on both sides (Fig. 2). Then, the supersensitive territory extended medially and laterally to cover an approximately 6 cm^2 cutaneous area just rostral to the thoracic cord transection. In contrast, no supersensitivity was detected behind the transection, and, indeed, SCT rats did not react even to a 100 g pressure exerted by von Frey filament applied within the cutaneous territory on the back, caudal to the transection.

Further assessment of supersensitivity to application of von Frey filaments within the 6 cm^2 area just rostral to the lesion led to identify three different aversive reactions: biting, shaking and escape (Fig. 3), in agreement with previous observations in SCI rats [5]. Determinations of pressure threshold values to trigger each of these behaviors showed parallel time-course decreases, down to very low levels that were reached 10–14 days after surgery and remained unchanged for the 7-weeks-observation period (Fig. 3).

Thermal Sensitivity

To make sure that no bias due to possible changes in skin temperature occurred in SCT- versus sham-operated rats, we first measured hindpaw skin temperature just prior performance of the paw immersion test, two weeks post surgery. Under controlled environmental conditions (with ambient temperature at 22±1°C; see Materials and Methods), hindpaw skin temperature was of 30.1±1.0°C and 29.8±0.5°C (means ± S.E.M. of 8 independent determinations in each group) in SCT- and sham-operated rats, respectively, indicating the lack of incidence of SCT on this parameter. However, clear-cut differences between SCT- and sham-operated rats were noted in withdrawal latencies after hindpaw immersion in cold (10°C) as well as hot (46°C) water. As shown in Figure 4A, SCT rats reacted with much shorter latencies compared to sham-operated animals, as expected of increased sensitivity to both cold and hot stimulation two weeks post SCT.

Further evaluation of cold hypersensitivity was made using the acetone drop test applied at the lesion site, where SCT rats developed mechanical allodynia (Fig. 2). As illustrated in Figure 4B, both the number of trunk shakes and the time spent in back licking and escape attempts for the first min after acetone drops application were significantly increased in SCT- compared to sham-operated animals (+67% and +400%, respectively).

Pharmacological Studies

Effects of Opioïdergic Drugs (Morphine and Tapentadol) on At-Level Mechanical Allodynia. As treatments with opioids were shown to reduce pain in humans with spinal cord lesions [27,28], we investigated whether morphine (1, 3 and 10 mg/kg s.c.) was effective to reduce at-level mechanical allodynia in SCT-rats. Acute treatment was performed 30 days after the surgery, when pressure threshold to elicit biting behavior in response to von Frey filament application had reached its minimum value (Fig. 3). As illustrated in Figure 5A, morphine exerted a dose-dependent effect: it was inactive at 1 mg/kg s.c., but increased pressure threshold value at higher doses, with complete suppression of allodynia-like response 30 and 60 min after administration of the highest dose tested (10 mg/kg s.c.). Confirmation of the anti-allodynic efficacy of opiate receptor activation was made with tapentadol, a mixed mu opioid receptor agonist and noradrenaline reuptake inhibitor with potent antalgic properties [29], which also reversed SCT-induced mechanical allodynia in a dose-dependent manner. As shown in Figure 5B, tapentadol at 10 mg/kg i.p. slightly increased the pressure threshold value, but the dose of 20 mg/kg i.p. completely suppressed allodynia-like response 30 and 60 min after its administration to SCT rats.

Effects of Ketamine on At-Level Mechanical Allodynia. Ketamine is well known to reduce pain in humans suffering from spinal cord injury, and its pain alleviating efficacy has also been reported in rat models of SCI, such as the one obtained by spinal cord contusion [30]. In SCT rats, acute administration of ketamine (50 mg/kg i.p.) induced a significant increase in pressure threshold value to trigger nocifensive response to von Frey filament application within the allodynic cutaneous area (Fig. 5C). At its maximum, 30 min after treatment, pressure threshold value reached 77.3±17.6 g (from 0.96 g±0.39 g before

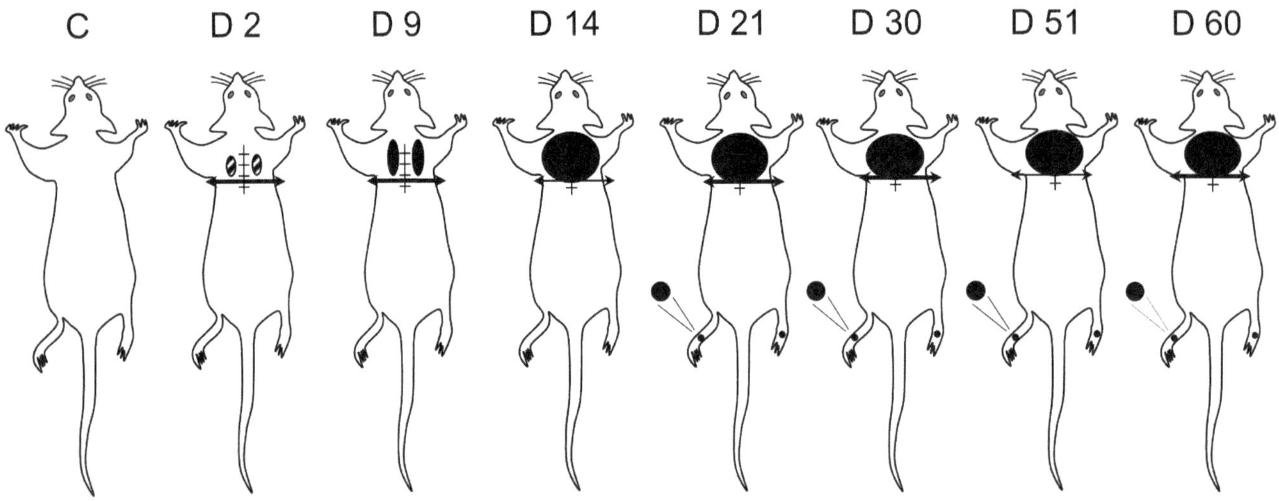

Figure 2. Body territories with increased mechanical sensitivity in spinal cord-transected rats. Pressure threshold values to trigger nocifensive responses were determined using a graded series of von Frey filaments applied throughout the body. Comparison with sham-operated rats (C) showed that pressure threshold values differed in SCT rats only in a limited territory (6 cm^2) bordering rostrally the spinal cord section (at T8–T9, horizontal bar with arrow heads) and in hindpaws (black areas tested), where reactions were obtained for pressure values significantly less than in controls. Time course (day 2 to day 60) changes in spinal cord transected rats showed that supersensitivity (allodynia) in the at-level area just rostral to the lesion was already detected at day 2 (D2) post-surgery, then extended and increased up to a plateau reached at D14 post-surgery. At hindpaw level, supersensitivity developed much later (from D21 post-surgery). Data were obtained in 8–14 rats at each time.

treatment, means ± S.E.M. of 6 determinations), which was not significantly different from the cut-off value corresponding to the non-allodynic state (in naïve rats, before surgery). However, this effect vanished rapidly because mechanical allodynia was completely restored 90 min after ketamine administration (Fig. 5C).

Effects of Baclofen on At-Level Mechanical Allodynia. Because baclofen, a GABA B receptor agonist, is often prescribed to reduce SCI-induced spasticity in humans, and is endowed with anti-neuropathic pain properties [31], we investigated whether this drug could reduce at-level mechanical allodynia in SCT rats. Indeed, baclofen induced a limited and transient increase ($p<0.05$) in pressure threshold value, from 0.6±0.4 g before treatment to 5.0±2.1 g 30 min after i.p. administration of this drug at 10 mg/kg (Fig. 5D).

Effects of Anticonvulsant Drugs on At-Level Mechanical Allodynia. The calcium channel blockers gabapentin and pregabalin and the benzodiazepine clonazepam are anticonvulsants endowed with anti-neuropathic pain properties both in humans [3,27] and in rodent models [32,33], and we tested whether these drugs also exerted anti-allodynic effects in SCT rats. In fact, acute treatments with either gabapentin (30 mg/kg i.p.), pregabalin (30 mg/kg i.p.) or clonazepam (0.25 mg/kg i.p.), at doses devoid of any inhibitory effect on locomotor coordination (as assessed using the rotarod test; not shown), had no significant effect on pressure threshold to trigger nocifensive response in SCT rats (Table 1). Some increase in pressure threshold values was noted with higher doses of clonazepam (2 mg/kg i.p.) and gabapentin

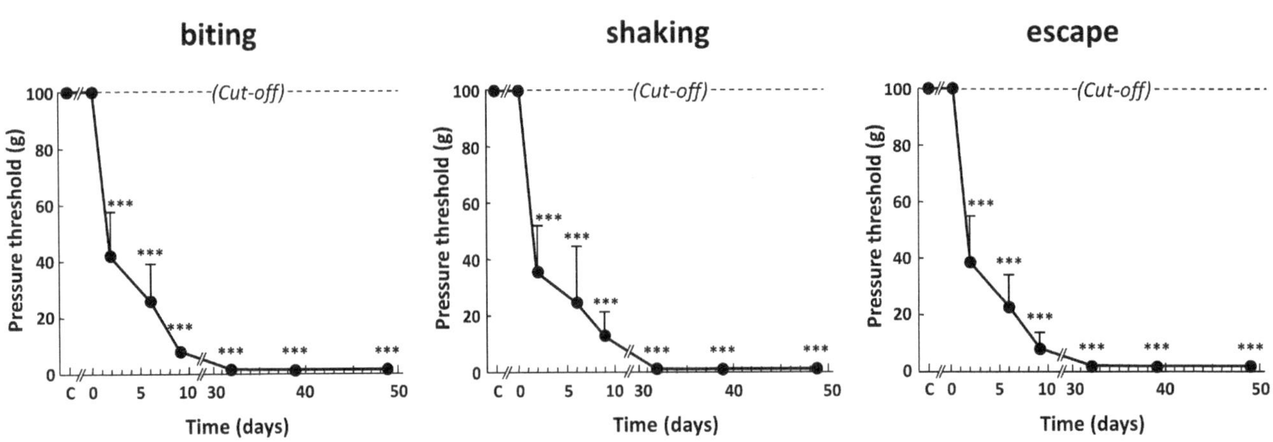

Figure 3. Time-course changes in nocifensive reactions to von Frey filaments application in the « at-level » allodynic territory rostral to the lesion in spinal cord-transected rats. Pressure threshold values to trigger biting (of the filament), shaking or escape were determined using the "up-down" method with a graded series of von Frey filaments applied onto the allodynic at-level area on the back at various times (in days) after surgery (0 on abscissa). Each bar is the mean + S.E.M. of independent determinations in 8 rats. *** $P<0.001$ compared to control (intact) rats (C on abscissa). One-way ANOVA for repeated measures followed by Dunnett's test.

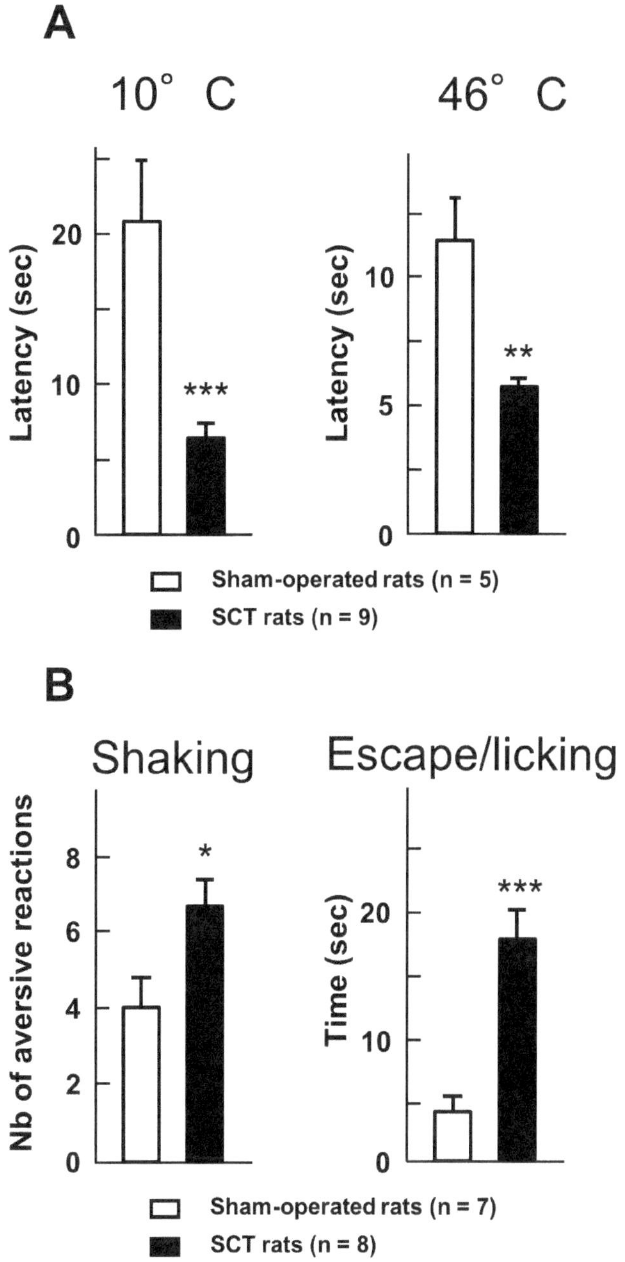

Figure 4. Hyper-responsiveness to thermal stimulation in spinal cord-transected rats. A – Latency (in sec) to hindpaw withdrawal was determined after paw immersion into a bath of hot (46°C) or cold (10°C) water, two weeks after the surgery. Each bar is the mean + S.E.M. of independent determinations in 9 SCT rats and 5 sham-operated rats. ** $P<0.01$, *** $P<0.001$ compared to respective values in sham-operated rats. Student's t test. **B** – Behavioral responses to the acetone drop test applied at the surgical scar two weeks after surgery. The number of shakes and the time (in sec) spent in escape attempts and licking of the back were measured for one minute after acetone drops application. Each bar is the mean + S.E.M. of independent determinations in 8 SCT rats and 7 sham-operated rats. * $P<0.05$, ** $P<0.01$ compared to respective values in sham-operated rats. Student's t test.

(100 and 300 mg/kg i.p.), but rats presented profound ataxia after such treatments (not shown).

Effects of Other Drugs on At-Level Mechanical Allodynia. As detailed in Table 1, the antidepressant amitriptyline, alone or combined with gabapentin, the anti-migraine drug naratriptan, the 5-$HT_{1A/7}$ receptor agonist 8-OH-DPAT, the 5-HT_3 receptor antagonist ondansetron, the BDNF-Trk B receptor blocker cyclotraxin B, at effective doses to reduce pain in validated neuropathic models in rodents [34–39], exerted no anti-allodynic effects up to 3 hours after acute administration in SCT rats.

Neuroinflammatory and Neuroplasticity Markers in Spinal Cord and DRG of SCT rats

Spinal Cord. A first series of determinations consisted of measuring the tissue concentrations of transcripts encoding the neuronal injury marker ATF3, the macrophage-microglial activation marker OX-42 and the astrocytic marker GFAP [21] in the dorsal and ventral halves of spinal cord segments just above (T6–T8) and just below (T9–T11) the surgery level in SCT- compared to sham-operated rats. Measurements were made at day 17 post surgery, when both mechanical (Fig.3) and thermal (Fig.4) allodynia had fully developed. As shown in Figure 6, expression of these three genes was markedly upregulated in both dorsal and ventral halves in segments above and below the section compared to sham-operated rats. Upregulation of ATF3 mRNA was slightly larger in dorsal spinal cord above and below SCT (×20.8- and ×21.1-fold, respectively) than in the corresponding ventral spinal cord segments (×15.7 and ×15.1-fold, respectively). On the other hand, no significant differences were noted between SCT-induced elevation of OX-42 mRNA and GFAP mRNA levels in the dorsal versus the ventral halves of spinal segments above and below SCT. Accordingly, no further distinction between the dorsal and ventral halves was made in subsequent experiments, and whole spinal cord segments were dissected out and processed for investigating the time-course changes in neuroinflammatory and neuroplasticity markers after thoracic cord transection.

As shown in Figure 7, already on day 2 post-surgery, ATF3 mRNA levels were 16.0- and 21.0-fold higher in thoracic spinal cord segments just caudal and rostral to the section, respectively, than in corresponding tissues from sham-operated rats. This up-regulation was long lasting as it persisted, but to a lower extent, up to the last observation day (×7.0 and 6.7 on day 60 post-surgery) (Fig. 7A). As illustrated in Figure 7A, a long lasting up regulation of ATF3 mRNA was also detected in both the cervical and lumbar enlargements of the spinal cord in SCT rats. However, this change was of much lower amplitude than in thoracic segments. OX42 mRNA levels were also markedly increased in thoracic segments of the spinal cord just caudal and rostral to the section on day 2 post-surgery (×6.2 and 4.8, respectively), and remained significantly elevated until day 60 (×2.8 and 2.5, respectively) (Fig. 7B). A long lasting up-regulation of OX-42 mRNA was also noted in both the cervical and lumbar enlargements of the spinal cord. However, it was of lower amplitude than in thoracic segments (Fig. 7B). The time course of SCT-induced changes in GFAP mRNA levels differed from those of the former two transcripts, as the observed up-regulation was delayed and relatively less pronounced (×3 at maximum) (Fig. 7C). However, these changes persisted to similar extents up to the last observation day (day 60 post surgery). In cervical and lumbar enlargements, only slight, generally non significant, increases in GFAP mRNA levels were observed in SCT rats, but they were also of long duration (Fig. 7C).

Concerning pro-inflammatory cytokines, a massive increase in IL-6 mRNA levels was observed as soon as 2 days after the section in thoracic segments bordering caudally (x 76.8 as compared to

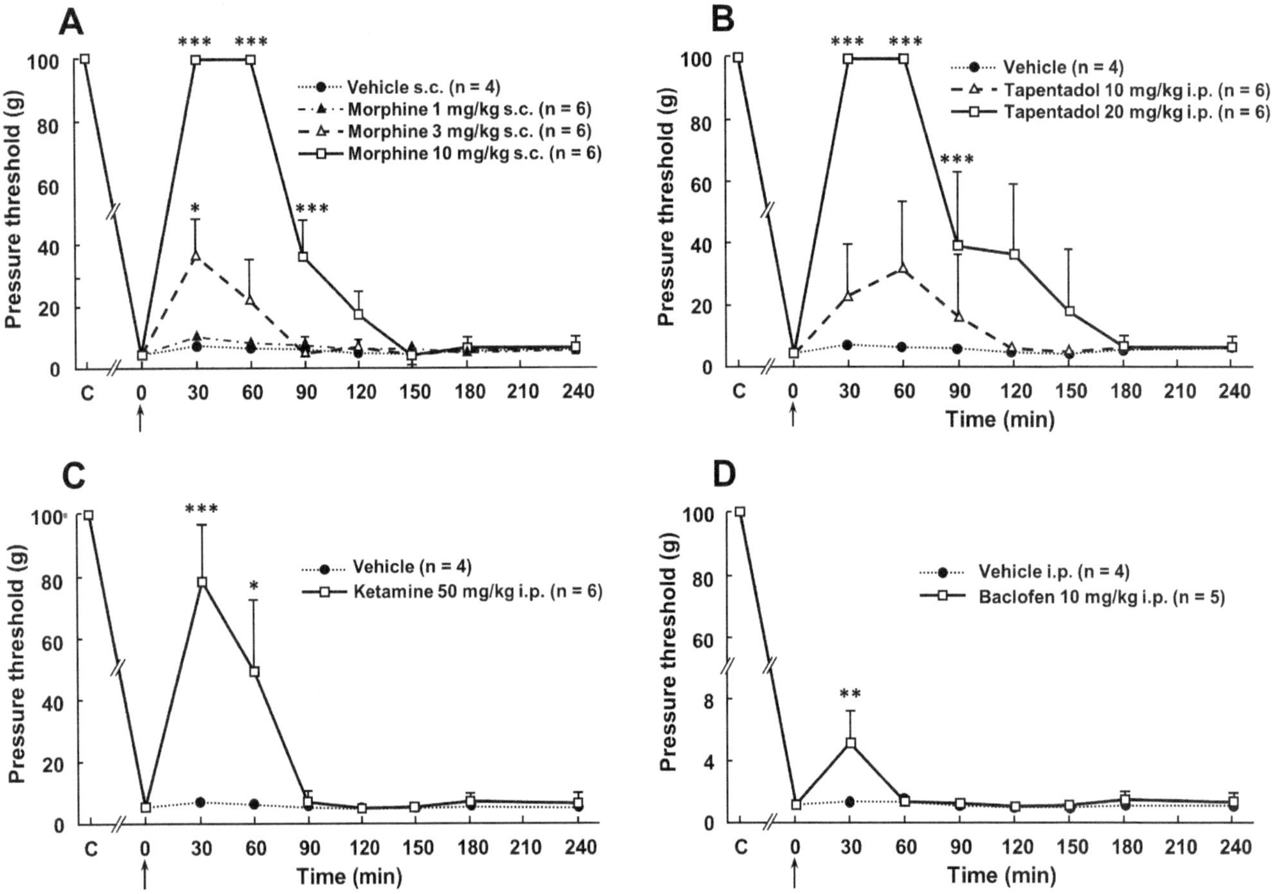

Figure 5. Anti-allodynic effects of acute administration of morphine (A), tapentadol (B), ketamine (C) or baclofen (D) in spinal cord-transected rats. Acute administration of morphine (1, 3 or 10 mg/kg s.c.), tapentadol (10 or 20 mg/kg i.p.), ketamine (50 mg/kg i.p.), baclofen (10 mg/kg i.p.) or their respective vehicle was performed (0 on abscissa, arrow) in rats whose spinal cord had been transected at T8–T9 level one month before. Pressure threshold values to trigger nocifensive biting were determined using von Frey filaments applied within the at-level allodynic territory at various times after treatment. Each point is the mean + S.E.M. of independent determinations in n rats. C on abscissa: Control (naive) rats (prior to surgery). P<0.05, ** P<0.01, *** P<0.001 compared to respective values in vehicle-treated rats. One-way ANOVA for repeated measures followed by Dunnett's test.

sham-operated rats) and rostrally (x 66.4) the section (Fig. 8A). A modest up-regulation was still observed on day 15 but not on day 60 post surgery. In contrast, no significant changes in IL-6 mRNA levels were detected in both the cervical and lumbar enlargements of the spinal cord at any time after SCT as compared to transcript levels measured in the same tissues of sham-operated rats (not shown).

The levels of IL-1β mRNA were also markedly increased 2 days after surgery in thoracic segments bordering caudally (x 172.2 as compared to sham-operated rats) and rostrally (x 98.6) the transection (Fig. 8B). Significant increases in IL-1β mRNA levels still persisted in caudal- and rostral-level segments on day 60 post-surgery, but to a much lower extent than on day 2. Similar but less pronounced changes in TNF-α mRNA levels were noted with a significant up-regulation in thoracic segments on day 2 post surgery (×3.0 caudally and ×1.9 rostrally to the section, respectively) (Fig. 8C). On day 60, a significant increase in TNF-α mRNA levels was still detected principally in thoracic segments rostral to the transection (x 1.9) (Fig. 8C). Finally, tissue concentrations of mRNA encoding the anti-inflammatory cytokine IL-10 were also markedly increased on day 2 after transection in both caudal-level (x 36.3) and rostral-level (x 38.7) thoracic segments, and an up-regulation of much lower amplitude was still detected on day 60 post surgery (Fig. 8D).

In contrast with the aforementioned transcripts, BDNF mRNA levels were reduced in spinal cord tissues of SCT rats, both on days 2 (−49% as compared to sham-operated rats, P<0.05) and 60 (−38%, P<0.05) post surgery in thoracic segments caudal to the section and on day 60 (−23%, P≤0.05) post surgery in thoracic segments rostral to the section (not shown). On the other hand, mRNAs encoding P2×4, P2×7 and TLR4 were upregulated in thoracic segments bordering caudally (×3.2, ×1.8 and ×3.8, respectively) and rostrally (×2.6, ×1.5 and ×3.6, respectively) the transection on day 2 post-surgery. This up-regulation was even more pronounced on post-surgery day 60 (×3.6, ×2.9 and ×4.5 caudal to the section, ×3.8, ×2.9 and ×5.6 rostral to the section, respectively) (Fig. 9A, 9B, 9C).

Dorsal Root Ganglia. Like that observed at spinal level, ATF3 mRNA was strongly up-regulated in DRG at T9–T11 caudal level as well as T6–T8 rostral level for the first two weeks after thoracic cord transection (Fig. 7A). Then, significant increases persisted up to the last observation day, two months after surgery, but to a lower extent, only in T6–T8 DRG (Fig. 7A). Transcripts encoding OX-42 (macrophages) and GFAP (satellite

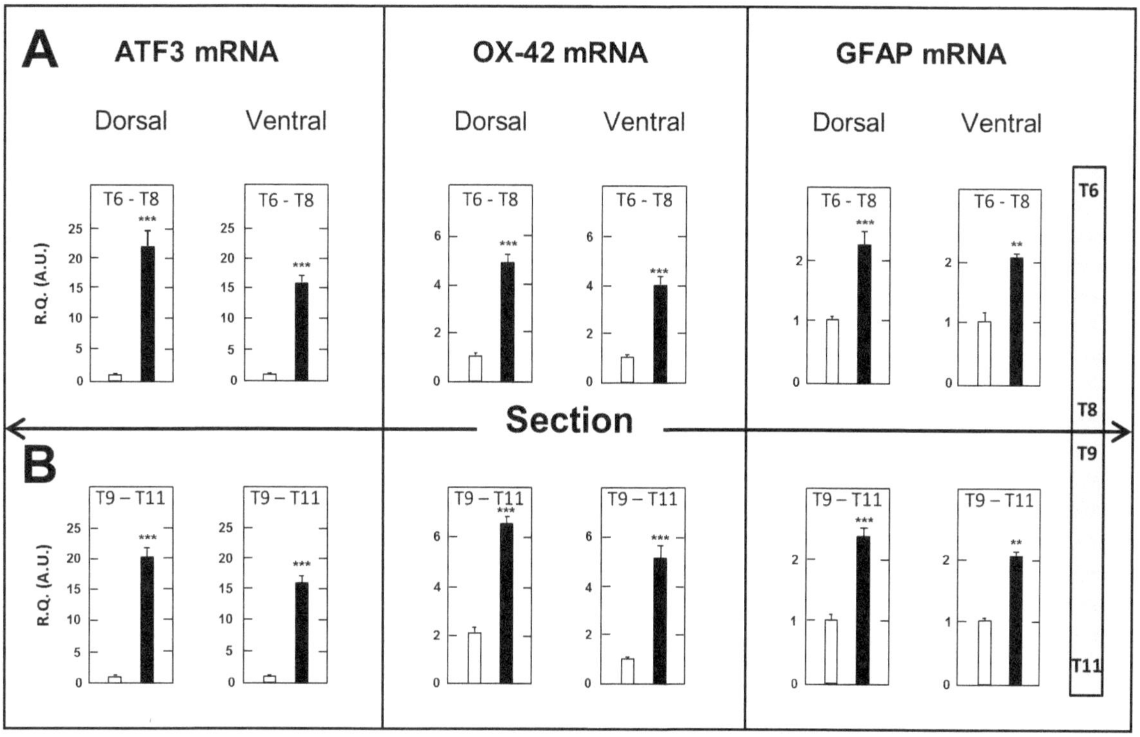

Figure 6. Increased expression of ATF3, OX-42 and GFAP mRNAs in the dorsal and ventral halves of spinal cord segments just above (T6–T8) and below (T9–T11) the surgery level in spinal cord-transected rats. Real time RT-qPCR determinations were made at day 17 after surgery. Data are expressed as the ratio of specific mRNA over GaPDH mRNA [R.Q.(A.U.)]. Each bar is the mean + S.E.M. of 10 independent determinations in both SCT (black bars) and sham-operated (empty bars) rats. *** P<0.001 compared to respective values in sham-operated rats. Two-way ANOVA followed by Bonferroni test.

glial cells) were also markedly up regulated in DRG at spinal cord segments caudal (T9–T11) and rostral (T6–T8) to the transection. However, this effect was transient, especially at rostral level (T6–T8) where significant increases in OX-42 and GFAP transcripts were noted on days 2–4 and up to day 9 post-surgery, respectively. At caudal level (T9–T11), up regulation of these transcripts lasted a few days more, but three weeks post-surgery, both OX-42 and GFAP transcripts no longer differed in thoracic DRG of SCT- versus sham-rats (Figs 7B,7C).

As illustrated in Figure 8A, mRNA encoding IL-6 also showed a dramatic up-regulation (x 65.6) in T9-T11 DRG at day 2 post surgery. Its levels then decreased rapidly, but remained significantly higher than in sham-operated rats up to day 9 post surgery (x 4.4; not shown). Interestingly, up-regulation of IL-6 mRNA was even larger at day 2 (x 145.0) and remained significant for a longer period (up to day 50 post surgery: ×1.6) in rostral level T6–T8 DRG (Fig. 8A, and data not shown). An up regulation of IL-1β mRNA was also noted in thoracic DRG at day 2 post-surgery (but not at day 60) in SCT rats (Fig. 8B), but this change was of much lower amplitude than that noted at spinal level. Also in sharp contrast with that previously noted at spinal level, TNF-α mRNA was not up-regulated in thoracic DRG of SCT rats, neither at day 2 nor at day 60 post-surgery (Fig. 8C). Finally, the levels of mRNA encoding the anti-inflammatory cytokine IL-10 were found to be slightly increased (x 3.1), but only in DRG caudal to the section (T9–T11) on day 2 post surgery, and at a markedly lower extent than in thoracic cord segments (Fig. 8D).

Further transcripts quantifications confirmed the existence of marked differences between DRG and spinal cord tissues. In particular, BDNF mRNA levels were significantly increased in caudal level T9–T11 DRG at both days 2 (×5.6, P<0.01) and 55 (×1.6, P≤0.05) post-surgery, but only at day 2 (×4.3, P<0.01) in rostral level T6–T8 DRG (not shown). On the other hand, mRNAs encoding P2×4, P2×7 and TLR4, which are all expressed by activated macrophages and satellite glial cells [40–42], showed no modification of their expression levels in T9–T11 DRG of SCT rats whatever the time after surgery. Similar negative results were noted in T6–T8 DRG except a modest but significant increase in P2×7 mRNA levels observed on day 2 post surgery (Fig. 9A, 9B, 9C).

Discussion

Spinal cord transection is a model widely used for the study of induced spasticity, hyper-reflexia and subsequent functional and structural plasticity underlying locomotor recovery under the control of the Central Pattern Generator [11–13]. Although neuropathic pain concerns a high proportion of SCI patients, only few investigations have been dedicated to alterations in pain signaling mechanisms in rats with complete SCT. Indeed, a large body of data has already been generated from studies in rodents with partial spinal cord lesion, but unavoidable interindividual variations in the severity and extent of lesion constitute serious limitations of such models (see Introduction). These considerations led us to thoroughly characterize the homogeneous model of complete transection of the spinal cord at thoracic level with regard to its possible relevance for studying central neuropathic pain, associated neuroplasticity changes and responses to drugs used to alleviate pain in SCI patients.

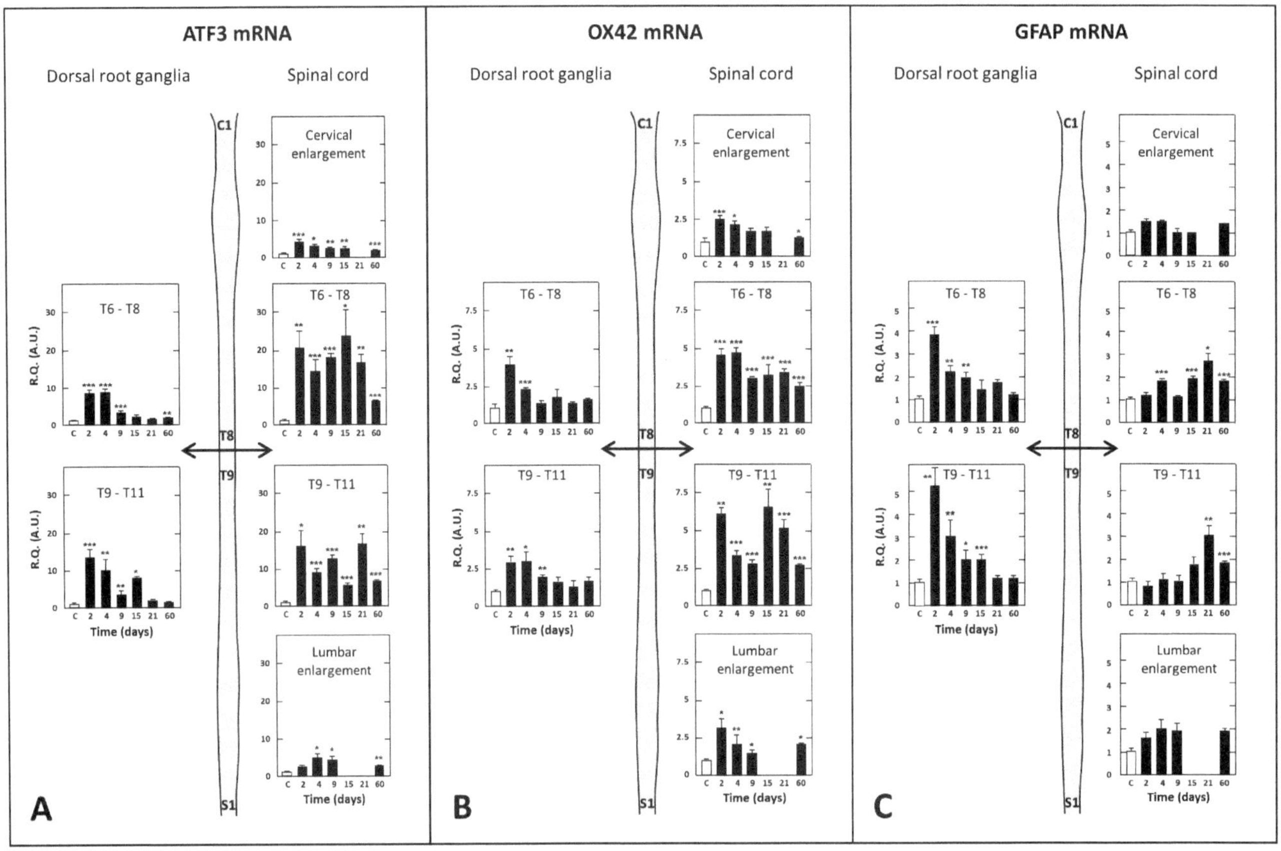

Figure 7. Time-course changes in tissue levels of transcripts encoding ATF3 (A), OX-42 (B) or GFAP (C) in dorsal root ganglia and spinal cord at various times after spinal cord transection. Real-time RT-qPCR determinations were made in T6–T8 and T9–T11 dorsal root ganglia, T6–T8 and T9–T11 spinal cord segments and the cervical and lumbar enlargements at various times (in days, D, abscissa) after spinal cord transection at T8–T9 level. Data are expressed as the ratio of specific mRNA over GaPDH mRNA [R.Q.(A.U.)]. Each bar is the mean + S.E.M. of n independent determinations (D2, D4, D9, D15, D21: n = 6; D60: n = 12). Sham values at every postoperative time are pooled under "C" (control) on abscissa. * P<0.05, * P<0.01, *** P<0.001 compared to respective values in sham-operated rats (C).Two-way ANOVA followed by Bonferroni test.

Clinical State of Spinal Cord Transected Rats

Despite complete transection of the spinal cord, rats showed a relatively good physiological state. The lack of micturition reflex and the hematuria, which are commonly encountered in paraplegic patients [43], usually resolved within 9 days post-surgery. Otherwise, their fur was clean, and very probably because they shared their cage with a congener, autotomia never occurred. Although rats lose weight for the first week after surgery, as a consequence of hindlimb muscles atrophy, they subsequently gained weight at the same rate as sham-operated rats, as expected from animals in good health [44].

Effects of Spinal Cord Transection on Hindlimb Sensitivity

Just after the lesion, hindlimbs no longer responded by a reflex motor reaction to cutaneous mechanical stimulation at high intensity (with the 100 g von Frey filament). Motor reaction then reappeared progressively up to a level corresponding to that found in control (unoperated) animals around the second week post-surgery. A marked hyper-reflexivity subsequently developed, along with spasticity, which reached their maximum approximately 7 weeks post-surgery and were still fully present on the last day (60) of our study. Marked alterations of motor reflexes also occur in humans with complete spinal cord transection, as evidenced by the exacerbated response in the H reflex of hindlimb muscles [45,46]. Such facilitated reflex responses may be due to α-motoneurons hyperexcitability [47]. Indeed, spinal cord transection causes an up-regulation of constitutively active 5-HT$_{2C}$ receptors expressed by motoneurons, and the reinforcement of their membrane depolarizing influence has been demonstrated to contribute to motoneuron hyperexcitability in lesioned rats [48]. On the other hand, spasticity could also be accounted for by a down regulation of the potassium-chloride cotransporter KCC2 within the lumbar spinal cord below transection [12]. Although spasticity can be painful in humans, and below-level pain exists in patients with extensive spinal cord injury [2,49], hyper-reflexivity and spasticity at hindlimb level could not be related to pain behavior in SCT rats because completeness of the lesion prevented the nociceptive messages to reach the sensory cortex where they can generate pain sensation.

Along with mechanical hypersensitivity, SCT rats also developed heat and cold hypersensitivity as shown by the reduced latency of hindpaw withdrawal after immersion in water at 46°C or 10°C (Fig.4). Heat hypersensitivity has already been described in mice after spinal cord contusion and transection [50], and cold hypersensitivity at hindpaw level has been well documented in rats with contused spinal cord [51]. Whether or not similar neuroplasticity mechanisms underlay thermal and mechanical hypersensitivity at hindpaw level in SCT rats is a pending question to be addressed in future studies. In particular, because thermal hypersensitivity was evidenced from a motor response (hindpaw

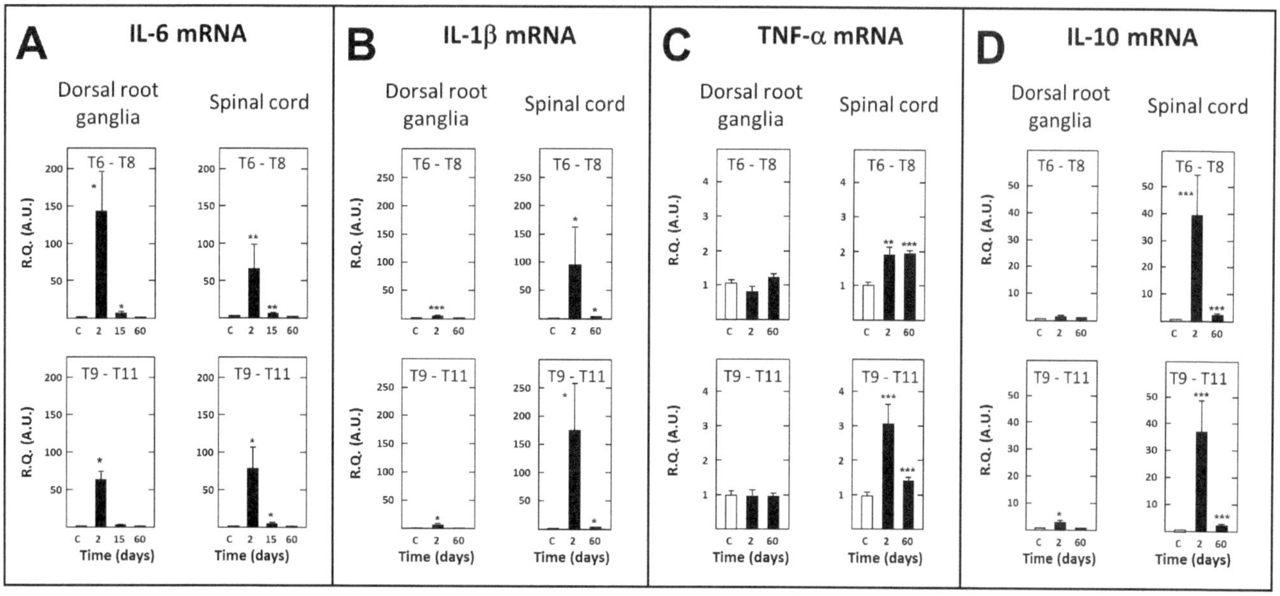

Figure 8. Short- and long-term changes in levels of transcripts encoding IL-6 (A), IL-1β (B), TNF-α (C) and IL-10 in dorsal root ganglia and spinal tissues in spinal cord-transected rats. Real-time RT-qPCR determinations were made in T6–T8 and T9–T11 dorsal root ganglia and T6–T8 and T9–T11 spinal segments at day (D) 2, 15 or 60 (abscissa) after spinal cord transection at T8–T9 level. Data are expressed as the ratio of specific mRNA over GaPDH mRNA [R.Q.(A.U.)]. Each bar is the mean + S.E.M. of n independent determinations (D2, D15: n=6; D60: n=12). Sham values at every postoperative time are pooled under "C" (control) on abscissa. * $P<0.05$, * $P<0.01$, *** $P<0.001$ compared to respective values in sham-operated rats (C). Two-way ANOVA followed by Bonferroni test.

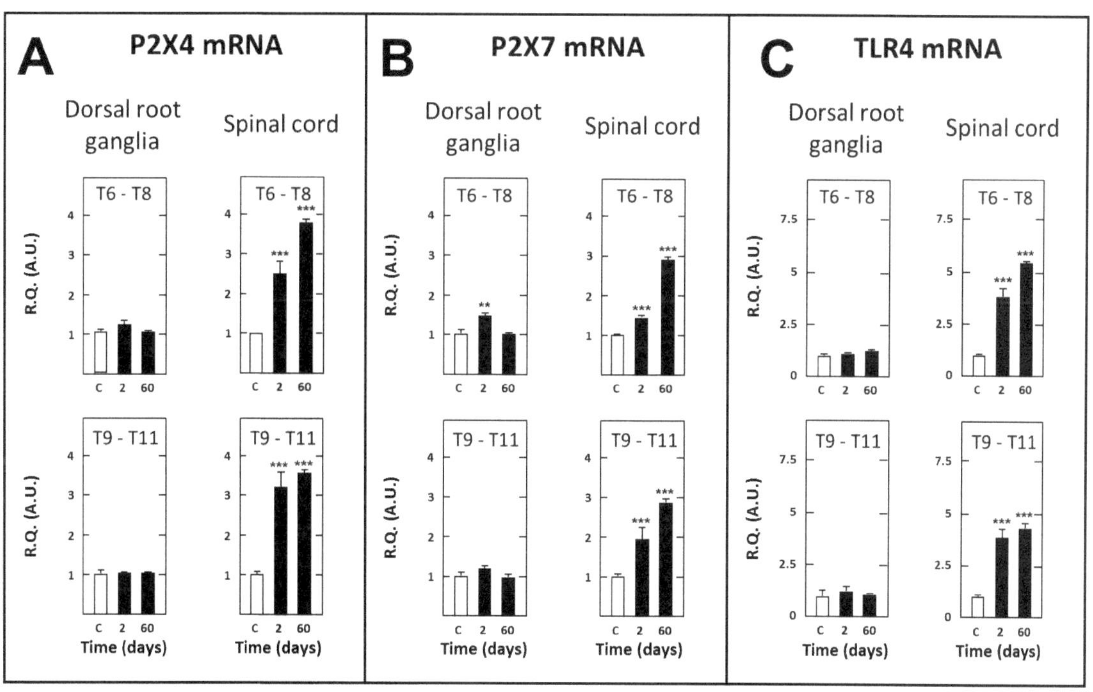

Figure 9. Short- and long-term changes in levels of transcripts encoding P2×4 (A), P2×7 (B) and TLR4 (C) in dorsal root ganglia and spinal tissues in spinal cord-transected rats. Real-time RT-qPCR determinations were made in T6–T8 and T9–T11 dorsal root ganglia and T6–T8 and T9–T11 spinal segments at day 2 or 60 (abscissa) after spinal cord transection at T8–T9 level. Data are expressed as the ratio of specific mRNA over GaPDH mRNA [R.Q.(A.U.)]. Each bar is the mean + S.E.M. of n independent determinations (D2: n=6; D60: n=12). Sham values at every postoperative time are pooled under "C" (control) on abscissa. ** $P<0.01$, *** $P<0.001$ compared to respective levels in sham-operated rats (C). Two-way ANOVA followed by Bonferroni test.

withdrawal), it might have also involved – at least in part - some α-motoneuron hyperexcitability as discussed above about SCT-induced mechanical hypersensitivity.

At-Level Allodynia

Whereas no behavioral reaction to the application of von Frey filaments within the trunk caudal to the lesion could be elicited in SCT rats, at-level allodynia-like reactions appeared relatively rapidly and reached a maximum 2–3 weeks after surgery. In particular, biting, which is considered as a brainstem response, and escape as a cortical response, were very probably associated with pain in SCT rats [5]. Since sham-operated rats did not develop such behaviors, we can exclude that they might have corresponded to musculoskeletal pain. Instead, at-level mechanical allodynia pain was very probably caused by spinal cord injury itself, as expected of neuropathic pain of central (spinal) origin [2]. Interestingly, 100% of SCT rats developed at-level allodynia, contrary to humans with spinal cord lesion and rats with spinal cord contusion as only a fraction of lesioned subjects suffer from such pain symptoms. Indeed, the prevalence for the rat/human to develop at-level pain depends on the extent of the lesion [52]. Such homogeneous data in SCT rats support the idea that the SCT model might be especially useful to assess the potential effects of drugs aimed at reducing centrally-evoked neuropathic pain and to investigate underlying physiopathological mechanisms.

Even though at-level cold allodynia is frequently seen in SCI patients [53], only few studies have reported this symptom in spinal cord lesioned rodents [5,54]. Indeed, according to Baastrup et al. [5], only 3% of the rats with contusion of the spinal cord exhibit clear-cut cold allodynia. In contrast, in our study, 100% of SCT rats presented at-level cold allodynia further emphasizing the usefulness of this model for improving experimental group homogeneity. A potential at-level heat allodynia could not be assessed in our studies because of the unavailability of appropriate equipment. Nevertheless, it can be recalled that using a Peltier device, Gao et al. [54] were unable to detect any heat allodynia in spinal cord contused rats.

Pharmacological Sensitivity of At-Level Mechanical Allodynia in SCT Rats

Only a few drugs among those tested were found to efficiently reduce at-level allodynia when injected acutely in SCT rats. The efficacy of morphine and tapentadol was probably underlain by the capacity of mu opioid receptor activation to inhibit the activity of wide dynamic range neurons in the dorsal horn of the spinal cord [55]. Interestingly, tapentadol had a somewhat more prolonged effect than morphine, may be because of its additional capacity to inhibit noradrenaline reuptake as this monoamine has been shown to be implicated in descending inhibitory control of neuropathic pain [56].

Ketamine also reversed at-level allodynia in SCT rats, in consistence with human data that demonstrated that this NMDA receptor antagonist is especially efficient to reduce allodynia in SCI patients [57]. This marked effect of ketamine, that may be sustained by a temporary inhibition of astrocyte activation, further supports the key role played by glutamate receptors, particularly NMDA receptors, in physiopathological mechanisms underlying neuropathic pain [58].

Finally, the last drug of the series tested which was found to exert some (but modest) anti-allodynic effects in SCT rats was the GABA B receptor agonist, baclofen, commonly used to suppress spasticity in spinal cord injured patients [59]. Spinal cord injury is known to be associated with a decreased tone of inhibitory GABAergic neurotransmission [7], and it can be proposed that baclofen transiently compensated for this deficit, thereby reducing allodynia in SCT rats. In contrast, clonazepam, which is used to alleviate SCI patients from neuropathic pain [27], was inefficient suggesting that GABA A receptor activation was ineffective to inhibit at-level allodynia in SCT rats.

Serotonin is known to play a major role in pain control via the activation of several receptor types [36]. Thus, F13640, a potent and selective 5-HT_{1A} receptor agonist, appeared to be especially effective to suppress allodynia in spinal cord lesioned rats [60]. In our hands, the prototypical 5-HT_{1A} receptor agonist, 8-OH-DPAT, did not reduce allodynia in SCT rats. Yet, this molecule is also an agonist at 5-HT_7 receptors, whose activation can result in effects opposite to that expected from 5-HT_{1A} receptor activation [61]. Further studies with selective 5-HT_{1A} and 5-HT_7 receptor ligands have therefore to be performed in order to reach a clear-cut conclusion regarding the potential modulations of at-level allodynia by serotonin acting at these receptors.

Because allodynia-like sensory dysfunctions are associated with migraine [62], we also investigated whether the anti-migraine drug, naratriptan, with potent 5-$HT_{1B/1D}$ receptor agonist properties [36], could alleviate at-level allodynia in SCT rats. Indeed, no effect was observed, possibly because triptans were found to selectively reduce neuropathic pain at cephalic level but not in extra-cephalic territories [35]. Finally, the last 5-HT receptor that we selected for our pharmacological investigations was the 5-HT_3 type whose implication in modulatory controls of neuropathic pain has been firmly established [63]. In contrast to the capacity of i.t. injection of ondansetron to attenuate neuropathic pain caused by spinal cord compression [64], this treatment was inactive in SCT rats, probably because complete transection of the spinal cord had suppressed the bulbo-spinal connections involved in 5-HT_3 receptor-mediated effects [38].

Under our acute treatment conditions, neither the antidepressant amitriptyline nor the anticonvulsants gabapentin and pregabalin, which are commonly used to reduce neuropathic pain in SCI patients [3], exerted any significant anti-allodynic effect in SCT rats (Table 1). Indeed, numerous studies showed that these drugs are effective only under chronic treatment conditions [39,65], and further experiments consisting of repeated administrations of antidepressants and anticonvulsants have to be performed before concluding about their effectiveness or ineffectiveness in the SCT rat model.

Finally, because BDNF and its receptor TrkB play key roles in physiopathological mechanisms underlying neuropathic pain [66,67], we investigated whether acute TrkB blockade by cyclotraxin B could affect allodynia in SCT rats. Indeed, Constandil et al. [34] reported that this drug can prevent and reverse neuropathic pain caused by peripheral nerve ligation in rats. In contrast, we found that cyclotraxin B was unable to reduce allodynia in SCT rats (Table 1), in line with RT-qPCR determinations which suggested that spinal BDNF expression would not be upregulated (in contrast to that observed in peripheral neuropathic pain models [66,67]) but rather downregulated after thoracic cord transection, as previously reported after other types of SCI in rats [68,69].

Neuroinflammation and Glial Activation in SCT Rats

The transcription factor ATF3 is induced when neurons are injured, and implicated in regeneration and plasticity [21]. Its role in the *maintenance* of central neuropathic pain is the matter of controversy, as it is no longer expressed when pain is still present after spinal cord injury [70]. However, ATF3 implication in the *induction* of central neuropathic pain is supported by data showing that it promotes the expression of the microglial/macrophage marker OX-42 and the astrocyte/satellite glial cell marker GFAP [71,72], two factors closely associated with neural lesion-evoked neuropathic pain [21,70,73–75]. Because ATF3 activation is triggered by cellular damages, and this transcription factor is able to repress its own promoter [71], the long lasting up-regulation of ATF3 transcript that occurred after SCT might reflect an ongoing neuronal damage associated with microglia activation. Convergent data in the literature showed that microglia activation is mediated, among others, by purinergic receptors [76] and Toll-Like Receptors [77]. Consistently, we observed, in thoracic cord segments just caudal (T9–T11) and rostral (T6–T8) to the transection, a long lasting (up to 60 days post-surgery) increase in the expression of mRNAs encoding P2XA, P2×7 and TLR4 receptors.

Numerous reports in the literature ascribe to activated microglia an important role in neuropathic pain consecutive to spinal cord injury [70,73,78], and the marked induction of OX42 mRNA in SCT rats is congruent with these data. In fact, IL-6, IL-1β, and TNF-α cytokines released from activated microglia can induce, by themselves, central (spinal) sensitization, thus maintaining neuropathic pain [79,80]. The huge induction of IL-6 and IL-1β that occurred on day 2 post-surgery suggests that these cytokines were involved more in the *induction* than in the *maintenance* of SCT-evoked neuropathic pain. In contrast, TNF-α would be more concerned by pain *maintenance* as SCT-induced up-regulation of its transcript in spinal T6–T8 segments was as pronounced at day 60 as at day 2 post-surgery. The strong increase in IL-10 mRNA that occurred shortly after the lesion might be linked to some inhibitory control of neuropathic pain for the first days after SCT, through the anti-inflammatory potency of this cytokine [81] and/or its neuroprotective effects in spinal cord injured models [82]. Overall, in contrast to that found in spinal tissues, none of the 11 genes studied were up-regulated beyond two weeks post-surgery in DRG above the lesion, supporting the idea that SCT-induced long lasting at-level allodynia did not involve some peripheral hypersensitivity but corresponded mainly, if not exclusively, to central neuropathic pain. Indeed, the short lasting induction of ATF3, OX-42, GFAP and cytokines encoding genes in DRG might have reflected some limited lesion of T8–T9 dorsal roots possibly occurring during surgery for thoracic cord transection. As a matter of fact, it has to be emphasized that our RT-qPCR determinations of time-course changes in mRNA levels will have to be completed by measurements of corresponding proteins in order to validate the inferences made above about the respective implications of pro-inflammatory cytokines and other neuroinflammatory markers in neuropathic pain-inducing mechanisms in SCT rats.

Within the spinal cord, GFAP mRNA up-regulation after SCT was delayed compared to that of transcripts encoding the pro-inflammatory cytokines IL-1β, IL-6 and TNF-α, in line with the idea that early production and release of these cytokines from microglial activation [83] leads to secondary induction of astrogliosis after injury [84]. That astrogliosis with an up-regulation of GFAP [74] - like that found in SCT rats - contributes to neuropathic pain after spinal cord injury is supported by the fact that pharmacological blockade of astroglia activation reduced pain in spinal cord-lesioned rats [73,85].

Conclusion

Spinal cord transection at thoracic level in rats appeared to generate a highly reproducible model of at-level neuropathic pain, mainly of central origin, suitable for pharmacological studies aimed at testing innovative treatments targeted specifically on spinal lesion-evoked neuropathic pain. Time course changes in mRNA levels of neuroinflammatory markers induced by the lesion supported the idea that both activated microglia and activated astroglia contributed to neuropathic pain in spinally transected rats. However, further investigations of these markers have to be made at protein level in order to determine more precisely the respective roles of both cell types in mechanisms underlying central allodynia in SCT rats.

Acknowledgments

We are grateful to pharmaceutical companies (Glaxo-Wellcome, Grünenthal) for generous gifts of drugs, and to Pr Guglielmo Foffani (Toledo, Spain) for helpful discussions.

Author Contributions

Conceived and designed the experiments: SM S. Bourgoin MH. Performed the experiments: SM S. Bourgoin VK S. Barthélémy CC FC DO. Analyzed the data: SM S. Bourgoin DO MH. Wrote the paper: SM MH.

References

1. Finnerup NB, Johannesen IL, Sindrup SH, Bach FW, Jensen TS (2001) Pain and dysesthesia in patients with spinal cord injury: A postal survey. Spinal Cord 39: 256–262.
2. Bryce TN, Biering-Sørensen F, Finnerup NB, Cardenas DD, Defrin R, et al. (2012) International spinal cord injury pain classification: part I. Background and description. March 6–7, 2009. Spinal Cord 50: 413–417.
3. Attal N, Cruccu G, Baron R, Haanpaa M, Hansson P, et al. (2010) EFNS guidelines on the pharmacological treatment of neuropathic pain: 2010 revision. Eur J Neurol 17: 1113–e1188.
4. Nakae A, Nakai K, Yano K, Hosokawa K, Shibata M, et al. (2011) The animal model of spinal cord injury as an experimental pain model. J Biomed Biotechnol 2011: 939023.
5. Baastrup C, Maersk-Moller CC, Nyengaard JR, Jensen TS, Finnerup NB (2010) Spinal-, brainstem- and cerebrally mediated responses at- and below-level of a spinal cord contusion in rats: evaluation of pain-like behavior. Pain 151: 670–679.
6. Baastrup C, Jensen TS, Finnerup NB (2011) Pregabalin attenuates place escape/avoidance behavior in a rat model of spinal cord injury. Brain Res 1370: 129–135.
7. Yezierski RP (2000) Pain following spinal cord injury: pathophysiology and central mechanisms. Prog Brain Res 129: 429–449.
8. Basso DM, Beattie MS, Bresnahan JC (1996) Graded histological and locomotor outcomes after spinal cord contusion using the NYU weight-drop device versus transection. Exp Neurol 139: 244–256.
9. Onifer SM, Rabchevsky AG, Scheff SW (2007) Rat models of traumatic spinal cord injury to assess motor recovery. ILAR J 48: 385–395.
10. Crown ED, Ye Z, Johnson KM, Xu GY, McAdoo DJ, et al. (2006) Increases in the activated forms of ERK 1/2, p38 MAPK, and CREB are correlated with the expression of at-level mechanical allodynia following spinal cord injury. Exp Neurol 199: 397–407.
11. Antri M, Barthe JY, Mouffle C, Orsal D (2005) Long-lasting recovery of locomotor function in chronic spinal rat following chronic combined pharmacological stimulation of serotonergic receptors with 8-OHDPAT and quipazine. Neurosci Lett 384: 162–167.
12. Boulenguez P, Liabeuf S, Bos R, Bras H, Jean-Xavier C, et al. (2010) Down-regulation of the potassium-chloride cotransporter KCC2 contributes to spasticity after spinal cord injury. Nat Med 16: 302–307.
13. Rossignol S, Frigon A (2011) Recovery of locomotion after spinal cord injury: some facts and mechanisms. Annu Rev Neurosci 34: 413–440.
14. Graziano A, Foffani G, Knudsen EB, Shumsky J, Moxon KA (2013) Passive exercise of the hind limbs after complete thoracic transection of the spinal cord promotes cortical reorganization. PLoS ONE 8(1):e54350.
15. Humanes-Valera D, Aguilar J, Foffani G (2013) Reorganization of the intact somatosensoty cortex immediately after spinal cord injury. PLoS ONE 8(7):e69655.
16. Santos-Nogueira E, Redondo Castro E, Mancuso R, Navarro X (2012) Randall-Selitto test: a new approach for the detection of neuropathic pain after spinal cord injury. J Neurotrauma 29: 898–904.

17. Hubscher CH, Kaddumi EG, Johnson RD (2008) Segmental neurtopathic pain does not develop in male rats with complete spinal transections. J Neurotrauma 25: 1241–1245.
18. Densmore VS, Kalous A, Keast JR, Osborne PB (2010) Above-level mechanical hyperalgesia in rats develops after incomplete spinal cord injury but not after cord transection, and is reversed by amitriptyline, morphine and gabapentin. Pain 151: 184–193.
19. Zimmermann M (1983) Ethical guidelines for investigations of experimental pain in conscious animals. Pain 16: 109–110.
20. Chaplan SR, Bach FW, Pogrel JW, Chung JM, Yaksh TL (1994) Quantitative assessment of tactile allodynia in the rat paw. J Neurosci Methods 53: 55–63.
21. Latrémolière A, Mauborgne A, Masson J, Bourgoin S, Kayser V, et al. (2008) Differential implication of proinflammatory cytokine interleukin-6 in the development of cephalic versus extracephalic neuropathic pain in rats. J Neurosci 28: 8489–8501.
22. Hole K, Tjølsen A (1993) The tail-flick and formalin tests in rodents: changes in skin temperature as a confounding factor. Pain 53: 247–254.
23. Kayser V, Elfassi IE, Aubel B, Melfort M, Julius D, et al. (2007) Mechanical, thermal and formalin-induced nociception is differentially altered in 5-HT1A-/-, 5-HT1B-/-, 5-HT2A-/-, 5-HT3A-/- and 5-HTT-/- knock-out male mice. Pain 130: 235–248.
24. Attal N, Jazat F, Kayser V, Guilbaud G (1990) Further evidence for 'pain-related' behaviours in a model of unilateral peripheral mononeuropathy. Pain 41: 235–251.
25. Mestre C, Pelissier T, Fialip J, Wilcox G, Eschalier A (1994) A method to perform direct transcutaneous intrathecal injection in rats. J Pharmacol Toxicol Methods 32: 197–200.
26. Schmittgen TD, Livak KJ (2008) Analyzing real-time PCR data by the comparative C(T) method. Nat Protoc 3: 1101–1108.
27. Fenollosa P, Pallares J, Cervera J, Pelegrin F, Inigo V, et al. (1993) Chronic pain in the spinal cord injured: statistical approach and pharmacological treatment. Paraplegia 31: 722–729.
28. Norrbrink C, Lundeberg T (2009) Tramadol in neuropathic pain after spinal cord injury: a randomized, double-blind, placebo-controlled trial. Clin J Pain 25: 177–184.
29. Tzschentke TM, Christoph T, Kogel B, Schiene K, Hennies HH, et al. (2007) (-)-(1R,2R)-3-(3-dimethylamino-1-ethyl-2-methyl-propyl)-phenol hydrochloride (tapentadol HCl): a novel mu-opioid receptor agonist/norepinephrine reuptake inhibitor with broad-spectrum analgesic properties. J Pharmacol Exp Ther 323: 265–276.
30. Bennett AD, Everhart AW, Hulsebosch CE (2000) Intrathecal administration of an NMDA or a non-NMDA receptor antagonist reduces mechanical but not thermal allodynia in a rodent model of chronic central pain after spinal cord injury. Brain Res 859: 72–82.
31. Gwak YS, Tan HY, Nam TS, Paik KS, Hulsebosch CE, et al. (2006) Activation of spinal GABA receptors attenuates chronic central neuropathic pain after spinal cord injury. J Neurotrauma 23: 1111–1124.
32. Yasuda T, Iwamoto T, Ohara M, Sato S, Kohri H, et al. (1999) The novel analgesic compound OT-700 (5-n-butyl-7-(3,4,5-trimethoxybenzoyl-amino)pyrazolo[1,5-a]pyrimidine) attenuates mechanical nociceptive responses in animal models of acute and peripheral neuropathic hyperalgesia. Jpn J Pharmacol 79: 65–73.
33. Wallin J, Cui JG, Yakhnitsa V, Schechtmann G, Meyerson BA, et al. (2002) Gabapentin and pregabalin suppress tactile allodynia and potentiate spinal cord stimulation in a model of neuropathy. Eur J Pain 6: 261–272.
34. Constandil L, Goich M, Hernàndez A, Bourgeais L, Cazorla M, et al. (2012) Cyclotraxin-B, a new TrkB antagonist, and glial blockade by propentofylline, equally prevent and reverse cold allodynia induced by BDNF or partial infraorbital nerve constriction in mice. J Pain 13: 579–589.
35. Kayser V, Aubel B, Hamon M, Bourgoin S (2002) The antimigraine 5-$HT_{1B/1D}$ receptor agonists, sumatriptan, zolmitriptan and dihydroergotamine, attenuate pain-related behavior in a rat model of trigeminal neuropathic pain. Br J Pharmacol 137: 1287–1297.
36. Kayser V, Bourgoin S, Viguier F, Michot B, Hamon M (2010) Toward deciphering the respective roles of multiple 5-HT receptors in the complex serotonin-mediated control of pain. In: Beaulieu P, Lussier D, Porreca F, Dickenson AH, editors. Pharmacology of pain. Seattle: IASP Press. pp. 185–206.
37. Kayser V, Latrémolière A, Hamon M, Bourgoin S (2011) N-methyl-D-aspartate receptor-mediated modulations of the anti-allodynic effects of 5-$HT_{1B/1D}$ receptor stimulation in a rat model of trigeminal neuropathic pain. Eur J Pain 15: 451–458.
38. Suzuki R, Rahman W, Hunt SP, Dickenson AH (2004) Descending facilitatory control of mechanically evoked responses is enhanced in deep dorsal horn neurons following peripheral nerve injury. Brain Res 1019: 68–76.
39. Vanelderen P, Rouwette T, Kozicz T, Heylen R, Van Zundert J, et al. (2013) Effects of chronic administration of amitriptyline, gabapentin and minocycline on spinal brain-derived neurotrophic factor expression and neuropathic pain behavior in a rat chronic constriction injury model. Reg Anesth Pain Med 38: 124–130.
40. Fellner L, Irschick R, Schanda K, Reindl M, Klimaschewski L, et al. (2013) Toll-like receptor 4 is required for α-synuclein dependent activation of microglia and astroglia. Glia 61: 349–360.
41. Inoue K (2002) Microglial activation by purines and pyrimidines. Glia 40: 156–163.
42. Inoue K (2006) The function of microglia through purinergic receptors: neuropathic pain and cytokine release. Pharmacol Ther 109: 210–226.
43. Singh R, Rohilla RK, Sangwan K, Siwach R, Magu NK, et al. (2011) Bladder management methods and urological complications in spinal cord injury patients. Indian J Orthop 45: 141–147.
44. Ramsey JB, Ramer LM, Inskip JA, Alan N, Ramer MS, et al. (2010) Care of rats with complete high-thoracic spinal cord injury. J Neurotrauma 27: 1709–1722.
45. Lotta S, Scelsi R, Alfonsi E, Saitta A, Nicolotti D, et al. (1991) Morphometric and neurophysiological analysis of skeletal muscle in paraplegic patients with traumatic cord lesion. Paraplegia 29: 247–252.
46. Calancie B, Broton JG, Klose KJ, Traad M, Difini J, et al. (1993) Evidence that alterations in presynaptic inhibition contribute to segmental hypo- and hyperexcitability after spinal cord injury in man. Electroencephalogr Clin Neurophysiol 89: 177–186.
47. Garrison MK, Yates CC, Reese NB, Skinner RD, Garcia-Rill E (2011) Wind-up of stretch reflexes as a measure of spasticity in chronic spinalized rats: The effects of passive exercise and modafinil. Exp Neurol 227: 104–109.
48. Murray KC, Nakae A, Stephens MJ, Rank M, D'Amico J, et al. (2010) Recovery of motoneuron and locomotor function after spinal cord injury depends on constitutive activity in 5-HT_{2C} receptors. Nat Med 16: 694–700.
49. L, Budh CN, Hultling C, Molander C (2004) Neuropathic pain after traumatic spinal cord injury - relations to gender, spinal level, completeness, and age at the time of injury. Spinal Cord 42: 665–673.
50. Hoschouer EL, Basso DM, Jakeman LB (2009) Aberrant sensory responses are dependent on lesion severity after spinal cord contusion injury in mice. Pain 148: 328–342.
51. Jung JI, Kim J, Hong SK, Yoon YW (2008) Long-term follow-up of cutaneous hypersensitivity in rats with a spinal cord contusion. Korean J Physiol Pharmacol 12: 299–306.
52. Hulsebosch CE, Hains BC, Crown ED, Carlton SM (2009) Mechanisms of chronic central neuropathic pain after spinal cord injury. Brain Res Rev 60: 202–213.
53. Finnerup NB, Norrbrink C, Trok K, Piehl F, Johannesen IL, et al. (2014) Phenotypes and predictors of pain following traumatic spinal cord injury: a prospective study. J Pain 15: 40–48.
54. Gao T, Hao JX, Wiesenfeld-Hallin Z, Xu XJ (2013) Quantitative test of responses to thermal stimulation in spinally injured rats using a Peltier thermode: a new approach to study cold allodynia. J Neurosci Methods 212: 317–321.
55. Wang J, Kawamata M, Namiki A (2005) Changes in properties of spinal dorsal horn neurons and their sensitivity to morphine after spinal cord injury in the rat. Anesthesiology 102: 152–164.
56. Millan MJ (2002) Descending control of pain. Prog Neurobiol 66: 355–474.
57. Kim K, Mishina M, Kokubo R, Nakajima T, Morimoto D, et al. (2013) Ketamine for acute neuropathic pain in patients with spinal cord injury. J Clin Neurosci 20: 804–807.
58. Niesters M, Dahan A (2012) Pharmacokinetic and pharmacodynamic considerations for NMDA receptor antagonists in the treatment of chronic neuropathic pain. Exp Opin Drug Metab Toxicol 8: 1409–1417.
59. Rekand T (2010) Clinical assessment and management of spasticity: a review. Acta Neurol Scand Suppl. 190: 62–66.
60. Colpaert FC, Wu WP, Hao JX, Royer I, Sautel F, et al. (2004) High-efficacy 5-HT_{1A} receptor activation causes a curative-like action on allodynia in rats with spinal cord injury. Eur J Pharmacol 497: 29–33.
61. Amaya-Castellanos E, Pineda-Farias JB, Castaneda-Corral G, Vidal-Cantu GC, Murbartian J, et al. (2011) Blockade of 5-HT_7 receptors reduces tactile allodynia in the rat. Pharmacol Biochem Behav 99: 591–597.
62. Aguggia M, Saracco MG, Cavallini M, Bussone G, Cortelli P (2013) Sensitization and pain. Neurol Sci 34 (Suppl 1): S37–40.
63. McCleane GJ, Suzuki R, Dickenson AH (2003) Does a single intravenous injection of the 5-HT_3 receptor antagonist ondansetron have an analgesic effect in neuropathic pain? A double-blinded, placebo-controlled cross-over study. Anesth Analg 97: 1474–1478.
64. Chen Y, Oatway MA, Weaver LC (2009) Blockade of the 5-HT_3 receptor for days causes sustained relief from mechanical allodynia following spinal cord injury. J Neurosci Res 87: 418–424.
65. Tzellos TG, Papazisis G, Amaniti E, Kouvelas D (2008) Efficacy of pregabalin and gabapentin for neuropathic pain in spinal-cord injury: an evidence-based evaluation of the literature. Eur J Clin Pharmacol 64: 851–858.
66. Merighi A, Salio C, Ghirri A, Lossi L, Ferrini F, et al. (2008) BDNF as a pain modulator. Progr Neurobiol 85: 297–317.
67. Trang T, Beggs S, Salter MW (2011) Brain-derived neurotrophic factor from microglia: a molecular substrate for neuropathic pain. Neuron Glia Biol 7: 99–108.
68. Hajebrahimi Z, Mowla SJ, Movahedin M, Tavallaei M (2008) Gene expression alterations of neurotrophins, their receptors and prohormone convertases in a rat model of spinal cord contusion. Neurosci Lett 441: 261–266.
69. Ying ZI, Roy RR, Edgerton VR, Gomez-Pinilla F (2005) Exercise restores levels of neurotrophins and synaptic plasticity following spinal cord injury. Exp Neurol 193: 411–419.
70. Carlton SM, Du J, Tan HY, Nesic O, Hargett GL, et al. (2009) Peripheral and central sensitization in remote spinal cord regions contribute to central neuropathic pain after spinal cord injury. Pain 147: 265–276.
71. Hai T, Hartman MG (2001) The molecular biology and nomenclature of the activating transcription factor/cAMP responsive element binding family of

transcription factors: activating transcription factor proteins and homeostasis. Gene 273: 1–11.
72. Block ML, Zecca L, Hong JS (2007) Microglia-mediated neurotoxicity: uncovering the molecular mechanisms. Nat Rev Neurosci 8: 57–69.
73. Gwak YS, Crown ED, Unabia GC, Hulsebosch CE (2008) Propentofylline attenuates allodynia, glial activation and modulates GABAergic tone after spinal cord injury in the rat. Pain 138: 410–422.
74. Gwak YS, Kang J, Unabia GC, Hulsebosch CE (2012) Spatial and temporal activation of spinal glial cells: role of gliopathy in central neuropathic pain following spinal cord injury in rats. Exp Neurol 234: 362–372.
75. Kim JY, Choi GS, Cho YW, Cho H, Hwang SJ, et al. (2013) Attenuation of spinal cord injury-induced astroglial and microglial activation by repetitive transcranial magnetic stimulation in rats. J Korean Med Sci 28: 295–299.
76. Marcillo A, Frydel B, Bramlett HM, Dietrich WD (2012) A reassessment of P2×7 receptor inhibition as a neuroprotective strategy in rat models of contusion injury. Exp Neurol 233: 687–692.
77. Kigerl KA, Lai W, Rivest S, Hart RP, Satoskar AR, et al. (2007) Toll-like receptor (TLR)-2 and TLR-4 regulate inflammation, gliosis, and myelin sparing after spinal cord injury. J Neurochem 102: 37–50.
78. Marchand F, Tsantoulas C, Singh D, Grist J, Clark AK, et al. (2009) Effects of etanercept and minocycline in a rat model of spinal cord injury. Pain 13: 673–681.
79. Chen K, Uchida K, Nakajima H, Yayama T, Hirai T, et al. (2011) Tumor necrosis factor-α antagonist reduces apoptosis of neurons and oligodendroglia in rat spinal cord injury. Spine 36: 1350–1358.
80. Guptarak J, Wanchoo S, Durham-Lee J, Wu Y, Zivadinovic D, et al. (2013) Inhibition of IL-6 signaling: A novel therapeutic approach to treating spinal cord injury pain. Pain 154: 1115–1128.
81. Genovese T, Esposito E, Mazzon E, Di Paola R, Caminiti R, et al. (2009) Absence of endogenous interleukin-10 enhances secondary inflammatory process after spinal cord compression injury in mice. J Neurochem 108: 1360–1372.
82. Zhou Z, Peng X, Insolera R, Fink DJ, Mata M (2009) IL-10 promotes neuronal survival following spinal cord injury. Exp Neurol 220: 183–190.
83. John GR, Lee SC, Brosnan CF (2003) Cytokines: powerful regulators of glial cell activation. Neuroscientist 9: 10–22.
84. Tian DS, Dong Q, Pan DJ, He Y, Yu ZY, et al. (2007) Attenuation of astrogliosis by suppressing of microglial proliferation with the cell cycle inhibitor olomoucine in rat spinal cord injury model. Brain Res 1154: 206–214.
85. Cronin M, Anderson PN, Cook JE, Green CR, Becker DL (2008) Blocking connexin43 expression reduces inflammation and improves functional recovery after spinal cord injury. Mol Cell Neurosci 39: 152–160.

Local and Systemic Cytokine Expression in Patients with Postherpetic Neuralgia

Nurcan Üçeyler[1]*, Michael Valet[2], Waldemar Kafke[1], Thomas R. Tölle[2], Claudia Sommer[1]

1 Department of Neurology, University of Würzburg, Würzburg, Germany, 2 Department of Neurology, Klinikum rechts der Isar, Technische Universität München, München, Germany

Abstract

Background: Postherpetic neuralgia (PHN) is the painful complication of a varicella zoster virus reactivation. We investigated the systemic and local gene expression of pro- and anti-inflammatory cytokine expression in patients with PHN.

Methods: Thirteen patients with PHN at the torso (Th4-S1) were recruited. Skin punch biopsies were obtained from the painful and the contralateral painless body area for intraepidermal nerve fiber density (IENFD) and cytokine profiling. Additionally, blood was withdrawn for systemic cytokine expression and compared to blood values of healthy controls. We analyzed the gene expression of selected pro- and anti-inflammatory cytokines (tumor necrosis factor-alpha [TNF] and interleukins [IL]-1β, IL-2, and IL-8).

Results: IENFD was lower in affected skin compared to unaffected skin ($p<0.05$), while local gene expression of pro- and anti-inflammatory cytokines did not differ except for two patients who had 7fold higher IL-6 and 10fold higher IL-10 gene expression in the affected skin compared to the contralateral unaffected skin sample. Also, the systemic expression of cytokines in patients with PHN and in healthy controls was similar.

Conclusion: While the systemic and local expression of the investigated pro- and anti-inflammatory cytokines was not different from controls, this may have been influenced by study limitations like the low number of patients and different disease durations. Furthermore, other cytokines or pain mediators need to be considered.

Editor: Thiago Mattar Cunha, University of Sao Paulo, Brazil

Funding: The study was supported by Bundesministerium für Bildung und Forschung (BMBF), Deutscher Forschungsverbund Neuropathischer Schmerz (DFNS). The publication of the authors' study was funded by the German Research Foundation (DFG) and the University of Würzburg in the funding programme Open Access Publishing. The funders had no role in study design, data collection and analysis, decision to publish, or preparation of the manuscript.

Competing Interests: The authors have declared that no competing interests exist.

* Email: ueceyler_n@ukw.de

Introduction

Postherpetic neuralgia (PHN) is the painful complication of a varizella zoster virus reactivation. Up to 30% of patients with acute herpes zoster develop PHN resulting in persistent pain that is often resistant to analgesic treatment [1,2]. The pathophysiology of pain in PHN is incompletely understood. High pain intensity during acute herpes zoster infection is one risk factor [3] and the question is why. One potential mechanism for the development of this localized pain syndrome with frequently associated severe allodynia and sometimes also itch [4] is the influence of algesic mediators such as pro-inflammatory cytokines, which might sensitize nociceptors locally.

Cytokines are pleiotropic small proteins that are key players in the induction and maintenance of neuropathic pain [5]. In several neuropathic pain conditions such as painful neuropathies, complex regional pain syndrome or small fiber neuropathy, an imbalance of systemic or local cytokine profiles has been reported e.g. for pro- and anti-inflammatory interleukins [6–9]. Although it is unclear if alterations in cytokine profiles are the cause or the consequence of neuropathic pain in these disorders, data from animal experiments give unequivocal evidence for the importance of cytokine homoeostasis as the basis for physiological pain perception [10]. In PHN, so far, only few and conflicting data on cytokine profiles are available. One study showed increased interleukin (IL)-8 concentrations in the cerebrospinal fluid of PHN patients [11], while in another study CSF levels of IL-8, IL-1α, IL-1β, IL-10, and tumor necrosis factor-alpha (TNF) were not different between patients with PHN and healthy controls [12]. In turn, long-term anti-TNF treatment (e.g. in patients with rheumatoid arthritis) while increasing the overall risk of herpes zoster, seems to reduce the incidence of PHN [13,14].

Here we investigated if pain in PHN is associated with alterations in systemic and local cytokine profiles. We hypothesized that patients with PHN have a local and systemic pro-inflammatory cytokine profile compared to healthy controls and compared to unaffected skin.

Methods

Patients and healthy controls

Between 2007 and 2010, 13 patients with PHN localized in the dermatomes Th4 to S1 of the torso were recruited at the Departments of Neurology of the Universities of Würzburg and Munich, Germany. The group consisted of five men and eight women with a median age of 68 years (range 36-88). All patients were seen and examined by a neurologist and the diagnosis was confirmed. Routine examination included standardized assessment of pain and in addition of depressive symptoms that were analyzed with the "Allgemeine Depressionsskala" (ADS, German version of the Centre for Epidemiologic Studies Depression Scale) [15]. For blood cytokine analysis a control group of eleven healthy volunteers without infectious disease, history of PHN, or pain at the time point of blood withdrawal was recruited. The control group consisted of three men and eight women with a median age of 61 years (range 37–73). Due to the diversity of the lesion site in PHN patients we did not perform respective skin biopsies in healthy controls. Subjects were excluded in case of current infectious diseases, heavy physical activity or alcohol consumption the day before. Our study was approved by the Würzburg and Munich Medical School Ethics Committees. Study participants were included after written informed consent was obtained.

Quantitative sensory testing

All patients underwent quantitative sensory testing (QST) according to the standardized protocol of the DFNS ("Deutscher Forschungsverbund Neuropathischer Schmerz", German Research Network of Neuropathic Pain) [16]. Thermal and mechanical detection and pain thresholds were determined in the affected painful area in comparison to a contralateral unaffected area. In patients with the unaffected area in the back we also compared individual QST results with published normative values [17]. Parameters included cold and warm detection thresholds (CDT, WDT), thermal sensory limen (TSL), cold and heat pain thresholds (CPT, HPT), mechanical detection threshold (MDT), mechanical pain threshold (MPT), mechanical pain sensitivity (MPS), vibration detection threshold (VDT) and pressure pain threshold (PPT). Based on the log transformed raw values for each item a z-score sensory profile was calculated. The presence of dynamic mechanical allodynia was determined by gentile brush of the respective area.

Blood withdrawal and RNA extraction

Five ml of venous whole blood was collected between 8 and 9 a.m. in PAXgene Blood RNA Tubes (PreAnalytics, BD, Hombrechtikon, Switzerland) after over-night fasting from all study participants. Blood samples were kept at room temperature for two hours before storage at −80°C. For RNA extraction the PAXgene Blood RNA MDx Kit (BD, Hombrechtikon, Switzerland) was used.

Skin punch biopsy

A 5-mm skin punch biopsy (Stiefel GmbH, Offenbach, Germany) was taken in local anesthesia from the affected painful and a corresponding contralateral unaffected site of patients with PHN as previously described [9]. Each skin specimen was divided into two pieces: one piece was incubated in 4% paraformaldehyde (PFA) for two hours at +4°C and was further processed for protein gene product 9.5 (PGP 9.5) staining; one piece was put in RNAlater RNA Stabilization Reagent (Qiagen, Hilden, Germany) and stored at -80°C before RNA extraction.

RNA extraction from skin samples

After thawing, the skin samples were homogenized in 1 ml TRIzol reagent (Invitrogen, Karlsruhe, Germany) and homogenized with an Ultraturrax homogenizer (Polytron PT 1600E, Kinematica, Luzern, Switzerland). After adding 200 µl of chloroform the samples were incubated at 25°C for 3 min and after spin down (12.000 g×15 min×4°C) the supernatant was mixed with 500 µl isopropanole. After incubation (25°C for 10 min) and another spin down (12.000 g×10 min×4°C) the pellet was washed with ethanol 75%. After another centrifugation step (7500 g×5 min×4°C) the samples were air-dried on ice for 5 min and the pellet was dissolved in water treated with diethylpyrocarbonate. Then the samples were incubated in a water bath at 55°C for 10 min.

Reverse transcription PCR

For reverse transcription of 750 ng of the extracted RNA, TaqMan Reverse Transcription Reagents (Applied Biosystems, Darmstadt, Germany) were used. The reaction was carried out at a total volume of 100 µl. Five µl of random hexameres were added to 750 ng RNA and the mixture was filled up with RNase free water to an end volume of 37.8 µl. After heat denaturation (85°C, 3 min), 2 µl of Oligo-dt, 10 µl 10× PCR-buffer, 6.25 µl Multiscribe reverse transcriptase, 2 µl RNase inhibitor, 22 µl $MgCl^2$, and 20 µl dNTPs were added. The PCR cycler conditions were as follows: annealing at 25°C for 10 min, reverse transcription at 48°C for 60 min and enzyme inactivation at 95°C for 5 min.

Quantitative real-time PCR

Five µl of cDNA were used for quantitative real-time PCR (qRT-PCR), which was performed in the GeneAmp 7700 sequence detection system (Applied Biosystems, Darmstadt, Germany) capable of fluorescence using TaqMan Universal Master Mix (Applied Biosystems, Darmstadt, Germany). Gene specific oligonucleotide primers and probes for human in IL-1β, IL-6, IL-8, tumor necrosis factor-alpha (TNF), and IL-10 as well as the endogenous control 18sRNA were obtained as TaqMan Assays (Applied Biosystems, Darmstadt, Germany; see Table 1 for Assay-ID). The reaction contained 12.5 µl TaqMan Master Mix and 1.25 µl of the specific primer in an end volume of 25 µl. The cycler conditions were as follows: incubation for 2 min at 50°C followed by another incubation step at 95°C for 10 min, afterwards 45 cycles with 15 sec at 95°C and 1 min at 60°C. In order to guarantee primer specificity and to exclude genomic contamination, negative controls without cDNA template were run on each qRT-PCR well plate. All samples were measured as triplicates, while the 18s-values were measured as duplicates.

For gene expression analysis in blood samples each qRT-PCR reaction plate contained a calibrator sample, which was the blood sample of the control person whose threshold cyclus (Ct)-values (i.e. qRT-PCR cyclus at which a significant signal was detected) were next to the calculated mean of all control blood samples specific for each primer. The evaluation of the obtained data was performed with the comparative ΔΔCt-method and data of PHN patients were compared with healthy controls. For gene expression analysis in skin samples the gene expression in the affected skin sample of the individual patients were compared with the gene expression in the respective unaffected skin sample. Again the ΔΔCt-method was used.

Table 1. Characteristics of the patient group.

#	Age [yrs]	Gender	Time since pain onset [yrs]	Affected body area	IEND affected area [fibers/mm]	IENFD unaffected contralateral area [fibers/mm]	Allodynia	Current pain intensity [NRS]	ADS score
1	69	F	15	Right thoracic Th5	2	28	no	8	13
2	79	M	4	Left paravertebral Th6	19	17	no	3	5
3	64	F	20	Right lumbosacral L5	0	6	no	5	37
4	36	M	3	Left paravertebral Th4	5	10	no	7	refused
5	62	F	4	Left paravertebral Th4	5	8	no	4	9
6	75	M	7	Left axillary Th4	1	6	yes	3	19
7	59	F	5	Left subaxillary Th4	5	5	yes	8	31
8	53	F	1	Left parasacral	7	15	yes	5	39
9	88	M	0.5	Left ventral Th5	0	8	no	8	refused
10	72	F	1	Left ventral Th4	2	19	yes	8	7
11	68	F	0,2	Left dorsal Th12	18	29	yes	7	12
12	70	F	0.1	Left thoracic Th12	21	26	yes	4	17
13	47	M	0.1	Right back L5	16	24	no	8	24

Abbreviations:
ADS: "Allgemeine Depressionsskala" (German version of the Centre for Epidemiologic Studies Depression Scale); F: female; M: male; IENFD: intraepidermal nerve fiber density; NRS: numeric rating scale from zero to ten (zero: no pain; ten: worst pain imaginable); yrs: years.

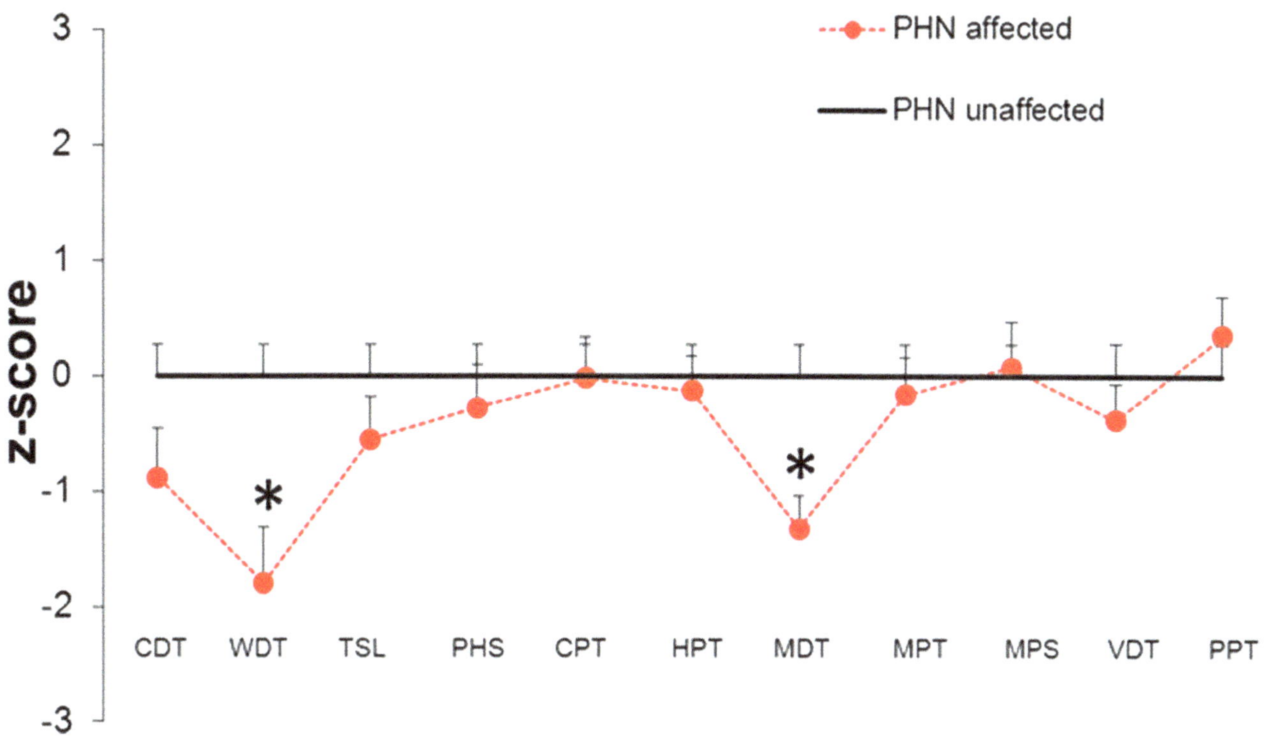

Figure 1. Sensory profile of patients with postherpetic neuralgia (PHN) assessed with quantitative sensory testing (QST), affected skin is compared to unaffected skin (zero line). In affected skin, patients showed elevated detection thresholds for warm and for tactile stimuli (*$p<0.05$). Abbreviations: CDT: cold detection threshold; CPT: cold pain threshold; HPT: warm pain threshold; MDT: mechanical detection threshold; MPS: mechanical pain sensitivity; MPT: mechanical pain threshold; PHS: paradoxical heat sensation; PPT: pressure pain threshold; TSL: thermal sensory limen; VDT: vibration detection threshold; WDT: warm detection threshold.

PGP 9.5 immunofluorescence for intraepidermal nerve fiber density

After fixation in 4% PFA (pH 7.4) for two hours at 4°C, skin samples were washed in 0.1 M phosphate buffer and transferred to 10% sucrose over-night. Afterwards tissue was embedded in Tissue Tek, frozen in 2-methylbutane cooled in liquid nitrogen and was stored at −80°C before further processing. Fifty-µm sections were cut with a microtome and were stained with rabbit polyclonal antibodies to human PGP 9.5 (Ultraclone, UK, 1:800; primary antibody) and goat anti-rabbit IgG labeled with cyanine 3.18 fluorescent probe (Amersham, USA, 1:100; Cy3, secondary antibody). A microscope (Axiophot 2, Zeiss, Jena, Germany) with a CCD camera (Visitron Systems, Tuchheim, Germany) and SPOT advanced software (Windows Version 4.5) were used for visualization. Nerve fibers were counted using a 40× objective according to standard criteria [18]. The average intraepidermal nerve fiber density (IENFD) per mm of epidermal length was calculated following international standards [19].

Assessment of inflammatory cells in the skin

We used 10 µm skin sections to visualize T-cells (CD-3, 1:200, Abcam, Germany), macrophages (CD-68, 1:3000, Abcam, Germany), and Langerhans cells (CD-1a, 1:500, Beckman Coulter, Krefeld, Germany). Stains were performed using a standard immunohistochemistry protocol (ABC kit, Vector, Germany) with diaminobenzidine as chromogen and hemalaun as a counterstain. Cells were assessed semiquantitatively by an investigator blinded to the diagnosis with regard to cell density: 0 = no cells; 1 = single cells; 2 = several cells; 3 = dense cell infiltrates.

Statistical analysis

Data were analyzed using IBM SPSS software (Version 21, Ehningen, Germany). qRT-PCR data did not display normal distribution in the Shapiro-Wilk-test, thus we used the Mann-Whitney-U-test for comparison of independent groups; the QST data were normally distributed and the t-test for independent groups was applied. We used the Levene test to check for equality in variance. Statistical significance was assumed at $p<0.05$.

Results

Characteristics of study population

Table 1 gives baseline data of the PHN patients. Seven patients were on analgesic medication with pregabalin (n = 5), amitriptyline, carbamazepine, duloxetine, fentanyl, flupirtine, lidocaine, and tilidine (n = 1 each) as monotherapy or in different combinations. The median duration of pain was four years (four months to 20 years) and the median current pain intensity on a numeric rating scale (0 = no pain, 10 = worst pain imaginable) was 7 (3–8). No correlation was found between depressive symptoms and pain.

Patients with PHN have hypoesthesia for warm and touch

QST showed that warm detection ($p<0.05$) and detection of mechanical stimulation ($p<0.05$) were impaired in the affected skin area compared the unaffected side in patients with PHN (Fig. 1). Dynamic mechanical allodynia was present in 6/13 (46%) patients in the affected area. QST parameters did not correlate with pain. Also, QST results of the unaffected contralateral area at

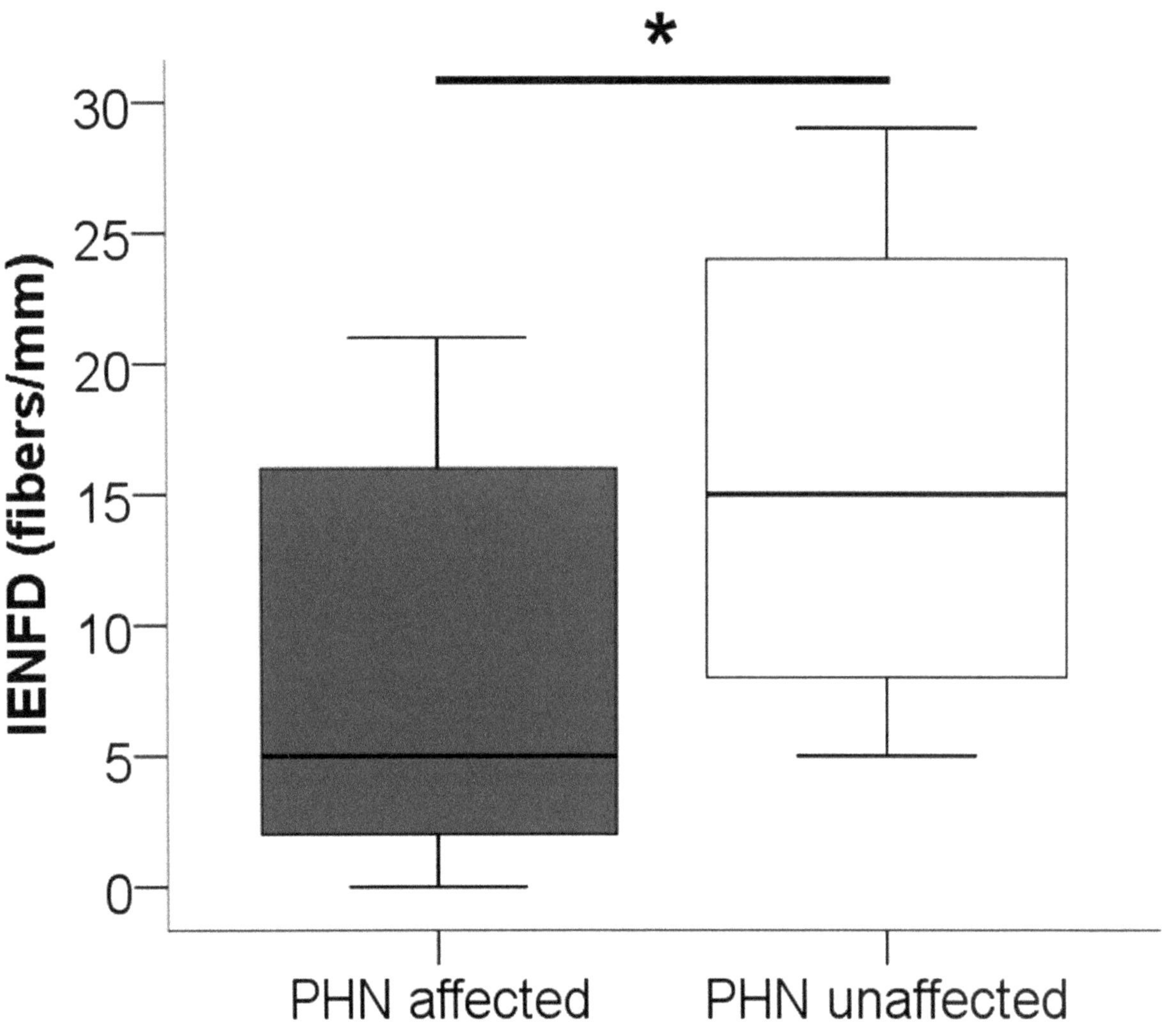

Figure 2. Boxplots show the intraepidermal nerve fiber density (IENFD) in affected versus unaffected skin of patients with postherpetic neuralgia (PHN). In affected skin IENFD is lower than in corresponding (contralateral) unaffected skin (*$p<0.05$). The horizontal black line in the box marks the median value.

the back (n = 5 patients, see Table 1) were not different from published normative values.

Cutaneous innervation is reduced in affected skin

In 11/13 (85%) patients with PHN the IENFD was lower in skin of the affected site compared to the unaffected contralateral side ($p<0.05$; Fig. 2). The median IENFD in affected skin was 5 fibers/mm (0–21 fibers/mm) and in unaffected skin 15 fibers/mm (5–29 fibers/mm). IENFD did not correlate with pain.

No inflammatory infiltrates are present in affected an unaffected skin

The semiquantitative assessment of dermal T-cells and macrophages and epidermal Langerhans cells did not reveal cellular infiltrates in the affected and unaffected skin (data not shown).

Systemic cytokine gene expression does not differ from controls

Systemic gene expression of the pro- and anti-inflammatory cytokines IL-1β, IL-6, IL-8, TNF, and IL-10 did not differ between patients with PHN and healthy controls (Fig. 3). Also, no difference was found when comparing patients with and without current analgesic medication.

Local cytokine gene expression does not differ between affected and unaffected sides

Local gene expression of the investigated markers was similar in affected and unaffected skin of patients with PHN (Fig. 4) for all investigated cytokines irrespective of current analgesic treatment. Also, patients with and without allodynia did not differ in cytokine expression patterns. In two patients IL-6 and IL-10 gene expression was very high in the affected skin (7fold higher IL-6 expression and 10fold higher IL-10 expression compared to unaffected skin area; patients #5 and #9 in Table 2).

Discussion

PHN is associated with severe localized pain of incompletely understood pathophysiology. We confirm the reduction of IENFD in affected skin compared to unaffected skin [20,21], however, in contrast to our hypothesis, we did not observe a pro-inflammatory cytokine profile in PHN patients. No changes were found in

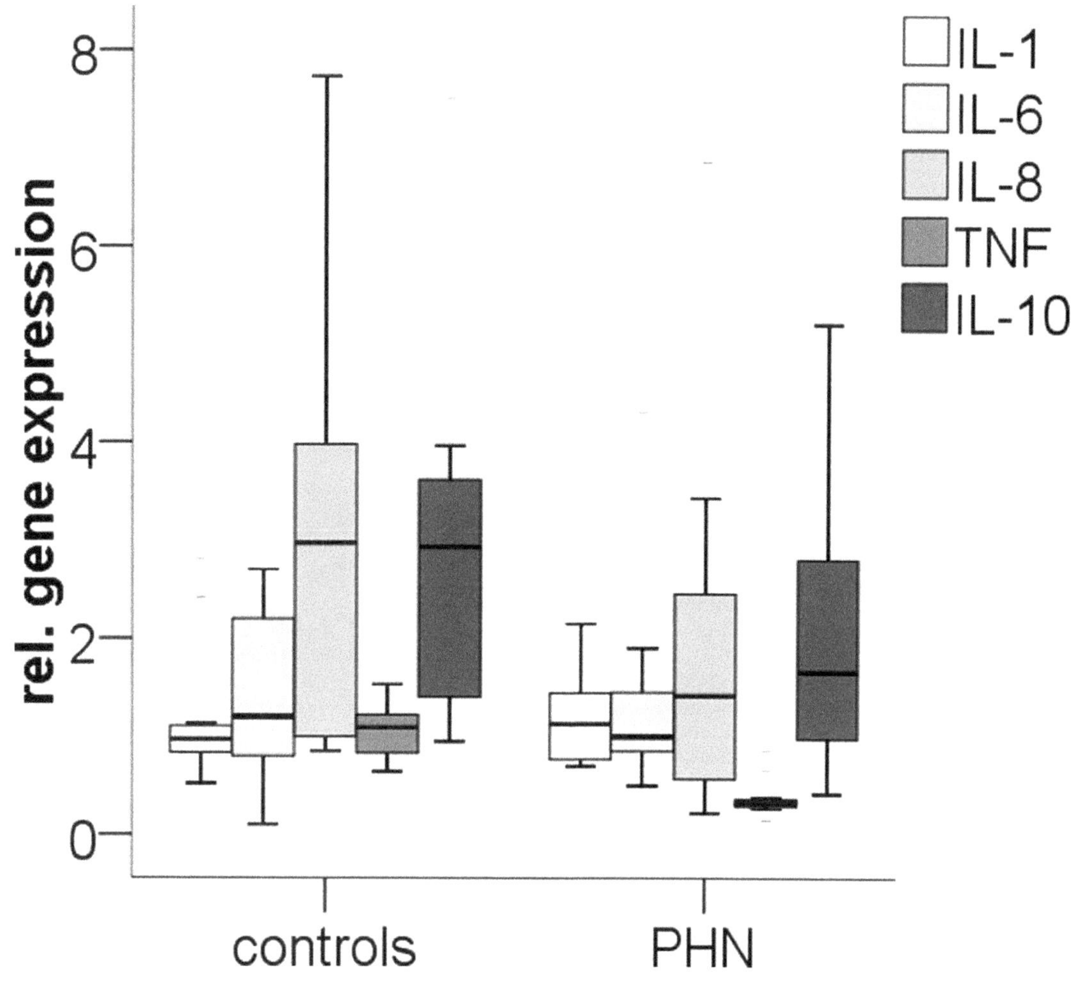

Figure 3. Boxplots illustrate the systemic (blood) relative gene expression of the pro- and anti-inflammatory cytokines interleukin-1β (IL-1β), IL-6, IL-8, tumor necrosis factor-alpha (TNF), and IL-10 comparing patients with postherpetic neuralgia (PHN) and healthy controls. No intergroup difference was found.

systemic and local cytokine gene expression profiles of patients with PHN compared to healthy controls and between affected and unaffected skin.

Cytokine measurements in PHN

Cytokines play a crucial role in neuropathic pain induction and maintenance [5,10]. This has been shown in a large number of different animal models and also in several human neuropathic pain disorders. Especially in localized pain states such as small fiber neuropathy and complex regional pain syndrome elevated cytokine levels have been reported [9,22]. A local increase in algesic pro-inflammatory cytokines was therefore assumed in PHN, however, it had not been studied so far.

In patients both with acute herpes zoster and PHN, cytokine levels have been investigated in the cerebrospinal fluid (CSF) [11,12] and in the blood [23] giving conflicting results. In the study by Kotani et al. control subjects had an IL-8 concentration of 18 μg/L (7 to 24 μg/L) in the CSF compared to 81 μg/L (57 to 380 μg/L) in patients with herpes zoster during rash and after rash healing (44 μg/L, 28 to 101 μg/L). An initially increased IL-8 CSF level was found to be an independent predictor of PHN [11]. In another study IL-1α, IL-1β, IL-10, TNF, MIP-1a, and fractalkine levels were below the detection limit in the majority of the investigated 25 PHN patients similar to controls and IL-8 levels were not different between groups [12]. This discrepancy might be explained by the fact that in the study by Rijsdijk et al. a PHN cohort had been examined that had a median pain duration of 24 months, thus IL-8 levels may have normalized in the meantime. Similarly, our patients had a median duration of pain of four years, and we cannot preclude that there might have been differences in cytokine expression earlier on. However, cytokine expression in our cohort did not correlate with disease duration (data not shown).

Zhu et al. showed that in serum samples of patients who already suffered from pain in the acute phase of herpes zoster IL-1β, IL-6, IL-8, TNF, and IL-10 protein levels were higher compared to healthy controls. In particular, IL-6 protein levels were higher in ten of the investigated 49 patients who later developed PHN and positively correlated with pain severity [23]. The observational period of this study was six months.

The assumption that changes in cytokine expression levels may be of pathophysiological importance in PHN induction and maintenance is supported by observations in patients that received anti-cytokine medication. In a retrospective analysis of patients with rheumatoid arthritis on anti-TNF treatment the number of PHN after herpes zoster was remarkably lower (only two cases out

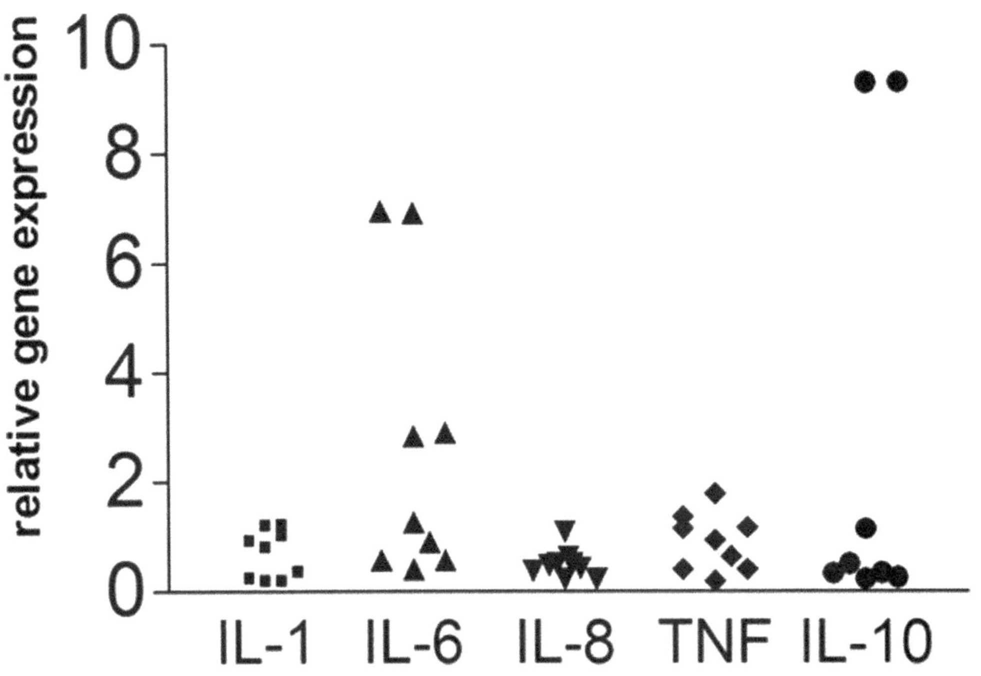

Figure 4. Scatter plots illustrate the local (skin) relative gene expression of the pro-inflammatory cytokines interleukin-1β (IL-1β), IL-6, IL-9, tumor necrosis factor-alpha (TNF) and the anti-inflammatory cytokine IL-10 in affected skin of patients with postherpetic neuralgia (PHN) compared to unaffected (contralateral) skin that is calibrated to a relative gene expression of 1.

of 206) compared to data of the general population [13]. In contrast, the development of severe PHN was reported after inadvertent infliximab administration [24]. In a prospective study assessing the risk of herpes zoster in more than 5000 patients with rheumatoid arthritis treated with anti-TNF drugs, 86 episodes of herpes zoster were recorded in 82 patients; in two of these patients PHN occurred [14].

In another study Zak-Prelich assessed serum cytokine levels and different subtypes of skin lymphocytes in patients with herpes zoster who did and did not develop PHN [25]. Interestingly, a reduced number of cellular infiltrates was found at the lesion sites of herpes zoster patients that developed PHN compared to those who did no without association with systemic cytokine levels. The authors suggested that an impaired immune response upon zoster infection resulted in an impaired containment of infection and more damage of the dermatome as the basis for neuralgia. Here, we did not find infiltrates of T-cells and macrophages in affected skin of PHN patients compared to unaffected skin, which may be due to the different duration of disease in our study until biopsy, while in the study by Zak-Prelich et al. patients were seen at standardized time points (within the first ten days of disease and one week later).

Table 2. Primers and Assay-IDs of the TaqMan assays used.

Primer	Assay-ID
IL-1β	Hs00174097_m1
IL-6	Hs00174131_m1
IL-8	Hs00174103_m1
TNF	Hs00174128_m1
IL-10	Hs00174086_m1

Abbreviations:
IL: interleukin; TNF: tumor necrosis factor-alpha.

Treatment of PHN

Since part of the pathology in PHN has been assumed to be located in the skin itself, also surgical excision of the lesioned skin has been tried. However, this approach did not lead to sustained pain relief [26], which indicates that the assumed pathology might be located upstream the pain pathway such as in dorsal root ganglia neurons. Interestingly, a recent case report described the analgesic effect of local laser therapy of the skin over a period of 13 months in a 73 year old women who had been suffering from PHN for 15 years [27]. The author suggested that the reducing effect of laser on local cytokine expression might be the underlying mechanism of this observation, however, cytokine levels were not investigated. In another case report the analgesic effect of anti-IL-2 that lasted throughout the three years of the follow-up period was described in a patient with PHN [28], but again cytokine levels were not measured before and after treatment.

Affected skin is denervated, unaffected skin is spared

Histological assessment of skin samples also revealed denervation of affected skin compared to unaffected contralateral skin in patients with PHN. This finding is in accordance with pervious findings. Petersen et al. reported a 40% reduction in painful skin compared to painless skin [21]. Similar results were found in the study of Buonocore et al. [20]. In accordance with these studies we also did not find a correlation between IENFD and the presence or absence of allodynia. As outlined in Table 1, IENFD of patients with and without allodynia ranged from normal to complete denervation. Also, no correlation was found between IENFD and patients' current pain intensity. Further studies are needed to decipher the underlying mechanisms that may range from hyperexcitable remaining nerve fibers causing allodyina while IENFD is normal, to hyperactive dorsal root ganglion neurons independent of peripheral nerve fiber density.

Limitations

The major limitation of our study is the relatively low number of patients and controls. Although we were recruiting at two centers, only 13 patients with PHN were seen during the study period of three years. This may be due to the fact that in the majority of cases patients with PHN are not hospitalized but treated as outpatients. Our patient group was inhomogeneous with regard to disease duration, which may have influenced our results such that we missed early changes in cytokine gene expression. We cannot exclude influence of current analgesic medication on the study results since the study cohort was small and those patients on analgesic medication used drugs from different pharmaceutical groups. We focused on cytokines as major algesic mediators, and due to limitations in bio-samples only a limited number of targets could be investigated. Also, no protein measurements were possible. Besides cytokines the assessment of further algesic mediators (e.g. chemokines, opioid receptors, neurotrophic factors) would have been desirable.

Acknowledgments

We thank H. Klüpfel, S. Mildner, and K. Stahl for expert technical assistance.

Author Contributions

Conceived and designed the experiments: NÜ TT CS. Performed the experiments: NÜ MV WK TT CS. Analyzed the data: NÜ MV WK TT CS. Contributed reagents/materials/analysis tools: NÜ MV WK TT CS. Contributed to the writing of the manuscript: NÜ MV WK TT CS.

References

1. Cohen JI (2013) Clinical practice: Herpes zoster. N Engl J Med 369: 255–263.
2. Dworkin RH, Gnann JW Jr, Oaklander AL, Raja SN, Schmader KE, et al. (2008) Diagnosis and assessment of pain associated with herpes zoster and postherpetic neuralgia. J Pain 9: S37–44.
3. Thyregod HG, Rowbotham MC, Peters M, Possehn J, Berro M, et al. (2007) Natural history of pain following herpes zoster. Pain 128: 148–156.
4. Oaklander AL (2008) Mechanisms of pain and itch caused by herpes zoster (shingles). J Pain 9: S10–18.
5. Üçeyler N, Schäfers M, Sommer C (2009) Mode of action of cytokines on nociceptive neurons. Exp Brain Res 196: 67–78.
6. Üçeyler N, Eberle T, Rolke R, Birklein F, Sommer C (2007) Differential expression patterns of cytokines in complex regional pain syndrome. Pain 132: 195–205.
7. Üçeyler N, Rogausch JP, Toyka KV, Sommer C (2007) Differential expression of cytokines in painful and painless neuropathies. Neurology 69: 42–49.
8. Alexander GM, Peterlin BL, Perreault MJ, Grothusen JR, Schwartzman RJ (2012) Changes in plasma cytokines and their soluble receptors in complex regional pain syndrome. J Pain 13: 10–20.
9. Üçeyler N, Kafke W, Riediger N, He L, Necula G, et al. (2010) Elevated proinflammatory cytokine expression in affected skin in small fiber neuropathy. Neurology 74: 1806–1813.
10. Austin PJ, Moalem-Taylor G (2010) The neuro-immune balance in neuropathic pain: involvement of inflammatory immune cells, immune-like glial cells and cytokines. J Neuroimmunol 229: 26–50.
11. Kotani N, Kudo R, Sakurai Y, Sawamura D, Sessler DI, et al. (2004) Cerebrospinal fluid interleukin 8 concentrations and the subsequent development of postherpetic neuralgia. Am J Med 116: 318–324.
12. Rijsdijk M, van Wijck AJ, Meulenhoff PC, Kavelaars A, van der Tweel I, et al. (2013) No beneficial effect of intrathecal methylprednisolone acetate in postherpetic neuralgia patients. Eur J Pain 17: 714–723.
13. Javed S, Kamili QU, Mendoza N, Tyring SK (2011) Possible association of lower rate of postherpetic neuralgia in patients on anti-tumor necrosis factor-alpha. J Med Virol 83: 2051–2055.
14. Strangfeld A, Listing J, Herzer P, Liebhaber A, Rockwitz K, et al. (2009) Risk of herpes zoster in patients with rheumatoid arthritis treated with anti-TNF-alpha agents. JAMA 301: 737–744.
15. Radloff LS (1977) The CES-D: a self-report symptom scale to detect depression in the general population. Appl Psychol Meas 3: 385–401.
16. Rolke R, Baron R, Maier C, Tölle TR, Treede RD, et al. (2006) Quantitative sensory testing in the German Research Network on Neuropathic Pain (DFNS): standardized protocol and reference values. Pain 123: 231–243.
17. Pfau DB, Krumova EK, Treede RD, Baron R, Toelle T, et al. (2014) Quantitative sensory testing in the German Research Network on Neuropathic Pain (DFNS): reference data for the trunk and application in patients with chronic postherpetic neuralgia. Pain 155: 1002–1015.
18. Kennedy WR, Wendelschafer-Crabb G, Polydefkis M, McArthur JC (2005) Pathology and quantitation of cutaneous nerves. In: Dyck PJ, Thomas PK, editors. Peripheral Neuropathy. Philadelphia: Elsevier Saunders. pp. 869–896.
19. Lauria G, Cornblath DR, Johansson O, McArthur JC, Mellgren SI, et al. (2005) EFNS guidelines on the use of skin biopsy in the diagnosis of peripheral neuropathy. Eur J Neurol 12: 747–758.
20. Buonocore M, Gatti AM, Amato G, Aloisi AM, Bonezzi C (2012) Allodynic skin in post-herpetic neuralgia: histological correlates. J Cell Physiol 227: 934–938.
21. Petersen KL, Rice FL, Farhadi M, Reda H, Rowbotham MC (2010) Natural history of cutaneous innervation following herpes zoster. Pain 150: 75–82.
22. Lenz M, Üçeyler N, Frettloh J, Hoffken O, Krumova EK, et al. (2013) Local cytokine changes in complex regional pain syndrome type I (CRPS I) resolve after 6 months. Pain 154: 2142–2149.
23. Zhu SM, Liu YM, An ED, Chen QL (2009) Influence of systemic immune and cytokine responses during the acute phase of zoster on the development of postherpetic neuralgia. J Zhejiang Univ Sci B 10: 625–630.
24. Failla V, Castronovo C, Meex C, Nikkels AF (2011) Protracted herpes zoster and severe postherpetic neuralgia after inadvertant infliximab administration. Eur J Dermatol 21: 782–783.
25. Zak-Prelich M, McKenzie RC, Sysa-Jedrzejowska A, Norval M (2003) Local immune responses and systemic cytokine responses in zoster: relationship to the development of postherpetic neuralgia. Clin Exp Immunol 131: 318–323.
26. Petersen KL, Rowbotham MC (2007) Relief of post-herpetic neuralgia by surgical removal of painful skin: 5 years later. Pain 131: 214–218.
27. Knapp DJ (2013) Postherpetic neuralgia: case study of class 4 laser therapy intervention. Clin J Pain 29: e6–9.
28. Rotty J, Heinzerling L, Schurmann D, Suttorp N (2006) Interleukin-2: a potential treatment option for postherpetic neuralgia? Clin Infect Dis 43: e109–110.

18

Subtle Alterations in Brain Anatomy May Change an Individual's Personality in Chronic Pain

Sylvia M. Gustin[1]*, Jamie G. McKay[2], Esben T. Petersen[3], Chris C. Peck[4], Greg M. Murray[4], Luke A. Henderson[2]

1 Neuroscience Research Australia, Randwick, NSW, Australia, **2** Department of Anatomy and Histology, University of Sydney, Sydney, NSW, Australia, **3** Departments of Radiology and Radiotherapy, University Medical Center Utrecht, Utrecht, The Netherlands, **4** Faculty of Dentistry, University of Sydney, Sydney, NSW, Australia

Abstract

It is well established that gross prefrontal cortex damage can affect an individual's personality. It is also possible that subtle prefrontal cortex changes associated with conditions such as chronic pain, and not detectable until recent advances in human brain imaging, may also result in subtle changes in an individual's personality. In an animal model of chronic neuropathic pain, subtle prefrontal cortex changes including altered basal dendritic length, resulted in altered decision making ability. Using multiple magnetic resonance imaging techniques, we found in humans, although gray matter volume and on-going activity were unaltered, chronic neuropathic pain was associated with reduced free and bound proton movement, indicators of subtle anatomical changes, in the medial prefrontal cortex, anterior cingulate cortex and mediodorsal thalamus. Furthermore, proton spectroscopy revealed an increase in neural integrity in the medial prefrontal cortex in neuropathic pain patients, the degree of which was significantly correlated to the personality temperament of novelty seeking. These data reveal that even subtle changes in prefrontal cortex anatomy may result in a significant change in an individual's personality.

Editor: Theodore J. Price, University of Texas at Dallas, United States of America

Funding: This research was supported by the National Health and Medical Research Council of Australia, the Australian Dental Research Foundation, Inc. and the Early Career Researchers/New Staff grant scheme of the University of Sydney. The funders had no role in study design, data collection and analysis, decision to publish, or preparation of the manuscript.

Competing Interests: The authors have declared that no competing interests exist.

* Email: sylvia.gustin@gmail.com

Introduction

It is well established that gross prefrontal cortex damage can alter an individual's personality. Less recognized is the possibility that in individuals with conditions such as chronic pain, subtle changes in prefrontal cortex anatomy associated with the condition, may also result in subtle changes in an individual's personality. The lack of recognition of a connection between personality and brain anatomy, likely stems from the fact that until recently, it was almost impossible to assess subtle changes in brain anatomy in living humans. The recent use of more sensitive brain imaging techniques has revealed that chronic pain is associated with subtle anatomical alterations in the thalamus, insular and cingulate cortices [1,2,3]. It is also evident that chronic pain is associated with subtle, less well known, cognitive changes. For example, subjects with chronic pain display impaired emotional-based decision making [4,5], that is, they have decreased ability to think clearly and make advantageous decisions. In addition, it has recently been reported that chronic pain subjects display altered personality temperaments such as increased harm avoidance, i.e. excessive worrying, and low novelty seeking, i.e. reduced appetite for new experiences and reduced impulsive decision making [6].

It has been proposed that cognitive changes associated with chronic pain may result from alterations in activity within cortical areas such as the prefrontal cortex [7,8,9,10]. In a recent animal investigation, Metz and colleagues [11] found that in the spared nerve injury model of neuropathic pain, basal dendrites of pyramidal neurons within the mPFC were longer and had more branches than in sham-operated rodents. In addition, pain was associated with increased spine density and increased contribution of the NMDA component of synaptic currents. If similar changes in mPFC anatomy occur in humans, they may underlie at least in part the altered temperament changes such as reduced novelty seeking and increased harm avoidance that occur in human subjects with chronic pain.

The study aims to explore anatomical and biochemical changes within the mPFC and related brain regions in individuals with chronic pain and to determine if any changes are associated with an individual's personality. Diffusion tensor imaging (DTI) and T2-relaxometry was used to detect subtle changes that indicate alterations in the physical organization and myelination and/or development of axons and dendrites [12,13]. Additionally, spectroscopy can reveal biochemical changes, e.g. N-acetyl aspartate (NAA), an indicator of neuronal viability [14]. We hypothesize that in chronic pain subjects, the mPFC will display decreased DTI and T2 relaxation parameters and increased NAA levels and that these changes will be significantly related to an individual's personality temperament of novelty seeking and harm avoidance. Such alterations would show that this region has undergone subtle changes in neuronal anatomy consistent with increased dendritic spine lengths, dendritic spine numbers and neuronal cell bodies.

Methods

Twenty two subjects with chronic pain (painful trigeminal neuropathy; 18 females, mean age 49.8±1.8 years [±SEM]) and 43 healthy controls without ongoing pain (35 females; mean age 46.4±2.7 years) were recruited at the University of Sydney, Australia. All chronic pain subjects were diagnosed with trigeminal neuropathy according to the Liverpool criteria [15]. After complete description of the study to the subjects, written informed consent was obtained for all procedures and the study was approved by Institutional Human Research Ethics Committees, University of Sydney. Some of the chronic pain subjects used in this study were also used in previous investigations [1,16,17,18,19].

Psychophysical Measures

Each chronic pain patient rated their on-going pain intensity with a vertical pencil stroke on a 10 cm horizontal line (visual analogue scale [VAS]; 0 cm = "no pain" to 10 cm = "maximum imaginable pain") three times a day for the week prior to the scanning session. These pain values were averaged to provide an indication of each subject's chronic pain rating. Each chronic pain subject also completed a McGill Pain Questionnaire and drew a distribution map of their on-going pain.

To assess individual subject's temperament, 19 chronic pain (16 females; mean age [±SEM]: 53±1.8) and 30 control subjects (24 females; age: 51±1.0) completed the revised version of the temperament and character inventory (TCI-R) [20]. Significant differences between these temperament measures in chronic pain subjects and controls were determined using t tests ($p<0.05$).

Table 1. Characteristics of chronic pain subjects.

Subject	Age	Gender	Duration of pain (years)	Site	Ongoing pain (10 cm VAS)	Analgesic Medication
1	51	M	3.5	right	2.1	Amitriptyline Hydrochloride
2	48	F	9.0	bilateral	2.5	Gabapentin
3	42	F	2.0	right	5.5	Neurontin
4	64	F	11.0	right	5.0	Gabapentin
5	52	F	3.5	right	4.5	none
6	47	F	5.0	left	1.1	none
7	53	F	2.5	right	1.5	none
8	52	F	1.5	bilateral	6.9	Gabapentin
						Oxycodone
						Paracetamol
9	55	F	2.0	left	5.2	Amitriptyline Hydrochloride
						Gabapentin
						Oxycodone Hydrochloride
						Paracetamol
10	46	M	9.0	bilateral	3.1	none
11	46	F	3.0	bilateral	6.5	Diazepam
						Paracetamol
						Ibuprofen (PRN)
12	42	F	11.0	bilateral	4.8	Carbamazepine
						Paracetamol
13	48	F	1.3	bilateral	2.6	Gabapentin
14	34	M	5.0	bilateral	3.5	Pregabalin Nortriptyline
15	59	F	5.0	left	3.3	Paracetamol
						Ibuprofen
16	54	F	2.0	right	1.6	Amitriptyline
17	44	F	6.5	bilateral	6.4	none
18	40	F	3.5	bilateral	4.0	Carbamazepine
19	67	F	14.0	left	8.4	none
20	43	M	16.0	left	5.8	Amitriptyline
21	44	F	7.0	bilateral	1.2	none
22	65	F	1.5	bilateral	2.5	none
Mean (±SEM)	49.8 (±1.8)		5.7 (±0.9)		4.0 (±0.4)	

PRN: *Pro re nata* – "as needed".

Table 2. T2 relaxation, mean diffusivity, grey matter volume and cerebral blood flow values within the contralateral medial prefrontal cortex (mPFC), anterior cingulate cortex (ACC), mediodorsal thalamus, ipsilateral posterior insula and contralateral primary somatosensory cortex (S1).

		contralateral mPFC	contralateral ACC	contralateral mediodorsal thalamus	ipsilateral posterior insula	contralateral S1
T2 relaxation	controls	151±4	125±2	143±6	149±4	126±4
time (ms±SEM)	chronic pain	132±4*	110±3*	118±7*	124±5*	104±4*
Mean diffusivity	controls	1.31±0.03	1.15±0.02	1.56±0.05	1.28±0.06	1.16±0.06
($mm^2/sx10^{-3}$±SEM)	chronic pain	1.16±0.03*	1.02±0.02*	1.36±0.04*	1.14±0.04	1.02±0.02*
Grey matter volume	controls	0.46±0.01	0.47±0.01	0.49±0.01	0.64±0.01	0.36±0.01
(prob*vol ±SEM)	chronic pain	0.46±0.01	0.45±0.01	0.48±0.02	0.64±0.02	0.38±0.01
Cerebral blood flow	controls	31.1±1.8	34.5±2.2	37.9±3.1	29.2±2.3	38.6±2.8
(ml/min/g ±SEM)	chronic pain	33.0±2.6	30.2±3.6	36.7±3.6	28.8±3.3	34.9±3.3

*significantly different to control subjects ($p<0.05$).

MRI Acquisition

In all subjects, three 3D T1-weighted anatomical image sets (echo time = 2.5 ms, repetition time [TR] = 5600 ms, flip angle = 8°, voxel size = 0.8×0.8×0.8 mm) and four high-resolution diffusion tensor image sets (TR = 8788ms; flip angle = 90°, voxel size = 2×2×2.5 mm, 32 directions, b = 0 and 1000 s/mm^2) covering the entire brain were collected using a 3T Philips Intera machine. Three T1-weighted images and 4 DTI series were collected separately for subsequent averaging. In 39 of the 43 control and 19 of the 22 chronic pain subjects, proton density and T2-weighted images covering the entire brain were also collected (TR = 4330 ms; echo times: 20, 40, 60, 80, 100 ms; voxel size = 2×2×2.5 mm). Multiple echo times were used to create multiple images for the subsequent calculation of T2-relaxation maps. In 24 controls and 18 chronic pain subjects, a quantitative arterial spin labelling (QASL) series, encompassing the entire brain was collected (TR/TE/DTI/TI1 = 4000/23/300/40 ms, 64×64 matrix, 14 slices, FOV = 240×240, flip-angle = 35/11.7°, SENSE = 2.5, V_{enc} = [∞, 4 cm/s], 82 (48 @ V_{enc} = 4 cm/s, 24 @ V_{enc} = ∞, 10 low flip angle, all implemented in a two separate sequences) [21]. In addition, a series of T1-weighted anatomical images, at the same slice locations as the QASL images were collected.

All neuropathic pain and healthy subjects were asked to return for a second scanning session. Twelve control (11 females; mean age±SEM: 53.4±3.1) and 11 neuropathic pain subjects (10 females; mean age±SEM: 53.5±2.8) returned for the second scanning session, the remaining subjects declined to return. Proton magnetic resonance spectroscopy (1H-MRS) was performed on the contralateral (to pain) mPFC and on the right mPFC in control subjects (TR = 2000 ms, echo time = 29 ms, 1024 acquisition points, spectral width of 2 kHz, total acquisition time = 9 min, voxel size 20×15×30 mm). The location of the region selected was based on the diffusion and T2 relaxometry results. Automatic shimming (pencilbeam auto first order option) was performed resulting in line widths of <10 Hz for all spectra. There were no significant differences in age ($p>0.05$, t-test) or gender composition ($p>0.05$; Chi2 test) in any of the MRI analyses.

MRI Analysis

DTI. All images were processed using SPM8 [22] and custom software. The diffusion-weighted images were motion corrected, coregistered to one another, averaged and diffusion tensors calculated [12]. Mean diffusivity maps were derived, spatially normalized and smoothed (6mm full-width-at-half-maximum [FWHM] Gaussian filter). Significant differences in mean diffusivity between controls and chronic pain subjects were determined ($p<0.05$, random effects, family wise error corrected for multiple comparisons, minimum cluster 30 voxels, age and gender nuisance variables). Mean diffusivity values of significantly different clusters were extracted and significance verified (2 sample t-tests, $p<0.05$). Significant correlations between mean diffusivity and pain intensity, pain duration, and temperament values (novelty seeking etc) were determined ($p<0.05$). Significant differences in r-values in chronic pain compared with controls were also determined using Fisher r-to-z transformation ($p<0.05$).

T2 relaxometry. The following equation was used to calculate T2 brain maps: $T_2 = (TE_2 - TE_1)/\ln(SI_1/SI_2)$ where TE_1 and TE_2 are the echo times for proton density and T2-weighted images, and SI_1, SI_2 represent proton density and T2-weighted image signal intensities, respectively. A ceiling threshold of 500 ms was applied to eliminate cerebrospinal fluid. In each subject, one of the T2-weighted images (TE = 60 ms) was spatially normalized and the parameters applied to the T2 map. The spatially normalized T2 map was smoothed (6 mm FWHM) and significant differences in T2 relaxation times between controls and chronic pain subjects determined ($p<0.05$, random effects, family wise error corrected for multiple comparisons, minimum cluster 30 voxels, age and gender nuisance variables). T2 relaxation times of significantly different clusters were extracted and significance verified (2 sample t-tests; $p<0.05$). Significant correlations between T2 relaxation times and pain intensity, pain duration, and temperament values (novelty seeking etc) were determined ($p<0.05$). Significant differences in r-values in chronic pain compared with controls were determined using Fisher r-to-z transformation ($p<0.05$).

Voxel based morphometry. T1-weighted anatomical image sets were coregistered to one another, averaged, modulated,

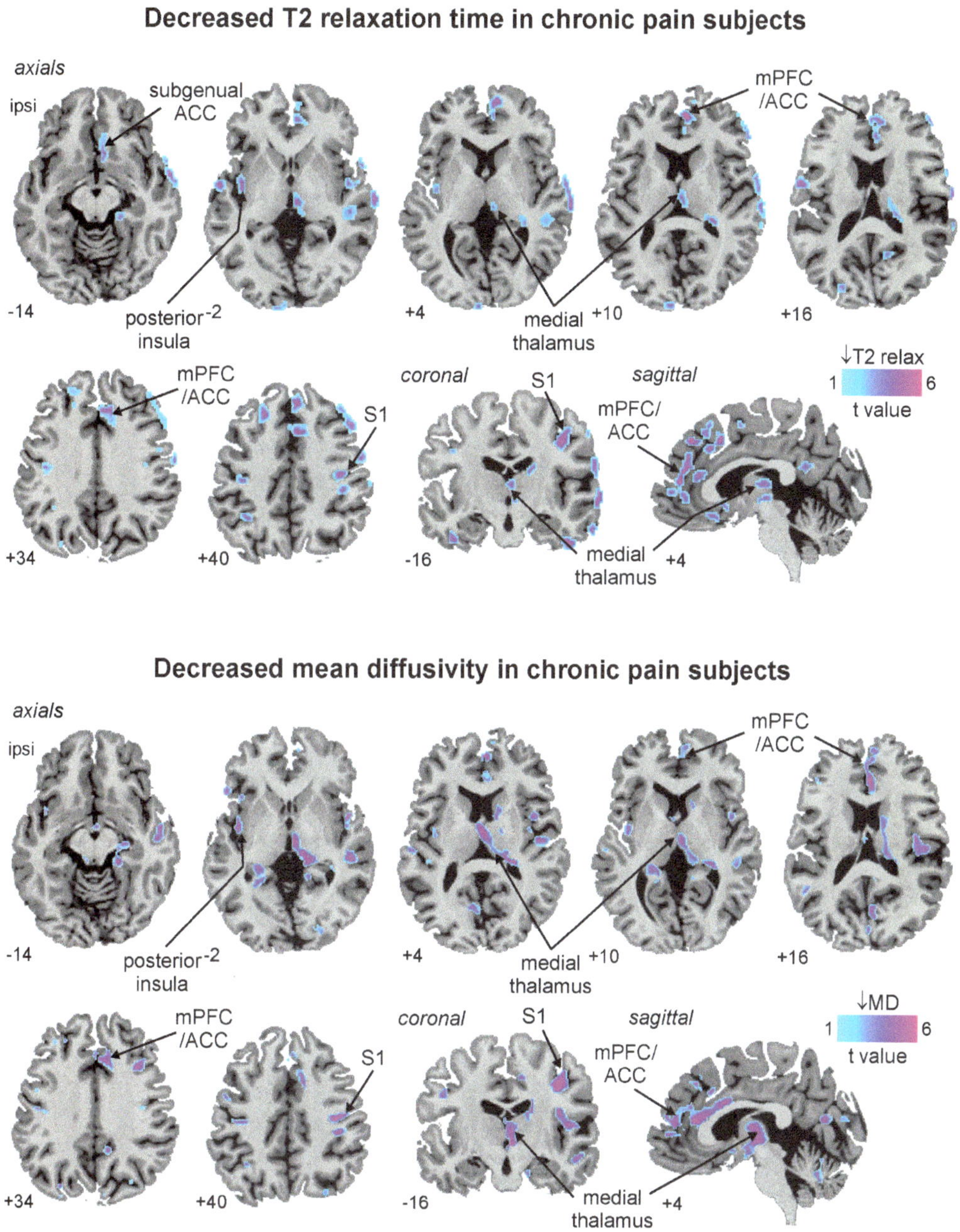

Figure 1. Brain regions in which T2-relaxation times (upper panel) or mean diffusivity values (lower panel) were significantly reduced in subjects with painful trigeminal neuropathy compared with pain-free, healthy controls. Significant reductions are colour-coded according to t-value and overlaid onto axial, coronal and sagittal sections of an individual subject's T1-weighted image set. Slice locations in Montreal Neurological Institute space are indicated at the lower left of each image. ACC: anterior cingulate cortex; ispi: ipsilateral to side of on-going pain; MD: mean diffusivity; mPFC: medial prefrontal cortex; S1: primary somatosensory cortex.

spatially normalized, segmented and smoothed (6 mm FWHM). Gray matter volumes from significant mean diffusivity and T2 relaxation clusters were extracted and compared between control and chronic pain subjects (2-tailed, 2-sample t-tests, $p<0.05$).

Quantitative arterial spin labelling. QASL images were opened [21] and cerebral blood flow (CBF) maps created. In addition, anatomical (gray/white) image sets were created from the CBF maps. These anatomical images were then co-registered to the T1-weighted anatomical image set collected at the same slice locations and the resulting parameters applied to the CBF maps. The T1-weighted anatomical images were then normalized and the parameters applied to CBF maps. CBF values from significant mean diffusivity and T2 relaxation clusters were extracted and compared between control and chronic pain subjects (2- tailed, 2-sample t-tests, $p<0.05$).

Proton magnetic resonance spectra (1H-MRS). MRS data were analyzed in the time domain using the Java-based magnetic resonance user's interface (jMRUI 4.1, European Union project). The dominant water resonance was removed using the Hankel Lanczos Singular Valve Decomposition algorithm. All metabolite resonances were quantified using QUEST (containing a 29 ms TE metabolite basis set including N-acetylaspartate

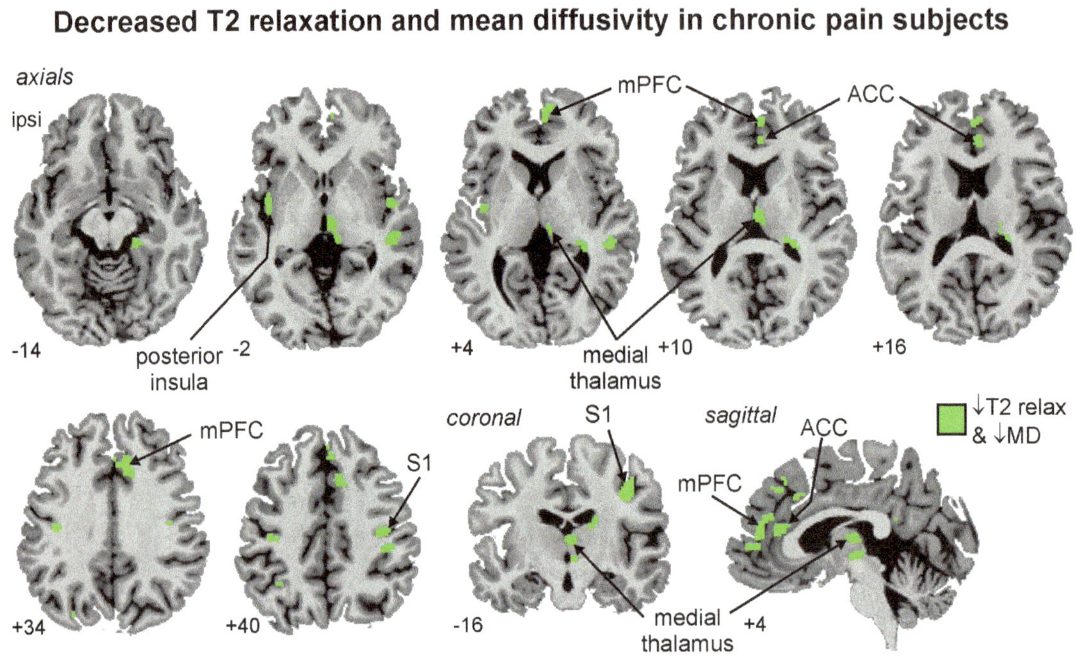

Figure 2. Brain regions in which both T2-relaxation times and mean diffusivity values (MD) were significantly reduced in subjects with painful trigeminal neuropathy compared with pain-free, healthy controls. Areas of significant reductions are shaded green and overlaid onto axial, coronal and sagittal sections of an individual subject's T1-weighted image set. Slice locations in Montreal Neurological Institute space are indicated at the lower left of each image. ACC: anterior cingulate cortex; ispi: ipsilateral to side of on-going pain; mPFC: medial prefrontal cortex; S1: primary somatosensory cortex.

(NAA), Creatine [23], Aspartate, Glutamate, Glutamine, Myo-Inositol (MI) and Glycerolphosphocholine). Ratios were calculated for NAA relative to Cr and MI relative to Cr. Significant differences in metabolite ratios between chronic pain subjects and healthy controls were determined (t-tests, $p<0.05$). One-tailed Pearson correlation test was used to determine significant ($p<0.05$) correlations between NAA/Cr ratios, MI/Cr ratios and pain intensity and pain duration.

Results

Pain and Temperament

Chronic pain subjects had on-going orofacial pain with mean pain intensity of 4.0±0.4 and mean pain duration of 5.7±0.9 years (Table 1). Chronic pain subjects had significantly lower mean novelty seeking values ([mean±SEM] controls: 102±2; chronic pain: 95±2) and significantly higher harm avoidance values (control: 89±3; chronic pain: 105±4) compared with controls. In contrast, there were no significant differences in temperament scores of reward dependence (control: 106±2; chronic pain), or persistence (control: 124±4; chronic pain: 117±5).

T2 relaxation times and mean diffusivity

Chronic pain subjects had reduced T2 relaxation times in the contralateral (to pain) subgenual anterior cingulate cortex (ACC), contralateral ACC and medial prefrontal cortices, ipsilateral posterior insula, contralateral medial thalamus and primary somatosensory cortex bilaterally (Figure 1, Table 2). Remarkably, whole brain analysis of mean diffusivity changes revealed significant decreases in these same regions apart from the subgenual ACC. Chronic pain subjects displayed significantly reduced mean diffusivity in the contralateral ACC, mPFC, ipsilateral posterior insula, contralateral medial thalamus (in the region of the mediodorsal nucleus) and primary somatosensory cortex bilaterally (Figure 1, Table 2). Brain regions where chronic pain subjects showed significant decreases in both T2 relaxation times and mean diffusivity are shown in Figure 2. Extraction of T2 relaxation times and mean diffusivity values from regions further confirmed these significant differences (Figure 3). Given the potential influence of medication we compared T2 relaxation times and mean diffusivity values within the mPFC, ACC and thalamus and found no significant differences between those chronic pain subjects taking medication ($n=8$) to those who were not ($n=14$). Furthermore, given the well-documented connections and functional interactions between the mediodorsal thalamus, mPFC and ACC [24], we restricted most of the remaining analysis on these three brain regions.

Gray matter volumes and baseline blood flow

Voxel based morphometry of T1-weighted anatomical images revealed that chronic pain was not associated with significant gray matter volume changes within the mPFC, ACC, mediodorsal thalamus, dorsal insula, or primary somatosensory cortex. Similarly, assessment of baseline regional cerebral blood flow using QASL revealed no significant difference in cerebral blood flow in chronic pain subjects compared with controls in the mPFC, ACC, mediodorsal thalamus, dorsal insula or primary somatosensory cortex (Figure 3, Table 2).

Proton magnetic resonance spectra (1H-MRS)

Finally, to assess biochemical changes within the mPFC, proton spectroscopy was performed. Within the contralateral mPFC, spectral analysis revealed that chronic pain subjects had significant elevated levels of N-acetyl aspartate/Creatine (NAA/Cr) compared to controls (mean±SEM NAA/Cr: controls: 1.16±0.03,

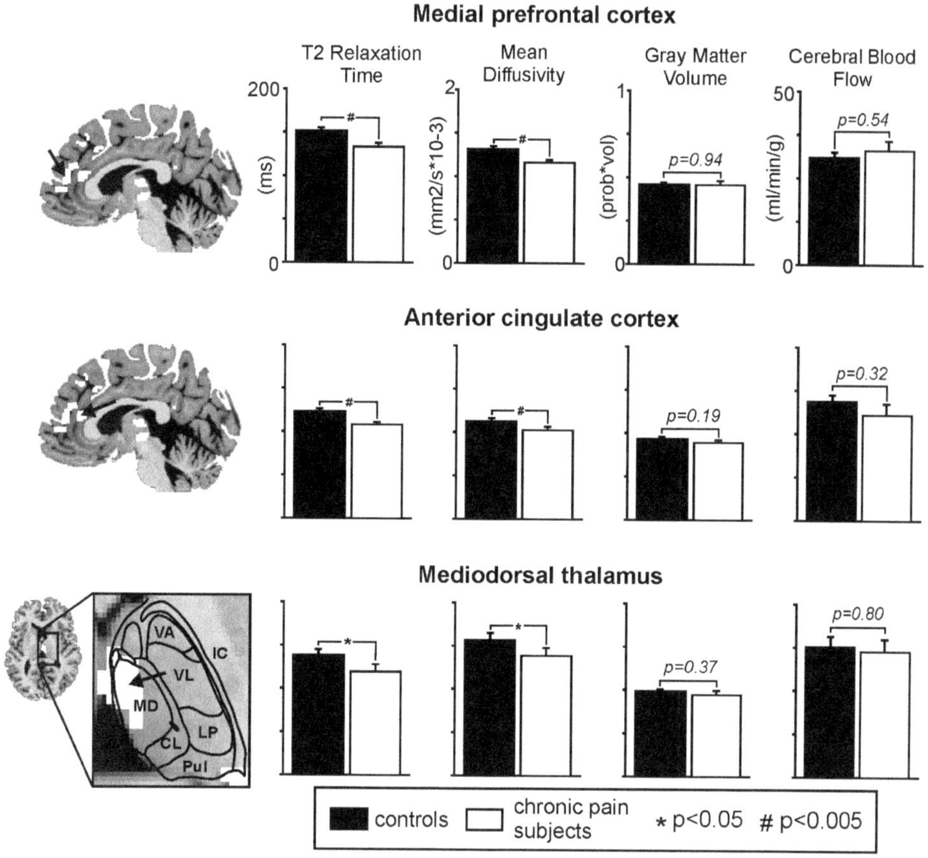

Figure 3. Plots of T2 relaxation times, mean diffusivity, gray matter volume and cerebral blood flow in three brain regions: the medial prefrontal cortex, anterior cingulate cortex and mediodorsal thalamus. Control subjects are shaded black and chronic pain subjects are shaded white. Note that although T2 relaxation times and mean diffusivity is reduced in all three regions, there are no significant changes in either gray matter volume or resting cerebral blood flow. Location of reductions in T2 relaxation times and mean diffusivity are shown to the left and indicated by an arrow. Note the thalamic reductions are located within the mediodorsal nucleus (MD). CL: centrolateral; IC: internal capsule; LP: lateral posterior; Pul: pulvinar; VA: ventral anterior; VL: ventral lateral.

chronic pain: 1.32±0.04; $p<0.005$) (Figure 4). No significant difference in myo-inositol/Cr (MI/Cr) was found in the mPFC of chronic pain subjects compared to controls (mean±SEM MI/Cr; controls: 0.78±0.03, chronic pain: 0.72±0.02; $p>0.05$).

Relationships with pain and temperament

Within the mPFC, ACC and thalamus, T2 relaxation times and mean diffusivity values in chronic pain subjects were not significantly correlated with either on-going pain intensity or pain duration. In contrast, within the mPFC and ACC, T2 relaxation

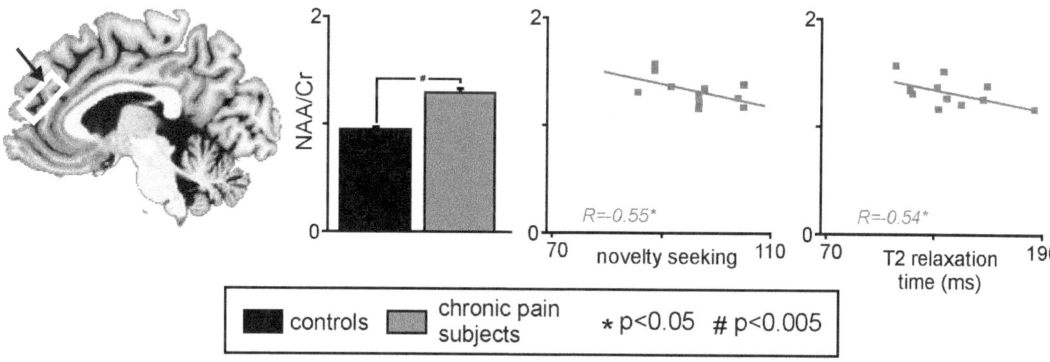

Figure 4. Sagittal slice showing location from which proton spectroscopy was performed in the contralateral medial prefrontal cortex (mPFC) of subjects with chronic pain and pain-free controls. The bar graph shows mean (±SEM) NAA/Cr values for chronic pain patients and healthy controls. To the right are two plots of novelty seeking against mPFC NAA/Cr and mPFC T2 relaxation times against mPFC NAA/Cr. Note that both novelty seeking and mPFC T2 relaxation times are significantly correlated to NAA/Cr within the mPFC. NAA: N-acetyl aspartate; Cr: creatine.

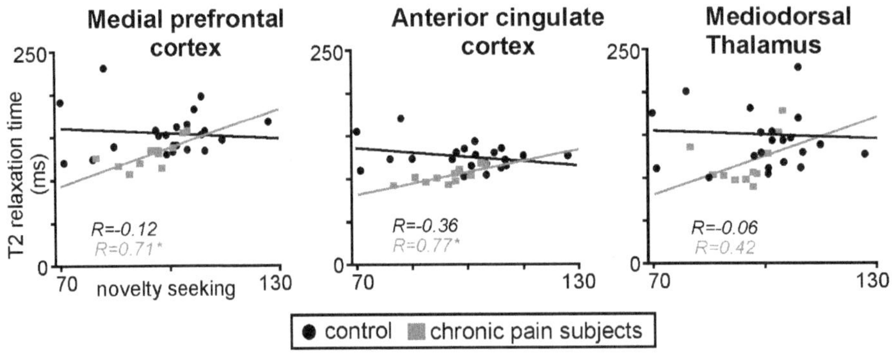

Figure 5. Plots of T2 relaxation times against novelty seeking temperament in control subjects (black circles) and in chronic pain subjects (gray squares) within the medial prefrontal cortex, anterior cingulate cortex and mediodorsal thalamus. Note that in chronic pain subjects, T2 relaxation times in the medial prefrontal and anterior cingulate cortices are significantly negatively correlated to novelty seeking. No such relationship was found in controls. *indicates significant difference in r values between controls and chronic pain subjects determined using Fisher r-to-z transformation.

times were positively correlated to novelty seeking (mPFC: r = 0.71; ACC: r = 0.77) (Figure 5). That is, the greater the decrease in T2 relaxation times, the lower the individual's novelty seeking score. In contrast, no significant relationship occurred between T2 relaxation times and novelty seeking within the thalamus (r = 0.42), or between T2 relaxation times and harm avoidance in all three regions (mPFC: r = −0.12; ACC: r = −0.36; mediodorsal thalamus: r = −0.06). In control subjects, no significant correlations were found between T2 relaxation times and either novelty seeking or harm avoidance in the mPFC, ACC or thalamus.

In chronic pain subjects NAA/Cr ratios within the mPFC were negatively correlated to novelty seeking (r = −0.55; Figure 5). That is, the greater the increase in NAA/Cr levels, the lower the individual's novelty seeking score. Furthermore, there was a significant negative correlation between mPFC NAA/Cr and T2 relaxation times within the mPFC (r = −0.54). That is the greater the neural viability, the lower the T2 relaxation time. No significant relationship occurred between mPFC NAA/Cr levels and harm avoidance (r = 0.02). In control subjects, no significant relationship occurred between mPFC NAA/Cr and MI/Cr ratios and either novelty seeking (NAA/Cr: r = 0.19; MI/Cr: r = −0.12), or harm avoidance (NAA/Cr: r = −0.18; MI/Cr: r = −0.04).

Discussion

Our results reveal that chronic pain is associated with significant anatomical changes within brain regions known to underpin an individual's personality traits, i.e. the mPFC, ACC and mediodorsal thalamus. Strikingly, in chronic pain subjects only, the anatomical and biochemical changes within the mPFC and ACC were significantly correlated to the personality temperament of novelty seeking, with greater anatomical change associated with reduced novelty seeking. These data suggest that subtle change in brain anatomy may alter an individual's personality characteristic.

Metz and colleagues [11] investigated the mPFC in the spared nerve injury model of neuropathic pain and reported that basal dendrites of pyramidal neurons in the contralateral mPFC, were longer, had more branches and had greater spine densities than those in sham-operated animals. Similar anatomical changes in humans would result in decreased mean diffusivity, since increased dendritic length and spine density would result in more restricted movement of free protons, and decreased T2 relaxation times, since axon and dendrite development results in increases in binding potential for protons of free water molecules to the surrounding macromolecules [13,25,26]. This is precisely what we found in our chronic pain subjects. Additionally, one would predict that such subtle changes in neuronal morphology would not result in a gross change in gray matter volume. Consistent with this we found that gray matter volume within the mPFC, as well as the ACC, and mediodorsal thalamus, did not display a significant change in chronic pain subjects compared with healthy pain-free controls.

Although taken alone, the mean diffusivity and T2 relaxation changes in our chronic pain subjects may reflect alterations in glia or blood vessels, our spectroscopy data reveals that these changes are also associated with increased NAA and no change in myoinositol. NAA occurs almost exclusively in neurons and is widely accepted as a marker of neuronal viability and synaptic health [27,28]. Increased NAA levels are associated with better cognitive test performance and reduced levels occur in neurodegenerative diseases [29,30]. In contrast, myoinositol is thought to be a glial marker, with elevated levels interpreted as gliosis in conditions such as Alzheimer's disease [31,32]. Although subject numbers of the spectroscopy scanning session were limited, we are confident that the changes in mean diffusivity and T2 relaxation reflect subtle neuronal changes such as altered basal dendritic length and spine density because we found increased levels of NAA and no change in myoinisotol within the mPFC.

It is becoming increasingly clear that chronic pain is characterized not only by an ongoing sensory and emotional experience, but also significant changes in an individual's cognitive ability. For example, it has been reported that chronic pain subjects display impaired decision making in the Iowa Gambling Task, making disadvantageous choices that gained high immediate monetary returns at the risk of higher future losses, i.e., they were less sensitive to future consequences [4,5]. Indeed, gross lesions of the mPFC and/or amygdala also result in decreased sensitivity to future consequences and poor performance on the Iowa Gambling Task [7,8,33]. Our chronic pain subjects had reduced novelty seeking and increased harm avoidance temperaments, a result consistent with a recent investigation, in which the personality profiles of over 200 chronic pain subjects were explored [6]. Furthermore, we found that novelty seeking, but not harm avoidance was significantly correlated to T2 relaxation times within the mPFC and ACC and NAA levels within the mPFC. Cloninger described novelty seeking as a "tendency toward intense exhilaration or excitement in response to novel stimuli … which leads to frequent exploratory activity in pursuit of potential rewards as well as active avoidance of monotony and potential punishment" [34]. The reduced novelty seeking in our chronic pain subjects implies that they are less likely to actively avoid monotony and potential punishment, which is consistent with being less sensitive to future consequences. Novelty seeking temperaments are thought to reflect the brain's "behavioural activation" system [35] which depends on the integrity of the mesolimbic dopaminergic pathway, of which the mPFC and ACC are integral parts [36,37]. In a number of psychiatric conditions, loss or impairment of PFC function is associated with cognitive deficits and conditions characterized by reduced dopaminergic activity such as Parkinson's disease, are associated with reduced novelty seeking temperaments [38,39].

The mPFC and ACC receive dopaminergic inputs directly from neurons within the ventral tegmental area. In experimental animals, ventral tegmental area lesions also result in cognitive deficits such as decreased exploration of environmental stimuli and reduced investigative behaviour [40]. Furthermore, dopamine depletion of the mPFC by 6-hydroxydopamine ventral tegmental area lesions, results in decreased basal dendritic lengths and spine densities of mPFC pyramidal cells [41]. Although in the opposite direction, these morphological changes are remarkably comparable in nature to those reported in the mPFC of experimental animals with neuropathic pain and supported by our MRI findings in humans with neuropathic pain. Importantly, given the unilateral nature of the mPFC anatomical changes that occur in the animal model of neuropathic pain (contralateral to injured nerve) and the unilateral nature of our MRI findings (contralateral to pain), it appears that the mPFC, ACC and thalamic anatomical changes associated with pain may result from the condition itself and may not pre-exist the injury/pain. It is possible that following neural injury, altered dopaminergic inputs result in increased basal dendrite lengths and increased spine densities of mPFC neurons, which in combination with inputs from other brain regions (e.g. amygdala), result in altered cognitive functions/temperaments such as novelty seeking and decision making ability. Interestingly, evidence is arising that chronic pain patients also have low Self-Directedness [6,42]. Indeed, a low value in self-directedness can predict the presence of a personality disorder [20]. Future research should examine the interaction of Novelty Seeking and Self-Directedness on brain biochemistry, structure and function, particularly within the mPFC.

Our data reveal that subtle neural changes in the mPFC and ACC of individuals with chronic pain are associated with subtle differences in an individual's personality profile. Of course it is well established that gross anatomical alterations in the prefrontal and cingulate cortices can drastically alter an individual's personality; the case of Phineas Gage is a prime example. Although our data cannot implicate causality, it may provide an indication that even subtle brain alterations can change an individual's personality. Interestingly, in healthy individuals the temperament Persistence has been shown to be associated with an overlapping circuit including the ACC, ventral striatum and the lateral orbital and mPFC [43,44]. As this association is lacking in pain patients, this may show that the reduction in Novelty Seeking involving reduced active avoidance may be an adaptive process generated by subtle brain alterations after the development of neuropathic pain. Since the recent advent of more sensitive structural magnetic resonance imaging techniques, it is now known that many relatively common medical conditions are associated with significant changes in brain anatomy, including changes within the mPFC and ACC. For example, gray matter volumes in the mPFC and ACC are significantly altered in subjects with respiratory disorders [45], diabetes [46], osteoarthritis [47] and even obesity [48]. Given this, it is likely that most individuals will experience at least some subtle change in brain anatomy over their life time that may potentially result in a change in their personality profile. The idea that an individual's personality is carried effectively unaltered throughout their adult life might need reconsideration.

Author Contributions

Conceived and designed the experiments: SG GM CP LH. Performed the experiments: SG GM CP LH. Analyzed the data: SG JM GM CP LH EP. Contributed reagents/materials/analysis tools: EP. Contributed to the writing of the manuscript: SG GM CP LH.

References

1. Gustin SM, Peck CC, Wilcox SL, Nash PG, Murray GM, et al. (2011) Different pain, different brain: thalamic anatomy in neuropathic and non-neuropathic chronic pain syndromes. J Neurosci 31: 5956–5964.
2. Burgmer M, Gaubitz M, Konrad C, Wrenger M, Hilgart S, et al. (2009) Decreased gray matter volumes in the cingulo-frontal cortex and the amygdala in patients with fibromyalgia. Psychosom Med 71: 566–573.
3. Younger JW, Shen YF, Goddard G, Mackey SC (2010) Chronic myofascial temporomandibular pain is associated with neural abnormalities in the trigeminal and limbic systems. Pain 149: 222–228.
4. Apkarian AV, Sosa Y, Krauss BR, Thomas PS, Fredrickson BE, et al. (2004) Chronic pain patients are impaired on an emotional decision-making task. Pain 108: 129–136.
5. Verdejo-Garcia A, Lopez-Torrecillas F, Calandre EP, Delgado-Rodriguez A, Bechara A (2009) Executive function and decision-making in women with fibromyalgia. Arch Clin Neuropsychol 24: 113–122.
6. Conrad R, Schilling G, Bausch C, Nadstawek J, Wartenberg HC, et al. (2007) Temperament and character personality profiles and personality disorders in chronic pain patients. Pain 133: 197–209.
7. Bechara A, Damasio H, Damasio AR, Lee GP (1999) Different contributions of the human amygdala and ventromedial prefrontal cortex to decision-making. J Neurosci 19: 5473–5481.
8. Bechara A, Dolan S, Denburg N, Hindes A, Anderson SW, et al. (2001) Decision-making deficits, linked to a dysfunctional ventromedial prefrontal cortex, revealed in alcohol and stimulant abusers. Neuropsychologia 39: 376–389.
9. Damasio H, Grabowski T, Frank R, Galaburda AM, Damasio AR (1994) The return of Phineas Gage: clues about the brain from the skull of a famous patient. Science 264: 1102–1105.
10. Schwarzbold M, Diaz A, Martins ET, Rufino A, Amante LN, et al. (2008) Psychiatric disorders and traumatic brain injury. Neuropsychiatr Dis Treat 4: 797–816.
11. Metz AE, Yau HJ, Centeno MV, Apkarian AV, Martina M (2009) Morphological and functional reorganization of rat medial prefrontal cortex in neuropathic pain. Proc Natl Acad Sci U S A 106: 2423–2428.
12. Basser PJ, Pierpaoli C (1996) Microstructural and physiological features of tissues elucidated by quantitative-diffusion-tensor MRI. J Magn Reson B 111: 209–219.
13. Mathur-De Vre R (1984) Biomedical implications of the relaxation behaviour of water related to NMR imaging. Br J Radiol 57: 955–976.
14. Barker PB (2001) N-acetyl aspartate–a neuronal marker? Ann Neurol 49: 423–424.
15. Nurmikko TJ, Eldridge PR (2001) Trigeminal neuralgia–pathophysiology, diagnosis and current treatment. Br J Anaesth 87: 117–132.
16. Gustin SM, Peck CC, Cheney LB, Macey PM, Murray GM, et al. (2012) Pain and Plasticity: Is Chronic Pain Always Associated with Somatosensory Cortex Activity and Reorganization? The Journal of Neuroscience 32: 14874–14884.
17. Gustin SM, Peck CC, Macey PM, Murray GM, Henderson LA (2013) Unraveling the Effects of Plasticity and Pain on Personality. The Journal of Pain 14: 1642–1652.
18. Henderson LA, Peck CC, Petersen ET, Rae CD, Youssef AM, et al. (2013) Chronic Pain: Lost Inhibition? The Journal of Neuroscience 33: 7574–7582.
19. Youssef AM, Gustin SM, Nash PG, Reeves JM, Petersen ET, et al. (2014) Differential brain activity in subjects with painful trigeminal neuropathy and painful temporomandibular disorder. PAIN 155: 467–475.
20. Cloninger R (1994) The temperament and character inventory (TCI): A guide to its development and use. St. Louis, MO: Washington University Center for Psychobiology of Personality.

21. Petersen ET, Lim T, Golay X (2006) Model-free arterial spin labeling quantification approach for perfusion MRI. Magn Reson Med 55: 219–232.
22. Friston KJ, Holmes AP, Poline JB, Grasby PJ, Williams SC, et al. (1995) Analysis of fMRI time-series revisited. Neuroimage 2: 45–53.
23. Zermatten A, Van der Linden M, d'Acremont M, Jermann F, Bechara A (2005) Impulsivity and decision making. J Nerv Ment Dis 193: 647–650.
24. Vogt BA, Gabriel M (1993) Anterior cingulate cortex and the medial pain system. Neurobiology of cingulate cortex and limbic thalamus; a comprehensive handbook. Boston: Birkhauser.
25. Dietrich RB, Bradley WG, Zaragoza EJt, Otto RJ, Taira RK, et al. (1988) MR evaluation of early myelination patterns in normal and developmentally delayed infants. AJR Am J Roentgenol 150: 889–896.
26. Ono J, Kodaka R, Imai K, Itagaki Y, Tanaka J, et al. (1993) Evaluation of myelination by means of the T2 value on magnetic resonance imaging. Brain Dev 15: 433–438.
27. Danielsen ER, Ross B (1999) Magnetic Resonance Spectroscopy Diagnosis of Neurological Diseases. New York, NY, USA: Marcel Dekker.
28. Urenjak J, Williams SR, Gadian DG, Noble M (1992) Specific expression of N-acetylaspartate in neurons, oligodendrocyte-type-2 astrocyte progenitors, and immature oligodendrocytes in vitro. J Neurochem 59: 55–61.
29. Clarke CE, Lowry M (2001) Systematic review of proton magnetic resonance spectroscopy of the striatum in parkinsonian syndromes. Eur J Neurol 8: 573–577.
30. Jung RE, Yeo RA, Chiulli SJ, Sibbitt WL Jr, Brooks WM (2000) Myths of neuropsychology: intelligence, neurometabolism, and cognitive ability. Clin Neuropsychol 14: 535–545.
31. Brand A, Richter-Landsberg C, Leibfritz D (1993) Multinuclear NMR studies on the energy metabolism of glial and neuronal cells. Dev Neurosci 15: 289–298.
32. Kantarci K, Jack CR Jr, Xu YC, Campeau NG, O'Brien PC, et al. (2000) Regional metabolic patterns in mild cognitive impairment and Alzheimer's disease: A 1H-MRS study. Neurology 55: 210–217.
33. Bechara A, Damasio AR, Damasio H, Anderson SW (1994) Insensitivity to future consequences following damage to human prefrontal cortex. Cognition 50: 7–15.
34. Cloninger CR (1987) A systematic method for clinical description and classification of personality variants. A proposal. Arch Gen Psychiatry 44: 573–588.
35. Cloninger CR (1986) A Unified Biosocial Theory of Personality and Its Role in the Development of Anxiety-States. Psychiatric Developments 4: 167–226.
36. Dellu F, Piazza PV, Mayo W, LeMoal M, Simon H (1996) Novelty-seeking in rats - Biobehavioral characteristics and possible relationship with the sensation-seeking trait in man. Neuropsychobiology 34: 136–145.
37. Iversen SD (1977) Brain dopamine systems and behavior. In: Iversen LL, Iversen SD, Snyder SH, editors. Handbook of Psychopharmacology. New York: Plenum. 333–374.
38. Goto Y, Yang CR, Otani S (2010) Functional and dysfunctional synaptic plasticity in prefrontal cortex: roles in psychiatric disorders. Biol Psychiatry 67: 199–207.
39. Menza MA, Golbe LI, Cody RA, Forman NE (1993) Dopamine-related personality traits in Parkinson's disease. Neurology 43: 505–508.
40. Stellar JR, Stellar E (1985) The neurobiology of motivation and reward. New York: Springer-Verlag.
41. Wang HD, Deutch AY (2008) Dopamine depletion of the prefrontal cortex induces dendritic spine loss: reversal by atypical antipsychotic drug treatment. Neuropsychopharmacology 33: 1276–1286.
42. Malmgren-Olsson E-B, Bergdahl J (2006) Temperament and Character Personality Dimensions in Patients With Nonspecific Musculoskeletal Disorders. The Clinical Journal of Pain 22: 625–631 610.1097/1001.ajp.0000210907.0000265170.a0000210903.
43. Cloninger CR, Zohar AH, Hirschmann S, Dahan D (2012) The psychological costs and benefits of being highly persistent: Personality profiles distinguish mood disorders from anxiety disorders. Journal of Affective Disorders 136: 758–766.
44. Gusnard DA, Ollinger JM, Shulman GL, Cloninger CR, Price JL, et al. (2003) Persistence and brain circuitry. Proceedings of the National Academy of Sciences 100: 3479–3484.
45. Macey PM, Henderson LA, Macey KE, Alger JR, Frysinger RC, et al. (2002) Brain morphology associated with obstructive sleep apnea. Am J Respir Crit Care Med 166: 1382–1387.
46. Musen G, Lyoo IK, Sparks CR, Weinger K, Hwang J, et al. (2006) Effects of type 1 diabetes on gray matter density as measured by voxel-based morphometry. Diabetes 55: 326–333.
47. Gwilym SE, Filippini N, Douaud G, Carr AJ, Tracey I (2010) Thalamic atrophy associated with painful osteoarthritis of the hip is reversible after arthroplasty: a longitudinal voxel-based morphometric study. Arthritis Rheum 62: 2930–2940.
48. Taki Y, Kinomura S, Sato K, Inoue K, Goto R, et al. (2008) Relationship between body mass index and gray matter volume in 1,428 healthy individuals. Obesity (Silver Spring) 16: 119–124.

19

Carbamazepine Potentiates the Effectiveness of Morphine in a Rodent Model of Neuropathic Pain

Michael R. Due[1], Xiao-Fang Yang[2], Yohance M. Allette[3], Aaron L. Randolph[1], Matthew S. Ripsch[1], Sarah M. Wilson[4], Erik T. Dustrude[3], Rajesh Khanna[2,5], Fletcher A. White[1,5]*

1 Department of Anesthesia, Indiana University School of Medicine, Indianapolis, Indiana, United States of America, **2** Department of Pharmacology, College of Medicine, University of Arizona, Tucson, Arizona, United States of America, **3** Department of Cell Biology and Anatomy, Indiana University School of Medicine, Indianapolis, Indiana, United States of America, **4** Program in Medical Neurosciences, Paul and Carole Stark Neurosciences Research Institute, Indiana University School of Medicine, Indianapolis, Indiana, United States of America, **5** Department of Pharmacology and Toxicology, Indiana University School of Medicine, Indianapolis, Indiana, United States of America

Abstract

Approximately 60% of morphine is glucuronidated to morphine-3-glucuronide (M3G) which may aggravate preexisting pain conditions. Accumulating evidence indicates that M3G signaling through neuronal Toll-like receptor 4 (TLR4) may be central to this proalgesic signaling event. These events are known to include elevated neuronal excitability, increased voltage-gated sodium (NaV) current, tactile allodynia and decreased opioid analgesic efficacy. Using an *in vitro* ratiometric-based calcium influx analysis of acutely dissociated small and medium-diameter neurons derived from lumbar dorsal root ganglion (DRG), we observed that M3G-sensitive neurons responded to lipopolysaccharide (LPS) and over 35% of these M3G/LPS-responsive cells exhibited sensitivity to capsaicin. In addition, M3G-exposed sensory neurons significantly increased excitatory activity and potentiated NaV current as measured by current and voltage clamp, when compared to baseline level measurements. The M3G-dependent excitability and potentiation of NaV current in these sensory neurons could be reversed by the addition of carbamazepine (CBZ), a known inhibitor of several NaV currents. We then compared the efficacy between CBZ and morphine as independent agents, to the combined treatment of both drugs simultaneously, in the tibial nerve injury (TNI) model of neuropathic pain. The potent anti-nociceptive effects of morphine (5 mg/kg, i.p.) were observed in TNI rodents at post-injury day (PID) 7–14 and absent at PID21–28, while administration of CBZ (10 mg/kg, i.p.) alone failed to produce anti-nociceptive effects at any time following TNI (PID 7–28). In contrast to either drug alone at PID28, the combination of morphine and CBZ completely attenuated tactile hyperalgesia in the rodent TNI model. The basis for the potentiation of morphine in combination with CBZ may be due to the effects of a latent upregulation of NaV1.7 in the DRG following TNI. Taken together, our observations demonstrate a potential therapeutic use of morphine and CBZ as a combinational treatment for neuropathic pain.

Editor: Thiago Mattar Cunha, University of Sao Paulo, Brazil

Funding: This work was supported by NIH NIDA R01DA026040 and NIDDK DK100905. The funders had no role in study design, data collection and analysis, decision to publish, or preparation of the manuscript.

Competing Interests: The authors have declared that no competing interests exist.

* Email: fawhite@iupui.edu

Introduction

Morphine is the cornerstone of pain management in a number of pain conditions. However, therapeutic administration of morphine or morphine equivalents for neuropathic pain is limited to the second or third line of medication due to multiple adverse effects including incomplete efficacy [1], respiratory depression, and induction of sedation, constipation, nausea, vomiting, addiction and tolerance [2]. It has also been reported both experimentally and clinically that exposure to morphine can elicit a paradoxical pain in regions of the body unrelated to the initial pain complaint, aggravating preexisting pain; opioid-induced hyperalgesia (OIH) [3]. However, the molecular mechanisms of OIH are largely unknown. Numerous groups have suggested that OIH may be due to tonic, descending facilitation in the spinal cord [4,5] or in the spinal cord dorsal horn [6,7] through changes in activity of NMDA receptors. Though neither of these modes of action can be completely ruled out, an alternative OIH mechanism involves functional activation of the innate immune receptor Toll-like receptor 4 (TLR4) known to exhibited by a subpopulation of nociceptive neurons [8,9].

TLR4 is a member of a fundamental family of receptors known for their ability to recognize pathogen-associated molecular patterns and facilitate the production of pro-inflammatory cytokines. TLR4 activation is not limited to pathogen detection; recent publications suggest that opioids and their glucuronide metabolites, among other ligands, can elicit TLR4-dependent activation in glial and neuronal cells [9,10,11,12,13,14]. Moreover, both pharmacological blockade of TLR4 signaling and the use of TLR4 knockout mice serve to prevent behavioral hyperalgesia due to morphine tolerance and potentiate acute morphine analgesia *in vivo* [9,15,16].

Molecular modeling of opioid receptors has provided key information regarding the affinity of a variety of opioid ligands. Yet relatively little is known regarding the opioid-mediated TLR4 receptor action on neurons associated with the nociceptive pathway. A recent investigation using the morphine metabolite, morphine-3-glucuronide (M3G) to study TLR4-mediated activation in small diameter nociceptive neurons revealed that the there is a substantial increase in the current density for voltage-gated sodium channels (NaV), NaV1.6, NaV1.7 and NaV1.9, but not NaV1.8. [9]. The fact that these Na^+ currents were influenced by a TLR4 agonist suggests that pharmacological targeting may provide mechanistic insights into both OIH and neuropathic disorders.

A suitable candidate to potentially diminish the neuronal TLR4 agonist-mediated signaling increases in excitation via sodium current modulation, is the anti-epileptic drug carbamazepine (CBZ) [17]. CBZ, a state-dependent channel blocker that inhibits sodium current within seconds when applied externally, [18] is known to stabilize the inactivated current state of NaV1.3, NaV1.7, and NaV1.8 without targeting resurgent sodium current [19,20]. Though the degree to which sodium channel blockade impacts TLR4 agonist-mediated effects is largely unknown, Black and colleagues have shown that phenytoin and tetrodotoxin substantially reduces phagocytic activity of microglia cells activated with the TLR4 agonist, lipopolysaccharide (LPS) [21]. Taken together, these TLR4-agonist-mediated events demonstrate that sodium channels may be possibly affiliated with TLR4 signaling as well as instrumental to the rapid induction of cellular activity in both immune cells and nociceptive sensory neurons.

The aim of this study was to assay the degree to which CBZ administration can diminish M3G/TLR4-induced neuronal activity *in vitro* and to characterize the potency of morphine, alone or in combination, with CBZ in the tibial nerve injury (TNI) model of neuropathic pain over time. We also determined the degree to which expression levels of NaV1.7 change following TNI paralleled changes in diminished morphine efficacy.

Materials and Methods

Pathogen-free, adult female and male Sprague-Dawley (S/D) rats (150–200 g; Harlan Laboratories, Madison, WI) were housed in temperature (23±3°C) and light (12-h light: 12-h dark cycle; lights on at 07:00 h) controlled rooms with standard rodent chow and autoclaved tap water available. Experiments were performed during the light cycle. Animals were randomly assigned to the treatment groups. All animal experiments were approved by the Institutional Animal Care and Use Committees of Indiana University School of Medicine and College of Medicine, University of Arizona. All procedures were conducted in accordance with the Guide for Care and Use of Laboratory Animals published by the National Institutes of Health and the ethical guidelines established by the International Association for the Study of Pain.

Tibial Nerve Injury

All rodents were anesthetized during the procedure with isoflurane (4% induction, 2% maintenance). To model neuropathic pain we performed a tibial nerve injury (TNI) as previously described [22,23,24,25]. Rodents were anesthetized using isoflurane at 4% induction and 2% maintenance. Under anesthesia, the right sciatic nerve was isolated under aseptic surgical conditions by blunt dissection of the femoral biceps muscle, without damaging the epimycium. The sciatic nerve and its three branches were isolated: the sural, common peroneal and tibial nerves and only the tibial nerve was tightly-ligated with 5-0 silk and transected distal to the ligation. The removal of an additional 2–4 mm of distal nerve stump was removed to prevent re-innervation by the proximal nerve. The overlying muscle and skin was then sutured in two separate layers.

Behavioral assessment

All rodents were habituated to testing chambers which were transparent plastic cages with a floor of wire mesh with ~1 cm×1 cm openings for at least two days and baseline testing occurred for each of three days before TNI to establish force threshold necessary for paw withdrawal using previously described techniques [26,27]. The incidence of foot withdrawal was expressed as a percentage of the 6 applications of each stimulus and the percentage of withdrawals was then plotted as a function of force. The von Frey withdrawal threshold was defined as the force that evoked a minimum detectable withdrawal observed on 50% of the tests given at the same force level. Following TNI, animal behavioral thresholds were assayed at least 30 minutes prior to drug administration and tested again following reagent administration.

Drugs and Administration

Carbamazepine (CBZ) was purchased from Sigma (St. Louis, MO). Morphine sulfate salt and morphine-3-glucuronoide (M3G) was provided by NIDA Drug Supply Program (Rockville, MD). For *in vitro* studies, a 75 mM solution of CBZ was made up in dimethyl sulphoxide (DMSO). A 2.67-µl aliquot was taken directly from this stock and put into the 2 ml of bathing solution for the population data to obtain a final concentration of 100 µM [DMSO, 0.1% (v/v)]. For *in vivo* studies, CBZ was suspended in 5% DMSO (% of final volume) in saline (0.9%). Morphine was freshly prepared on the day of the experiment in saline such that the final dose was dissolved in 1 mL and administered by intraperitoneal (i.p.) injections.

RNA isolation and RT-qPCR

Lumbar dorsal root ganglia (DRG; L4-L5) were dissected from adult Sprague Dawley rats, frozen in liquid nitrogen, and maintained at −80°C until processed for RNA extraction. Total RNA was extracted from the samples using the RNeasy RNA extraction and purification kit (Qiagen). Single stranded cDNA was synthesized using reverse transcriptase (Bioline) with oligo-dT primers. Quantitative PCR was performed as previously described [28]. Briefly, resultant cDNA samples were amplified on an ABI PRISM 7900 HT Sequence Detection System (Applied Biosystems) using the reporter, SYBR Green. The PCR reaction was as follows: 1x, 50°C, 2 min; 1x, 95°C, 10 min; 45x, 95°C, 15 s, 60°C, 1 min; 1x, 25°C, hold. To check for DNA contamination, PCR was run using an L27 (ribosomal housekeeping gene) primer pair, whose PCR product crosses an intron. The mRNA level for each gene (x) relative to L27 mRNA (internal control) was calculated using the following equation where Ct refers to threshold cycles: $\text{mRNA (x\%)} = 2^{Ct(L27)-Ct(x)} \times 100$.

Nav 1.7 For GAGAGCGGAGAGATGGATTC

Nav 1.7 Rev GCTTCAGTGGTTGTGATG

Preparation of acutely dissociated dorsal root ganglion neurons

The L4–L6 DRGs were acutely dissociated using methods described by Ma and LaMotte [29]. Briefly, L4–L6 DRGs were removed from naive animals. The cells were then dissociated by mechanical trituration in culture media containing 1 mg/ml bovine serum albumin and trypsin inhibitor (Worthington Biochemical, Lakewood, NJ). The culture media was Ham's F-12 mixture, DMEM, supplemented with 10% fetal bovine serum, penicillin and streptomycin (100 µg/ml and 100 U/ml) and N2 (Life Technologies). The cells were then plated on coverslips coated with poly-L lysine and laminin (BD bioscience) and incubated for 2–3 h before more culture media was added to the wells. The cells were then allowed to sit undisturbed for 12–15 h to adhere at 37°C (with 5% CO2).

Intracellular calcium imaging

Acute dissociation of lumbar DRG and ratiometric Fura 2-AM based intracellular calcium imaging was performed between 20–26°C using methods previously described [27]. Sterile solution was applied to cells prior to LPS followed by M3G application, and any cells that responded to buffer alone were not used. Compounds were applied directly into the coverslip bathing solution as a static solution. LPS (1 µg/mL) was applied first, followed by M3G (3 µM), after which capsaicin (3 nM; Sigma-Aldrich) was added (at least 100 cells were assayed from three rodents). Additional experiments utilizing at least 50 cells reversed the order of LPS and M3G. Only calcium imaging traces that reflected at least a 50% increase over baseline were included in the analysis. At least three minutes were allowed to pass between ligand inductions in order to allow neurons to return to a manifested baseline of calcium flux, to maintain the integrity of the results. If the neuron was unable to return to a baseline level, it was omitted from the study. All data were analyzed by two independent analyzers and only responses that were in agreement between the two individuals were used in the responsive cell counts.

Electrophysiology

Sharp-electrode intracellular recordings were obtained from 4 to 18 hours after acute dissociation of lumbar DRG and current clamp protocols were performed using methods previously described [9,22]. A neuron was accepted for study only when it exhibited a resting membrane potential (RMP) more negative than −45 mV. For each neuron isolated for study, a continuous recording was obtained for 1 minute without the delivery of any external stimulus. Neuronal excitability of small and medium diameter dissociated DRG sensory neurons was measured by injecting 1-s current pulses into the soma every 30 s. Current was adjusted in order to elicit 1–2 action potentials per current injection under baseline conditions. Following control current injections, M3G (3 µM) was applied to the coverslip and current injections continued every 30 s. Neuronal excitability was measured as number of action potentials elicited per current pulse before and immediately after addition of M3G (15 and 45 s, respectively). If M3G increased neuronal excitability, CBZ (2 mM) or vehicle was added to the bath to determine if M3G-elicited neuronal excitation could be reversed.

Whole cell voltage-clamp recordings were made from small- and medium-diameter DRG neurons (25 µm<DRG diameter < 45 µm) using HEKA EPC10 amplifier (Germany). Electrodes were pulled from Warner Instruments thin walled borosilicate glass (Hamden, CT) with a Sutter P-97 electrode puller (Novato, CA) to produce 1–2 megaohm resistant pipets when filled with internal solutions. Recordings were performed in a reduced sodium solution to ensure fidelity of the voltage-clamp. External solution concentrations (in mM): 70 NaCl, 60 Choline-Cl, 30 TEA-Cl, 3 KCl, $1 CaCl_2$, 1 $MgCl_2$, 0.05 $CdCl_2$, 10 HEPES, 10 Glucose (pH 7.3) (310–320 mOsm/L). Internal solution concentrations (in mM): 140 CsCl, 5 $MgSO_4$, 10 EGTA, 4 ATP Na_2-ATP, 25 HEPES (pH 7.2) (290–310 mOsm/L). Whole cell capacitance and series resistance were compensated by the amplifier, and linear leak currents were digitally subtracted by P/4. Analysis was performed using HEKA FitMaster (Germany) and Origin 9.1 (Northhampton, MA).

Statistics

GraphPad Software (LaJolla, CA) was used to determine the statistical significance. Results were expressed as mean ± SEM. When only two groups were compared, Student t test was used. Multiple comparisons were evaluated by Tukey's multiple comparison tests after one-way ANOVA. $p<0.05$ was considered to be statistically significant.

Results

TLR4 agonist-induced intracellular calcium mobilization in dissociated sensory neurons

It is known that LPS can elicit excitation in sensory neurons in culture [9] and can contribute to the release of CGRP from capsaicin sensitive neurons [30]. Some reports suggest that this relatively fast neuronal activation may be dependent on both TLR4 and TRPV1 channels [8]. We therefore examined the effects of the known TLR4 agonists, LPS and M3G on $[Ca^{2+}]_i$ in cultured rat DRG neurons as a screen for the presence of functional receptors. Calcium mobilization was used in this instance strictly as an indication of TLR4 receptor activation and does not necessarily imply a role for this phenomenon in the other physiological effects of TLR4 agonists. The concentration of M3G and LPS used in this experiment was based on our previous observations of their effects on Ca mobilization in sensory neurons [9]. The application of vehicle at the beginning of experiment (i.e., 10 µl of 0.1% BSA/PBS in 1 ml of BSS) did not alter $[Ca^{2+}]_i$ (data not shown). Bath application of M3G followed by LPS exposure increased $[Ca^{2+}]_i$ in a large number of DRG neurons (**Fig 1** and **Table 1**). Many of these DRG neurons also responded to capsaicin (**Table 1**). These observations were maintained and

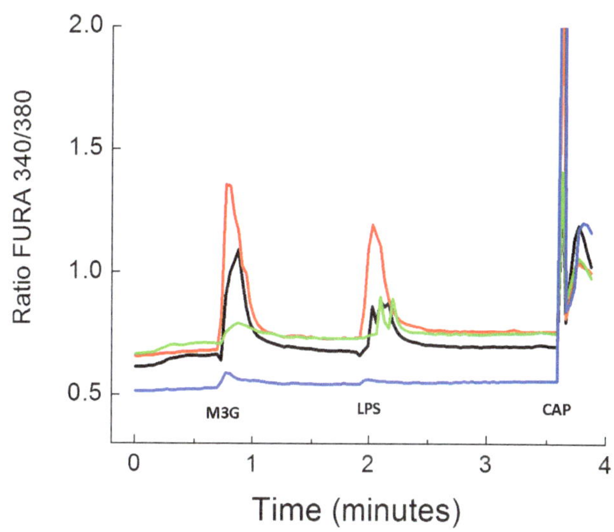

Figure 1. Description of calcium imaging. LPS-induced calcium flux in acutely dissociated small to medium diameter sensory neurons. Fura-2 loaded primary afferent neurons were stimulated with bath applications of morphine metabolite, morphine 3 glucuronide (M3G), the TLR4 agonist LPS, and capsaicin (CAP). [Ca2+]I levels were measured as ratio fluorscence of excitation at 340/380 nm over time. Four cells were assayed in this experiment and were represented by the blue, black green and red traces. The red and black traces clearly exhibited significant calcium flux after both M3G and LPS exposure while the green and blue traces exhibited only mild to moderate responses to these exogenous stimuli. All four traces exhibited robust calcium flux responses to capsaicin.

Table 1.

Total Number of cells: 122

Treatment	Cell Number	Percentage
LPS responsive cells	(45/122)	36.89%
LPS/Capsaicin-sensitive cells	(21/45)	46.67%
M3G responsive cells	(19/122)	15.57%
M3G/LPS responsive cells	(18/19)	94.73%
M3G/LPS + Capsaicin-sensitive cells	(7/18)	38.88%

supported regardless of whether the cells were first subjected to M3G followed by LPS, or vice versa.

Morphine-3-glucuronide-induced sensory neuron excitation *in vitro* is blocked by carbamazepine

Activation of TLR4-mediated neuronal excitation by M3G selectively elicits increased density in the voltage-gated sodium currents NaV1.6, NaV1.7 and NaV1.9 [9] and CBZ is known to produce a differential block of NaV1.7 [20]. To investigate the degree to which M3G-induced neuronal excitation is affected by exposure to CBZ, we subjected sensory neurons to bath-applied M3G, followed by administration of CBZ. Not unlike our previous published observations [9], repeated current pulse combined with M3G administration produced a significant increase in the excitability of small- to medium-diameter sensory neurons when compared to baseline levels. Less than 18% of total neurons responded to M3G administration. We also observed 1.53±0.2 APs in cells under control conditions compared to 5.75±0.5 APs in cells subjected to M3G (n = 28) (Fig. 2A). Subsequent treatment with CBZ completely blocked M3G-dependent excitability in all sensory neurons that responded to M3G (1.13±0.3 APs for CBZ, n = 10; ANOVA, interaction F = 45.35, $p<0.05$; Dunnett's multiple comparison test, $P<0.05$) (Fig. 2B).

Morphine-3-glucuronide-induced potentiation is dependent on voltage-gated sodium channels

Treatment with M3G potentiates currents in dorsal root ganglia cells [9]. CBZ has also been shown to inhibit voltage-gated sodium channel currents via hyperpolarizing shift in the voltage dependence of steady-state fast inactivation [20]. Here, we verify that the observed potentiation is dependent on voltage-gated sodium channels using whole-cell patch clamp technique and voltage step depolarizations from −80 mV to record isolated sodium currents and current densities from primary afferent sensory neurons (**Fig. 3A**). Sensory neurons were treated with an exposure to vehicle, 500 ug CBZ, 3 μM M3G, or a combination of both 3 μM M3G and 500 ug CBZ and current densities were compared between treatment groups (**Fig. 3B**; n = 24). CBZ treated cells measured 95.7±15.2 pA/pF, a ~70% decrease in current density (**Fig. 3C**). M3G treated cells measured 430.0±48.3 pA/pF compared to 283.0±38.8 pA/pF for vehicle treated cells, a ~50% increase in current density (**Fig. 3C**). Treatment with both M3G and CBZ measured 111.3±25.1 pA/pF, a ~60% decrease in current density (**Fig. 3C**). Potentiation and reduction of current density by all treatment groups was measured to be statistically significant by one-way ANOVA and Tukey's post-hoc test. Thus, the potentiation of voltage gated sodium current mediated by M3G was attenuated by treatment with CBZ. Treatment with CBZ produced a characteristic hyperpolarizing shift in the voltage dependence of steady-state fast inactivation, −82.9±3.6 mV compared to −50.3±1.5 mV in vehicle treated cells (**Fig. 3C**). Treatment with both M3G and CBZ prevented this shift (**Table 2**).

Effect of Morphine on TNI-induced tactile allodynia at post-injury day 7–28

Opioids such as morphine are the most effective broad spectrum analgesics available for moderate to severe pain acute pain

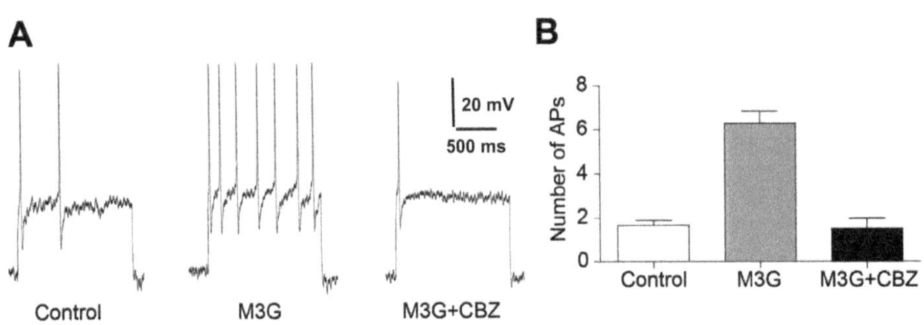

Figure 2. Morphine-3-glucuronide (M3G) increased excitability of nociceptive dorsal root ganglion neurons is reversed in the presence of carbamazepine (CBZ). (A) Current clamp recordings were performed on small (≥30 μm) to medium (≥40 μm) dorsal root ganglion (DRG) neurons (L1-6) from naïve rats. Firing of two to four action potentials (APs) was elicited by a 1 second depolarizing current injection (ranging from 0.1 to 0.6 nA depending on the cell) every 30 seconds. Representative recordings demonstrating that application of 3 μg/mL M3G increases the number of elicited APs. Bath applied CBZ reversed the effect of M3G-increased excitability. (B) Group data showing that M3G caused a significant increase in DRG AP firing that is reversed by CBZ (*$P<0.05$).

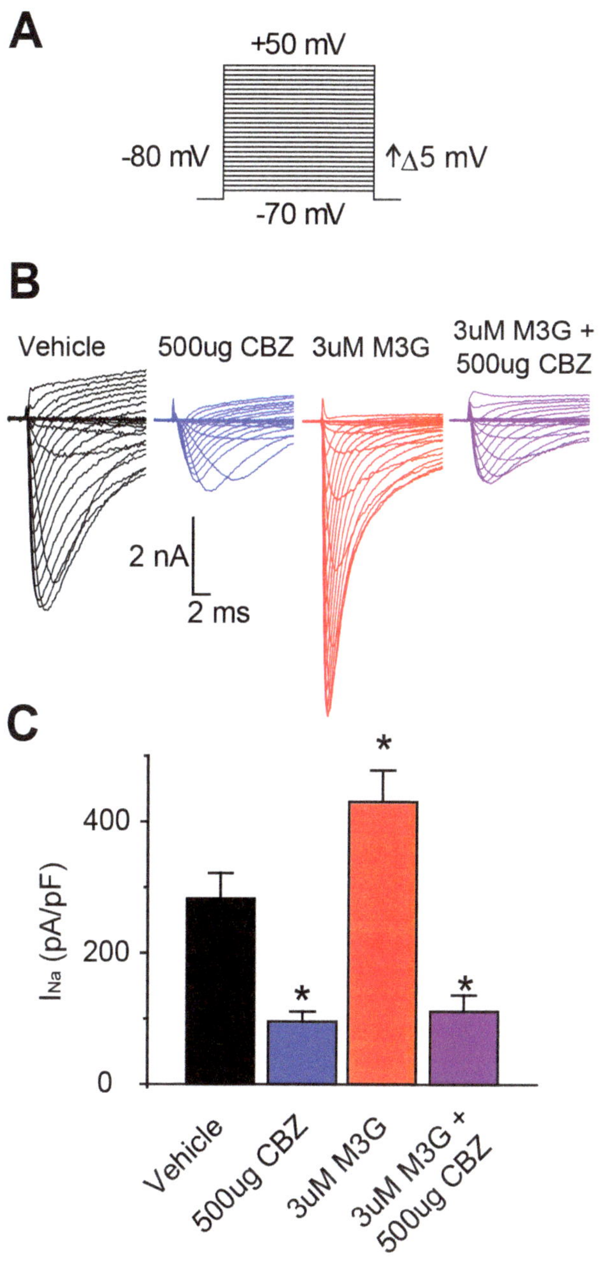

Figure 3. Morphine-3-glucuronide (M3G) potentiation of sodium currents is blocked by carbamazepine (CBZ). A, currents were elicited by performing voltage steps from a holding potential of −80 mV, in 5 mV increments, from −70 mV to +50 mV. B, representative traces from dorsal root ganglia cells treated with either 0.1% DMSO (Vehicle), 500 ug CBZ, 3 μM M3G, or both 3 μM M3G and 500 ug CBZ. C, peak currents (pA) were normalized to cell capacitance (pF) to measure current density (pA/pF). Asterisks indicate statistically significant differences between treatment groups and vehicle group (*$P<0.05$, one way ANOVA with Tukey's post-hoc test). Bars represent mean ± S.E.

conditions, however neuropathic pain tends to be less responsive to opioids. The ability of morphine to evoke pain relief diminishes over time and may be partially due to the ability of the opioid and the metabolite M3G to act through non-classic opioid receptors [31]. To identify the limits of morphine to reduce hypernociception following induction of a rodent neuropathic pain model, rats were subjected to a TNI procedure and tested at post-injury day 7 (PID7). All tested animals demonstrated signs of mechanical allodynia with ipsilateral threshold values of 28.7±2.5 mN compared with pre-surgery withdrawal threshold values of 72.1±5.0 mN ($n=64$; $p<0.001$) (**Fig. 4A**). The injured animals continued to exhibit mechanical allodynia for as long as they were monitored. Body weight and general welfare (grooming/socialization) of the animals were routinely observed and appeared to be unaffected by the nerve injury.

The dose-response function for the morphine reversal of TNI pain at PID7 was determined using a within-subjects design. Rats were habituated and baseline testing conducted as described in the methods. Not unlike previous work by Erichsen and Blackburn-Monro [32], systemic administration of low dose morphine (0.5 or 1 mg/kg, i.p.) had no effect on withdrawal threshold up to 120 min post-injection for the ipsilateral hindlimb compared with either the pre-injection withdrawal threshold or with vehicle-treated animals at the corresponding time points. In contrast, i.p. injection of morphine at 5 mg/kg significantly increased withdrawal threshold of the ipsilateral hindlimb 30 min after injection to 73±1.6 mN ($F=12.81$, $p<0.05$), compared with baseline and vehicle), and this effect continued up to 90 min, before returning to a level of sensitivity comparable with baseline and vehicle at 120 min (**Fig. 4A**).

To test the degree to which the 5 mg/kg (i.p.) concentration of morphine is effective for the reversal of TNI-induced tactile allodynia across time, independent groups of injured rats at PID 14 ($n=8$), 21 ($n=8$), and 28 ($n=8$) were also assayed for mechanical allodynia following morphine administration. At a dosage of 5 mg/kg of morphine in the rodents, tactile allodynia was reversed in PID 14 animals. However, this dosage proved ineffective at PID 21 or 28, with no significant differences in pain behavior ($F=48.14$, $p<0.05$, **Fig. 4B**).

Combination of morphine and carbamazepine reverses TNI-induced tactile allodynia at post-injury day 28 in a dose dependent manner

It is known that administration of M3G can induce tactile allodynia through a TLR4-mediated mechanism in the absence of nerve injury [9]. That neuronal exposure to M3G and the associated potentiation of NaV currents in vitro can be reversed by CBZ suggests a potential benefit of a combination pharmacotherapy approach using morphine and CBZ *in vivo* for TNI-induced tactile allodynia. To first determine whether CBZ alone is effective for TNI-induced tactile allodynia, we administered CBZ 10 mg/kg i.p. to TNI rodents at PID28 and compared the outcomes to similar injections of morphine 5 mg/kg i.p. at PID 28. Neither drug negated the injury-induced behavior ($F=19.2$, $p<0.05$, **Fig. 5A**).

The potential impact of NaV1.7 in the injured peripheral nervous system may be pain syndrome specific as determined by NaV1.7 knockout mouse strains [33] and gain of NaV1.7 function appears to result in congenital insensitivity to pain or lead to severe familial pain disorders [34]. However diminishing the off-target effects of morphine directly or via its metabolite M3G may offer increased analgesic value for the widely used clinical opioid. As a proof-of-concept, morphine was combined with CBZ to produce a novel combination pharmacotherapy. In the 2-drug-combination studies, morphine plus CBZ completely attenuated mechanical allodynia at 5 mg/kg and 1 mg/kg concentration ($F=19.2$, $p<0.05$, **Fig. 5B**). Additional analysis revealed that there was increased efficacy with the combination pharmacotherapy of 5 mg/kg morphine and 10 mg/kg CBZ as PWTs following administration of both drugs did not return to pre-injury levels for

Table 2.

Condition	Activation		Fast Inactivation	
	V1/2	k	V1/2	k
Vehicle	−17.4±2.1 (n = 4)	6.7±0.7 (n = 4)	−50.3±1.5 (n = 4)	14.8±1.4 (n = 4)
500 ug CBZ	−12.4±1.7 (n = 5)	5.4±0.5 (n = 5)	−82.9±3.6 (n = 4)	17.7±2.7 (n = 4)
3 μM M3G	−17.0±2.1 (n = 5)	6.7±0.7 (n = 5)	−52.7±1.9 (n = 5)	18.5±2.3 (n = 5)
3 μM M3G + 500 ug CBZ	−21.4±0.4 (n = 3)	3.0±0.3 (n = 3)	−45.7±3.0 (n = 3)	11.1±2.1 (n = 3)

at least 240 minutes in the PID28 rodent group. Similar observations were present in age-matched male rodents subjected to TNI (data not shown; n = 6–8 per post injury time point).

Increased NaV1.7 expression following tibial nerve injury by post-injury day 28

Given the relative selectivity of CBZ for the NaV1.7 current state [20] and a recent report by Laedermann and colleagues which describes spared nerve injury-induced increases in NaV1.7 [35,36], we sought to determine the degree to which TNI changes in NaV1.7 correspond with morphine efficacy across time. Based on a quantitative real time PCR analysis, it appears that rodents subjected to TNI exhibited substantial increases in NaV1.7 mRNA by day 28 compared to naïve tissue levels, whereas post-injury day 14 values did not reach statistical significance (**Fig. 6**; n = 4, ANOVA, F = 5.571; $p < 0.05$).

Discussion

It is known that opioids such as morphine and opioid metabolites induce glial-associated inflammatory responses within the brain and spinal cord via the non-classical opioid receptor, TLR4 [12]. Ligand activation of neuronal TLR4 has also been observed in the nervous system [8,10,37] and may play a direct role in the diminished efficacy of opioids in neuropathic pain conditions. The present set of multidisciplinary studies provide converging lines of evidence that TLR4-mediated increased neuronal excitation is likely dependent upon the CBZ-sensitive sodium current, and that the latent increase in NaV1.7 mRNA expression in sensory ganglia following TNI contributes to decreased opioid efficacy in a rodent model of neuropathic pain.

The use of opioids such as morphine to treat neuropathic pain is controversial due to the mixed results of clinical studies and is considered to be a second or third tier of treatment at best [38] [39]. Pre-clinical evidence indeed supports the observation that the analgesic effects of morphine are greatly diminished in the setting of neuropathic pain and quite often necessitates greater concentrations of morphine to provide pain relief. The mechanisms associated with these changes in opioid efficacy are often attributed to opioid tolerance. However, clear examples of the loss of morphine analgesia are evident in models of neuropathic pain such as spared nerve injury. Erichsen and Blackburn-Monro first demonstrated that this type of injury model required systemic doses of up to 6 mg/kg morphine for nociceptive pain relief at day 7 [32]. In contrast, doses of morphine as high as 10–30 mg/kg are necessary to provide relief for neuropathic pain at post-injury day 14 [40,41]. A comparison of the opioid dose needed to reverse mechanical allodynia in the present study appear to parallel these previous observations as the efficacy of the morphine dose that provided opioid analgesia up to day 14 was completely lacking at injury day 21 or 28. Together, these data readily indicate that the efficacy of morphine alone in attenuation of tactile allodynia is refractory over time following injury-induced changes in the neurobiology of the rodent.

Though the analgesic mechanism of opioids is largely thought to modulate transmission of pain sensation at the level of the spinal cord or by altering the perception of painful stimulus/stimulus-independent pain at cortical regions [42], it is conceivable that cell membrane bound receptors other than opioid receptors in either the spinal cord or the peripheral nervous system may contribute to the diminished efficacy of opioids in neuropathic pain conditions over time. For example, numerous lines of evidence suggest that the pathogenesis of neuropathic pain is dependent in part on abnormal spontaneous activity within sensory neurons [29,43,44]. As this spontaneous activity is likely dependent on NaVs for the generation and conduction of action potentials, it is conceivable that neuronal hyperexcitability after injury is dependent on injury-induced changes in specific isoforms of NaV channels including NaV1.7 [45]. Molecular mechanisms which may contribute to the latent changes in sodium channel expression include the ubiquitin protein ligase known as neuronal precursor cell expressed developmentally downregulated-4 type 2 or NEDD4-2 [35]. NEDD4-2 was recently identified as a posttranslational regulator of a number of different sodium channels including NaV1.7 [35]. Subsequently reduced levels of NEDD4-2 due to peripheral nerve injury may contribute to the development of both neuropathic pain disorders and diminished analgesic efficacy of opioids.

Expression of both Navl.7 and TLR4 may endow small nociceptive neurons with rapid repriming abilities that contribute to spontaneous discharge or hyperexcitability in the presence of opioids or opioid metabolites. To potentially control for the off-target effect of morphine or its metabolite M3G, we utilized CBZ in combination with morphine. CBZ is known to produce a substantial block of electrical activity associated with NaV current in sensory neurons and stably transfected human embryonic kidney 293 cells expressing wild-type NaV1.7 independent of resurgent currents [19,20]. Given the apparent effects of CBZ blockade of NaV current, it is reasonable to conclude that the combination of morphine with CBZ diminishes opioid-induced enhancement of electrical activity potentially associated with NaV1.7 in nociceptive sensory neurons while the central nervous system effects of morphine elicits analgesia sufficient to influence nociceptive behavior in the TNI model of neuropathic pain. However, evidence contained herein also suggests that responsive neurons elicit a range of current changes following exposure to M3G, all of which are greater that the averaged control value. This range of effects may be dependent on varying extents of expression of necessary pathway proteins in the heterogeneous system [9,46]. Although not tested in this study, it is unlikely that other anti-epileptic drugs such as gabapentin and pregabalin elicit

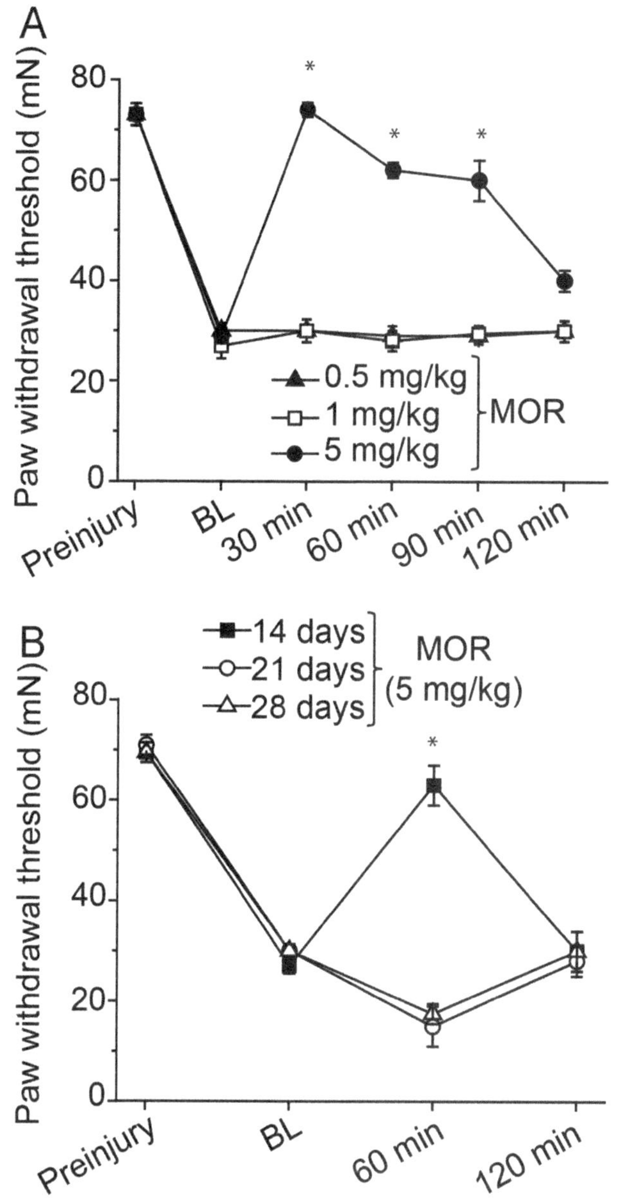

Figure 4. Dose- and time-effects of intraperitoneally administered morphine (MOR) on tactile allodynia in the tibial nerve injury (TNI) model at post-injury day 7. (A) The ability of MOR to attenuate tactile allodynia induced by TNI in a dose-dependent fashion was limited to 5 mg/kg. Each line represents the groups mean and SEM of 6–10 female rats. Drug group behavior at 30, 60, 90, or 120 minute vs TNI baseline (BL) behavior. (B) Time-dependent effects of intraperitoneally administered morphine (MOR) on tactile allodynia in the tibial nerve injury (TNI) model at post-injury day (PID) 14, 21 and 28. The ability of MOR to attenuate tactile allodynia induced by TNI was evident in PID 14 rats but not animals at PID21 or 28. Each line represents the groups mean and SEM of 6–10 rats. Drug group behavior at 60 minute or 120 minute vs TNI baseline (BL) behavior (*$P<0.05$).

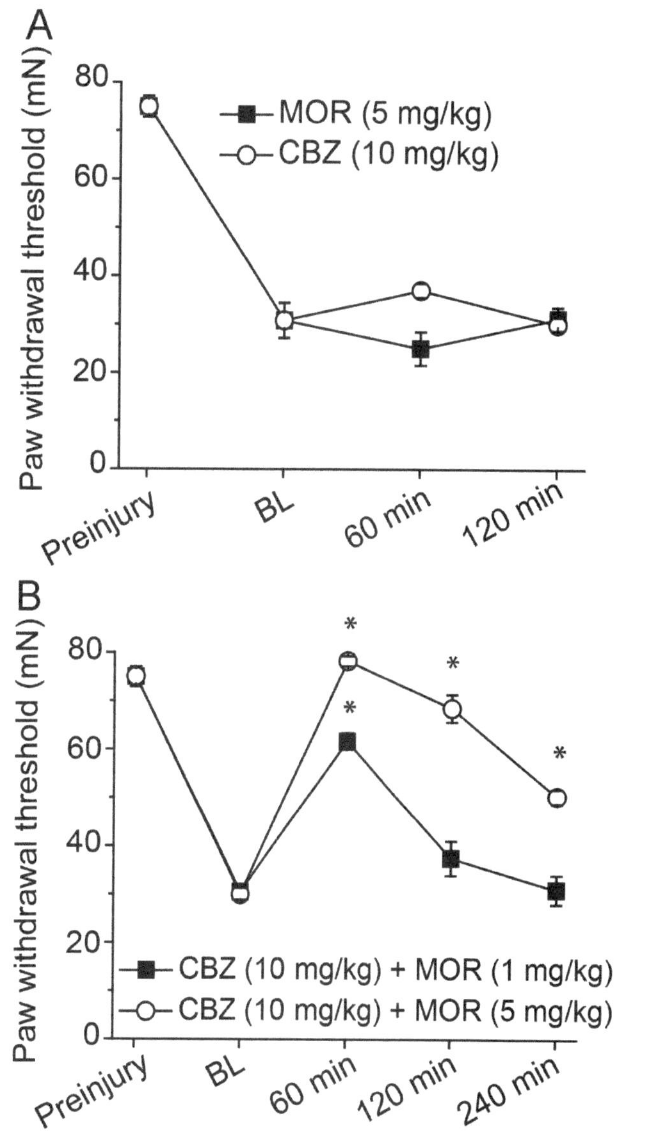

Figure 5. The effect of intraperitoneally administered morphine (MOR), carbamazepine (CBZ) or combination of MOR/CBZ on tactile allodynia in the tibial nerve injury (TNI) model at post-injury day (PID) 28. (A) Neither MOR or CBZ affect tactile allodynia induced by TNI. Each line represents the groups mean and SEM of 6–10 female rats. Drug group behavior at 60 minute or 120 minute vs TNI baseline (BL) behavior. (B) Effect of co-administered MOR and CBZ on tactile allodynia in the tibial nerve injury (TNI) model at post-injury day 28. The ability of MOR/CBZ to attenuate tactile allodynia induced by TNI was dose-dependent. Each line represents the groups mean and SEM of 6–10 rats. (*$P<0.05$; combination therapy group vs TNI baseline (BL) behavior).

similar effects as neither compound directly affects sodium current in a similar fashion [47].

The neuronal excitability mediated by opioids or their metabolites via TLR4 could also be influenced by signaling downstream of the receptor and may influence both capsaicin and non-capsaicin sensitive neurons. For example, it is possible that coordinated interactions between TLR4 ligands and sensory neurons could evoke TNFα-dependent tactile hypersensitivity and may be indicative of signaling dependent on the MyD88 signaling pathway [48]. Other proinflammatory cytokines which could conceivably be altered by the neuronal TLR4/MyD88 pathway including interleukin-1β [49] and deserves further investigation. However, the observed M3G-related neuronal signaling events are rapid and may be independent of signal transcription factors. Alternatively, the assembly of TLR adapter signaling proteins and activation of phospholipids in neurons may

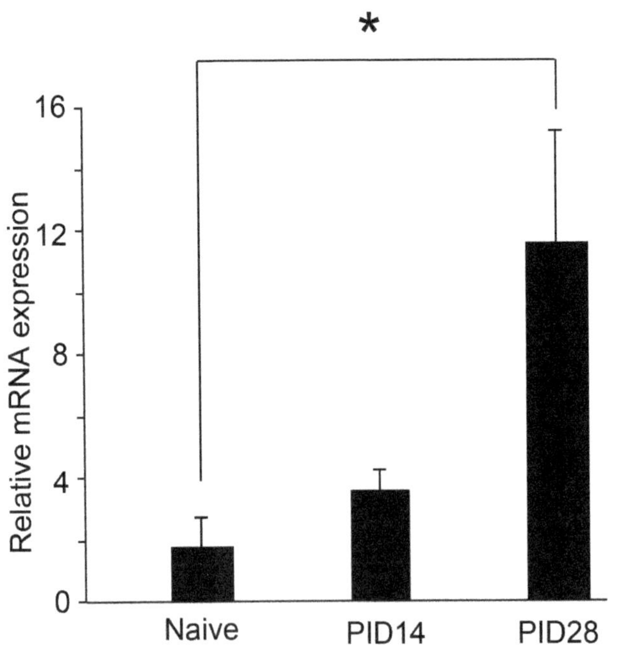

Figure 6. Tibal Nerve Injury (TNI) alters the expression of neuronal transcripts in rat dorsal root ganglion (DRG). RT-PCR analysis showing the mRNA expression profile of NaV1.7 in the DRG derived from naïve animal and at different time points following TNI; post injury day (PID) 14 and PID 28 (n = 3). RT-PCR data were analyzed using the Ct method and mRNA expression levels are expressed relative to L27- ribosomal housekeeping gene. (*P<0.05; TNI gene expression vs naive threshold baseline).

only require activation of a signal-transduction pathway leading to the observed increase in NaV current [50]. Additional studies are also underway to determine the degree to which hormonal regulation of neuronal TLR4 responses serve to influence neuropathic pain states alone or in combination with opioids [48,51].

The apparent lack of morphine efficacy *in vivo* may depend on the increased expression of NaV1.7 in the rat DRG following injury to the peripheral nerve. Given the negligible change of gene expression change up to PID14, morphine administration serves as an effective means by which to transiently reverse TNI-induced mechanical allodynia. However, the observed pronounced increase in NaV1.7 expression observed by PID28 in the rat supports the functional change in the inability of morphine to attenuate mechanical allodynia. The degree to which injury produces similar effects in murine spared nerve injury models is unknown and may vary from species to species [36].

It is likely that abnormal functioning of sodium channels in the peripheral nervous system is a key event in both the etiology of neuropathic pain [52] and opioid-induced hyperalgesia [9]. Subsequently, there are potential avenues for the use of morphine in combination with several FDA-approved partial seizure therapeutics currently known to affect the NaV1.7 current; lacosamide [20] or rufinamide [53] or possibly the anti-depressant duloxetine [54]. Oxcarbazepine, as a structural derivative of CBZ, may also affect NaV1.7 and serve as a suitable combinatorial therapeutic in combination with morphine for chronic pain (see Clinical Trials Registry No. NCT02078089). In contrast, anti-convulsive therapeutics that target focal seizure disorders by acting on voltage-sensitive calcium channels may not be able to diminish the off-target effects of opioids or provide enhanced opioid efficacy [55].

Together, the increased neuronal excitability via opioid-metabolite mediated neuronal TLR4 signaling increased NaV current in sensory neurons may serve as a robust signal to dampen the analgesic effects of morphine over time. However, here we show that the dampening of the analgesic effects of morphine on neuropathic pain behavior in vivo can be countered with the addition of CBZ. Thus, the same peripheral sensory neurons may possess opposing properties that elicit a critical interplay of mechanisms which may be central to the understanding of tolerance and paradoxical allodynia that can occur with opioid-based therapies.

Acknowledgments

We gratefully acknowledge Drs. Theodore Cummins and Zhiyong Tan for valuable discussion and critical reading of the manuscript. This work was supported by the NIH (DA026040 to FAW; DK100905 to FAW and RK); the National Scientist Development from the American Heart Association (SDG5280023 to RK); the Neurofibromatosis New Investigator Award from the DOD/CDMRP (NF1000099 to RK). Additional support for YMA as an Indiana CTSI Predoctoral trainee was provided by UL1 TR001107, NIH/NCATS (A. Shekhar, PI). The authors declare no conflicts of interest.

Author Contributions

Conceived and designed the experiments: MRD RK FAW. Performed the experiments: MRD XFY ALR MSR ETD YMA SMW. Analyzed the data: MRD YMA RK FAW. Contributed reagents/materials/analysis tools: YMA MRD RK FAW. Wrote the paper: MRD YMA RK FAW. Behavior/Physiology experiments: YMA MRD MSR XFY ETD SMW ALR.

References

1. Watson CP, Moulin D, Watt-Watson J, Gordon A, Eisenhoffer J (2003) Controlled-release oxycodone relieves neuropathic pain: a randomized controlled trial in painful diabetic neuropathy. Pain 105: 71–78.
2. Inturrisi CE, Lipman AG (2010) Opioid Analgesics; Fishman SM, Ballantyne JC, Rathmell JP, editors. Philadelphia: Lippincott Williams & Wilkins.
3. Angst MS, Clark JD (2006) Opioid-induced hyperalgesia: a qualitative systematic review. Anesthesiology 104: 570–587.
4. Ossipov MH, Lai J, King T, Vanderah TW, Malan TP Jr, et al. (2004) Antinociceptive and nociceptive actions of opioids. J Neurobiol 61: 126–148.
5. Vanderah TW, Suenaga NM, Ossipov MH, Malan TP Jr, Lai J, et al. (2001) Tonic descending facilitation from the rostral ventromedial medulla mediates opioid-induced abnormal pain and antinociceptive tolerance. J Neurosci 21: 279–286.
6. Drdla R, Gassner M, Gingl E, Sandkuhler J (2009) Induction of synaptic long-term potentiation after opioid withdrawal. Science 325: 207–210.
7. Heinl C, Drdla-Schutting R, Xanthos DN, Sandkuhler J (2011) Distinct mechanisms underlying pronociceptive effects of opioids. J Neurosci 31: 16748–16756.
8. Diogenes A, Ferraz CC, Akopian AN, Henry MA, Hargreaves KM (2011) LPS Sensitizes TRPV1 via Activation of TLR4 in Trigeminal Sensory Neurons. J Dent Res Jun; 90(6): 759–764.
9. Due MR, Piekarz AD, Wilson N, Feldman P, Ripsch MS, et al. (2012) Neuroexcitatory effects of morphine-3-glucuronide are dependent on Toll-like receptor 4 signaling. J Neuroinflammation 9: 200.
10. Maroso M, Balosso S, Ravizza T, Liu J, Aronica E, et al. (2010) Toll-like receptor 4 and high-mobility group box-1 are involved in ictogenesis and can be targeted to reduce seizures. Nat Med 16: 413–419.
11. Yaksh TL, Harty GJ, Onofrio BM (1986) High dose of spinal morphine produce a nonopiate receptor-mediated hyperesthesia: clinical and theoretic implications. Anesthesiology 64: 590–597.

12. Wang X, Loram LC, Ramos K, de Jesus AJ, Thomas J, et al. (2012) Morphine activates neuroinflammation in a manner parallel to endotoxin. Proc Natl Acad Sci U S A 109: 6325–6330.
13. Alfonso-Loeches S, Pascual-Lucas M, Blanco AM, Sanchez-Vera I, Guerri C (2010) Pivotal role of TLR4 receptors in alcohol-induced neuroinflammation and brain damage. J Neurosci 30: 8285–8295.
14. Lewis SS, Hutchinson MR, Zhang Y, Hund DK, Maier SF, et al. (2013) Glucuronic acid and the ethanol metabolite ethyl-glucuronide cause toll-like receptor 4 activation and enhanced pain. Brain Behav Immun 30: 24–32.
15. Hutchinson MR, Zhang Y, Shridhar M, Evans JH, Buchanan MM, et al. (2010) Evidence that opioids may have toll-like receptor 4 and MD-2 effects. Brain Behav Immun 24: 83–95.
16. Eidson LN, Murphy AZ (2013) Blockade of Toll-like receptor 4 attenuates morphine tolerance and facilitates the pain relieving properties of morphine. J Neurosci 33: 15952–15963.
17. Fischer TZ, Gilmore ES, Estacion M, Eastman E, Taylor S, et al. (2009) A novel Nav1.7 mutation producing carbamazepine-responsive erythromelalgia. Ann Neurol 65: 733–741.
18. Jo S, Bean BP (2014) Sidedness of carbamazepine accessibility to voltage-gated sodium channels. Mol Pharmacol 85: 381–387.
19. Theile JW, Cummins TR (2011) Inhibition of Navbeta4 peptide-mediated resurgent sodium currents in Nav1.7 channels by carbamazepine, riluzole, and anandamide. Mol Pharmacol 80: 724–734.
20. Sheets PL, Heers C, Stoehr T, Cummins TR (2008) Differential block of sensory neuronal voltage-gated sodium channels by lacosamide [(2R)-2-(acetylamino)-N-benzyl-3-methoxypropanamide], lidocaine, and carbamazepine. J Pharmacol Exp Ther 326: 89–99.
21. Black JA, Liu S, Waxman SG (2009) Sodium channel activity modulates multiple functions in microglia. Glia 57: 1072–1081.
22. Feldman P, Due MR, Ripsch MS, Khanna R, White FA (2012) The persistent release of HMGB1 contributes to tactile hyperalgesia in a rodent model of neuropathic pain. J Neuroinflammation 9: 180.
23. Wang Y, Wilson SM, Brittain JM, Ripsch MS, Salome C, et al. (2011) Merging Structural Motifs of Functionalized Amino Acids and alpha-Aminoamides Results in Novel Anticonvulsant Compounds with Significant Effects on Slow and Fast Inactivation of Voltage-gated Sodium Channels and in the Treatment of Neuropathic Pain. ACS Chem Neurosci 2: 317–322.
24. Lee BH, Won R, Baik EJ, Lee SH, Moon CH (2000) An animal model of neuropathic pain employing injury to the sciatic nerve branches. Neuroreport 11: 657–661.
25. Ju W, Li Q, Allette YM, Ripsch MS, White FA, et al. (2012) Suppression of pain-related behavior in two distinct rodent models of peripheral neuropathy by a homopolyarginine-conjugated CRMP2 peptide. J Neurochem Oct 26. doi: 10.1111/jnc.12070. [Epub ahead of print].
26. Ma C, Shu Y, Zheng Z, Chen Y, Yao H, et al. (2003) Similar Electrophysiological Changes in Axotomized and Neighboring Intact Dorsal Root Ganglion Neurons. J Neurophysiol 89: 1588–1602.
27. Bhangoo S, Ren D, Miller RJ, Henry KJ, Lineswala J, et al. (2007) Delayed functional expression of neuronal chemokine receptors following focal nerve demyelination in the rat: a mechanism for the development of chronic sensitization of peripheral nociceptors. Mol Pain 3: 38.
28. Brittain JM, Duarte DB, Wilson SM, Zhu W, Ballard C, et al. (2011) Suppression of inflammatory and neuropathic pain by uncoupling CRMP-2 from the presynaptic Ca(2)(+) channel complex. Nat Med 17: 822–829.
29. Ma C, LaMotte RH (2005) Enhanced excitability of dissociated primary sensory neurons after chronic compression of the dorsal root ganglion in the rat. Pain 113: 106–112.
30. Hou L, Wang X (2001) PKC and PKA, but not PKG mediate LPS-induced CGRP release and [Ca(2+)](i) elevation in DRG neurons of neonatal rats. J Neurosci Res 66: 592–600.
31. Hutchinson MR, Shavit Y, Grace PM, Rice KC, Maier SF, et al. (2011) Exploring the neuroimmunopharmacology of opioids: an integrative review of mechanisms of central immune signaling and their implications for opioid analgesia. Pharmacol Rev 63: 772–810.
32. Erichsen HK, Blackburn-Munro G (2002) Pharmacological characterisation of the spared nerve injury model of neuropathic pain. Pain 98: 151–161.
33. Minett MS, Falk S, Santana-Varela S, Bogdanov YD, Nassar MA, et al. (2014) Pain without nociceptors? Nav1.7-independent pain mechanisms. Cell Rep 6: 301–312.
34. Raouf R, Rugiero F, Kiesewetter H, Hatch R, Hummler E, et al. (2012) Sodium channels and mammalian sensory mechanotransduction. Mol Pain 8: 21.
35. Laedermann CJ, Cachemaille M, Kirschmann G, Pertin M, Gosselin RD, et al. (2013) Dysregulation of voltage-gated sodium channels by ubiquitin ligase NEDD4-2 in neuropathic pain. J Clin Invest 123: 3002–3013.
36. Laedermann CJ, Pertin M, Suter MR, Decosterd I (2014) Voltage-gated sodium channel expression in mouse DRG after SNI leads to re-evaluation of projections of injured fibers. Mol Pain 10: 19.
37. Ochoa-Cortes F, Ramos-Lomas T, Miranda-Morales M, Spreadbury I, Ibeakanma C, et al. (2010) Bacterial cell products signal to mouse colonic nociceptive dorsal root ganglia neurons. Am J Physiol Gastrointest Liver Physiol 299: G723–732.
38. O'Connor AB, Dworkin RH (2009) Treatment of neuropathic pain: an overview of recent guidelines. Am J Med 122: S22–32.
39. Eisenberg E, McNicol ED, Carr DB (2005) Efficacy and safety of opioid agonists in the treatment of neuropathic pain of nonmalignant origin: systematic review and meta-analysis of randomized controlled trials. JAMA 293: 3043–3052.
40. Miyazaki R, Yamamoto T (2012) The efficacy of morphine, pregabalin, gabapentin, and duloxetine on mechanical allodynia is different from that on neuroma pain in the rat neuropathic pain model. Anesth Analg 115: 182–188.
41. Decosterd I, Allchorne A, Woolf CJ (2004) Differential analgesic sensitivity of two distinct neuropathic pain models. Anesth Analg 99: 457–463.
42. Ossipov MH, Lai J, King T, Vanderah TW, Porreca F (2005) Underlying mechanisms of pronociceptive consequences of prolonged morphine exposure. Biopolymers 80: 319–324.
43. Devor M (2006) Sodium channels and mechanisms of neuropathic pain. J Pain 7: S3–S12.
44. Ma C, LaMotte RH (2007) Multiple sites for generation of ectopic spontaneous activity in neurons of the chronically compressed dorsal root ganglion. J Neurosci 27: 14059–14068.
45. Dib-Hajj SD, Yang Y, Black JA, Waxman SG (2013) The Na(V)1.7 sodium channel: from molecule to man. Nat Rev Neurosci 14: 49–62.
46. Allette YM, Due MR, Wilson SM, Feldman P, Ripsch MS, et al. (2014) Identification of a functional interaction of HMGB1 with Receptor for Advanced Glycation End-products in a model of neuropathic pain. Brain Behav Immun. 10.1016/j.bbi.2014.06.199.
47. Zhang JL, Yang JP, Zhang JR, Li RQ, Wang J, et al. (2013) Gabapentin reduces allodynia and hyperalgesia in painful diabetic neuropathy rats by decreasing expression level of Nav1.7 and p-ERK1/2 in DRG neurons. Brain Res 1493: 13–18.
48. Stokes JA, Cheung J, Eddinger K, Corr M, Yaksh TL (2013) Toll-like receptor signaling adapter proteins govern spread of neuropathic pain and recovery following nerve injury in male mice. J Neuroinflammation 10: 148.
49. Tse KH, Chow KB, Leung WK, Wong YH, Wise H (2014) Lipopolysaccharide differentially modulates expression of cytokines and cyclooxygenases in dorsal root ganglion cells via Toll-like receptor-4 dependent pathways. Neuroscience 267: 241–251.
50. Kagan JC, Medzhitov R (2006) Phosphoinositide-mediated adaptor recruitment controls Toll-like receptor signaling. Cell 125: 943–955.
51. Sorge RE, LaCroix-Fralish ML, Tuttle AH, Sotocinal SG, Austin JS, et al. (2011) Spinal cord Toll-like receptor 4 mediates inflammatory and neuropathic hypersensitivity in male but not female mice. J Neurosci 31: 15450–15454.
52. Waxman SG, Zamponi GW (2014) Regulating excitability of peripheral afferents: emerging ion channel targets. Nat Neurosci 17: 153–163.
53. Suter MR, Kirschmann G, Laedermann CJ, Abriel H, Decosterd I (2013) Rufinamide attenuates mechanical allodynia in a model of neuropathic pain in the mouse and stabilizes voltage-gated sodium channel inactivated state. Anesthesiology 118: 160–172.
54. Wang SY, Calderon J, Kuo Wang G (2010) Block of neuronal Na+ channels by antidepressant duloxetine in a state-dependent manner. Anesthesiology 113: 655–665.
55. Gilron I, Bailey JM, Tu D, Holden RR, Weaver DF, et al. (2005) Morphine, gabapentin, or their combination for neuropathic pain. N Engl J Med 352: 1324–1334.

A Capsaicin (8%) Patch in the Treatment of Severe Persistent Inguinal Postherniorrhaphy Pain: A Randomized, Double-Blind, Placebo-Controlled Trial

Joakim M. Bischoff[1]*, Thomas K. Ringsted[1], Marian Petersen[1], Claudia Sommer[2], Nurcan Üçeyler[2], Mads U. Werner[1]

1 Multidisciplinary Pain Center 7612, Neuroscience Center, Rigshospitalet, Copenhagen University, Copenhagen, Denmark, 2 Department of Neurology, University Hospital of Würzburg, Würzburg, Germany

Abstract

Background: Persistent pain after inguinal herniorrhaphy is a disabling condition with a lack of evidence-based pharmacological treatment options. This randomized placebo-controlled trial investigated the efficacy of a capsaicin 8% cutaneous patch in the treatment of severe persistent inguinal postherniorrhaphy pain.

Methods: Forty-six patients with persistent inguinal postherniorrhaphy pain were randomized to receive either a capsaicin 8% patch or a placebo patch. Pain intensity (Numerical Rating Scale [NRS 0–10]) was evaluated under standardized conditions (at rest, during movement, and during pressure) at baseline and at 1, 2 and 3 months after patch application. Skin punch biopsies for intraepidermal nerve fiber density (IENFD) measurements were taken at baseline and 1 month after patch application. Quantitative sensory testing was performed at baseline and at 1, 2, and 3 months after patch application. The primary outcome was comparisons of summed pain intensity differences (SPIDs) between capsaicin and placebo treatments at 1, 2 and 3 months after patch application (significance level $P<0.01$).

Results: The maximum difference in SPID, between capsaicin and placebo treatments, was observed at 1 month after patch application, but the pain reduction was not significant (NRS, mean difference [95% CI]: 5.0 [0.09 to 9.9]; $P=0.046$). No differences in SPID between treatments were observed at 2 and 3 months after patch application. Changes in IENFD on the pain side, from baseline to 1 month after patch application, did not differ between capsaicin and placebo treatment: 1.9 [−0.1 to 3.9] and 0.6 [−1.2 to 2.5] fibers/mm, respectively ($P=0.32$). No significant changes in sensory function, sleep quality or psychological factors were associated with capsaicin patch treatment.

Conclusions: The study did not demonstrate significant differences in pain relief between capsaicin and placebo treatment, although a trend toward pain improvement in capsaicin treated patients was observed 1 month after patch application.

Trial Registration: Clinicaltrialsregister.eu 2012-001540-22 ClinicalTrials.gov NCT01699854

Editor: T. Mark Doherty, Glaxo Smith Kline, Denmark

Funding: The study was supported by an unrestricted research grant from Astellas Pharma a/s, Kastrup, Denmark (http://www.astellas.dk/). The funders had no role in study design, data collection and analysis, decision to publish, or preparation of the manuscript.

Competing Interests: The authors have read the journal's policy and have the following conflicts: JMB and MW have received an unrestricted research grant from Grünenthal GmbH, Aachen, Germany. CS and NÜ have been speakers for Astellas GmbH, Germany and NÜ has received travel grants from Astellas GmbH, Germany.

* Email: jomutahi@hotmail.com

Introduction

Inguinal herniorrhaphy is a common surgical procedure with more than 800.000 repairs annually in the United States [1]. Persistent severe pain affecting daily activities is present in 5% of patients [2,3] and in spite of exploratory surgery including selective neurectomy [4,5], that has been associated with a satisfactory outcome, the invasive nature of the procedure requires availability of medical treatment options for patients reluctant to undergo repeat surgery or not fit for a surgical procedure. The evidence-base for pharmacological treatment of persistent pain following inguinal hernia repair is nearly non-existent and therefore it is of considerable clinical relevance to identify the efficaciousness of drug therapy.

The capsaicin 8% cutaneous patch is used in the treatment of peripheral neuropathic pain and significant pain-relief for up to 12 weeks has been observed in randomized, controlled trials in post-herpetic neuralgia and HIV-related distal neuropathy [6–10]. Capsaicin is a selective agonist for the transient receptor potential vanilloid (TRPV1) receptor residing on nociceptive peripheral nerve fibers and keratinocytes [11]. The effect of capsaicin is assumed to be mediated by a reversible defunctionalization of cutaneous nociceptors thereby inhibiting transmission of nociceptive signals [12,13]. The long lasting pain relieving effect, up to three months after a single capsaicin 8% patch application, is of particular clinical interest. From a pharmacodynamic view, the localized action of the capsaicin patch confers a reduced risk of systemic side effects and a lessened potential for drug interactions. In an un-controlled prospective study (n = 1,044) the capsaicin 8% patch relieved pain and improved sleep quality in patients with various peripheral neuropathic pain states [14]. Interestingly, in this cohort 23% of the patients experienced persistent postsurgical pain of differing etiologies. However, the efficacy of capsaicin 8% patch treatment has never been evaluated in a randomized controlled trial in persistent postsurgical pain. Purified capsaicin has been shown to reduce acute postoperative pain following inguinal hernia repair. In a randomized placebo-controlled trial intraoperative wound instillation of purified capsaicin significantly reduced pain scores in the capsaicin group during the first 4 days after inguinal hernia repair [15].

In the present study we tested the hypothesis that capsaicin 8% patch treatment would be associated with a higher analgesic efficacy compared to placebo in patients suffering from severe persistent inguinal postherniorrhaphy pain.

Since changes in intraepidermal nerve fiber density (IENFD) have been observed following capsaicin 8% patch application in healthy volunteers [16,17], we investigated the effect of capsaicin on IENFD and sensory function, assessed by thermal and mechanical thresholds, as secondary outcomes. Additional secondary outcomes were changes in ratings of sleep quality, catastrophizing behaviour, anxiety and depression, associated with capsaicin 8% patch treatment.

Materials and Methods

A randomized, double-blind, placebo-controlled, parallel-group study was conducted at the Multidisciplinary Pain Center, Rigshospitalet, Copenhagen with patients recruitment from August 2012 to May 2013 and follow-up from September 2012 to September 2013. Study approval was obtained from the Committee on Health Research Ethics of the Capital Region of Denmark (H-4-2012-055), the Danish Data Protection Agency, the Danish Medicines Agency (EudraCT-Nr. 2012-001540-22) and the study was registered at ClinicalTrials.gov (NCT01699854). The study was conducted in accordance with Good Clinical Practice (GCP) Guidelines and was monitored by the Copenhagen University Hospital GCP Unit. The protocol for this trial and supporting CONSORT checklist are available as supporting information; see Checklist S1 and Protocol S1.

Patients eligible in the study were referred to the Multidisciplinary Pain Center by a surgeon or a general practitioner and written informed consent was obtained from all patients. Patients were ≥18 years with severe unilateral persistent inguinal postherniorrhaphy pain (numerical rating scale [NRS, 0–10] ≥ 5) for more than 6 months. Concomitant analgesic medication was allowed if patients had maintained a stable regimen for at least 4 weeks prior to study entry and stayed on stable doses throughout the study period. Exclusion criteria were allergy to capsaicin or vehicle-ingredients in the patch, skin lesions or inflamed skin at the application site, bilateral groin pain, severe cardiac impairment, known diseases impairing nervous system function, alcohol or drug abuse, inability to understand Danish, and in female patients lactation or pregnancy (negative pregnancy test required for females of fertile age).

Randomization

Randomization was done by Herning Hospital Pharmacy according to a computer-generated randomization list (http://randomization.com/) and a block-size of four was used.

Pain assessment

Patients evaluated pain intensities (NRS) every morning and evening, at rest in the supine position, during transition from supine to standing position, and during the patient's palpation of the point of maximum pain in the groin. Assessments were made in the 3 days preceding the patch treatment (baseline) and in the 3 days preceding the clinical visits at 1, 2 and 3 months after patch application.

Questionnaires

Questionnaires were completed at baseline and at 1, 2 and 3 months after patch application. Anxiety and depression were evaluated with the Hospital Anxiety and Depression Scale (HADS) [18] and the level of catastrophizing behaviour with the Pain

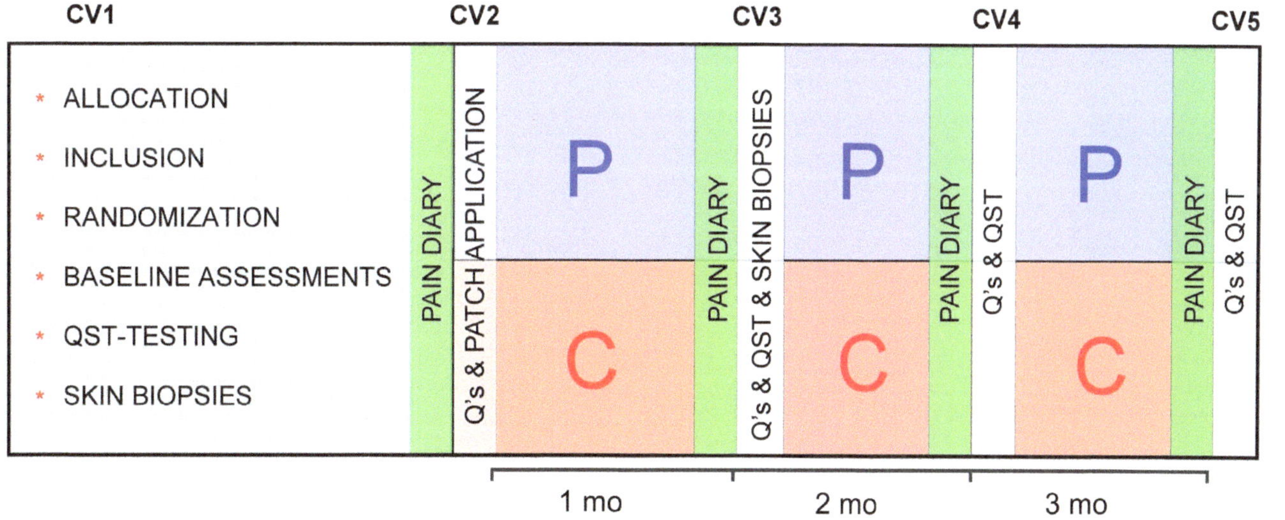

Figure 1. Study algorithm, CV = Clinical visit, Q's = Questionnaires.

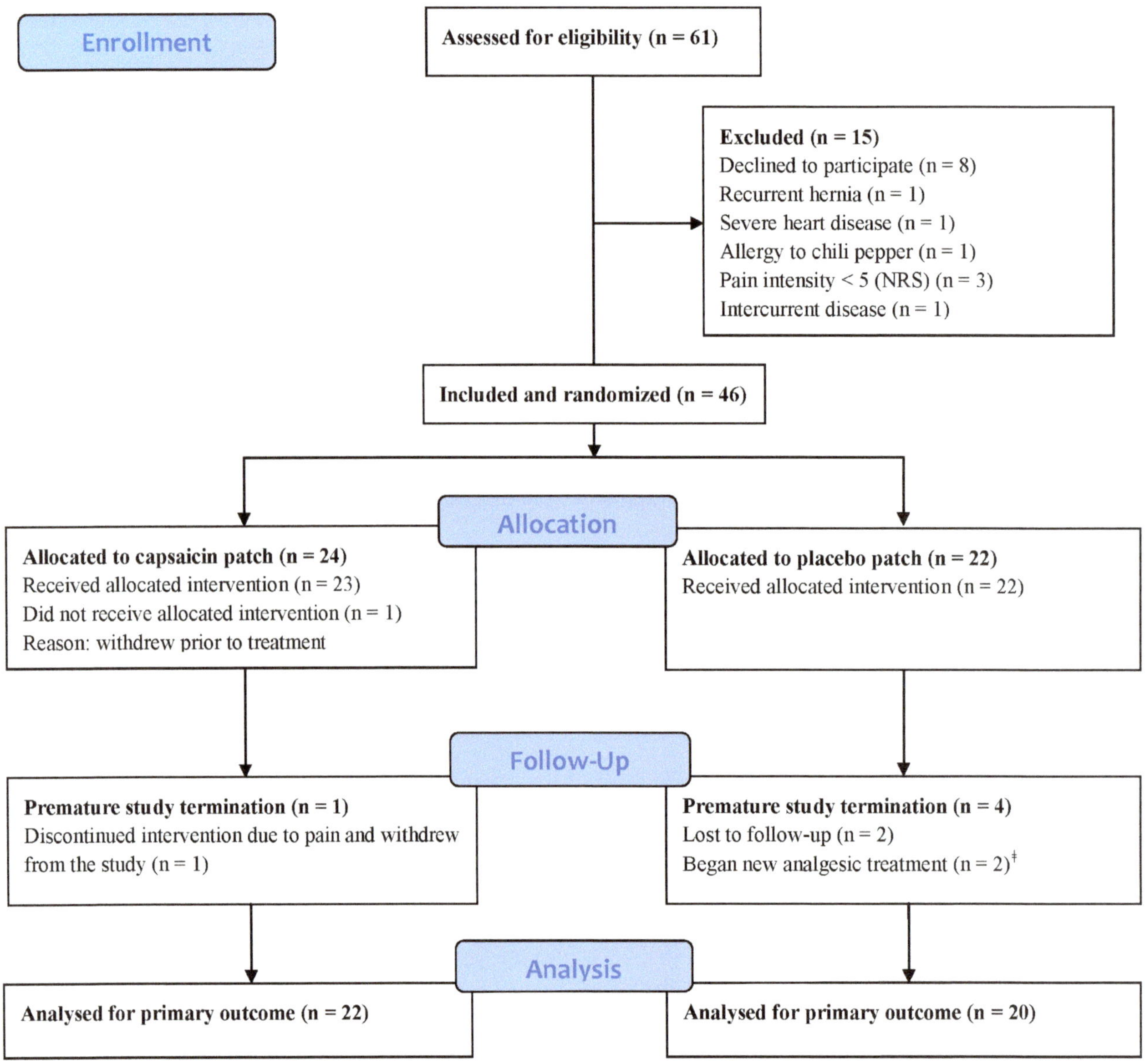

Figure 2. Flow diagram of patients in the study. ‡ Data from these two patients were included in the analyses up to the time of the medication violation. NRS = Numerical Rating Scale.

Catastrophizing Scale (PCS) [19]. Pain-related sleep interference was evaluated with the Daily Sleep Interference Scale (DSIS [0–10, 0 = pain did not interfere with sleep, 10 = pain completely interfered with sleep]) [20]. The self-report version of the Leeds Assessment of Neuropathic Symptoms and Signs pain scale (S-LANSS) was used for assessment of neuropathic pain components [21].

Quantitative sensory testing (QST)

Prior to the QST, hair growth in the inguinal and suprapubic areas was carefully trimmed using a surgical clipper (3M-9671, St. Paul, MN). The QST assessments were performed in accordance with previous studies in persistent inguinal postherniorrhaphy pain [22,23]. The sensory testing area on the pain side included the point of maximum pain and in addition the contralateral inguinal region was used as a control area. The warmth and cool detection thresholds (WDT, CDT) and the heat pain threshold (HPT) were determined using a computer controlled thermode (Somedic AB, Hörby, Sweden; contact area 2.5×5.0 cm^2). The baseline temperature was 32°C and thermal stimuli were delivered with a ramp rate of ±1°C/s with cut-off values of 50°C for heat, and 5°C for cold stimuli. The pressure pain threshold (PPT) was assessed at the point of maximum pain using a handheld pressure algometer (Somedic AB, Hörby, Sweden; 1 cm^2 felt-tipped probe) applied perpendicularly to the skin, until the pressure was perceived as painful or exceeded the cut-off value of 350 kPa. A heat stimulus (5 s at 47°C, ramp rate 1°C/s) was delivered at the point of maximum pain to evaluate the suprathreshold heat pain perception (STH) rated by the patient (NRS). All QST parameters were assessed three times and the median values were used. The QST was performed at baseline and at the clinical visits: at 1 month (day 30–36), 2 months (day 60–66), and 3 months (day 90–96) after patch application (fig. 1).

Table 1. Baseline patient characteristics.

	Capsaicin (n = 24)	Placebo (n = 22)
Age (yrs)[†]	52 (17)	55 (14)
Sex (male/female)	20/4	22/0
BMI (kg/m^2) [‡]	25 (23–30)	26 (23–28)
Duration of pain (mo)[‡]	37 (22–58)	39 (18–63)
Primary/recurrent operation[§], *n*	20/4	20/2
Open mesh/laparoscopic[§], *n*	21/3	17/5
Unilaterally/bilaterally operated, *n*	23/1	17/5
Exploratory surgery for pain, yes/no, *n*	10/14	7/15
Concomitant pain medication, yes/no, *n*	11/13	13/9
- Acetaminophen, *n*	7	7
- NSAIDs, *n*	3	7
- Gabapentin, *n*	2	4
- Tricyclic antidepressants, *n*	1	2
- Opioids, *n*	2	2
Baseline pain ratings[¶]		
- Pain at rest (NRS)	4 (3–7)	4 (3–6)
- Pain during movement (NRS)	5 (4–7)	6 (3–7)
- Pain during palpation (NRS)	7 (5–9)	7 (5–8)

[†]Mean (standard deviation).
[‡]Median (25–75% interquartile range).
[§]Pain-generating inguinal hernia operation.
[¶]Pain ratings at baseline assessed at rest in the supine position, during transition from supine to standing position, and during the patient's palpation of the point of maximum pain in the groin. Values are medians (25–75% interquartile range). Two patients who withdrew early from the study and one patient who was lost to follow-up did not report baseline pain ratings and were not included in the analyses of pain ratings.
BMI = Body Mass Index, NRS = Numerical Rating Scale (0–10), NSAIDs = Non-steroidal Anti-inflammatory Drugs.

Skin biopsies

At baseline and at the clinical visit at 1 month after patch application two 3-mm skin punch biopsies (disposable biopsy punch, Miltex, York, PA) were performed, using a sterile technique, at the point of maximum pain in the groin and on the contralateral control side. Prior to biopsies, the skin areas were anesthetized with 1–2 ml of mepivacaine (10 mg/ml, AstraZeneca AB, Södertälje, Sweden). The IENFD was estimated in agreement with previously described methods [23,24]. After fixation with 4% paraformaldehyde, the biopsies were washed in phosphate buffer and then stored in 10% sucrose with 0.1 M phosphate buffer at 4°C, until analysis. Sections of 50-μm thickness were immunostained with the pan-neuronal marker PGP-9.5 (1:800, Ultraclone, Wellow, UK) and visualized with Cy3-coupled anti-rabbit antibodies (1:100, Amersham Biosciences, Piscataway, NJ). Intraepidermal nerve fiber counting was performed with a light-microscope (Zeiss Axiophot 2, Wetzlar, Germany) and Spot advanced software (Windows Version 4.5, Sterling Heights, MI). The skin biopsies were analyzed blinded in regard to side.

Treatment procedure and blinding method

The research nurse and the physician responsible for the intervention did only meet the patient on the day of treatment and were not further involved in the study. The research nurse delineated the patch area corresponding to the inguinal pain distribution including the point of maximum pain. Patients were pre-treated with a topical local anesthetic cream (EMLA, lidocaine/prilocaine 25 mg/25 g, AstraZeneca AB, Södertälje, Sweden) 60 min before patch application. The patch application, patch removal, and skin cleansing were done by a physician. During this procedure the research nurse was not allowed presence in the treatment room since minute quantities of aerosolized capsaicin-particles during patch handling could have led to accidental un-blinding of the research nurse.

The capsaicin patches (capsaicin 640 μg/cm^2, 8% w/w; Astellas Pharma Europe B.V., Leiderdorp, The Netherlands) and the inactive placebo patches were identical in appearance and composition (in regard to vehicle substances). An inactive placebo patch was used since an active placebo patch was not obtainable from the manufacturer of the capsaicin patch. The patients were informed that they might experience pain during and after the patch application. The patches were applied in the groin area for 60 min. After patch removal a cleansing gel (Astellas Pharma Europe B.V., Leiderdorp, The Netherlands) was applied in order to remove capsaicin residues. In order to decrease local irritation of the skin cool packs (assistCo AS, Rjukan, Norway) were administered for 45–60 minutes after patch removal. Patients were told to use oral acetaminophen 1 g every 6 h and ibuprofen 400 mg every 6 h for up to 3 days as needed after patch application. The patients and investigators were blinded to the treatment allocation throughout the study. At the clinical visit 1 month after patch application patients were asked to report if they had experienced application site skin reactions (erythema, pain, burning sensation) or any other adverse events. To evaluate patient blinding we asked patients at the clinical visit 1 month after patch application to verbally report which treatment they had received.

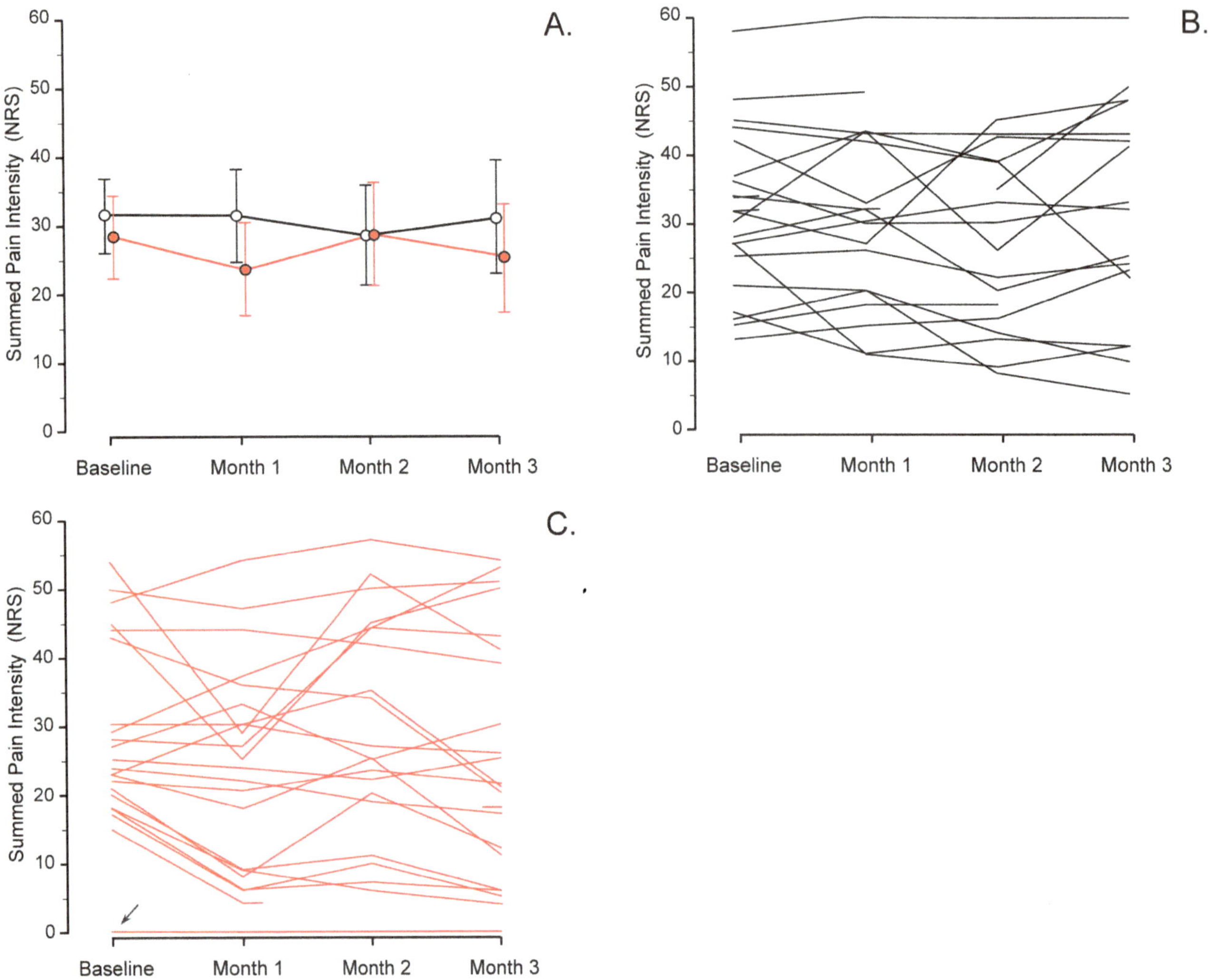

Figure 3. Panel A. Summed pain intensity (SPI) values assessed on a Numerical Rating Scale (NRS) at baseline and at 1, 2 and 3 months after patch application. Each SPI-value contains six median values (pain assessments twice daily for three days) and the maximum SPI-value is 60 NRS units. Values are mean (95% confidence interval). Black line (○) placebo treated patients. Red line (●) capsaicin treated patients. Individual time profiles are displayed for placebo treated patients (panel B, black lines) and capsaicin treated patients (panel C, red lines). The arrow (panel C) indicates patient #10 with baseline median NRS-value of 0 (see text for explanation).

Statistical analyses

The pain intensities during the 3 standardized conditions (at rest, during movement and pressure evoked), were evaluated twice daily in the 3 days preceding patch treatment (baseline) and in the 3 days preceding the clinical visit at 1, 2 and 3 months after patch application. The median value of the 3 standardized pain assessments was used to calculate the summed pain intensity (SPI) values (containing 6 median values [pain assessments twice daily for 3 days]) in accordance with a previously described method [23]. The summed pain intensity differences (SPID) were

Table 2. Changes in pain intensity between baseline and 1 month after patch application presented as SPID for capsaicin and placebo patch treatments, and the mean difference.

	Capsaicin (n = 22)	Placebo (n = 20)	Difference	*P*-value
SPID (NRS)	4.8 (1.4 to 8.2)	−0.2 (−3.8 to 3.4)	5.0 (0.09 to 9.9)	0.046
SPID %	19.8 (7.5 to 32.1)	−1.0 (−14.1 to 12.1)	20.9 (2.9 to 38.9)	0.024

The SPID was calculated as the difference between the baseline SPI-value and the SPI-value at 1 month after patch application. Each SPI- value contains six median values (pain assessments twice daily for three days). Values are mean (95% CI). Positive values of SPID indicate pain reduction after treatment. *P*-values indicate comparisons of SPID (capsaicin *vs.* placebo).
NRS = Numerical Rating Scale (0–10), SPID = Summed pain intensity difference, SPI = summed pain intensity.

Table 3. Differences in quantitative sensory assessments on the pain side from baseline to 1 month after patch application.

Δ-value	Capsaicin (n = 21)	Placebo (n = 19)	*P*-value
ΔWDT[§] (°C)	0.2 (−0.9 to 1.2)	0.6 (−0.1 to 1.3)	0.52[‡]
ΔCDT (°C)	0.0 (−0.8 to 0.7)	−0.1 (−0.7 to 0.8)	0.96
ΔHPT (°C)	0.3 (−0.4 to 1.5)	0.3 (−0.2 to 1.2)	0.91
ΔPPT[§] (kPa)	1.5 (−24.8 to 27.8)	−0.4 (−23.2 to 22.4)	0.91[‡]
ΔSTH (NRS)	0.0 (−1.0 to 0.0)	0.0 (−1.0 to 1.0)	0.56

Values are mean (95% CI)[§] or median (95% CI). Δ value = post-treatment minus baseline value. *P*-values indicate comparisons of Δ-values (capsaicin *vs.* placebo [unpaired t-test[‡] or the Mann-Whitney test). Positive Δ-values for WDT, HPT, PPT and CDT indicate increased thresholds after treatment.
WDT = warmth detection threshold, CDT = cool detection threshold, HPT = heat pain threshold, PPT = pressure pain threshold, STH = suprathreshold heat pain perception, NRS = Numerical Rating Scale (0–10).

calculated for 1, 2 and 3 months after patch application, as the difference between the baseline SPI-value and the post-treatment SPI-value. The primary outcome was comparisons of SPIDs between capsaicin and placebo treatments at 1, 2 and 3 months after patch application. No data from previous studies were available and the *a priori* sample size calculation was therefore based on the best estimates for the study cohort. Based on a significance level of 0.01 (α), a power of 0.9 (β = 0.1), an estimated standard deviation for the SPI assessments of 3.1 (NRS), and a minimal relevant difference for the six SPI assessments of 4.5 (NRS), the estimated number of patients needed in each group were 24 (48 in total). In order to compensate for dropouts the number of patients was set to 50. Due to uncertainties in the power calculation an interim analysis by an independent statistician was planned *a priori* following completion of the first 32 patients.

Linear regression analyses for repeated measures (a mixed model method) were used to evaluate the treatment effects over time. The summed pain intensity difference (SPID) was the outcome variable and treatment group (capsaicin or placebo) and time (1, 2 and 3 months after patch application) were explanatory variables. While measurements taken at different time points were expected to correlate, we also assumed that measurements taken at adjacent time points were more correlated than measurements further apart, and therefore we used an unstructured covariance structure (all covariance parameters are freely estimated). We used the PROC MIXED procedure and the repeated statement in SAS software (9.3, SAS Institute Inc., Cary, NC) to estimate the model. We included the interaction because we were interested in testing whether potential group differences changed over time. The mixed model is dealing with missing longitudinal measures and the analysis included all patients with at least one SPID-value. For secondary outcomes, including QST variables and questionnaire scores (DSIS, HADS, PCS, S-LANNS), differences (Δ) between post-treatment follow-up and baseline values were used to compare capsaicin and placebo patch treatments. The numbers of patients included in the data analyses vary for different outcome measures and are indicated in the tables for each analysis.

The normality of data was assessed with the Kolmogorov-Smirnov test and visual estimation of relevant residual distribution plots. Comparisons between treatment groups were performed with unpaired t-tests (normally distributed data) and the Mann-Whitney tests (non-normally distributed data). Fischer's exact test was used to compare proportions. Statistical analyses were conducted using SPSS software (SPSS 20.0, Chicago, IL) and MedCalc Software (12.3.0.0, Mariakerke, Belgium). The linear regression analyses for repeated measures were performed with SAS software. Due to the three statistical tests performed (comparisons 1, 2 and 3 months after patch application) and the planned interim analysis, thus increasing the probability of a type I error, all results were considered significant at $P<0.01$ (two-tailed).

Results

A total of 46 patients were randomized (fig. 2). Baseline patient characteristics and pain ratings are shown in table 1. In one patient (#46) severe pain at the application site necessitated premature patch removal leading to study withdrawal. In two patients (#16, #34) add-on treatment with other analgesics was initiated during the study. Data from these two patients were included in the analyses only up to the time of the violation of the medication criterion. One patient (#10) reported severe pain (NRS ≥5) at the first clinical visit and was thus included in the study in accordance with the protocol. However, in the pain diary evaluations preceding the patch application the patient only reported pain during palpation (NRS = 5), and, no pain (NRS = 0) at rest and during movement Therefore, the median NRS-value of the three standardized pain assessments at baseline was 0 for this patient (indicated in Fig. 3C). Five patients had one or more missing SPID values. Three patients (#4, #15, #49) had one

Table 4. Assessments of intraepidermal nerve fiber density (IENFD) on the pain side at baseline and at 1 month after patch application.

	Baseline (IENFD/mm)	1 month (IENFD/mm)	Δ value	*P*-value
Capsaicin (n = 18)	4.8 (2.5 to 7.2)	2.9 (1.2 to 4.7)	1.9 (−0.1 to 3.9)	0.32
Placebo (n = 20)	5.8 (3.2 to 8.3)	5.2 (2.2 to 8.1)	0.6 (−1.2 to 2.5)	

Values are mean (95% CI). The *P*-value indicates comparison of Δ values (capsaicin *vs.* placebo unpaired t-test). Δ value = baseline −1 month value. Δ values are normally distributed while baseline and 1 month IENFD values are non-normally distributed.

Table 5. Skin reactions at application site.

	Capsaicin (n = 23)	Placebo (n = 20)
Any application site reaction, *n* (%)	17 (74)	6 (30)
- Erythema, *n*	9	3
- Pain, *n*	12	6
- Burning sensation, *n*	12	1

missing SPID value and two patients (#2, #34) had two missing SPID values.

As previously mentioned, an interim analysis was planned for the first 32 patients, but due to a lower patient-recruitment rate than anticipated and a premature expiry date of the placebo patches (May 2013) an interim analysis could not be performed. The interim analysis would have impeded study progression and prolonged the study for an estimated period of at least three months (time from patch application to study completion; fig. 1). Therefore, it was decided to continue the study without an interim analysis and to recruit patients until the expiration date of the placebo patch: the actual number of randomized patients (n = 46) in the study were thus lower than the originally estimated sample size of 50 patients.

Pain

The summed pain intensity (SPI) values (NRS) at baseline and at 1, 2 and 3 months after patch application are presented in (fig. 3). A linear regression analysis for repeated measures with SPID as outcome variable and treatment group (capsaicin [n = 22] or placebo [n = 20]) and time (1, 2 and 3 months after patch application) as explanatory variables revealed a significant interaction for group * time ($F_{2,37.4} = 5.53$, $P = 0.008$). The analysis showed that the maximum difference in SPID between capsaicin and placebo treated patients was observed at 1 month after patch application, although statistical significance at the 0.01 level was not achieved. The mean difference [95% CI] in SPID at 1 month after patch application was (5.0 [0.09 to 9.9] NRS-units; $P = 0.046$, table 2), corresponding to a mean difference [95% CI] in SPID percentage of (20.9% [2.9 to 38.9%]; $P = 0.024$). Similarly, there were no significant differences in SPID between capsaicin and placebo patch treatments at 2 months after patch application (mean difference [95% CI]: −1.7 [−6.4 to 3.1] NRS-units; $P = 0.48$) or at 3 months after patch application (mean difference [95% CI]: 3.6 [−3.1 to 10.2] NRS-units; $P = 0.29$).

Sensory Function

Analyses of changes in QST assessments from baseline to 1 month after treatment are presented in table 3. No significant differences between capsaicin and placebo patch treated patients for thermal thresholds, suprathreshold heat pain perception, and pressure pain thresholds were observed.

Skin innervation

The median (95% CI) IENFD at baseline was significantly lower on the pain side, i.e. 4.3 (1.5 to 6.8) fibers/mm compared with the non-pain side 8.6 (7.4 to 11.0) fibers/mm, ($P<0.0001$, Wilcoxon signed rank test). Changes in IENFD, from baseline to 1 month after patch application on the pain side, did not differ between capsaicin and placebo treated patients ($P = 0.32$, table 4).

S-LANSS, Sleep Quality and Psychological Factors

At baseline the median (95% CI) S-LANSS score was 15 (10 to 17) and 26 of 42 patients (62%) reported a S-LANSS score of ≥12 indicating pain components of predominantly neuropathic origin [21]. Changes from baseline to 1 month after patch application with regard to sleep quality, PCS, S-LANSS, and HADS scores did not differ between capsaicin and placebo treated patients.

Adverse Events

Seventeen of 23 (74%) capsaicin treated patients and 6 of 20 (30%) placebo treated patients reported one or more skin reactions on the application site ($P = 0.006$, Fischer's exact test, table 5). No other adverse events or complications were observed in the study.

Patient Blinding

Sixteen of 23 patients (70%) treated with the capsaicin patch and 17 of 21 patients (81%) treated with the placebo patch correctly identified their treatment allocation ($P = 0.49$, Fischer's exact test).

Discussion

The present study in patients with severe persistent inguinal postherniorrhaphy pain, comparing the pain relief of a capsaicin 8% patch with an inactive placebo patch, was not able to demonstrate significant differences in pain reduction during standardized testing conditions. In addition, we did not observe any changes in secondary outcome variables including sensory function, IENFD, sleep quality, catastrophizing behaviour (PCS), or anxiety and depression (HADS) scores associated with capsaicin patch treatment.

Statistical Issues

Interpretation of the study's main finding should consider the *a priori* assigned significance level of 0.01. The authors regarded this conservative statistical measure a precaution against the introduction of type I errors due to the use of multiple comparisons and interim analysis. However, the statistical comparisons of SPID-scores, one month after patch application, yielding *P*-values of 0.024 and 0.046, indicated a trend of an improved pain relief in capsaicin treated patients. A potential contributing factor to the non-significant findings is obviously the premature discontinuation of the study after 46 randomized patients compared to the *a priori* estimated sample size of 50 patients. This circumstance may have introduced a type II error. A post hoc power calculation could be considered but is generally not recommended [25].

Skin innervation

The study corroborates our previous findings of a reduced IENFD on the pain side compared to the contralateral side in persistent inguinal postherniorrhaphy pain patients, most likely caused by surgical nerve injury [23,26]. Several studies in healthy volunteers have demonstrated a 60–80% reduction in IENFD one week after capsaicin 8% patch treatment [16,17,27]. The current study, the first to evaluate changes in IENFD following capsaicin patch treatment in patients, failed to show a significant difference in IENFD between treatment groups. A plausible explanation is the low baseline IENFD on the pain side in postherniorrhaphy pain patients compared to healthy volunteers, making it difficult to demonstrate a further reduction in IENFD following capsaicin treatment. The small group size may be another reason why the observed reduction of IENFD in the capsaicin group did not reach significance. However, it should be emphasized that none of the studies investigating IENFD after application of an 8% capsaicin patch in healthy volunteers provide data at 4 weeks after application [16,17,27], and it cannot be excluded that partial regeneration of nerve fibers already may have taken place [28].

Sensory Assessments

The QST assessment did not demonstrate any differences in cutaneous (thermal) or deep tissue (mechanical) sensory function between capsaicin and placebo treatment. A possible explanation is the previously mentioned lack of a significant reduction in IENFD after capsaicin treatment. In addition, sensory nerve endings not expressing TRPV1 receptors, i.e. Aβ-fibers, the majority of Aδ-fibers, and a subgroup of C-fibers, remain intact after capsaicin treatment and are thus still capable of transmitting sensory stimuli [12]. Accordingly, previous studies in neuropathic pain patients have failed to demonstrate sensory impairment after capsaicin patch treatment. In painful HIV-related neuropathy no differences in thermal and vibration detection thresholds were observed between capsaicin treated patients and controls at 4 and 12 weeks after patch application [9]. Furthermore, no differences between treatment groups were found in two studies investigating detection thresholds for brush, punctate stimulation, vibration and warmth in patients with post-herpetic neuralgia at 4 and 12 weeks after patch application [8,29].

Limitations

A confounding factor for the study is the patient-blinding. The higher incidence of local side effects experienced by patients in the capsaicin group (74%) compared to the placebo group (30%), and the correspondingly high proportion of patients who correctly identified their treatment allocation, indicate an insufficient blinding-technique. Therefore, it cannot be excluded that the potential analgesic effect experienced by the capsaicin treatment may in fact represent a placebo effect. The short duration of the potential analgesic effect (i.e. one month) also may connote to a placebo effect. The study thus supports the use of an active placebo (e.g. low-dose of capsaicin) in order to ensure adequate blinding in future studies assessing the effects of topical capsaicin.

Pathophysiological Mechanism

Pain relief up to 12 weeks after capsaicin patch application has been observed in previous randomized, controlled trials in post-herpetic neuralgia and HIV-related distal neuropathy [6–10]. The lack of a significant analgesic effect in the present study may be explained by a different pain mechanism in persistent inguinal postherniorrhaphy pain. The S-LANNS findings in the present study and the QST results in previous studies [30,31] point towards neuropathic pain components in this patient cohort, which is also underscored by the reduced IENFD on the painful side, specifying a small-fiber neuropathy. However, a number of postherniorrhaphy pain patients demonstrate decreased pain thresholds to pressure algometry indicating increased deep tissue sensitivity and suggesting deep pain components that may be caused by an untoward inflammatory reaction to the implanted mesh [31]. The negative findings in our study suggest that interruption of cutaneous nerve transmission alone may be insufficient to relieve pain substantially in these patients and seem to indicate that nerve injury, as well as deep tissue inflammation, may contribute to the development and maintenance of persistent postherniorrhaphy pain. Further studies are needed to elucidate the pathophysiological contributors in persistent postherniorrhaphy pain in order to guide future treatment strategies.

In conclusion capsaicin patch 8% did not significantly reduce combined static and dynamic pain components compared to placebo in persistent inguinal postherniorrhaphy pain, albeit a trend towards pain relief was observed 1 month after capsaicin patch application.

Supporting Information

Checklist S1 CONSORT Checklist.

Protocol S1 Trial Protocol.

Acknowledgments

The authors would like to thank Morten Aagaard Petersen, M.Sc., Department of Palliative Medicine, Bispebjerg Hospital, Copenhagen University Hospitals, DENMARK for statistical assistance, Manuel Pedro Pereira M.D., Department of Anaesthesia, Center of Head and Orthopaedics, Rigshospitalet, Copenhagen University Hospitals, DENMARK for assistance during patch application and Kathleen Stahl, Department of Neurology, University Hospital of Würzburg, GERMANY, for technical help during skin biopsy staining.

Author Contributions

Wrote the paper: JMB MW. Critically revising the manuscript: TR MP CS NÜ. Conceived and designed the experiments: JMB MW CS NÜ. Performed the experiments: JMB TR MP. Analyzed the data: JMB MW. Contributed reagents/materials/analysis tools: MW CS NÜ.

References

1. Rutkow IM (2003) Demographic and socioeconomic aspects of hernia repair in the United States in 2003. Surg Clin North Am 83: 1045-10vi. S0039-6109(03)00132-4 [pii]; 10.1016/S0039-6109(03)00132-4 [doi].
2. Franneby U, Sandblom G, Nordin P, Nyren O, Gunnarsson U (2006) Risk factors for long-term pain after hernia surgery. Ann Surg 244: 212–219.
3. Kalliomaki ML, Meyerson J, Gunnarsson U, Gordh T, Sandblom G (2008) Long-term pain after inguinal hernia repair in a population-based cohort; risk factors and interference with daily activities. Eur J Pain 12: 214–225.
4. Chen DC, Hiatt JR, Amid PK (2013) Operative management of refractory neuropathic inguinodynia by a laparoscopic retroperitoneal approach. JAMA Surg 148: 962–967. 1722800 [pii]; 10.1001/jamasurg.2013.3189 [doi].
5. Bischoff JM, Enghuus C, Werner MU, Kehlet H (2013) Long-term follow-up after mesh removal and selective neurectomy for persistent inguinal postherniorrhaphy pain. Hernia 17: 339–345. 10.1007/s10029-013-1073-z [doi].
6. Derry S, Sven-Rice A, Cole P, Tan T, Moore RA (2013) Topical capsaicin (high concentration) for chronic neuropathic pain in adults. Cochrane Database Syst Rev 2: CD007393. 10.1002/14651858.CD007393.pub3 [doi].
7. Backonja M, Wallace MS, Blonsky ER, Cutler BJ, Malan P Jr, et al. (2008) NGX-4010, a high-concentration capsaicin patch, for the treatment of postherpetic neuralgia: a randomised, double-blind study. Lancet Neurol 7: 1106–1112. S1474-4422(08)70228-X [pii]; 10.1016/S1474-4422(08)70228-X [doi].
8. Irving GA, Backonja MM, Dunteman E, Blonsky ER, Vanhove GF, et al.(2011) A multicenter, randomized, double-blind, controlled study of NGX-4010, a

high-concentration capsaicin patch, for the treatment of postherpetic neuralgia. Pain Med 12: 99-109. 10.1111/j.1526-4637.2010.01004.x [doi].

9. Simpson DM, Brown S, Tobias J (2008) Controlled trial of high-concentration capsaicin patch for treatment of painful HIV neuropathy. Neurology 70: 2305–2313. 70/24/2305 [pii]; 10.1212/01.wnl.0000314647.35825.9c [doi].
10. Webster LR, Malan TP, Tuchman MM, Mollen MD, Tobias JK, et al. (2010) A multicenter, randomized, double-blind, controlled dose finding study of NGX-4010, a high-concentration capsaicin patch, for the treatment of postherpetic neuralgia. J Pain 11: 972–982. S1526-5900(10)00296-8 [pii]; 10.1016/j.jpain.2010.01.270 [doi].
11. Ringkamp M, Raja SN, Campbell JN, Meyer RA (2013) Peripheral mechanisms of cutaneous nociception. In: McMahon SB, Koltzenburg M, Tracey I, Turk DC, editors. Wall and Melzack's textbook of pain. Elsevier Saunders. pp. 1–30.
12. Anand P, Bley K (2011) Topical capsaicin for pain management: therapeutic potential and mechanisms of action of the new high-concentration capsaicin 8% patch. Br J Anaesth 107: 490–502. aer260 [pii]; 10.1093/bja/aer260 [doi].
13. Treede RD, Wagner T, Kern KU, Husstedt IW, Arendt G, et al. (2013) Mechanism- and experience-based strategies to optimize treatment response to the capsaicin 8% cutaneous patch in patients with localized neuropathic pain. Curr Med Res Opin 29: 527–538. 10.1185/03007995.2013.781019 [doi].
14. Maihofner C, Heskamp ML (2013) Prospective, non-interventional study on the tolerability and analgesic effectiveness over 12 weeks after a single application of capsaicin 8% cutaneous patch in 1044 patients with peripheral neuropathic pain: first results of the QUEPP study. Curr Med Res Opin 29: 673–683. 10.1185/03007995.2013.792246 [doi].
15. Aasvang EK, Hansen JB, Malmstrom J, Asmussen T, Gennevois D, et al. (2008) The effect of wound instillation of a novel purified capsaicin formulation on postherniotomy pain: a double-blind, randomized, placebo-controlled study. Anesth Analg 107: 282–291.
16. Malmberg AB, Mizisin AP, Calcutt NA, von ST, Robbins WR, et al. (2004) Reduced heat sensitivity and epidermal nerve fiber immunostaining following single applications of a high-concentration capsaicin patch. Pain 111: 360–367. 10.1016/j.pain.2004.07.017 [doi];S0304-3959(04)00344-6 [pii].
17. Kennedy WR, Vanhove GF, Lu SP, Tobias J, Bley KR, et al. (2010) A randomized, controlled, open-label study of the long-term effects of NGX-4010, a high-concentration capsaicin patch, on epidermal nerve fiber density and sensory function in healthy volunteers. J Pain 11: 579–587.
18. Zigmond AS, Snaith RP (1983) The hospital anxiety and depression scale. Acta Psychiatr Scand 67: 361–370.
19. Sullivan MJL, Bishop SR, Kivik J (1995) The pain catastrophizing scale: development and validation. Psych Assess 7: 524–532.
20. Vernon MK, Brandenburg NA, Alvir JM, Griesing T, Revicki DA (2008) Reliability, validity, and responsiveness of the daily sleep interference scale among diabetic peripheral neuropathy and postherpetic neuralgia patients. J Pain Symptom Manage 36: 54–68.
21. Bennett MI, Smith BH, Torrance N, Potter J (2005) The S-LANSS score for identifying pain of predominantly neuropathic origin: validation for use in clinical and postal research. J Pain 6: 149–158.
22. Bischoff JM, Koscielniak-Nielsen ZJ, Kehlet H, Werner MU (2012) Ultrasound-guided ilioinguinal/iliohypogastric nerve blocks for persistent inguinal post-herniorrhaphy pain: a randomized, double-blind, placebo-controlled, crossover trial. Anesth Analg 114: 1323–1329. ANE.0b013e31824d6168 [pii]; 10.1213/ANE.0b013e31824d6168 [doi].
23. Bischoff JM, Petersen M, Uceyler N, Sommer C, Kehlet H, et al. (2013) Lidocaine Patch (5%) in Treatment of Persistent Inguinal Postherniorrhaphy Pain: A Randomized, Double-blind, Placebo-controlled, Crossover Trial. Anesthesiology 119: 1444–1452. 10.1097/ALN.0b013e3182a2a243 [doi].
24. Torvin MA, Winther BF, Feldt-Rasmussen U, Rasmussen A, Hasholt L, et al. (2009) Functional and structural nerve fiber findings in heterozygote patients with Fabry disease. Pain 145: 237–245.
25. Moher D, Hopewell S, Schulz KF, Montori V, Gotzsche PC, et al. (2010) CONSORT 2010 explanation and elaboration: updated guidelines for reporting parallel group randomised trials. BMJ 340: c869.
26. Kehlet H, Jensen TS, Woolf CJ (2006) Persistent postsurgical pain: risk factors and prevention. Lancet 367: 1618–1625.
27. Knolle E, Zadrazil M, Kovacs GG, Medwed S, Scharbert G, et al. (2013) Comparison of cooling and EMLA to reduce the burning pain during capsaicin 8% patch application: a randomized, double-blind, placebo-controlled study. Pain 154: 2729–2736. S0304-3959(13)00437-5 [pii]; 10.1016/j.pain.2013.08.001 [doi].
28. Rage M, Van AN, Facer P, Shenoy R, Knaapen MW, et al. (2010) The time course of CO2 laser-evoked responses and of skin nerve fibre markers after topical capsaicin in human volunteers. Clin Neurophysiol 121: 1256–1266. S1388-2457(10)00263-4 [pii]; 10.1016/j.clinph.2010.02.159 [doi].
29. Webster LR, Tark M, Rauck R, Tobias JK, Vanhove GF (2010) Effect of duration of postherpetic neuralgia on efficacy analyses in a multicenter, randomized, controlled study of NGX-4010, an 8% capsaicin patch evaluated for the treatment of postherpetic neuralgia. BMC Neurol 10: 92. 1471-2377-10-92 [pii]; 10.1186/1471-2377-10-92 [doi].
30. Mikkelsen T, Werner MU, Lassen B, Kehlet H (2004) Pain and sensory dysfunction 6 to 12 months after inguinal herniotomy. Anesth Analg 99: 146–151.
31. Aasvang EK, Brandsborg B, Jensen TS, Kehlet H (2010) Heterogeneous sensory processing in persistent postherniotomy pain. Pain 150: 237–242.

21

Spinal Autofluorescent Flavoprotein Imaging in a Rat Model of Nerve Injury-Induced Pain and the Effect of Spinal Cord Stimulation

Joost L. M. Jongen[1]*, Helwin Smits[2], Tiziana Pederzani[3], Malik Bechakra[3], Mehdi Hossaini[3], Sebastiaan K. Koekkoek[3], Frank J. P. M. Huygen[4], Chris I. De Zeeuw[3,5], Jan C. Holstege[3], Elbert A. J. Joosten[2]

1 Dept. of Neurology, Erasmus MC, Rotterdam, the Netherlands, **2** Pain Management and Research Center, UMC+, Maastricht, the Netherlands, **3** Dept. of Neuroscience, Erasmus MC, Rotterdam, the Netherlands, **4** Dept. of Pain Medicine, Erasmus MC, Rotterdam, the Netherlands, **5** Netherlands Institute for Neuroscience, Royal Academy for Arts and Sciences, Amsterdam, the Netherlands

Abstract

Nerve injury may cause neuropathic pain, which involves hyperexcitability of spinal dorsal horn neurons. The mechanisms of action of spinal cord stimulation (SCS), an established treatment for intractable neuropathic pain, are only partially understood. We used Autofluorescent Flavoprotein Imaging (AFI) to study changes in spinal dorsal horn metabolic activity. In the Seltzer model of nerve-injury induced pain, hypersensitivity was confirmed using the von Frey and hotplate test. 14 Days after nerve-injury, rats were anesthetized, a bipolar electrode was placed around the affected sciatic nerve and the spinal cord was exposed by a laminectomy at T13. AFI recordings were obtained in neuropathic rats and a control group of naïve rats following 10 seconds of electrical stimulation of the sciatic nerve at C-fiber strength, or following non-noxious palpation. Neuropathic rats were then treated with 30 minutes of SCS or sham stimulation and AFI recordings were obtained for up to 60 minutes after cessation of SCS/sham. Although AFI responses to noxious electrical stimulation were similar in neuropathic and naïve rats, only neuropathic rats demonstrated an AFI-response to palpation. Secondly, an immediate, short-lasting, but strong reduction in AFI intensity and area of excitation occurred following SCS, but not following sham stimulation. Our data confirm that AFI can be used to directly visualize changes in spinal metabolic activity following nerve injury and they imply that SCS acts through rapid modulation of nociceptive processing at the spinal level.

Editor: David D McKemy, University of South California, United States of America

Funding: The development of this manuscript was supported by research grants from the Pain Knowledge Center Rotterdam/Dutch Ministry of Health (JJ), the TREND consortium (HS), the BSIK program from the Dutch government (HS), the Dutch Organization for Medical Sciences (CDZ), Life Sciences (CDZ), Senter (Neuro-Basic; CDZ), the Prinses Beatrix Fonds (CDZ), and the European Union (CDZ). The funders had no role in study design, data collection and analysis, decision to publish, or preparation of the manuscript.

Competing Interests: The authors have declared that no competing interests exist.

* Email: j.jongen@erasmusmc.nl

Introduction

Flavoproteins are involved in a wide array of biological processes, among which adenosine triphosphate production via the mitochondrial electron transport chain. During this process the flavoprotein moieties of respiratory chain complexes I and II are oxidized, resulting in green fluorescence when illuminated with blue-spectrum light. This oxidation is followed by a reduction when the energy demand of a cell has been met, overall resulting in a bi-phasic fluorescence response. The light phase of flavoprotein autofluorescence may be used as a marker for neuronal (metabolic) activity [1]. We and others have demonstrated a linear relationship between the intensity of the neuronal stimulus and flavoprotein autofluorescence [2,3].

Since autofluorescent flavoprotein imaging (AFI) is an optical method, it is suitable to monitor activity in superficial areas of the nervous system such as the somatosensory cortex [4–8], auditory cortex [9,10], visual cortex [11,12], cerebellar cortex [13,14] and superficial dorsal horn of the spinal cord [3]. A major advantage is that it enables imaging of large areas at high-resolution in both the spatial (down to10×10 μm) and temporal (up to 100 frames/second) domain simultaneously. Furthermore, AFI directly represents neuronal metabolic activity, in contrast to intrinsic optical imaging [15] or fMRI using the BOLD signal [16]. AFI, however, does not allow imaging of deep structures like the deep dorsal horn of the spinal cord and has a relatively low signal-to-noise ratio [3].

Peripheral nerve injury often induces pain, which is, among others, driven by sensitization mechanisms within the spinal cord [17]. These sensitization mechanisms may be accurately monitored using autofluorescent flavoprotein imaging of the superficial spinal dorsal horn, as was shown previously using intraplantar capsaicin injection [3,18]. The Seltzer model consists of partial ligation of the proximal part of the sciatic nerve, which generates pain behavior in rats, closely resembling the clinical condition of Complex regional Pain Syndrome (CRPS) type 2 in humans [19].

CRPS type 2 in turn has many characteristics of painful neuropathy, including spontaneous and evoked pain [20,21]. Therefore, the Seltzer model may be considered a relevant model of nerve injury induced pain [22].

Painful neuropathy and CRPS are frequently refractory to pharmacological treatment and physical therapy. Spinal cord stimulation (SCS) is a generally accepted therapy in patients with CRPS [23–25] and recently SCS has yielded promising results in patients with painful diabetic neuropathy [26,27]. SCS is based on the gate-control theory from the 1960's [28], although the exact mechanism of action is still only partially clarified [29]. Probably, GABA-ergic interneurons, situated in the substantia gelatinosa, are of major importance in SCS treatment of chronic neuropathic pain [30]. It should be stressed, however, that the latter evidence is based on data obtained after dialysis of the spinal dorsal horn [31] or immunohistochemical visualization [32]. Hence, these data present only indirect evidence on the exact spatial and temporal changes of SCS in the spinal superficial dorsal horn.

We first set out experiments to study the mechanisms of sensitization in the superficial spinal dorsal horn by applying AFI to the Seltzer model. Subsequently, changes in nociceptive transmission in the superficial dorsal horn of chronic neuropathic rats brought about by SCS were visualized at a high spatial and temporal resolution using the same AFI imaging technology.

Materials and Methods

Animal preparation

All animal experimentation conformed to the guidelines laid out in the Guide for the Care and Use of Laboratory Animals (National Academy of Sciences) and was approved by the Institutional Animal Ethics Committee of Erasmus MC Rotterdam (EMCnr. 115-08-26). Recordings were obtained from a total number of 18 young adult male Sprague Dawley rats from Harlan or Charles River, the Netherlands, weighing 250–300 g. Neuropathic pain was induced by partial ligation of the sciatic nerve as described by Seltzer et al [19]. Recordings from 20 Wistar rats with similar age/weight from previous experiments [3] were used as controls.

Behavioral tests

Behavioral testing took place before the Seltzer operation and at post-operative days 10, 12 and 14. Every time before behavioral testing, rats were habituated to the experimenter (T.P. or M.B.), the room in which the behavioral experiments took place and the transparent chamber used for von Frey testing, for at least half an hour. Mechanical sensitivity was assessed by testing the withdrawal response to increasing in thickness von Frey filaments (Stoelting Co., Wood Dale, IL). The threshold was set at three out of five withdrawal responses. After testing for mechanical sensitivity, thermal thresholds were assessed by the hotplate test. The surface of the hot plate was heated to a constant temperature of 51°C. Rats were placed on the hot plate (25.4 cm×25.4 cm) (Ugo Basile Srl., Comerio, VA, Italy), which was surrounded by a transparent plexiglas chamber with an open top, and the latency to respond with either a hind paw lick or hind paw flick was measured. Immediately after a response rats were removed from the hotplate. Rats were also removed if they did not respond after 30 seconds, to prevent tissue injury.

Autofluorescent Flavoprotein Imaging in rats with nerve injury

After behavioral testing at day 14, rats were anesthetized and surgery and image acquisition for autofluorescent flavoprotein imaging of the spinal cord was performed as previously described [3], using a high speed 16-bit CCD camera with 512×512 pixel resolution (Roper Scientific, Evry, France). A silicon cuff containing a bipolar electrode was placed around the left sciatic nerve proximal to the knee, i.e. just distal to the suture from the partial nerve ligation. As a measure of fluorescence, generally ΔF/F is used. ΔF/F represents the change in fluorescence intensity of each pixel during registration relative to the mean fluorescence intensity of these pixels in frames preceding electrical stimulation (see also [3]). AFI responses were expressed as the maximal ΔF/F change in fluorescence following stimulation (AFI intensity), or as the area with an AFI intensity above a predefined ΔF/F level (area of excitation). This predefined ΔF/F level was always kept constant. Recordings using 2.5 mA, 10 Hz electrical stimulation of the left sciatic nerve lasting 10 seconds were obtained in 13 Sprague Dawley rats that had undergone partial sciatic nerve ligation and compared with recordings from 20 naïve Wistar rats from previous experiments [3], using the same electrical stimulus. A similar experiment was carried out in rats ($n = 5+5$) using a 10 seconds lasting 1 Hz innocuous palpation of the plantar surface of the left hind paw [3].

Autofluorescent Flavoprotein Imaging in rats with nerve injury undergoing SCS or sham stimulation

Following "before treatment" AFI recordings in neuropathic Sprague Dawley rats (see above), a monopolar stimulation system with a 3.0×1.0×0.1 mm platinum-iridium rectangular plate micro cathode was placed in the dorsal epidural space at the T12-T13 vertebral level, while the anode was placed in a subcutaneous pocket on the back, and rats underwent 50 Hz, amplitude 2/3 of motor threshold SCS ($n = 7$) or no electrical stimulation (sham; $n = 6$) for 30 minutes, as previously described [33]. Immediately following SCS or sham the micro cathode was removed and AFI responses to left sciatic nerve electrical stimulation (same stimulus as baseline) were recorded at T = 0 after SCS or sham and then every 5 minutes for up to an hour. Both the intensity of the AFI response (expressed as ΔF/F of the light phase) and the area with an AFI intensity above a predefined ΔF/F level was calculated and expressed as a percentage of ΔF/F before treatment. At the end of the experiment, rats were euthanized with an overdose of intraperitoneal urethane.

Statistical analysis and presentation of the figures

Statistical analyses were performed using GraphPad Prism version 6.0e and SPSS statistics version 21 software. For a comparison of means of behavioral responses, a repeated-measures ANOVA was used. For an overall comparison of means of AFI intensities and areas of excitation between naïve and neuropathic rats and between sides, two-way ANOVAs were used. For a comparison of means of AFI intensities following non-noxious palpation in naïve and neuropathic rats, an unpaired t-test was used. For comparing the effect of SCS versus sham on AFI intensities and area of excitation, paired t-tests were used, Pearson's correlation coefficients were calculated and a linear regression analysis was performed. The data in the figures are expressed as mean ± SEM. Figures were composed in Photoshop CS6 software version 13.0.6. Adjustments were made only to brightness and contrast and applied evenly to all panels of a figure.

Results

Following partial ligation of the left sciatic nerve in the thigh, all 18 Sprague Dawley rats used in this study developed mechanical and thermal hypersensitivity characteristic of the Seltzer model

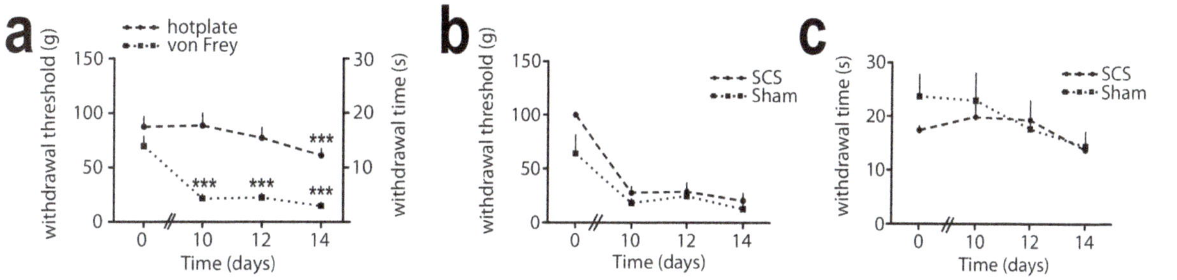

Figure 1. Behavioral data of rats that underwent partial ligation of the proximal sciatic nerve (Seltzer model). (A) Combined results of the von Frey withdrawal thresholds and hotplate latencies, at baseline and 10, 12 and 14 days after nerve ligation, from al 18 rats in the study, demonstrating tactile and thermal hyperalgesia. Error bars indicate SEM. $p<0.01$; repeated measures ANOVAs, source of variation timepoint; ***$p<0.01$; pairwise comparisons of day 0 versus day 10, 12 and 14, using Bonferroni correction. (B,C) Von Frey withdrawal thresholds (B) and hotplate latencies (C) from 7 neuropathic rats that subsequently underwent SCS and 6 neuropathic rats that subsequently underwent sham stimulation, demonstrating a similar degree of tactile and thermal hyperalgesia in both groups. Error bars indicate SEM. $p>0.06$; repeated measures ANOVAs, source of variation treatment.

(Table S1) [19]. Repeated-measures ANOVAs (source of variation timepoint) demonstrated that the decrease in von Frey thresholds and hotplate latencies was statistically significant (Fig. 1A; $p<0.01$).

We then set out to capture AFI responses in these neuropathic Sprague Dawley rats. A typical AFI recording of a 10 s, 2.5 mA, 10 Hz electrical stimulation of the left sciatic nerve showed a steep increase in spinal fluorescence (light phase) immediately after the start of the stimulation, followed by a decrease below baseline (dark phase) (Fig. 2; Movie S1). This pattern of activity is typical of autofluorescent flavoprotein imaging in the brain and spinal cord. In the rest of this paper we only use the light phase for analysis, since this is the default measure of activity in AFI.

Next, we compared mean AFI intensities and areas of excitation following 10 s, 2.5 mA, 10 Hz electrical stimulation of 13 Sprague Dawley rats with partial nerve ligation, with those from 20 naïve Wistar rats from a previous study [3], that had undergone exactly the same electrical stimulation protocol (Fig. 3; Table S2). The main effects of both type of animal (naïve Wistar versus neuropathic Sprague-Dawley rats) and side (ipsilateral versus contralateral) on AFI intensity and area of excitation were not significantly different, nor were the interactions between type of

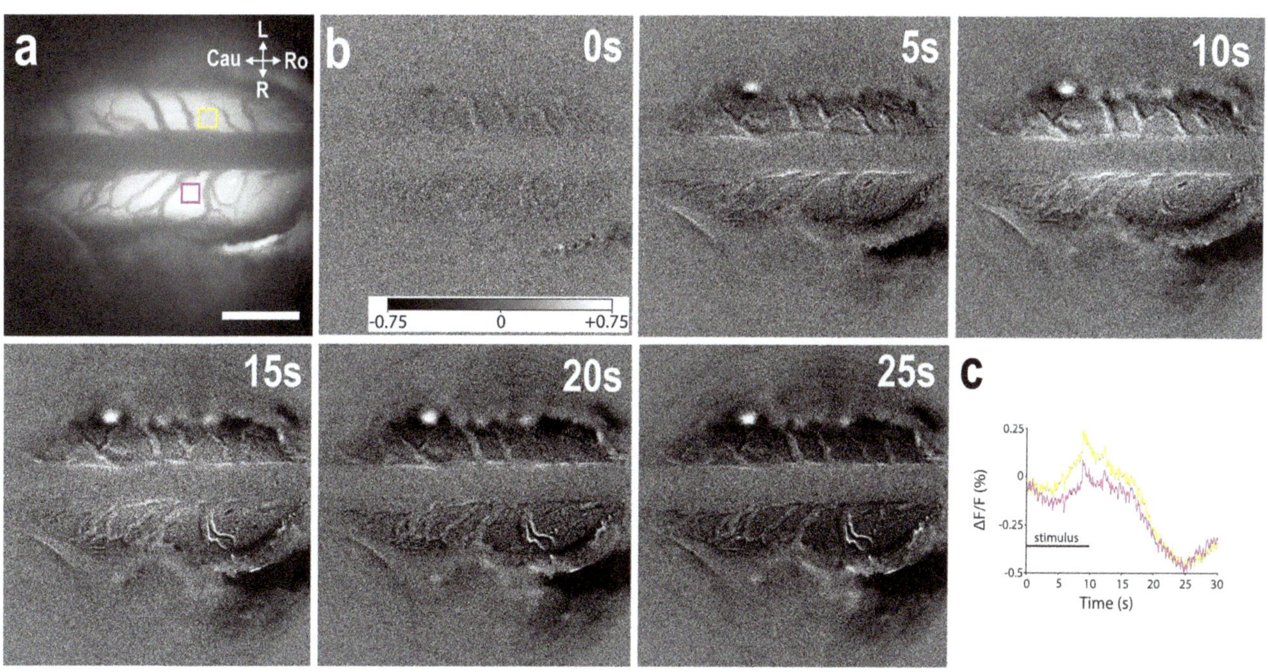

Figure 2. Spinal cord AFI signal following nociceptive electrical stimulation of the sciatic nerve, in a rat with partial ligation of the proximal sciatic nerve (Seltzer model). (A) Image of background fluorescence showing the dorsal surface of the spinal cord at the T13 vertebral level. The upper half is left, the lower half is right, the dark structure in the center is a dural vein. (B) Subtracted ΔF/F images at various time points after start of electrical stimulation (2.5 mA, 10 Hz) of the left sciatic nerve. (C) Graph showing the time course of ΔF/F in the yellow (left, i.e. ipsilateral or stimulated side) and purple (right, i.e. contralateral side) 20×20 pixel square selections in (A). Scale bar, 1 mm. Gray scale bar ranging from −0.75% (black) to +0.75% (white) of the 16-bit range; Cau = caudal, Ro = rostral, L = left, R = right.

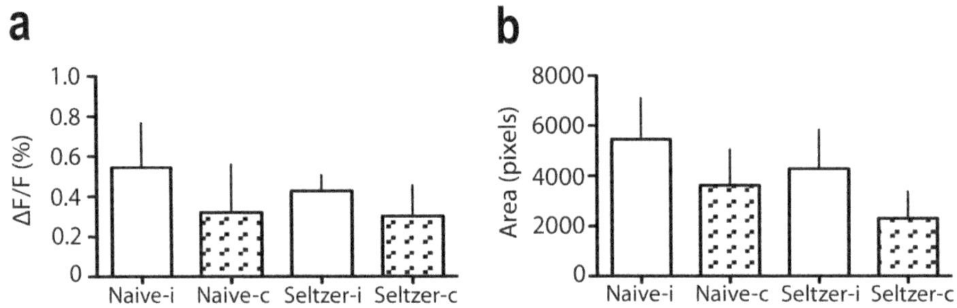

Figure 3. Mean intensity of the AFI signal (A) and area of excitation (B) following nociceptive electrical stimulation of the sciatic nerve, in naïve versus neuropathic rats (Seltzer model), on the ipsilateral (i) and contralateral (c) side of the nerve injury and nerve stimulation. Error bars indicate SEM; $n = 20$ naïve rats, $n = 13$ neuropathic rats.

animal and side on AFI intensity and area of excitation ($p > 0.23$; two-way ANOVAs).

Since it is known [17,19] that in neuropathic pain states also innocuous stimuli may elicit nociceptive activity in the superficial dorsal horn, we investigated AFI responses to 10 s, 1 Hz innocuous palpation of the left hind paw. We compared AFI intensities in 5 neuropathic Sprague Dawley rats with those from 5 naïve Wistar rats from our previous study (Fig. 4; Movie S2, Table S3). While we have demonstrated that after innocuous palpation in naïve rats AFI intensity is not different from recordings without stimulation, there was a robust increase in AFI intensity following palpation in neuropathic rats on the ipsilateral side, which was statistically significantly different from naïve rats ($p = 0.03$; unpaired t-test). Results on the contralateral side of naïve and neuropathic rats were not statistically significantly different ($p = 0.7$; unpaired t-test).

Finally, the effect of spinal cord stimulation on AFI responses in neuropathic Sprague Dawley rats was investigated. Prior to stimulation, neuropathic pain behavior was not statistically significantly different between rats that underwent SCS ($n = 7$) or sham ($n = 6$) stimulation (Fig. 1B and 1C; $p > 0.06$; repeated-measures ANOVA, source of variation treatment). We then studied relative AFI responses, expressed as a percentage of the "before treatment" AFI response, in 7 neuropathic rats after 30 minutes 50 Hz spinal cord stimulation, using a platinum cathode at the T12-T13 vertebral level, and in 6 neuropathic rats that underwent sham stimulation, i.e. with cathode placement but without the 50 Hz electrical stimulus (Table S4). In rats with SCS there was a strong and statistically significant reduction in AFI

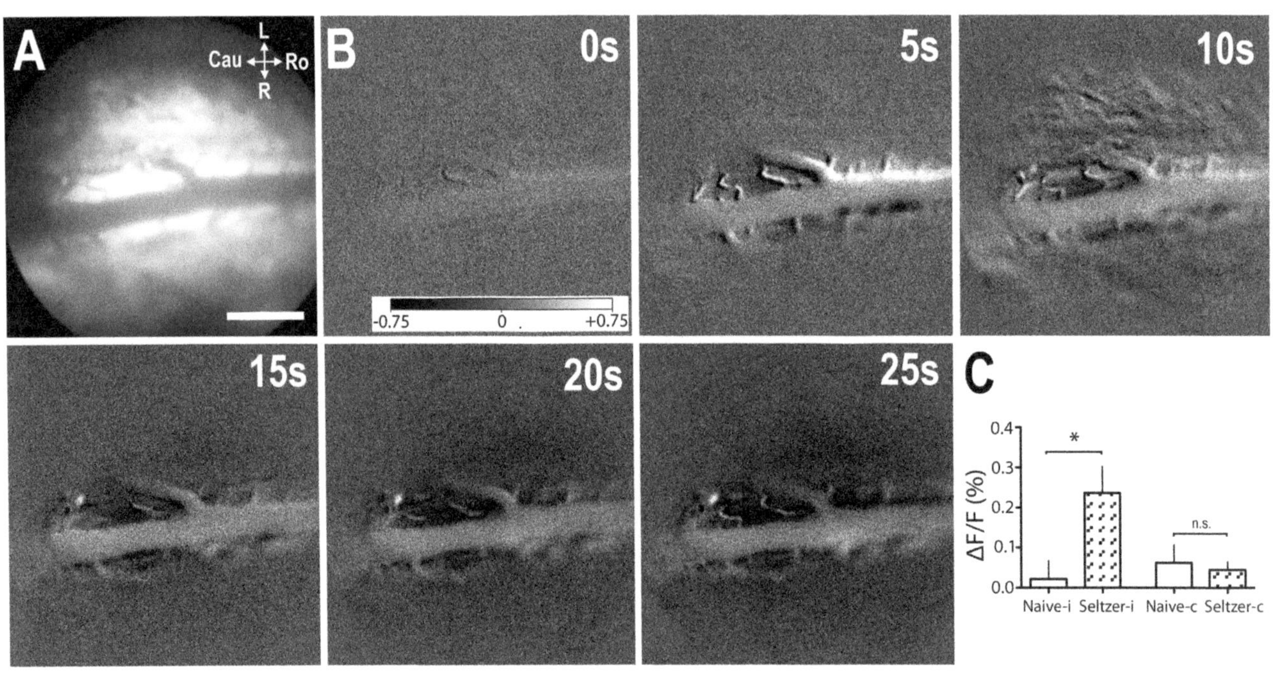

Figure 4. Intensity of the AFI signal, following innocuous palpation in naïve rats and rats with partial ligation of the proximal sciatic nerve (Seltzer model). (A) Image of background fluorescence of the dorsal surface of the spinal cord at T13. (B) Subtracted ΔF/F images at various time points after start of 10 seconds, 1 Hz innocuous palpation of the plantar surface of the left hindpaw. (C) Mean ΔF/F of the light phase in 20×20 pixel square selections on the ipsi-(i) and contralateral (c) side at the L4-6 spinal level, in naïve rats from our previous experiments [3] and in rats with partial ligation of the proximal sciatic nerve (Seltzer model). Scale bar, 1 mm. Gray scale bar ranging from −0.75% (black) to +0.75% (white) of the 16-bit range. Error bars indicate SEM; $^*p < 0.05$; unpaired t-test; $n = 5$ naïve rats, $n = 5$ neuropathic rats.

intensity as well as area of activation directly after cessation of SCS on the ipsilateral side (Fig. 5; $p = 0.049$ and $p = 0.041$ respectively; paired t-test), while in rats that underwent sham stimulation there was no statistically significant reduction ($p>0.8$; paired t-test). In the period from T = 0 to T = 60 minutes following cessation of SCS, there was a statistically significant linear increase in AFI intensity on the ipsilateral side in the rats with SCS (slope 0.92%ΔF/F *min^{-1}; $p = 0.021$; Pearson's correlation coefficient and linear regression analysis), indicating a reducing efficacy of SCS at these later time-points. In the rats with sham stimulation the slope was not statistically significant non-zero (slope 0.19%ΔF/F *min^{-1}; $p = 0.72$; Pearson's correlation coefficient and linear regression analysis), indicating no treatment effect in the rats that underwent sham stimulation.

Discussion

Nerve injury-induced pain is a complex disorder, which is driven by a multitude of plastic changes, like sensitization of (peripheral) nociceptors [34,35], increased excitability of spinal cord projection neurons [36], decreased propriospinal [37] and descending [38] spinal inhibition, spinal glia activation [39] and changes in the transmission of nociceptive signals in the brainstem and neocortex [40]. In this study we focused on changes following nerve injury in (metabolic) activity in the superficial dorsal horn, a major relay station in the transmission of the nociceptive signal to higher brain centers. Using the Seltzer model of nerve injury-induced pain and AFI, we first demonstrate that although neuropathic rats did not have an increased activation following nociceptive electrical stimulation compared to naïve rats, they express a robust ipsilateral response to non-noxious palpation, which is not present in naïve rats. Secondly, we used AFI to study the effect of spinal cord stimulation on nociceptive activity in the superficial dorsal horn in neuropathic animals. AFI shows an immediate and pronounced, but short-lasting reduction in intensity and area of spinal nociceptive activity following SCS, which was not observed following sham stimulation.

We have previously put forward, that the spinal cord AFI response following primary afferent stimulation is generated by projection neurons and local interneurons in the superficial laminae of the spinal dorsal horn [16]. Secondly, we have shown that spinal AFI is suitable to study plastic changes in this area following an intraplantar capsaicin injection [3]. In this study we have used a similar approach to study changes in spinal nociceptive activity following nerve-injury. Behavioral studies in experimental animals [19,41] and psychophysical studies [42,43] in humans with nerve injury consistently demonstrate pain (behavior) evoked by stimuli that are not painful under normal conditions, e.g. tactile allodynia. Similarly, in the Seltzer model of nerve injury-induced pain we now demonstrate a strong ipsilateral AFI response to innocuous palpation, which was not present in naïve animals.

There were no statistically significant differences between naïve and neuropathic rats following a nociceptive 2.5 mA electrical stimulus. Although hyperalgesia to nociceptive stimuli does exist both in experimental and clinical neuropathic conditions, a strong enough electrical stimulus may saturate metabolic activity of superficial spinal dorsal horn neurons, i.e. the AFI signal. The electrical stimulus intensity that we used here is almost three times C-fiber threshold and generates a response that is close to the maximal AFI intensity that we found previously in naïve animals

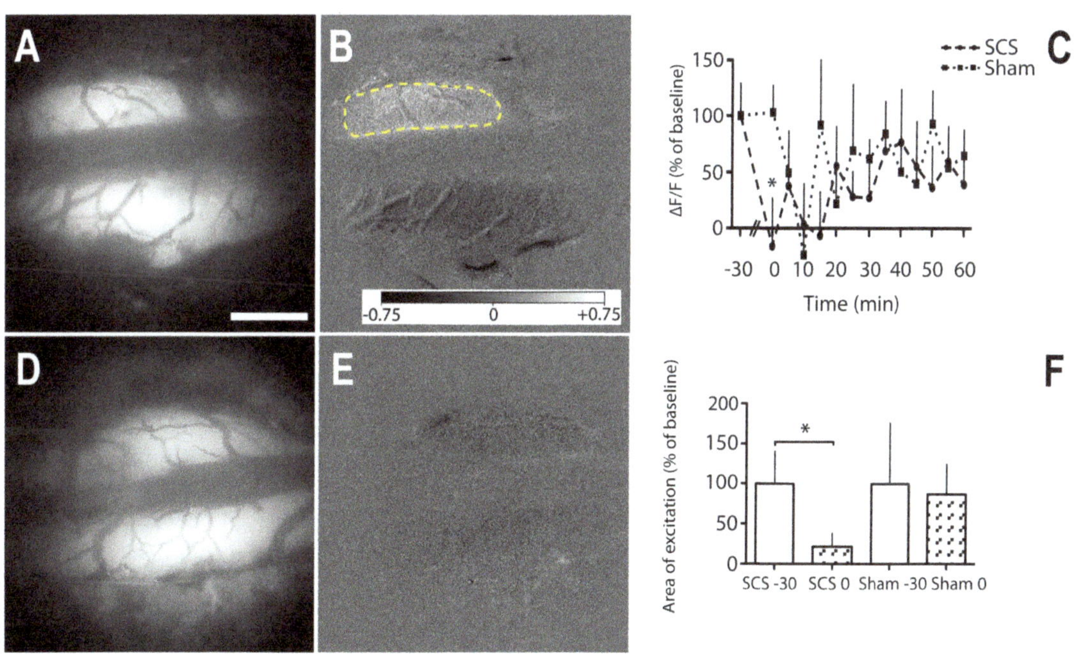

Figure 5. Effect of 30 minutes SCS or sham stimulation on the intensity of the AFI signal and area of excitation in response to sciatic nerve electrical stimulation, in rats with partial ligation of the proximal sciatic nerve (Seltzer model). (A,D) Images of background fluorescence of the dorsal surface of the spinal cord at T13 of a sham (A) and SCS treated rat (D). (B,E) Area of excitation (yellow) on the ipsilateral side, directly after sham stimulation (B); after SCS, in this rat, there is no area exceeding the predefined ΔF/F level (E). (C) Time course of the intensity of the AFI signal after SCS or sham stimulation (T = 0 min), as a percentage of ΔF/F before treatment (T = -30 min), in 20×20 pixel square selections on the ipsilateral side at the L4-L6 spinal level. (F) Mean areas of excitation on the ipsilateral side directly after SCS or sham stimulation (T = 0 min), as a percentage of the areas before treatment (T = -30 min). Scale bar, 1 mm; Grayscale bar ranging from −0.75% (black) to +0.75% (white) of the 16-bit range; Error bars indicate SEM; *$p<0.05$; paired t-tests; $n = 7$ SCS, $n = 6$ sham stimulation.

[3]. Although this response could be further enhanced in the acute situation by intraplantar capsaicin injection [3], the same may not be true in chronic neuropathy. Similarly, c-Fos expression, another marker of spinal nociceptive activity, is not increased in animals with chronic neuropathy compared to naïve animals, following nociceptive stimulation [44].

To reduce the number of experimental animals, we used naïve rats from a previous study [3] as controls. These animals were Wistar rats, i.e. not the same strain as the Sprague-Dawley rats that were used here because of the Seltzer model. One may therefore argue that the above-described lack of a difference in AFI activity following nociceptive electrical stimulation between naïve and neuropathic rats could be the result of a genetic difference in sensitivity to nociceptive stimuli. However, at least behaviorally Sprague-Dawley rats demonstrate a hyperalgesic phenotype in comparison to other rat strains, including Wistar rats [45,46]. In addition, it is highly unlikely that non-noxious palpation would induce an AFI response in naïve Sprague-Dawley rats (as opposed to Wistar rats), since metabolic activity solely in the deep dorsal horn cannot be visualized by AFI. We therefore conclude that the strain differences in our study do not affect our conclusions regarding spinal nociceptive processing in nerve injury-induced pain.

Regarding our second aim, to study mechanisms of action of SCS, this is the first report directly demonstrating reduced activity in the superficial dorsal horn *in vivo* following SCS. We used the AFI response to a 2.5 mA electrical stimulus as outcome measure, since in our hands this stimulus generates the most robust and consistent AFI responses. Others have also used nociceptive stimulation to study the effect of SCS [47].

Previous studies measuring peptides involved in antinociception [31,48] or using pharmacological approaches [49,50] present only indirect evidence of reduced spinal nociceptive activity. Furthermore, studies of electrophysiological activity in wide dynamic range neurons in the deep dorsal horn [51] focus on an area that may not be decisive in generating the neuropathic pain phenotype [52,53] and that may not be the locus of "gate control", which instead is postulated to be the substantia gelatinosa in the superficial dorsal horn [28]. Our finding of decreased activity in the superficial dorsal horn is in line with two reports [54,55] demonstrating a significant increase in c-Fos expression in the superficial dorsal horn following SCS in rats with nerve injury, which was larger than the increase in the deep dorsal horn. These c-Fos expressing neurons presumably represent inhibitory interneurons [37], considering the decrease in neuronal metabolic activity in the superficial dorsal horn. Indeed, a double immunohistochemical staining procedure revealed the presence of c-Fos positive GABA-immunoreactive neurons in the superficial dorsal horn of SCS-treated chronic neuropathic rats [32]. The latter report and that of Cui et al. [31] stress the role of GABA-ergic interneurons in the mechanism underlying SCS in chronic neuropathic pain. Nevertheless, so far no direct changes in the spatial and temporal domain related to the effect of SCS on nociceptive transmission in the superficial dorsal horn of chronic neuropathic rats have been studied. Our findings therefore provide the first direct evidence that SCS acts through modulation of nociceptive processing at the spinal segmental level.

The effect of SCS on nociceptive activity in the superficial dorsal horn that we describe here is rather short lasting, as demonstrated by a linear decrease of efficacy from SCS directly following cessation of stimulation (i.e. T = 0 min) and a lack of statistical significance between SCS and sham animals at time-points T = 5 minutes or later after SCS. A lack of statistical significance at those later time-points may be caused by a relatively low signal-to-noise ratio and technical challenges of spinal cord AFI that were discussed previously [3], resulting in large variation between recordings within the same animal and between animals. However, behavioral effects of SCS also do not outlast the duration of SCS [33]. The relatively short duration of an initially significant effect of SCS does not preclude a clinical meaningful effect of SCS in patients with nerve injury-induced pain or CRPS, since in patients spinal cord stimulators deliver continuous stimulation. Continuous stimulation during AFI recording was not feasible due to our experimental setup, as the spinal electrode prevented imaging of the spinal cord.

In conclusion, we demonstrated changes in neuronal metabolic activity in the superficial dorsal horn following nerve injury, which may reflect mechanisms of hyperalgesia in patients with neuropathic pain syndromes. Secondly, our study provides a rationale for spinal cord stimulation in neuropathic pain patients.

Supporting Information

Movie S1 Typical AFI recording in a neuropathic rat, following nociceptive electrical stimulation. The video shows a stack of subtracted ΔF/F images of the dorsal surface of the spinal cord at the T13 vertebral level, before, during and after nociceptive electrical stimulation of the left sciatic nerve.

Movie S2 Typical AFI recording in a neuropathic rat, following innocuous palpation. The video shows a stack of subtracted ΔF/F images of the dorsal surface of the spinal cord at the T13 vertebral level, before, during and after innocuous palpation of the left hindpaw.

Table S1 Behavioral data of neuropathic Sprague-Dawley rats. VF0 = Von Frey threshold at day 0, etc.; HP0 = Hotplate at day 0 etc.; SCS = rats undergoing spinal cord stimulation; sham = rats undergoing sham stimulation; palpation = rats undergoing innocuous palpation.

Table S2 AFI intensity and AFI area of naïve Wistar and neuropathic Sprague-Dawley (SD) rats on the ipsilateral (i.e. left) and contralateral (i.e. right) side of the spinal cord, following nociceptive electrical stimulation of the left sciatic nerve.

Table S3 AFI intensity of naïve Wistar and neuropathic (i.e. Seltzer) Sprague-Dawley (SD) rats on the ipsilateral (ipsi) and contralateral (contra) side of the spinal cord, following innocuous palpation of the left hindpaw.

Table S4 AFI intensities and AFI areas following spinal cord versus sham stimulation. SCS vs Sham deltaFF: AFI intensities of 7 SCS and 6 Sham rats as a percentage of mean ΔF/F before treatment, up to one hour (T = 60) following cessation of SCS or Sham; SCS and Sham deltaFF bf vs T0: AFI intensities of 7 SCS and 6 Sham rats as a percentage of mean ΔF/F before treatment, before and directly following cessation (T = 0) of SCS of Sham; SCS and Sham area% bef vs T = 0: AFI areas of 7 SCS and 6 Sham rats as a percentage of mean area before treatment, before and directly following cessation (T = 0) of SCS or Sham; Linear regression = mean relative AFI intensities of 7 SCS and 6 Sham rats, from directly following cessation of SCS or Sham (T = 0) to one hour (T = 60).

Acknowledgments

The authors would like to thank Johannes van der Burg (Dept. of Neuroscience, Erasmus MC, Rotterdam, the Netherlands) for technical support. The Medtronic Bakken Research Center in Maastricht deserves gratitude for developing and supplying the electrodes (special regards to Paul van Venrooij and Victor Duysens).

Author Contributions

Conceived and designed the experiments: JJ HS TP. Performed the experiments: JJ HS TP MB. Analyzed the data: JJ TP MB. Contributed reagents/materials/analysis tools: SK MH. Wrote the paper: JJ FH CZ JH EJ.

References

1. Reinert KC, Gao W, Chen G, Ebner TJ (2007) Flavoprotein autofluorescence imaging in the cerebellar cortex in vivo. J Neurosci Res 85: 3221–3232.
2. Reinert KC, Dunbar RL, Gao W, Chen G, Ebner TJ (2004) Flavoprotein autofluorescence imaging of neuronal activation in the cerebellar cortex in vivo. J Neurophysiol 92: 199–211.
3. Jongen JL, Pederzani T, Koekkoek SK, Shapiro J, van der Burg J, et al. (2010) Autofluorescent flavoprotein imaging of spinal nociceptive activity. J Neurosci 30: 4081–4087.
4. Shibuki K, Hishida R, Murakami H, Kudoh M, Kawaguchi T, et al. (2003) Dynamic imaging of somatosensory cortical activity in the rat visualized by flavoprotein autofluorescence. J Physiol 549: 919–927.
5. Murakami H, Kamatani D, Hishida R, Takao T, Kudoh M, et al. (2004) Short-term plasticity visualized with flavoprotein autofluorescence in the somatosensory cortex of anaesthetized rats. Eur J Neurosci 19: 1352–1360.
6. Weber B, Burger C, Wyss MT, von Schulthess GK, Scheffold F, et al. (2004) Optical imaging of the spatiotemporal dynamics of cerebral blood flow and oxidative metabolism in the rat barrel cortex. Eur J Neurosci 20: 2664–2670.
7. Komagata S, Chen S, Suzuki A, Yamashita H, Hishida R, et al. (2011) Initial phase of neuropathic pain within a few hours after nerve injury in mice. J Neurosci 31: 4896–4905.
8. Yamashita H, Chen S, Komagata S, Hishida R, Iwasato T, et al. (2012) Restoration of contralateral representation in the mouse somatosensory cortex after crossing nerve transfer. PloS one 7: e35676.
9. Takahashi K, Hishida R, Kubota Y, Kudoh M, Takahashi S, et al. (2006) Transcranial fluorescence imaging of auditory cortical plasticity regulated by acoustic environments in mice. Eur J Neurosci 23: 1365–1376.
10. Kubota Y, Kamatani D, Tsukano H, Ohshima S, Takahashi K, et al. (2008) Transcranial photo-inactivation of neural activities in the mouse auditory cortex. Neurosci Res 60: 422–430.
11. Tohmi M, Takahashi K, Kubota Y, Hishida R, Shibuki K (2009) Transcranial flavoprotein fluorescence imaging of mouse cortical activity and plasticity. J Neurochem 109 Suppl 1: 3–9.
12. Husson TR, Mallik AK, Zhang JX, Issa NP (2007) Functional imaging of primary visual cortex using flavoprotein autofluorescence. J Neurosci 27: 8665–8675.
13. Barnes JA, Ebner BA, Duvick LA, Gao W, Chen G, et al. (2011) Abnormalities in the climbing fiber-Purkinje cell circuitry contribute to neuronal dysfunction in ATXN1[82Q] mice. J Neurosci 31: 12778–12789.
14. Wang X, Chen G, Gao W, Ebner TJ (2011) Parasagittally aligned, mGluR1-dependent patches are evoked at long latencies by parallel fiber stimulation in the mouse cerebellar cortex in vivo. J Neurophysiol 105: 1732–1746.
15. Sasaki S, Yazawa I, Miyakawa N, Mochida H, Shinomiya K, et al. (2002) Optical imaging of intrinsic signals induced by peripheral nerve stimulation in the in vivo rat spinal cord. Neuroimage 17: 1240–1255.
16. Jongen JL, Holstege JC (2012) Propagation of spinal nociceptive activity in the spatial and temporal domains. The Neuroscientist: 18: 8–14.
17. Latremoliere A, Woolf CJ (2009) Central sensitization: a generator of pain hypersensitivity by central neural plasticity. J Pain 10: 895–926.
18. Latremoliere A, Woolf CJ (2010) Synaptic plasticity and central sensitization: author reply. J Pain 11: 801–803.
19. Seltzer Z, Dubner R, Shir Y (1990) A novel behavioral model of neuropathic pain disorders produced in rats by partial sciatic nerve injury. Pain 43: 205–218.
20. Shir Y, Seltzer Z (1991) Effects of sympathectomy in a model of causalgiform pain produced by partial sciatic nerve injury in rats. Pain 45: 309–320.
21. Oaklander AL, Rissmiller JG, Gelman LB, Zheng L, Chang Y, et al. (2006) Evidence of focal small-fiber axonal degeneration in complex regional pain syndrome-I (reflex sympathetic dystrophy). Pain 120: 235–243.
22. Doth AH, Hansson PT, Jensen MP, Taylor RS (2010) The burden of neuropathic pain: a systematic review and meta-analysis of health utilities. Pain 149: 338–344.
23. Kemler MA, Barendse GA, van Kleef M, de Vet HC, Rijks CP, et al. (2000) Spinal cord stimulation in patients with chronic reflex sympathetic dystrophy. N Engl J Med 343: 618–624.
24. Kemler MA, de Vet HC, Barendse GA, van den Wildenberg FA, van Kleef M (2006) Spinal cord stimulation for chronic reflex sympathetic dystrophy–five-year follow-up. N Engl J Med 354: 2394–2396.
25. Cruccu G, Aziz TZ, Garcia-Larrea L, Hansson P, Jensen TS, et al. (2007) EFNS guidelines on neurostimulation therapy for neuropathic pain. Eur J Neurol 14: 952–970.
26. de Vos CC, Rajan V, Steenbergen W, van der Aa HE, Buschman HP (2009) Effect and safety of spinal cord stimulation for treatment of chronic pain caused by diabetic neuropathy. J Diabetes Complicat 23: 40–45.
27. Pluijms WA, Slangen R, Bakkers M, Faber CG, Merkies IS, et al. (2012) Pain relief and quality-of-life improvement after spinal cord stimulation in painful diabetic polyneuropathy: a pilot study. Brit J Anaesth 109: 623–629.
28. Moayedi M, Davis KD (2013) Theories of pain: from Specificity to Gate Control. J Neurophysiol 109: 5–12.
29. Geurts JW, Smits H, Kemler MA, Brunner F, Kessels AG, et al. (2013) Spinal Cord Stimulation for Complex Regional Pain Syndrome Type I: A Prospective Cohort Study With Long-Term Follow-Up. Neuromodulation 16: 523–529
30. Smits H, van Kleef M, Joosten EA (2012) Spinal cord stimulation of dorsal columns in a rat model of neuropathic pain: evidence for a segmental spinal mechanism of pain relief. Pain 153: 177–183.
31. Cui JG, O'Connor WT, Ungerstedt U, Linderoth B, Meyerson BA (1997) Spinal cord stimulation attenuates augmented dorsal horn release of excitatory amino acids in mononeuropathy via a GABAergic mechanism. Pain 73: 87–95.
32. Janssen SP, Gerard S, Raijmakers ME, Truin M, Van Kleef M, et al. (2012) Decreased intracellular GABA levels contribute to spinal cord stimulation-induced analgesia in rats suffering from painful peripheral neuropathy: the role of KCC2 and GABA(A) receptor-mediated inhibition. Neurochem Int 60: 21–30.
33. Smits H, Ultenius C, Deumens R, Koopmans GC, Honig WM, et al. (2006) Effect of spinal cord stimulation in an animal model of neuropathic pain relates to degree of tactile "allodynia". Neuroscience 143: 541–546.
34. Bennett DL, Koltzenburg M, Priestley JV, Shelton DL, McMahon SB (1998) Endogenous nerve growth factor regulates the sensitivity of nociceptors in the adult rat. Eur J Neurosci 10: 1282–1291.
35. Woolf CJ, Ma Q (2007) Nociceptors—noxious stimulus detectors. Neuron 55: 353–364.
36. Schoffnegger D, Ruscheweyh R, Sandkuhler J (2008) Spread of excitation across modality borders in spinal dorsal horn of neuropathic rats. Pain 135: 300–310.
37. Hossaini M, Duraku LS, Sarac C, Jongen JL, Holstege JC (2010) Differential distribution of activated spinal neurons containing glycine and/or GABA and expressing c-fos in acute and chronic pain models. Pain 151: 356–365.
38. Hossaini M, Goos JA, Kohli SK, Holstege JC (2012) Distribution of glycine/GABA neurons in the ventromedial medulla with descending spinal projections and evidence for an ascending glycine/GABA projection. PloS one 7: e35293.
39. Coull JA, Beggs S, Boudreau D, Boivin D, Tsuda M, et al. (2005) BDNF from microglia causes the shift in neuronal anion gradient underlying neuropathic pain. Nature 438: 1017–1021.
40. Tracey I, Mantyh PW (2007) The cerebral signature for pain perception and its modulation. Neuron 55: 377–391.
41. Costigan M, Scholz J, Woolf CJ (2009) Neuropathic Pain: A Maladaptive Response of the Nervous System to Damage. Annu Rev Neurosci 32: 1–32.
42. Ochoa JL, Yarnitsky D (1993) Mechanical hyperalgesias in neuropathic pain patients: dynamic and static subtypes. Ann Neurol 33: 465–472.
43. Rowbotham MC, Fields HL (1996) The relationship of pain, allodynia and thermal sensation in post-herpetic neuralgia. Brain 119(2): 347–354.
44. Catheline G, Le Guen S, Honore P, Besson JM (1999) Are there long-term changes in the basal or evoked Fos expression in the dorsal horn of the spinal cord of the mononeuropathic rat? Pain 80: 347–357.
45. Mogil JS (1999) The genetic mediation of individual differences in sensitivity to pain and its inhibition. Proc Natl Acad Sci U S A 96: 7744–7751.
46. LaCroix-Fralish ML, Rutkowski MD, Weinstein JN, Mogil JS, Deleo JA (2005) The magnitude of mechanical allodynia in a rodent model of lumbar radiculopathy is dependent on strain and sex. Spine 30: 1821–1827.
47. Shechter R, Yang F, Xu Q, Cheong YK, He SQ, et al. (2013) Conventional and Kilohertz-frequency Spinal Cord Stimulation Produces Intensity- and Frequency-dependent Inhibition of Mechanical Hypersensitivity in a Rat Model of Neuropathic Pain. Anesthesiology 119: 422–432.
48. Schechtmann G, Song Z, Ultenius C, Meyerson BA, Linderoth B (2008) Cholinergic mechanisms involved in the pain relieving effect of spinal cord stimulation in a model of neuropathy. Pain 139: 136–145.
49. Song Z, Meyerson BA, Linderoth B (2011) Spinal 5-HT receptors that contribute to the pain-relieving effects of spinal cord stimulation in a rat model of neuropathy. Pain 152: 1666–1673.
50. Barchini J, Tchachaghian S, Shamaa F, Jabbur SJ, Meyerson BA, et al. (2012) Spinal segmental and supraspinal mechanisms underlying the pain-relieving effects of spinal cord stimulation: an experimental study in a rat model of neuropathy. Neuroscience 215: 196–208.
51. Guan Y, Wacnik PW, Yang F, Carteret AF, Chung CY, et al. (2010) Spinal cord stimulation-induced analgesia: electrical stimulation of dorsal column and dorsal roots attenuates dorsal horn neuronal excitability in neuropathic rats. Anesthesiology 113: 1392–1405.

52. Craig AD (2003) Pain mechanisms: labeled lines versus convergence in central processing. Annu Rev Neurosci 26: 1–30.
53. Craig AD (2004) Lamina I, but not lamina V, spinothalamic neurons exhibit responses that correspond with burning pain. J Neurophysiol 92: 2604–2609.
54. Smits H, Kleef MV, Honig W, Gerver J, Gobrecht P, et al. (2009) Spinal cord stimulation induces c-Fos expression in the dorsal horn in rats with neuropathic pain after partial sciatic nerve injury. Neurosci Lett 450: 70–73.
55. Maeda Y, Ikeuchi M, Wacnik P, Sluka KA (2009) Increased c-fos immunoreactivity in the spinal cord and brain following spinal cord stimulation is frequency-dependent. Brain Res 1259: 40–50.

Permissions

All chapters in this book were first published in PLOS ONE, by The Public Library of Science; hereby published with permission under the Creative Commons Attribution License or equivalent. Every chapter published in this book has been scrutinized by our experts. Their significance has been extensively debated. The topics covered herein carry significant findings which will fuel the growth of the discipline. They may even be implemented as practical applications or may be referred to as a beginning point for another development.

The contributors of this book come from diverse backgrounds, making this book a truly international effort. This book will bring forth new frontiers with its revolutionizing research information and detailed analysis of the nascent developments around the world.

We would like to thank all the contributing authors for lending their expertise to make the book truly unique. They have played a crucial role in the development of this book. Without their invaluable contributions this book wouldn't have been possible. They have made vital efforts to compile up to date information on the varied aspects of this subject to make this book a valuable addition to the collection of many professionals and students.

This book was conceptualized with the vision of imparting up-to-date information and advanced data in this field. To ensure the same, a matchless editorial board was set up. Every individual on the board went through rigorous rounds of assessment to prove their worth. After which they invested a large part of their time researching and compiling the most relevant data for our readers.

The editorial board has been involved in producing this book since its inception. They have spent rigorous hours researching and exploring the diverse topics which have resulted in the successful publishing of this book. They have passed on their knowledge of decades through this book. To expedite this challenging task, the publisher supported the team at every step. A small team of assistant editors was also appointed to further simplify the editing procedure and attain best results for the readers.

Apart from the editorial board, the designing team has also invested a significant amount of their time in understanding the subject and creating the most relevant covers. They scrutinized every image to scout for the most suitable representation of the subject and create an appropriate cover for the book.

The publishing team has been an ardent support to the editorial, designing and production team. Their endless efforts to recruit the best for this project, has resulted in the accomplishment of this book. They are a veteran in the field of academics and their pool of knowledge is as vast as their experience in printing. Their expertise and guidance has proved useful at every step. Their uncompromising quality standards have made this book an exceptional effort. Their encouragement from time to time has been an inspiration for everyone.

The publisher and the editorial board hope that this book will prove to be a valuable piece of knowledge for researchers, students, practitioners and scholars across the globe.

List of Contributors

Yanhu Ge
Department of Anesthesiology, Eastern Hepatobiliary Surgery Hospital, Changhai Hospital, Second Military Medical University, Shanghai, China
Department of Anesthesiology, 309th Hospital of CPLA, Beijing, China

Feixiang Wu, Liqun Yang, Zhijie Lu, Yuming Sun and Wei-Feng Yu
Department of Anesthesiology, Eastern Hepatobiliary Surgery Hospital, Changhai Hospital, Second Military Medical University, Shanghai, China

Xuejun Sun
Department of Diving Medicine, Faculty of Naval Medicine, Second Military Medical University, Shanghai, China

Zhenghua Xiang
Department of Neurobiology, Second Military Medical University, Shanghai, China

Shengdong Huang
Department of Cardiothoracic Surgery, Changhai Hospital, Second Military Medical University, Shanghai, China

An-Kuo Chou
Department of Anesthesiology, Kaohsiung Chang Gung Memorial Hospital and Chang Gung University College of Medicine, Kaohsiung, Taiwan, R.O.C.

Ming-Chang Yang
Department of Biological Sciences, National Sun Yat-Sen University, Kaohsiung, Taiwan, R.O.C.
Department of Biochemistry, Faculty of Medicine, College of Medicine, Kaohsiung Medical University, Kaohsiung, Taiwan, R.O.C.
Laboratory of Medical Research, Kaohsiung Armed Forces General Hospital, Kaohsiung, Taiwan, R.O.C.

Hung-Pei Tsai
Graduate Institute of Medicine, College of Medicine, Kaohsiung Medical University, Kaohsiung, Taiwan, R.O.C.

Chee-Yin Chai
Department of Pathology, Kaohsiung Medical University Chung-Ho Memorial Hospital, Kaohsiung, Taiwan, R.O.C.

Ming-Hong Tai
Institute of Biomedical Science, National Sun Yat-sen University, Kaohsiung, Taiwan, R.O.C.

Aij-Li Kwan
Graduate Institute of Medicine, College of Medicine, Kaohsiung Medical University, Kaohsiung, Taiwan, R.O.C.
Department of Neurosurgery, Kaohsiung Medical University Chung-Ho Memorial Hospital, Kaohsiung, Taiwan, R.O.C.

Yi-Ren Hong
Department of Biological Sciences, National Sun Yat-Sen University, Kaohsiung, Taiwan, R.O.C.
Department of Biochemistry, Faculty of Medicine, College of Medicine, Kaohsiung Medical University, Kaohsiung, Taiwan, R.O.C.
Graduate Institute of Medicine, College of Medicine, Kaohsiung Medical University, Kaohsiung, Taiwan, R.O.C.

Ikuko Suzuki, Yoshiyuki Tsuboi, Masamichi Shinoda, Kazuo Shibuta, Ayano Katagiri and Masaaki Kiyomoto
Department of Physiology, Nihon University School of Dentistry, Chiyoda-ku Tokyo, Japan

Kuniya Honda
Department of Physiology, Nihon University School of Dentistry, Chiyoda-ku Tokyo, Japan
Department of Oral and Maxillofacial Surgery, Nihon University School of Dentistry, Chiyoda-ku Tokyo, Japan

Barry J. Sessle
Department of Oral Physiology, Faculty of Dentistry, University of Toronto, Toronto, Ontario, Canada

Shingo Matsuura and Kinuyo Ohara
Department of Endodontics, Nihon University School of Dentistry, Chiyoda-ku Tokyo, Japan

Kentaro Urata
Department of Prosthodontics, Nihon University School of Dentistry, Chiyoda-ku Tokyo, Japan

Koichi Iwata
Department of Physiology, Nihon University School of Dentistry, Chiyoda-ku Tokyo, Japan
Division of Functional Morphology, Dental Research Center, Nihon University School of Dentistry, Tokyo, Japan
Division of Applied System Neuroscience Advanced Medical Research Center, Nihon University Graduate School of Medical Science, Tokyo, Japan

Yang Yang, Ji- Dong Liu, Hui Liu, Li Li and Jian-Hua Chen
Department of Neurosurgery, The Zhumadian City Center Hospital, Zhumadian, P.R. China

Yong-Gang Zhang
Department of ICU, The Zhumadian City Center Hospital, Zhumadian, P.R. China

Guo-An Lin
Department of Burn, The 159th Hospital of PLA, Zhumadian, P.R. China

He-Qiu Xie
Department of Pain, The Zhumadian City Center Hospital, Zhumadian, P.R. China

Hai-Tao Pan
School of Statistics, Xi'an University of Finance and Economics, Xi'an, P.R. China

Ben-Qing Huang
Department of Oncology, The 159th Hospital of PLA, Zhumadian, P.R. China

Nan Zhang
Department of student affairs, Xinxiang Medical University, Xinxiang, P.R. China

Karine Thibault
Brain Plasticity Unit, ESPCI-ParisTech, Paris, France
Centre National de la Recherche Scientifique, UMR 8249, Paris, France
Neurorestoration Group, The Wolfson Centre for Age-Related Diseases, King's College London, London, United Kingdom

Bernard Calvino, Sophie Dubacq and Sophie Pezet
Brain Plasticity Unit, ESPCI-ParisTech, Paris, France
Centre National de la Recherche Scientifique, UMR 8249, Paris, France

Isabelle Rivals
Equipe de Statistique Appliquée, ESPCI-ParisTech, Paris, France

Fabien Marchand
Institut National de la Santé et de la Recherche Médicale, Unité 1107, NEURO-DOL, Clermont-Ferrand, France
Clermont Université , Université d'Auvergne, Pharmacologie Fondamentale et Clinique de la Douleur, Clermont-Ferrand, France

Stephen B. McMahon
Neurorestoration Group, The Wolfson Centre for Age-Related Diseases, King's College London, London, United Kingdom

Masanori Kawaguchi, Yasushi Satoh, Yukiko Otsubo and Tomiei Kazama
Department of Anesthesiology, National Defense Medical College, Tokorozawa, Saitama, Japan

Aldric T. Hama, Matthew S. Varghese and Jacqueline Sagen
Miami Project to Cure Paralysis, University of Miami Miller School of Medicine, Miami, Florida, United States of America

Peter Germano, G. Todd Milne and James P. Pearson
Ironwood Pharmaceuticals, Inc., Cambridge, Massachusetts, United States of America

Benjamin F. Cravatt
Department of Chemical Physiology, The Skaggs Institute for Chemical Biology, The Scripps Research Institute, La Jolla, California, United States of America

Kiran Vasudeva, Karl Andersen, Bree Zeyzus-Johns, John A. Pollock
Biological Sciences, Bayer School of Natural and Environmental Sciences, and Chronic Pain Research Consortium, Duquesne University, Pittsburgh, Pennsylvania, United States of America

T. Kevin Hitchens
NMR Center for Biomedical Research, Carnegie Mellon University, Pittsburgh, Pennsylvania, United States of America

Sravan Kumar Patel and Jelena M. Janjic
Graduate School of Pharmaceutical Sciences, Mylan School of Pharmacy, and Chronic Pain Research Consortium, Duquesne University, Pittsburgh, Pennsylvania, United States of America

Anthony Balducci
Department of Research and Development, Celsense, Inc., Pittsburgh, Pennsylvania, Unite States of America

Courtney L. Donica, Yan Cui and Shanping Shi
Department of Anesthesiology, The University of Texas - MD Anderson Cancer Center, Houston, Texas, United States of America

Howard B. Gutstein
Department of Anesthesiology, The University of Texas - MD Anderson Cancer Center, Houston, Texas, United States of America
Department of Biochemistry and Molecular Biology, Genes and Development Graduate Program, The University of Texas - MD Anderson Cancer Center, Houston, Texas, United States of America

Katsuyuki Iwatsuki, Tetsuya Arai, Hideyuki Ota, Shuichi Kato, Tadahiro Natsume, Shigeru Kurimoto, Michiro Yamamoto and Hitoshi Hirata
Department of Hand Surgery, Nagoya University Graduate School of Medicine, Showa-ku, Nagoya, Japan

Junya Yokobe, Masaki Kitahara and Shoichi Uezono
Department of Anesthesiology, The Jikei University School of Medicine, Minato, Tokyo, Japan

Masato Matsushima
Division of Clinical Epidemiology, The Jikei University School of Medicine, Minato, Tokyo, Japan

Xin Luo, Wai Lydia Tai, Liting Sun and Qiu Qiu
Department of Anaesthesiology, The University of Hong Kong, HKSAR, China
Laboratory and Clinical Research Institute for Pain, The University of Hong Kong, HKSAR, China

Zhengyuan Xia
Department of Anaesthesiology, The University of Hong Kong, HKSAR, China
Research Center of Heart, Brain, Hormone and Healthy Aging, The University of Hong Kong, HKSAR, China

Sookja Kim Chung
Department of Anatomy, The University of Hong Kong, HKSAR, China
Research Center of Heart, Brain, Hormone and Healthy Aging, The University of Hong Kong, HKSAR, China
Laboratory and Clinical Research Institute for Pain, The University of Hong Kong, HKSAR, China

Chi Wai Cheung
Department of Anaesthesiology, The University of Hong Kong, HKSAR, China
Research Center of Heart, Brain, Hormone and Healthy Aging, The University of Hong Kong, HKSAR, China
Laboratory and Clinical Research Institute for Pain, The University of Hong Kong, HKSAR, China

Hans Jürgen Solinski, Kathrin Rothe, Ingrid Boekhoff, Thomas Gudermann and Andreas Breit
Walther-Straub-Institut für Pharmakologie und Toxikologie, Ludwig-Maximilians-Universität München, Munich, Germany

Franziska Petermann
Department of Neurology, Klinikum rechts der Isar, Technical University Munich, Munich, Germany

Haijun Shao, Qingsheng Xue, Fujun Zhang, Yan Luo, Xiaoqing Zhang and Buwei Yu
Department of Anesthesiology, Ruijin Hospital, School of Medicine, Shanghai Jiao Tong University, Shanghai, PR China

Hao Zhu and Wenlong Ding
Department of Anatomy, School of Medicine, Shanghai Jiao Tong University, Shanghai, PR China

Honghai Zhang
Department of Anesthesiology, Hangzhou First People's Hospital, Nanjing Medical University, Zhejiang, PR China

Katsuya Morita
Department of Pharmacology, Faculty of Nursing, Hiroshima Bunka Gakuen University, Hiroshima, Japan

Seiji Shiraishi
Cancer Pathophysiology, Division National Cancer Center Research Institute, Tokyo, Japan

Naoyo Motoyama
Cancer Pathophysiology, Division National Cancer Center Research Institute, Tokyo, Japan
Department of Dental Science for Health Promotion, Division of Integrated Health Sciences, Institute of Biomedical and Health Sciences, Hiroshima University, Hiroshima, Japan

Tomoya Kitayama and Takashi Kanematsu
Department of Cell and Molecular Pharmacology, Division of Basic Life Science, Institute of Biomedical and Health Sciences, Hiroshima University, Hiroshima, Japan

Yasuhito Uezono
Cancer Pathophysiology, Division National Cancer Center Research Institute, Tokyo, Japan

Toshihiro Dohi
Department of Pharmacotherapy, Pharmaceutical Sciences, Nihon Pharmaceutical University, Saitama, Japan

Saïd M'Dahoma, Sylvie Bourgoin, Valérie Kayser, Sandrine Barthélémy, Caroline Chevarin
Centre de Psychiatrie et Neurosciences, Institut National de la Santéet de la Recherche Médicale, INSERM U894, Université Paris Descartes, Paris, France
Neuropsychopharmacologie, Faculté de Médecine Pierre et Marie Curie, site Pitié-Salpêtrière, Paris, France

Farah Chali and Didier Orsal
Laboratoire de Neurobiologie des Signaux Intercellulaires, Centre National de la Recherche Scientifique, CNRS UMR 7101, Université Pierre et Marie Curie, Paris, France

Michel Hamon
Centre de Psychiatrie et Neurosciences, Institut National de la Santé et de la Recherche Médicale, INSERM U894, Université Paris Descartes, Paris, France
Neuropsychopharmacologie, Faculté de Médecine Pierre et Marie Curie, site Pitié-Salpêtrière, Paris, France

Nurcan Üçeyler, Waldemar Kafke and Claudia Sommer
Department of Neurology, University of Würzburg, Würzburg, Germany

Michael Valet and Thomas R. Tölle
Department of Neurology, Klinikum rechts der Isar, Technische Universität München, München, Germany

Sylvia M. Gustin
Neuroscience Research Australia, Randwick, NSW, Australia

Jamie G. McKay
Department of Anatomy and Histology, University of Sydney, Sydney, NSW, Australia

Esben T. Petersen
Departments of Radiology and Radiotherapy, University Medical Center Utrecht, Utrecht, The Netherlands

Chris C. Peck and Greg M. Murray
Faculty of Dentistry, University of Sydney, Sydney, NSW, Australia

Luke A. Henderson
Department of Anatomy and Histology, University of Sydney, Sydney, NSW, Australia

Michael R. Due, Aaron L. Randolph and Matthew S. Ripsch
Department of Anesthesia, Indiana University School of Medicine, Indianapolis, Indiana, United States of America

Xiao-Fang Yang
Department of Pharmacology, College of Medicine, University of Arizona, Tucson, Arizona, United States of America

Yohance M. Allette and Erik T. Dustrude
Department of Cell Biology and Anatomy, Indiana University School of Medicine, Indianapolis, Indiana, United States of America

Sarah M. Wilson
Program in Medical Neurosciences, Paul and Carole Stark Neurosciences Research Institute, Indiana University School of Medicine, Indianapolis, Indiana, United States of America

Rajesh Khanna
Department of Pharmacology, College of Medicine, University of Arizona, Tucson, Arizona, United States of America
Department of Pharmacology and Toxicology, Indiana University School of Medicine, Indianapolis, Indiana, United States of America

Fletcher A. White
Department of Anesthesia, Indiana University School of Medicine, Indianapolis, Indiana, United States of America
Department of Pharmacology and Toxicology, Indiana University School of Medicine, Indianapolis, Indiana, United States of America

Joakim M. Bischoff, Thomas K. Ringsted, Marian Petersen and Mads U. Werner
Multidisciplinary Pain Center 7612, Neuroscience Center, Rigshospitalet, Copenhagen University, Copenhagen, Denmark

Claudia Sommer and Nurcan Üçeyler
Department of Neurology, University Hospital of Würzburg, Würzburg, Germany

Joost L. M. Jongen
Dept. of Neurology, Erasmus MC, Rotterdam, the Netherlands

Helwin Smits and Elbert A. J. Joosten
Pain Management and Research Center, UMC+, Maastricht, the Netherlands

Tiziana Pederzani, Malik Bechakra, Mehdi Hossaini, Sebastiaan K. Koekkoek and Jan C. Holstege
Dept. of Neuroscience, Erasmus MC, Rotterdam, the Netherlands

Frank J. P. M. Huygen
Dept. of Pain Medicine, Erasmus MC, Rotterdam, the Netherlands

Chris I. De Zeeuw
Dept. of Neuroscience, Erasmus MC, Rotterdam, the Netherlands
Netherlands Institute for Neuroscience, Royal Academy for Arts and Sciences, Amsterdam, the Netherlands

Index